GENETICS AND ETIOLOGY OF DOWN SYNDROME

Edited by **Subrata Dey**

Genetics and Etiology of Down Syndrome
Edited by Subrata Dey

Published by InTech
Janeza Trdine 9, 51000 Rijeka, Croatia

Publishing Process Manager Romina Krebel

Technical Editor Teodora Smiljanic

Cover Designer InTech Design Team

Additional hard copies can be obtained from orders@intechopen.com

Genetics and Etiology of Down Syndrome, Edited by Subrata Dey
p. cm.
ISBN 978-953-307-631-7

Meet the editor

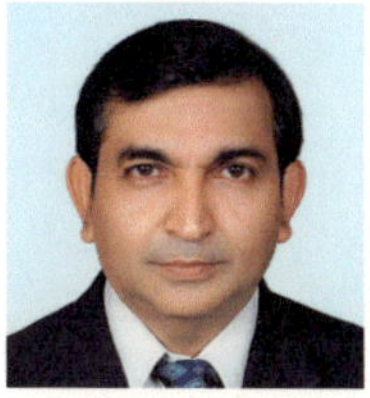

Subrata Dey was born in India and grew up in the state of Assam. He received his Ph.D. from the University of Kalyani, West Bengal. He joined the faculty of West Bengal University of Technology as Professor of Biotechnology in 2005. In 2006 he became the Director of the School of Biotechnology and Biological Sciences. His laboratory has long been involved in research on Genetics of Down syndrome & other congenital disorders, Genetics of Alzheimer's disease, radiation induced genomic instability, radioprotection by antioxidants & stem cell biology. He has been teaching courses in Genetics, Molecular Biology, Evolution & Developmental Biology for more than thirty years. Prof. Dey received golden jubilee award of excellence from Presidency College (Presidency University), Kolkata, in recognition of his contributions to undergraduate and post graduate teaching. He is also the founder Director of the Centre for Genetic Counselling. Prof. Dey is the author of many scientific papers resulting from research funded by University Grants Commission, Council of Scientific & Industrial Research, Inter-University Accelerator Centre, National Tea Research Foundation & Department of Biotechnology.

Contents

Preface

This book provides the recent developments and advances in research on Down syndrome. It also covers a wide range of topics, including investigations on neurologic, urologic, dental and allergic disorders in Down syndrome. Chromosomal aneuploidy is the leading cause of fetal death in our species and the information about chromosomal nondisjunction in man largely comes from studies in trisomy 21 or Down syndrome, the most frequent of the autosomal trisomies in liveborns. The cause of nondisjunction of chromosome 21 remains largely unknown. Accurate investigations on meiotic nondisjunction have been made possible in recent years by the development and utilization of microsatellite markers. Although several hypotheses have been put forward, it is still unclear as to whether particular gene loci on chromosome 21 are sufficient to cause Down syndrome and its associated features. For over two decades trisomy 21 has represented a prototype disorder for the study of human aneuploidy and copy-number variation, but the genes responsible for most Down syndrome phenotypes are still unknown. The genetic mechanism by which wide variability in the phenotypes arise is not understood, additional complexity may exist due to possible epigenetic changes that may act differently on Down syndrome. Consequently, gene-disease links have often been based on indirect evidence from cellular or animal models. Numerous mouse models with features reminiscent of those seen in individuals with Down syndrome have been produced and studied in some depth, and these have added considerable insight into possible genetic mechanisms by which trisomy 21 leads to Down syndrome.

The book is organized into four sections. All sections include chapters on recent advances in Down syndrome research.

Section I deals with our present knowledge on the genetics and etiology of Down syndrome.

Section II discusses the utility of using mouse model for in depth study of Down syndrome. Down syndrome could be used as model for understanding the genetics of Alzheimer's disease.

Section III describes the etiology and clinical aspects of some common disorders of Down syndrome patients such as neurologic, urologic, dental and allergic disorders.

Section IV focuses on prenatal diagnosis and screening of Down syndrome.

This book provides a concise yet comprehensive source of current information on Down syndrome. Research workers, scientists, medical graduates and paediatricians will find it an excellent source for reference and review.

Acknowledgements

The editor wants to acknowledge the superb assistance of staff members and management of InTech Publisher. In particular, Ms. Romina Krebel for her co-ordination and editorial assistance. We are grateful to all contributing authors and scientists who made this book possible by providing valuable research and review papers.

Subrata Dey
Salt Lake City, Kolkata,
India

Part 1

Genetics and Etiology

1

Genetics of Down Syndrome

Thomas Eggermann[1] and Gesa Schwanitz[2]
[1]*Institute of Human Genetics, RWTH Aachen*
[2]*Institute of Human Genetics, University of Bonn*
Germany

1. Introduction

1.1 Morphology

According to the International System for Human Cytogenetic Nomenclature (ISCN) human chromosomes (2n=46) are divided into two groups (Shaffer et al., 2009). These are the two sex chromosomes or gonosomes (X,Y) and the 44 non-sex chromosomes or autosomes, respectively. Chromosomes of the latter group are numbered as 1 to 22, according to their decreasing size. Autosomes in somatic cells are comprised of two homologous, genetically identical chromosomes.

The time of the first conference for nomenclature in 1959 is called the pre-banding area. Individual chromosomes could not yet be ascertained beyond reasonable doubt. Thus it happened that the second smallest chromosome, chromosome 21, which had been analysed three times in the patient's karyotype, was believed to cause Down Syndrome (DS). Later studies showed that DS is trisomic in the smallest chromosome. To avoid conflict between previous and subsequent publications, the position of the two smallest chromosomes (21 and 22) was switched, resulting in the definition of DS as trisomy 21.

The relative length of chromosome 21 is 1.9 ± 0.17 % of the total length of the human genome, and its size is approximately 60 Mb. Chromosome 21 belongs to the acrocentric chromosomes, i.e. the centromere is localised closer to the end of the short arm (p). The short arm 21p is heterochromatic but consists of different types of repetitive DNA (Figure 1)(Wyandt and Tonk, 2004).

The relative length of the short arm of chromosome 21 comprises 30 % of its total length (Figure 1). Variants in brilliant fluorescence after QFQ-staining are diagnosed in 2.0 % of band p11.2 and 10.0 % of band p13. Duplications in p12 show a frequency of 0.7-1.3 % and 0.1 % in the satellites of p13. Deletions in all three regions (p11.2, p12, p13) are rare (Kalz et al., 2004).

These frequencies are derived from population studies based on Europeans. Significant differences in comparison to other ethnic groups have been observed (Kalz et al., 2005). The polymorphic regions in the short arm of chromosome 21 allowed the first studies on the parental origin of trisomy 21 (Mikkelsen et al., 1980).

The long arm (q) of chromosome 21 is euchromatic, with the exception of the peri-centromeric region q11.1 and the distal telomere.

Chromosomes are usually presented and analysed in the metaphase of mitosis after *in vitro* cultivation, which is not identical to their appearance *in vivo*. Among the differentiated cells,

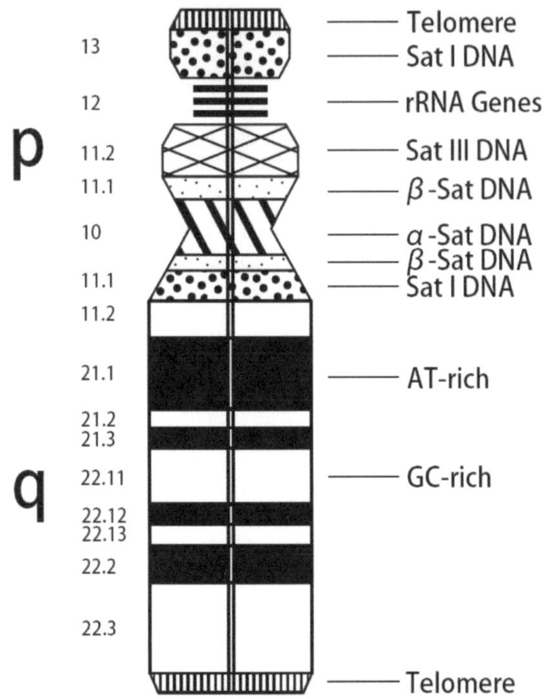

Fig. 1. Structure and morphology of chromosome 21. Ideogram according to the ISCN (Shaffer et al., 2009).

only some (i.e. T-lymphocytes in a blood sample) can be stimulated *in vitro* to enter the cell cycle again and thus represent a selected cell population. In addition, cells are treated with colcemid. This substance arrests the chromosomes in the c-metaphase of mitosis and, at the same time, increases the contraction of chromosomes, rendering the centromeres and the fissure between the two chromatids visible (Figure 2a).

1.2 Structure

The central part of the centromere of chromosome 21 consists of α-satellite DNA that is almost identical to the centromere of chromosome 13 (homology 99.7%)(Figure 1). On both sides α-satellite DNA is flanked by β-satellite DNA. These two non-coding regions can vary significantly in size through duplication or deletion. They are irrelevant for the carrier, unless their length is less than 20 % of the average length of the region and thus prevents the normal development of the kinetochores. This would result in the failure of exact separation of the chromatids in the anaphase of mitosis (Waye et al., 1989; Mitchell et al., 1992).

Distal of the β-satellite DNA, satellite DNA class III is situated on the short arm (p11.2). Significantly varying in size, this band shows a specific absorption of DNA-dyes. Therefore, it is defined as a polymorphic region. It is followed in the short arm by the band p12, which is also named the nucleolus organising region (NOR) and contains the ribosomal RNA-genes. It is characterised by its slightly lateral expansion (satellite stalks). It is polymorphic and can be deleted or amplified (Tagarro et al., 1994a). The most distal regions of the short arms are the satellites (p13 or s), consisting of Sat I DNA with the telomeres at the ends

(Tagarro et al., 1994b). Satellites are also polymorphic varying in size and staining characteristics. They also have the ability to duplicate.
In describing the structure of the short arm of chromosome 21, only the main components of the different bands are mentioned. Especially p11.1, p11.2, and p13 contain further subgroups of repetitive DNA.

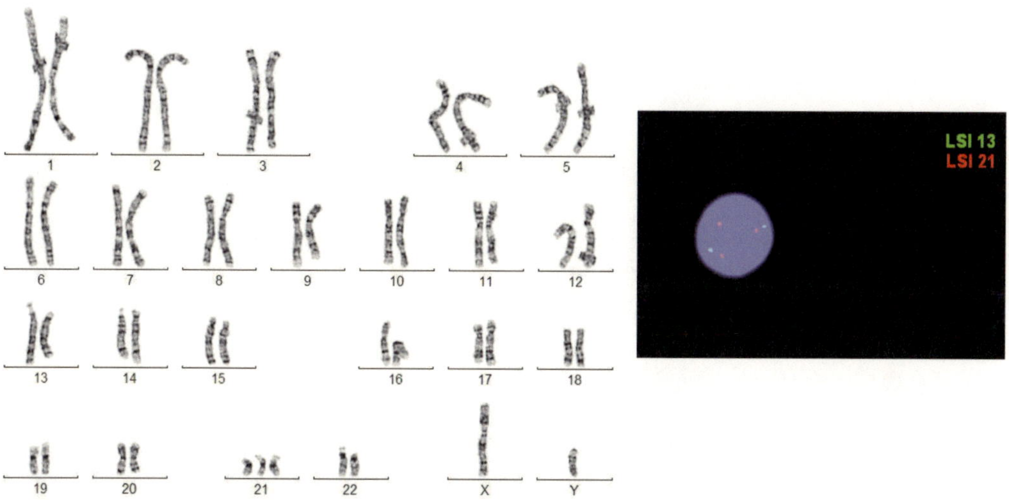

a) b)

Fig. 2. Routine diagnostic workup for identification of trisomy 21. **a)** Standard karyotype (47,XY,+21) by GTG banding (by kind courtesy of U. Mau-Holzmann, Tübingen). **b)** Interphase FISH showing three signals of chromosome 21 and two of chromosome 13 (LSI21:21q22.13q22.2; AneuVysion multicolor DNA probe Kit, Vysis).

According to the literature, the proximal heterochromatic region of the long arm (q11.1) of chromosome 21 consists of β-satellite DNA boarding the central α-satellite DNA and followed distal by Sat I DNA (Waye et al., 1989; Mitchell et al., 1992; Tagarro et al., 1994a, 1994b). The main part of the long arm is euchromatic. AT- and GC-rich bands have characteristic sequences and can be differentiated by their typical staining features (figure 1). These bands of single copy DNA are interspersed by non-coding repetitive DNA (SINEs and LINEs).

1.3 Aneuploidy and gene content

A complete or partially aneuploid chromosome is associated with a pathologic phenotype in the carrier, the expression of which depends on the type and amount of the aberrant genetic material.
In contrast to chromosome 22, chromosome 21 consists of a high number of AT sequences which contain a smaller amount of vitality-determining genes than the GC-rich ones.
GC-rich or housekeeping genes are expressed in most cell types. They lead to proteins that carry out various metabolic and structural functions. In contrast, the AT-rich genes are tissue-specific and are only active in certain cell types while being inactivated in others by methylation. This gene inactivation is accompanied by a more condensed structure of the

chromatin and, consequently, the DNA of these genes is not accessible to the transcription factors. These AT-rich DNA regions show a higher staining intensity and can thus be localised by chromosome analysis.

Because of its high content of AT-rich regions, trisomy 21 is compatible with life, and in the majority of cases, leads only to retardation in the development of the carrier and not, as in trisomy 22, to lethality.

The gene map of chromosome 21 was initially constructed by combining the analyses of small structural aberrations with the results of different gene product analyses (dosage effect). Chromosome 21 was sequenced in 2000 (Hattori et al., 2000), and 225 loci (genes) were identified, which was less than expected. This might explain the relatively mild phenotype of the carriers.

In the following years, a high number of small regions in 21q has been analysed in order to localise the DS critical region (Figure 3)(Wong, 2011), but recent investigations revealed in contrast to the first assumptions that a direct genotype-phenotype correlation does not exist, since a large number of gene products from chromosome 21 also influences gene products and their function on heterologous chromosomes (Gardner and Sutherland, 2004; Weinhaeusel et al., 2011).

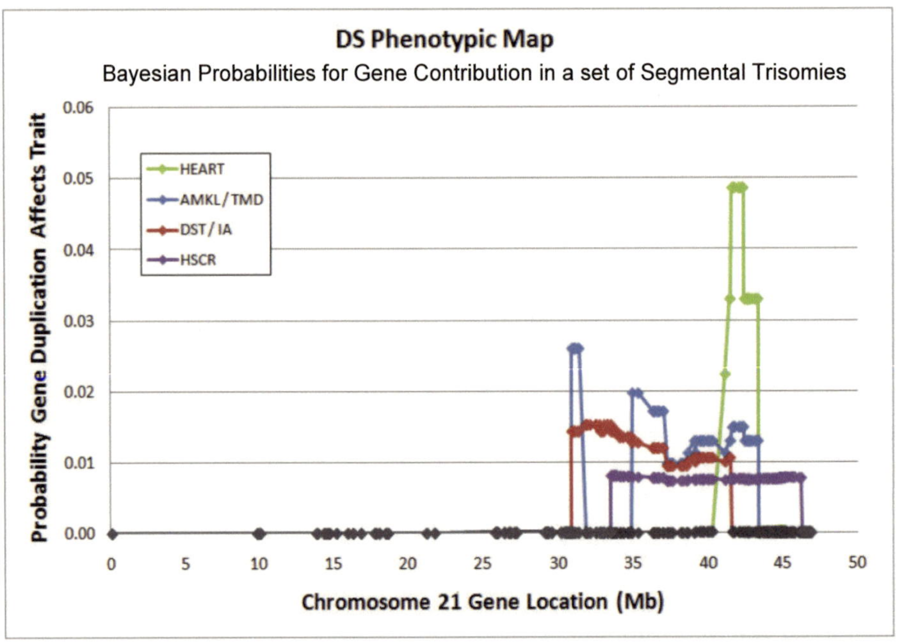

(AMKL acute megakaryocytic leukemia; TMD transient myeloproliferative disorder; DST duodenal stenosis; IA inperforate anus; HSCR Hirschsprung disease)

Fig. 3. Genotype-phenotype correlation in trisomy 21 based on partial trisomy 21 cases (from Korbel et al., 2009). (with kind permission of J.R. Korenberg)

2. Historic development of the cytogenetics of DS

DS was the first malformation complex that could be delineated as a chromosome abnormality in 1959. This was enabled by the new technology to prepare chromosomes in

the metaphase of mitosis. In the early years, mitoses were analysed after direct preparations of bone marrow cells and long term cell cultures of tissue biopsies. Starting in 1960, the lymphocyte culture of peripheral blood was established. Thereby screening of handicapped persons on a large scale became possible. At the beginning of the 1980s, prenatal diagnoses were started for high-risk groups.
Any extension of the spectrum of investigations, any more precise definition of the localisation of the aberration and characterisation of the patients´ symptoms were combined with an improvement of the investigation methods.
The direct preparation of meristematic somatic cells was followed by long-term and short-term cell cultures of differentiated somatic cells removed postpartum, by the culture of amniotic fluid specimen and biopsy of chorionic villi, as well as the analysis of germ cells and their precursor stages in certain special cases, of polar bodies and early postzygotic stages like morula and gastrula in preimplantation diagnostics.
Initially, the presentation of chromosomes was only possible through homogeneous staining, which was succeeded by application of radioactive markers and subsequently of the differentiated characterisation of the chromosomal banding patterns (GTG, GAG, QFQ, RBG, RBA, CBG, and others).
Today, a necessary requirement in diagnostic investigations is a high differentiation of the euchromatin (usually 550 bands per genome). By that way, structural aberrations of chromosome 21 can be safely detected microscopically, starting with a minimal length of 5 Mb. In the 1980s, fluorescence-in-situ hybridisation (FISH) as a new technique was introduced (Figure 2b). By FISH the characterisation of either the entire euchromatin or the centromeric areas or selected euchromatic bands with specific DNA-probes became possible. Simultaneously, this allowed the analysis of cells in interphase and the rapid investigation of larger amounts of cells without cell culture. This so-called rapid aneuploidy testing is especially important for prenatal diagnostics.
Further improvement of the investigation spectrum provided the development of the comparative genomic hybridisation (CGH) with the advancement to the microarray, which has been depicting an improvement and specification of diagnostics on the molecular-genetic level through development of specific tiling arrays.
The newest development is next-generation sequencing. This method is still known to be in trial tests, and its establishment in diagnostics is to be expected.
The various methods of investigation are often combined to improve diagnostics.

3. Types and frequencies of chromosome 21 aberrations

In addition to the predominance of standard trisomy 21 as the cause of DS, further types of aberrations exist. They differ in relation to the type of abnormality, and they lead to different prognoses as to the chances of development of the carrier and recurrence risks for the relatives of a carrier.
Therefore, the indication for a chromosome analysis is always given in the presence of the distinct phenotype of DS.

3.1 Standard trisomy 21

In this type of aberration, the carrier has 47 chromosomes, including three chromosomes 21. It accounts for nearly 90% of DS cases. Standard trisomy 21 typically occurs sporadically, therefore the recurrence risk is low.

The majority of free trisomy 21 cases (85-90%) originates from errors in maternal meiosis. In particular, maternal meiosis I is the most frequently affected stage of nondisjunction (>75%), whereas maternal meiosis II errors account for >20%. In 5% of free trisomy 21, paternal meiotic errors can be observed, here meiosis II nondisjunction is more frequent than meiosis I errors. In addition, postzygotic mitotic errors have also been reported (5%). The predominant influence of disturbed maternal meiosis is reflected by the decreased number of of chiasmata in meiosis I increasing with maternal age. Indeed, the reason for this association is unknown, however numerous hypotheses have been proposed (for review: Hultén et al., 2010).

3.2 Robertsonian translocations

Trisomy 21 due to an unbalanced translocation of chromosome 21 with a hetero- or homologous acrocentric, satellite-bearing chromosome (13, 14, 15, 21, 22) is called a Robertsonian translocation. However, the frequency of translocation partners varies and is a result of homologies in the heterochromatin of the short arm, thus leading to failures in the pairing of meisosis I. The resulting fusion products can be monocentric or dicentric with an inactive centromere.

In monocentric translocation chromosomes, the centromere can derive from each of the two partners or can be a hybrid structure originating from both of them.

Robertsonian translocations involve about 5% of the cases of trisomy 21. Approximately 75% are formed de-novo in the carrier , and 25% are familial (for review: Gardner and Sutherland, 2004). Among these, translocation 21/21 is an unusual rearrangement, but in the majority of cases, it is not a fusion of homologous but the formation of an isochromosome.

In general rule, carriers of the balanced Robertsonian translocation display only 45 chromosomes, the unbalanced ones show 46, as in the majority of carriers, and two short-arm regions are lost. The loss of two NOR-regions does not lead to clinical symptoms in the carriers of balanced translocations.

Among the different heterologous translocations of the acrocentric chromosomes with chromosome 21, the combination with chromosome 14 (rob(14q21q)) is the most frequent one with about 60%. This is followed by the translocation rob(21q21q) or by the formation of isochromosome i(21q21q), respectively, in 35% of the cases. The other translocations are rare and do not exceed 5%. (for review: Gardner and Sutherland, 2004)

Current studies of meiosis are leading to new insights on frequency of formation and postzygotic selection of Robertsonian translocations in familial cases. These studies are largely based on analyses of translocation rob(14q21q) as the most common subgroup. According to these, women with a balanced translocation have an aberrant karyotype in about 20 % of their polar bodies as well as in the oocytes and men in 10-15% of their sperms. These frequencies decrease postzygotically in the course of the development of the embryo, therefore the risk of a child with heterologous translocation trisomy 21 amounts to only 8% if the mother is the carrier and to 4 % with the father (for review: Gardner and Sutherland, 2004).

It is noticeable that in families with translocations, children with a normal phenotype carry a balanced translocation more often than the normal karyotype if the origin is maternal (60:40), while the ratio is equal with paternal origin (50:50).

3.3 Reciprocal translocations

Reciprocal translocations are caused by the exchange of euchromatic regions of chromosome 21 with the euchromatin of different autosomes or gonosomes. In addition to trisomic regions in various length and location of chromosome 21, unbalanced forms at the same time show partial monosomy for the exchanged regions of the second translocation chromosome. As a result, the phenotype in the carriers of unbalanced translocations is not consistent.

Caused by the rare occurrence of these translocations, there are no reliable data for their incidence, a frequency of less than 1:1000 standard trisomies can be assumed. According to the literature, the most common partners for a reciprocal translocation seem to be the chromosomes 18 and 22 (Schinzel, 2001).

3.4 Duplications

This type of aberration is always formed de-novo in carriers with a noticeable pathologic phenotype. If the duplicated segment is only of small size or originated from a postzygotic mosaic, the impairment of the carrier may be mild, and he might have an almost unrestricted life opening the possibility of inheriting the duplication to his offsprings.

A duplication in the cells of the carrier can be caused by an unequal pairing of homologous chromosomes in the pachytene of meiosis I and an aberrant crossing-over as the consequence.

A paracentric inversion in the long arm of a parental chromosome 21 may present an increased risk for the formation of a duplication. According to published cases, the size of the duplicated region can vary significantly, and so far, no preferential sites for the exchange have been documented. With the few existing case reports, no data concerning the frequency of duplications can be given.

3.5 Submicroscopic aberrations

Investigations with FISH probes and applications of molecular-genetic methods for small euchromatic regions enabled the detection of structural aberrations in chromosome 21 in a size of less than 5 Mb. The amount of disorders that can be attributed to small duplications and deletions of chromosome 21 therefore has risen significantly within the last years. The phenotype of the carriers is predominantly not characteristic for the DS.

3.6 Gene mutations

Meanwhile, extensive genotype-phenotype correlations on the basis of structural aberrations of chromosome 21 have been reported, which help to narrow down the DS critical regions (Figures 3, 4)(for review: Korbel et al., 2009). A small number of genes has been proposed to cause the specific DS features, and among them are: DSCR1, DYRK1A or APP (for further details see other chapters of this book).

3.7 Mosaicism

The frequency of trisomy 21 mosaics after chromosomal analysis is about 3-5 %. This number is most likely too small since tissue-specific mosaics cannot always be detected.

Mosaics always originate from mitotic aberrations during the early postzygotic development of the conceptus. Their formation may be caused by an aberrant zygote loosing one of the three chromosomes 21 of a standard trisomy in a portion of the cells. Alternatively, the zygote can have a normal karyotype, but in a postzygotic mitosis, nondisjunction of chromosomes 21 takes place.

Structural aberrations of chromosome 21 as mosaics are always caused by postzygotic rearrangements. Carriers of mosaics with the aberrant cells occuring only in the gonads have an increased risk compared to the general population of the same age for the birth of a child with the aberration in all cells.
The risk of mosaic carriers for a retardation or affected offspring can not be specified because of the different types of aberrant karyotypes and their unequal distribution in the organism.
If the percentage of trisomic cells in all somatic tissues is small (0.5 – 5 %), the phenotype of the carrier can be normal.
Carriers with mosaics have a better prognosis than carriers of non-mosaic trisomies, but there is always a risk of uneven distribution of pathologic cells in the various tissues. Therefore, only the analyses of cells type stemming from different germ layers can lead to a reliable prognosis concerning the development of the patient.

3.8 Tetrasomy 21

A specific type of hyperploidy 21 is the tetrasomy where the chromosome 21 is present for four times. In the literature, only single cases have been published (Gardner and Sutherland, 2004). This abnormality can either consist of four free chromosomes 21 or of two normal chromosomes and in addition an isochromosome 21. The aberration is usually lethal in the conceptus in early pregnancy, but a mosaic constitution has been diagnosed in patients postnatally.

4. Techniques for DS testing

Many different cytogenetic as well as molecular-genetic techniques have been developed in the past to detect standard trisomy 21 and structural aberrations of chromosome 21. Whereas the "simple" detection of genomic imbalances can be performed with numerous molecular techniques (short tandem repeat typing, MLPA, molecular karyotyping), information on structural rearrangements is usually up till now achieved by classical microscopic methods, e.g. chromosome analysis and FISH. In future the development of high resolution next generation sequencing techniques will allow a nearly complete overview on all numerical and unbalanced structural rearrangements in one molecular assay.

4.1 Chromosome analyses

Chromosome investigation is the conventional cytogenetic method based on cells undergoing mitosis to obtain metaphase spreads. The chromosomes can be pre-treated and stained according to different protocols to induce specific banding patterns. By karyotyping, the specifically banded chromosomes can be arranged into seven groups (A to G) based on descending order of size and of the position of the centromere. According to the type of induced banding pattern, two subtypes can be defined: a) those resulting in bands distributed along the length of the whole chromosome, such as G-, Q- and R-bands, and b) those that stain specific chromosome structures (e.g. C-bands, nucleolus organizing regions, telomeric bands)(Shaffer et al., 2009).
The advantage of classical cytogenetics is that both unbalanced as well as balanced chromosomal aberrations are detectable. However, the technique is limited by the microscopic solution. Therefore, imbalances <5 Mb are not analysable by routine cytogenetics. Another disadvantage is that the majority of cell types has to be cultured in vitro either as a short-term

or long-term culture. The long culture times bear the risk of *in-vitro* chromosomal changes. The direct preparation of mitoses is only possible when analysing meristematic cells (bone marrow biopsies, trophoblast cells, germ cells and their precursors). This mehtod has the advantage that the chromosomal analysis reflects the situation in-vivo.
Chromosome analyses are mainly done after lymphocyte culture from peripheral blood samples. The cells are easily obtained and stimulated to mitosis, and the time of cultivation is only 48-72h.
The chromosomes are arranged in a formal karyotype, according to their size, centromere position, and banding pattern (Figure 2a) following the International System for Human Cytogenetic Nomenclature (ISCN; Shaffer et al. 2009).

4.2 Fluorescence-in-situ-hybridization (FISH)

FISH is a widely used method to analyse different target DNA sequences by supplying specific DNA - probes. It combines cytogenetic and molecular genetic techniques. The principle of FISH is the interaction of a labelled single-stranded DNA with a denatured metaphase or interphase.
Since a much higher resolution than chromosome analysis, FISH is used to identify and characterise small structural chromosome aberrations in clinical cytogenetics, including microdeletions and microduplications. A precise and detailed breakpoint analysis is possible. However, a FISH investigation is only applicable if the aberration in question is suspected.
At first this technique was restricted to metaphase analysis, meanwhile, it has gained importance in interphase diagnostics as well. In particular the latter procedure is extremely helpful to detect low-level mosaicism. Furthermore, it has enabled rapid prenatal testing for the frequent aneuploidies in the fetus, including trisomy 21 (for review: Caine et al., 2005).

4.3 Microsatellite typing

Short tandem repeat markers (STRs, microsatellites) are highly informative molecular markers which are easy to handle. STRs have been described as an abundant class of DNA - polymorphisms in the human genome, consisting of highly repetitive short DNA - sequences. They can be typed by using PCR and single-copy primers flanking the repeats, followed by denaturing on a high resolution gel or by capillary electrophoresis. In 1991, Petersen and co-workers were the first to describe the application of these markers in order to determine the parental origin of the extra chromosome in families with a trisomy 21 patient. Meanwhile, numerous studies on the origin of unbalanced chromosomal aberrations have been published.
It is the advantage of microsatellite analysis that it needs only minimal amounts of genomic DNA. Furthermore, it is a fast and simple method which is widely established. It is therefore not amazing that this technique is one of the most frequently used methods for rapid prenatal aneuploidy testing (Mann et al., 2004). It circumvents time-consuming cell cultivation and needs approximately 6-8 h from taking the sample to final report. In addition, the comparison of the allelic distribution of a fetus and his parents allows the exclusion of a maternal contamination in fetal DNA - samples.
However, the technique does not allow the detection of balanced rearrangements. Furthermore, a reduced informativity of microsatellite markers might hamper the interpretation. In particular in case of parental consanguinity, the informativity might be reduced.

4.4 Multiplex Ligation-dependent Probe Amplification (MLPA)

Multiplex Ligation-dependent Probe Amplification (MLPA) is a simple, high throughput method that allows detection of DNA copy number changes of up to 40 sequences in a single reaction. It is based on the semi-quantitative polymerase chain reaction principle and can be applied for detecting copy number changes and has been developed by MRC Holland (http://www.mlpa.com/). MLPA has rapidly gained acceptance in genetic diagnostic laboratories due to its simplicity compared to other methods, its relatively low costs, the capacity for high throughput, and its robustness. Typical for the MLPA is that not target sequences are amplified but MLPA probes that hybridise to the target sequence. In contrast to a standard multiplex PCR, a single pair of PCR primers is used for MLPA amplification. The resulting amplification products of an MLPA assay range between 130 and 480 nucleotides in length and can be analysed by capillary electrophoresis. By comparing the peak pattern obtained to that of reference samples it can be delineated which sequences have aberrant copy numbers. The MLPA reaction can be divided into five major steps: 1) DNA denaturation and hybridisation of MLPA probes; 2) ligation reaction; 3) PCR reaction; 4) separation of amplification products by electrophoresis; and 5) data analysis. For trisomy 21 and further frequent aneuploidies (trisomies 13 and 18), an aneuploidy MLPA kit is commercially available.

The advantage of MLPA is indeed the low amount of genomic DNA needed for genotyping and the fact that that parental samples are not necessary for comparison. However, the procedure is time-consuming and needs at least two days.

4.5 Array analysis

Molecular karyotyping is meanwhile a well established method to identify genomic imbalances. In particular the resolution is much better than that of conventional cytogenetics. While chromosome analysis detects imbalances (deletions and duplications) >5 Mb, array typing has a resolution of <100 kb (figure 4). Microarray analysis allows the identification of any type of segmental imbalance by virtue of its design, but it does not allow the identification of balanced rearrangements or small mosaics.

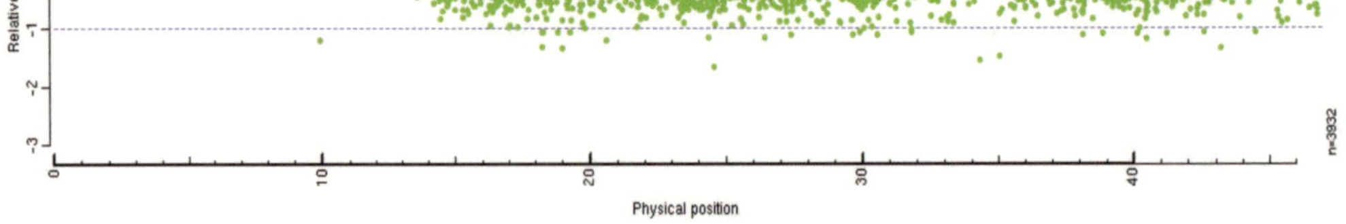

Fig. 4. Example of Micro-array based characterisation of a partial trisomy 21 in a patient affected by Silver-Russell syndrome (Eggermann et al., 2010). The patient did not exhibit any symptoms of DS, thus the trisomic region could be excluded to be involved in the specific phenotypic expression of DS.

As a large number of strategies and platforms are commercially available and cannot be covered here, we strongly emphasize checking the updated literature. Dependent on the array type, molecular karyotyping allows the detection of imbalances with a size of a few kb. And thus the detection rate for chromosomal aberrations in patients with mental retardation could be increased impressively (for review: Shaffer and Bejjani, 2010). However, the interpretation of microarray data is currently hampered by the large genomic instability mainly in non-coding regions, resulting in the analysis of a growing number of copy number variations (CNVs).
Nevertheless, first guidelines for molecular karyotyping have recently been published (Vermeesch et al., 2010).

4.6 Next generation sequencing

Due to the development of genome-wide sequencing (next generation sequencing) the cheap and accurate characterisation of whole genomes in a short time has become possible. Indeed, the methods and applications are extremely manifold and can be merely covered in this short paragraph (for review: Metzker, 2010). Of course, it is too early to apply this complex technology for characterisation of whole chromosome aberrations like trisomy 21. However, target assays will be developed, and it has to be considered that next generation sequencing will allow to rapidly identify and reliably characterise genomic disturbances - balanced as well as unbalanced - and breakpoints in cases of structural rearrangements.

5. Probability for the birth of a child with DS

As the clinical symptoms of a child with the phenotype of DS cannot be considered as a reliable classification, the diagnosis must always be accompanied by a chromosome analysis. The occurrence of trisomy 21 in young mothers lead to screening investigations to ascertain whether exogeneous factors might play a role in the aetiology of trisomy 21 besides the well-known genetic risk factors.

5.1 Subjects for discussion on exogeneous risk factors

Different substances known as mutagens, co-mutagens, and teratogens have been investigated in detail.
The atomic bomb blasts in Japan at the end of the World War Two and the explosion of the atomic reactor in Chernobyl in 1986 are well-known examples of exposures and have been thoroughly explored. However, they did not lead to an increased birth of children with DS (Dean et al., 2000).
Furthermore, neither contact with different organic substances or heavy metals nor an increased consumption of caffeine, alcohol, or nicotine could be shown to increase the number of births of children with trisomy 21 or other chromosome aberrations.

5.2 Endogeneous risk factors

This group encloses carriers of balanced and unbalanced chromosome 21 aberrations and includes the risk of advanced maternal age at pregnancy as well.

5.2.1 Carriers of standard trisomy 21

Adequate therapy has increased the life expectancy of carriers of trisomy 21 significantly within the last decades. Furthermore, a largerly normal life by a specific support of motor and

mental abilities has become possible for many DS individuals. This leads to pregnancies in DS women and makes adequate genetic counselling necessary. The theoretical risk for a woman with trisomy 21 to have a child with trisomy 21 is 50%, but it is reduced by the high amount of abortions in early pregnancy. An empirical risk of 30-40% can therefore be delineated.
However, genetic counselling has also to take into account the risks of a pregnancy in a DS woman suffering from malformations such as heart defects or kidney anomalies. Males with a trisomy 21 are usually sterile.

5.2.2 Recurrence risk in carriers of mosaic trisomy 21

In mosaic cases, the risk of a female or male in rare cases carrier to have a child with full trisomy 21 cannot be estimated precisely, because only the amount of trisomic cells in the somatic tissues can be analysed but not the one in the gonads. The ratio of trisomic cells may even be 100% in the ovaries and testes, leading to the same risk factor as in carriers with a full trisomy.
A special situation is given if the carrier has a normal karyotype in all somatic cells investigated, and the trisomic cells are restricted to the gonads (parental germline mosaicism). In these cases the empiric recurrence risk is delineated as 1-2%, but in two cases of two or more pregnancies with trisomy 21 it is estimated to be much higher (empirical value of more than 10%) (Warburton et al., 2001).
Mosaics are usually found in free trisomy 21 but mosaicism of translocation trisomy 21 has also been observed.

5.2.3 Carriers of a balanced heterologous Robertsonian translocation

Significant differences concerning risk factors have been observed for female and male carriers of heterologous translocations. In female carriers, the empiric risk of having a child with an unbalanced translocation is about 10%, and in males it is only 1-2% (Ferguson-Smith, 1983; Daniel et al., 1989). In both sexes, the translocations rob(14q21q) and rob(15q21q) harbour the additional risk of uniparental disomy 14 or 15 as a consequence of trisomic rescue (Kotzot and Utermann, 2005) which is associated with specific clinical syndromes.

5.2.4 Robertsonian translocation rob(21q21q) and isochromosome 21

Balanced carriers of these two types of rearrangements have a risk of 100% that the offspring will inherit a translocation trisomy 21, regardless of the sex.

5.2.5 Parents with a balanced reciprocal translocation

In the rare group of parents carrying a balanced chromosome rearrangement affecting whole or partial 21q, the risk of having a child with a complete or partial trisomy 21 is relatively high, with about 20% in females and 10% in males. If the translocation chromosomes and their normal homologous show pairing difficulties in meiosis I, the additional risk of a 3:1 segregation has to be taken into account, leading to a recurrence risk of up to 30%. Offspring with an unbalanced translocation show monosomy of the heterologous chromosomal segment, in addition to the complete or partial trisomy 21. As a result, the phenotype will be complex and heterogeneous, depending on the origin of the second translocation chromosome.

5.2.6 Parents with normal karyotype having a child with DS

This is the main group of consultants. The maternal age at pregnancy is significantly elevated in the majority of cases, and therefore, an increased risk for elder women can be

delineated (risk of 1:1667 at 20 years and 1:32 at 45 years (Morris et al., 2002). There is a second slight increase of risk in very young mothers (1:1000 at 15 years). The probability for a child with DS is not correlated with paternal age.
However, in a small cohort of families an age independent high risk for pregnancies with different trisomies has been observed (Munné et al., 2004; Baart et al., 2006).
Molecular investigations made it probable that in these cases the increased aneuploidy rate is caused by an autosomal recessive mutation. To identify this group of carriers a thorough pedigree analysis is necessary, cytogenetic karyotyping is indicated for the consultants and their offspring - children and miscarriages. Failures from pregnancy induction by IVF (in-vitro fertilisation) have to be included in the risk estimation. These couples are usually recommended to a special IVF program for a further pregnancy, and preimplantation-testing procedures might be considered (Stumm et al., 2006).

5.2.7 Siblings and 3rd degree relatives of a patient with DS

Healthy relatives of a patient with a free trisomy 21 have no increased risk for the birth of a child with trisomy 21 when compared to the average population of the same age.
Relatives of a proband with DS caused by an unbalanced structural rearrangement have an increased risk if they are balanced carriers of the translocation (see above). The risk factor depends on the type of rearrangement and on the sex of the carrier.

5.2.8 Prenatal findings of symptoms characteristic for DS detectable by ultrasound

At the end of the first trimester of pregnancy (10th to 12th week,) ultrasound investigations are routinely recommended. At that age, the majority of fetuses with trisomy 21 show a number of characteristic features. These include nuchal translucency, absence of nasal bone, heart defect and growth retardation. In the second trimester, the main symptoms detectable by ultrasonography are a flat occiput, a flat profile of the face, small nose, dysmorphic and deep seated ears, receding chin and short neck, malformations of the internal organs, and growth retardation.
These observations by ultrasound are an indication for prenatal chromosome analysis either by chorionic villi sampling (CVS) or by amniocentesis (AC).

5.2.9 Comparison of invasive and non-invasive prenatal investigations

Non-invasive methods

The main technique in prenatal diagnostics is ultrasound. In Germany, it is usually applied three times during pregnancy. Ultrasound can meanwhile be regarded as a prerequisite for CVS, AC, or fetal blood sampling (FBS) since morphologic abnormalities are caused by a pathologic karyotype in 20-50% of the cases (personal observation).
A second group of non-invasive parameters are specific biochemical factors (AFP, β-HCG, estriol) analysed from maternal blood. They are combined with the risk delineated from the given maternal age. If the result differs from expectation and corresponds to an increased risk for DS, invasive methods to determine the karyotype are applied.
A third possibility for non-invasive investigations in pregnancy is the analysis of fetal cells and fetal DNA in the maternal blood. By special procedures, fetal DNA can be isolated and enriched from maternal blood, however, this method is still under development and is currently not applied in routine prenatal testing.

Invasive prenatal investigations

Three different methods are usually applied: CVS in the first trimester, AC in the second, and AC, FBS, and placenta biopsy in the third.
All three methods generally include an investigation risk of about 1%. Therefore, these methods should only be applied if the genetic risk is higher than the risk of investigation.
Sometimes different methods have to be combined to receive a diagnosis. However, this increases the time of investigation and prolongs the psychological stress of the parents (Geskas et al., 2011).
Usually, a reliable, final diagnosis can only be achieved by invasive investigations but the non-invasive methods enable the investigator to get information of an increased or decreased extent of the pre-existing risk in the individual pregnancy.

6. Comparison of type and contretype of DS

As a full monosomy 21 is lethal in life-born children and also exceedingly rare in spontaneous abortions, the phenotype of carriers of this aberration is delineated from mosaic cases and partial deletions. The clinical findings revealed a number of symptoms, especially facial dysmorphic features that can be defined as opposite type or "contretype" to patients with trisomy 21 (Table 1).

Trisomy 21	**Partial monosomy 21**
Muscular hypotonia	Muscular hypertonia
Overextension of joints	Spasticity
Hyperflexible fingers	Camptodactyly
Flat occiput	Protuberant occiput
Upslanting palpebral fissures	Downslanting palpebral fissures
Small round ears	Large ears
Aplastic nasal bridge	Protuberant nasal bridge

Table 1. Phenotypes of trisomy and (partial or mosaic) monosomy 21. (Schinzel, 2001)

7. DS and uniparental disomy

As trisomic rescue is the most frequent way of uniparental disomy formation, this type of cytogenetic aberration has to be discussed in context with trisomy 21. Uniparental disomy (UPD) is the inheritance of both homologous of a chromosome pair from only one parent. The concept of UPD was first postulated to cause specific phenotypes in the eighties (Engel, 1980). This hypothesis was then confirmed by UPD of different chromosomes in association with typical syndromes. The best examples of this type of aberration are maternal UPD15 (upd(15)mat) in Prader-Willi and paternal UPD15 (upd(15)pat) in Angelman syndrome.
Different mechanisms may lead to UPD (Spence et al., 1988): each of them includes at least two errors either during meiosis or in postzygotic mitoses. During meiosis, a nondisjunction of two homologous chromosomes occurs, which leads to a trisomy in the zygote. In most cases, this zygote will not be viable, unless a correction or a "trisomic rescue" happens. Statistically, in one third of cases, the chromosome of the parent who did not contribute to the trisomy is lost, thus resulting in UPD.

A cytogenetic hint for a trisomy rescue is the confined placental mosaicism (CPM), which describes the presence of a partial chromosomal aberration (usually a trisomy mosaic) in the placenta but not in the fetus. This constitution can be diagnosed in approximately 1-2% of chorionic villous samples (Kalousek et al., 1989). CPM can have relevant clinical consequences since it may lead to placental insufficiency and then induces intrauterine growth retardation.

Clinical features in context with UPD can be caused by:

a. hidden chromosomal mosaicism originating by the UPD formation via trisomy rescue;
b. by the imbalanced expression of imprinted genes in the respective chromosomal region resulting in a specific imprinting disorder;
c. homozygosity for recessive mutations. Interestingly, this phenomenon led to the detection of the first case of UPD. Spence et al. (1988) reported a patient suffering from cystic fibrosis who was homozygous for the mutation F508del in the CFTR gene. Only his mother was a heterozygous carrier for F508del transmitting the mutant gene copy twice to her child. Therefore, UPD always involves the usually unpredictable risk for homozygosity of mutant genes in addition to imprinted gene effects.

Due to the frequency of trisomy 21, UPD of this chromosome should be a well-known aberration. Indeed, maternal as well as paternal UPD21 (upd(21)mat, upd(21)pat) have been reported for several times (for review: Kotzot and Utermann, 2005), including healthy carriers. Based on the latter finding, it can be decided that the clinical course of upd(21)mat or upd(21)pat carriers is rather caused by a hidden chromosomal mosaicism which can be delineated from the UPD formation mechanism or by homozygosity of a recessive allele than by the UPD itself. Imprinted genes involved in the aetiology of imprinting disorders are not localised on chromosome 21. A different epigenetic effect was shown by recent investigations.

It could be demonstrated that trisomy 21 affects the methylation pattern of different heterologous chromosomes by decreasing their extent of methylation (Weinhaeusel et al., 2011) and thus leas to clinical abnormalitiesof the carrier.

8. The simultaneous occurrence of trisomy 21 and other chromosomal aberrations

This group of combined aberrations comprises numerical and structural abnormalities which present as pathologic karyotype in all cells of an organism or as different types of mosaicism. Investigations usually rely on conventional chromosome analyses of spontaneous abortions as in this group the frequency among conceptus with pathological karyotype is about 25% compared to life-born children with 0.2% (own investigations and findings from the literature).

8.1 Double aneuploidies

Trisomy 21 can be combined with aneuploidies of different heterologous chromosomes (Micale et al., 2010). The maternal age of a pregnancy with a conceptus showing a double aneuploidy is on average higher than that with a single trisomy. The life expectance of the carrier is lower in prenatal and postnatal period than in single trisomies. Double trisomies of autosomes show a higher lethality than combinations of autosomes and gonosomes.

8.1.1 Combinations with gonosome aberrations

Gonosomal aneuploidies in patients with an additional trisomy 21 were diagnosed in the four possible combinations with monosomy X, XXY, XYY and XXX. The most frequent gonosome aberration in this context is XXY. Monosomy X often presents as mosaic.

The phenotype of the patients usually corresponds to that of trisomy 21. The reason might be the inactivation of more than one X chromsome and the low number of genes on the Y chromosome. The combinations of these double aneuploidies are more frequent than the total amount of the two single trisomies, or the trisomy combined with that of monosomy X.

8.1.2 Combinations with heterologous autosome aberrations

In life-born children, only three combinations of trisomy 21 with additional heterologous chromosomes have been observed: +8, +13, +18, and trisomy 8 is always occurring as mosaic. The double trisomy 21 and 18 seems to be the most frequent combination with an average of 1:1000 among trisomy 21 carriers. The frequency of this combination is much higher in spontaneous abortions with about 2.5 in 100 trisomies. This is explained by the high and early lethality of conceptus with a double autosomal trisomy.

Clinical investigations reveal a heterogenous picture: The carrier can show the phenotype of one of the 2 trisomies or a combination of both. The majority of double trisomies presents as a mosaic with one or two trisomic cell lines.

8.2 Trisomy 21 in combination with structural aberrations

The most frequent aberration is a trisomy 21 in combination with a balanced Robertsonian translocation rob(13q14q). It has been hypothesized that a familial translocation rob(13q14q) induces frequently errors of pairing of heterologous chromosomes in the prophase of meiosis I leading to an aneuploid gamete (interchromosomal effect). Recent investigations could not prove this hypothesis. It is nowadays assumed that the reduced fertility of the translocation carriers is the reason for pregnancies at increased maternal age, which leads to an elevated risk for pregnancies with trisomy 21.

Further single cases of trisomy 21 combined with structural aberrations comprise unbalanced and balanced reciprocal translocations, deletions, and sub-microscopic aberrations.

9. Differential diagnoses

Carriers of trisomy 21 are characterised by a number of clinical symptoms caused by disturbances during early embryonic development. This abnormal course of differentiation can also occur in other syndromes based on an aberrant embryogenesis.

These syndromes can be caused by other chromosome abnormalities, by monogenic mutations, and by exogeneous factors or teratogenic agents.

Chromosome syndromes with a phenotype that, especially in early childhood, resembles that of children with trisomy 21 are the two poly-X syndromes, penta-X syndrome in the female, and XXXXY in the male.

A monogenic disease with a phenotype similar to that of trisomy 21 is hypothyroidism.

The best-known differential diagnosis to trisomy 21 though, is fetal alcohol syndrome.

The similarity between them is so high and the facial dysmorphic features are so characteristic for both that even in the general population the typical phenotype is well-known but often misinterpreted. Therefore, it may happen that a child with DS is wrongly mistaken as one with fetal alcohol syndrome and which can lead to discrimination of the family.

The possibility that the phenotype of DS may be caused by other diseases than trisomy 21 makes it necessary for all patients with the clinical diagnosis of DS to be investigated cytogenetically because otherwise prognosis, therapy, and estimation of recurrence risk might not be correct.

10. Acknowledgement

We thank U. Mau-Holzmann for providing us with Figure 2a and J.R. Korenberg for the kind permission to use the data included in Figure 3.

11. References

Baart, E.B., Martini, E., van den Berg, I., Macklon, N.S., Galjaard, R.J., Fauser, B.C., Van Opstal, D. (2006) Preimplantation genetic screening reveals a high incidence of aneuploidy and mosaicism in embryos from young women undergoing IVF. *Hum Reprod,* Vol.21: pp. 223-233.

Caine, A.; Maltby, A.E.; Parkin, C.A.; Waters, J.J.; Crolla, J.A. (2005) Association of Clinical Cytogeneticists (ACC). Prenatal detection of Down's syndrome by rapid aneuploidy testing for chromosomes 13, 18, and 21 by FISH or PCR without a full karyotype: a cytogenetic risk assessment. *Lancet,* Vol.366: pp. 123-128.

Daniel, A., Hook, E.B., Wulf, G. (1989) Risks of unbalanced progeny at amniocentesis to carriers of chromosome rearrangements: data from United States and Canadian laboratories. *Am J Med Genet,* Vol.33: pp. 14-53.

Dean, G., Nevin, N.C., Mikkelsen, M., Karadima, G., Petersen, M.B., Kelly, M., O'Sullivan, J. (2000) Investigation of a cluster of children with Down's syndrome born to mothers who had attended a school in Dundalk, Ireland. *Occup Environ Med,* Vol.57: pp. 793-804.

Eggermann, T., Schönherr, N., Spengler, S., Jäger, S., Denecke, B., Binder, G., Baudis, M. (2010) Identification of a 21q22 duplication in a Silver-Russell syndrome patient further narrows down the DS critical region. *Am J Med Genet,* Vo.152A: pp. 356-359.

Engel, E. (1980) A new genetic concept: uniparental disomy and its potential effect, isodisomy. *Am J Med Genet,* Vol. 6: pp. 137-143.

Ferguson-Smith, M.A. (1983) Prenatal chromosome analysis and its impact on the birth incidence of chromosome disorders. *Br Med Bull,* Vol.39: pp. 355-364.

Gardner, R.J.M., Sutherland, G.R. (2004) Chromosome abnormalities and genetic counselling. Oxford University Press (3rd ed.)

Gekas, J., van den Berg, D.G., Durand, A., Vallée, M., WilDSchut, H.I., Bujold, E., Forest, J.C., Rousseau, F., Reinharz, D. (2011) Rapid testing versus karyotyping in Down's syndrome screening: cost-effectiveness and detection of clinically significant chromosome abnormalities. *Eur J Hum Genet,* Vol.19: pp. 3-9.

Hattori, M., Fujiyama, A., Taylor, T.D., Watanabe, H., Yada, T., Park, H.S., Toyoda, A., Ishii, K., Totoki, Y., Choi, D.K., Groner, Y., Soeda, E., Ohki, M., Takagi, T., Sakaki,

Y., Taudien, S., Blechschmidt, K., Polley, A., Menzel, U., Delabar, J., Kumpf, K., Lehmann, R., Patterson, D., Reichwald, K., Rump, A., Schillhabel, M., Schudy, A., Zimmermann, W., Rosenthal, A., Kudoh, J., Schibuya, K., Kawasaki, K., Asakawa, S., Shintani, A., Sasaki, T., Nagamine, K., Mitsuyama, S., Antonarakis, S.E., Minoshima, S., Shimizu, N., NorDSiek, G., Hornischer, K., Brant, P., Scharfe, M., Schon, O., Desario, A., Reichelt, J., Kauer, G., Blocker, H., Ramser, J., Beck, A., Klages, S., Hennig, S., Riesselmann, L., Dagand, E., Haaf, T., Wehrmeyer, S., Borzym, K., Gardiner, K., Nizetic, D., Francis, F., Lehrach, H., Reinhardt, R., Yaspo, M.L. (2000) The DNA sequence of chromosome 21. *Nature,* Vol.405: pp. 311-319.

Hultén, M.A., Patel, S., Jonasson, J., Iwarsson, E. (2010) On the origin of the maternal age effect in trisomy 21 DS: the Oocyte Mosaicism Selection model. *Reproduction,* Vol.139: pp. 1-9.

Kalousek, D.K., Barrett, I.J., McGillivray, B.C. (1989) Placental mosaicism and intrauterine survival of trisomies 13 and 18. *Am J Hum Genet,* Vol.44: pp. 338-343.

Kalz, L., Schwanitz, G. (2004) Characterisation of constitutive heterochromatin, in particular of fluorescence polymorphisms, in a central European population. *Int J Hum Genet,* Vol.4: pp. 1-10.

Kalz, L., Kalz-Füller, B.. Hegde, S., Schwanitz, G. (2005) Polymorphisms of Q-band heterochromatin: qualitative and quantitative analyses of features in 3 ethnic groups (Europeans, Indians and Turks). *Int J Hum Genet,* Vol.5: pp. 153-163.

Korbel, J.O., Tirosh-Wagner, T., Urban, A.E., Chen, X.N., Kasowski, M., Dai, L., Grubert, F., Erdman, C., Gao, M.C., Lange, K., Sobel, E.M., Barlow, G.M., Aylsworth, A.S., Carpenter, N.J., Clark, R.D., Cohen, M.Y., Doran, E., Falik-Zaccai T., Lewin, S.O., Lott, I.T., McGillivray, B.C., Moeschler, J.B., Pettenati, M.J., Pueschel, S.M., Rao, K.W., Shaffer, L.G., Shohat, M., Van Riper, A.J., Warburton, D., Weissman, S., Gerstein, M.B., Snyder, M., Korenberg, J.R. (2009) The genetic architecture of DS phenotypes revealed by high-resolution analysis of human segmental trisomies. *Proc Natl Acad Sci U S A,* Vol.106: pp. 12031-12036.

Kotzot, D., Utermann, G. (2005) Uniparental disomy (UPD) other than 15: phenotypes and bibliography updated. *Am J Med Genet A,* Vol.136: pp. 287-305.

Mann, K., Donaghue, C., Fox, S.P., Docherty, Z., Ogilvie, C.M. (2004) Strategies for the rapid prenatal diagnosis of chromosome aneuploidy. *Eur J Hum Genet,* Vol.12: pp. 907-915.

Metzker, M.L. (2010) Sequencing technologies - the next generation. *Nat Rev Genet,* Vol.11 : pp. 31-46.

Micale, M., Insko, J., Ebrahim, S.A., Adeyinka, A., Runke, C., Van Dyke, D.L. (2010) Double trisomy revisited – a multicenter experience. *Prenat Diagn* Vol.30: pp. 173-176.

Mikkelsen, M., Poulsen, H., Grinsted, J., Lange, A. (1980) Nondisjunction in trisomy 21: study of chromosomal heteromorphisms in 110 families. *Ann Hum Genet* Vol.44: pp. 17-28.

Mitchell, A., Jeppesen, P., Hanratty, D., Gosden, J. (1992) The organisation of repetitive DNA sequences on human chromosomes with respect to the kinetochore analysed using a combination of oligonucleotide primers and CREST anticentromere serum. *Chromosoma* Vol.101: pp. 333-341.

Morris, J.K., Mutton, D.E., Alberman, E. (2002) Revised estimates of the maternal age specific live birth prevalence of Down's syndrome. *J Med Screen*, Vol.9: pp. 2-6.

Munné, S., Sandalinas, M., Magli, C., Gianaroli, L., Cohen, J., Warburton, D. (2004) Increased rate of aneuploid embryos in young women with previous aneuploid conceptions. *Prenat Diagn*, Vol.24: pp. 638-643.

Petersen, M.B., Schinzel, A.A., Binkert, F., Tranebjaerg, L., Mikkelsen, M., Collins, F.A., Economou, E.P., Antonarakis, S.E. (1991) Use of short sequence repeat DNA polymorphisms after PCR amplification to detect the parental origin of the additional chromosome 21 in DS. *Am J Hum Genet*, Vol.48: pp. 65-71.

Schinzel, A. (2001) Catalogue of unbalanced chromosome aberrations in man. De Gruyter, Berlin (2nd ed.)

Shaffer, L., Slowak, M.L., Campbell, L.J. (eDS.)(2009) ISCN: An international system for human cytogenetic nomenclature. S. Karger, Basel.

Shaffer, L.G., Bejjani, B.A. (2010) Development of new postnatal diagnostic methods for chromosome disorders. *Semin Fetal Neonatal Med* [Epub ahead of print].

Spence, E.J., Periaccante, R.G., Greig, G.M., Willard, H.F., Ledbetter, D.J., Hejtmancik, J.F., Pollack, M.S., O´Brian, W.E., Beaudet, A.L. (1988) Uniparental disomy as a mechanism for human genetic disease. *Am J Hum Genet*, Vol.42: pp. 217-226.

Stumm, M., Wegner, R.D., Bloechle, M., Eckel, H. (2006) Interphase M-FISH applications using commercial probes in prenatal and PGD diagnostics. *Cytogenet Genome Res*, Vol.114: pp. 296-301.

Tagarro, I., Fernández-Peralta, A.M., González-Aguilera, J.J. (1994a) Chromosomal localisation of human satellites 2 and 3 by a FISH method using oligonucleotides as probes. *Hum Genet*, Vol.93: pp. 383-388.

Tagarro, I., Wiegantm, J., Raap, A.K., González-Aguilera, J.J., Fernández-Peralta, A.M. (1994b) Assignment of human satellite 1 DNA as revealed by fluorescent in situ hybridisation with oligonucleotides. *Hum Genet*, Vol.93: pp. 125-128.

Vermeesch, J.R., Fiegler, H., de Leeuw, N., Szuhai, K., Schoumans, J., Ciccone, R., Speleman, F., Rauch, A., Clayton-Smith, J., Van Ravenswaaij, C., Sanlaville, D., Patsalis, P.C., Firth, H., Devriendt, K., Zuffardi, O. (2007) Guidelines for molecular karyotyping in constitutional genetic diagnosis. *Eur J Hum Genet*, Vol.15: pp. 1105-1114.

Warburton, D., Garniez, J., Dallaire, L., Thangavelu, M., Ross, L., Anaya D., Pargas, C., Kline, J. (2001) Trisomy recurrence: a reconsideration based on North American data. *Am J Hum Genet*, Vol.69(Supp): p. 232.

Waye, J.S., Willard, H.F. (1989) Human beta satellite DNA: genomic organization and sequence definition of a class of highly repetitive tandem DNA. *Proc Natl Acad Sci U S A*, Vol.86: pp. 6250-6254.

Weinhaeusel, A., Plessl, T., Senger, G., Pulverer, W., Wielscher, M., Pichler, R., Kriegner, A., Gencik, M., Noehammer, C. (2011) DNA methylation alterations in trisomy 21. *Medgen*, Vol. 23: p. 199.

Wong, B.K.Y. (2011) Cognitive deficits in Down syndrome: narrowing „Down" to Olig 1 and Olig 2. *Clin Genet* Vol.79: pp .47-48.

Wyandt, H.E., Tonk, V.S. (2004) Atlas of human chromosome heteromorphisms. Kluwer Academic Publishers, Dordrecht/NL

2

Etiology of Down Syndrome: Risk of Advanced Maternal Age and Altered Meiotic Recombination for Chromosome 21 Nondisjunction

Subrata Kumar Dey[1] and Sujoy Ghosh[1,2]
[1]*School of Biotechnology & Biological Sciences, West Bengal University of Technology,*
[2]*Department of Zoology, Sundarban Hazi Desarat College, Pathankhali, West Bengal,*
India

1. Introduction

Down Syndrome (DS) is the most frequent live born aneuploidy and recognizable form of mental retardation among all the ethnic groups of human population across the globe. The overwhelming majority of this birth defect is caused by trisomy 21 due to nondisjunction (NDJ), i.e., failure of chromosomes to separate properly during meiosis at parental gametogenesis and the fact was initially reported by Lejeune et al. (1959). Since that time attempts were made to explore the etiologic factors that are associated with the underlying mechanism of NDJ of chromosome 21(Ch21). Like that of other autosomal aneuploidy, the errors during maternal oogenesis accounts for about 90% of DS births (Antonarakis, 1991; Freeman et al. 2007), of which majority occurs at first meiotic division(MI) (Antonarakis et al. 1992; Yoon et al. 1996). In searching the maternal risk factors for DS birth, researchers have identified advanced maternal age (Hassold and Chiu, 1985) and altered meiotic recombination (Warren at al. 1987; Sherman et al. 1991) as two strong correlates associated with underlying mechanism of Ch21 NDJ in oocyte and the risk factors are preferentially present in oocyte due to its mode of development in the lifetime of women.

The meiosis in fetal ovary initiates at about 11-12 weeks of gestation (Gondos et al. 1986) and becomes arrested at late prophase I following pairing, synapsis and recombination. The process resumes at the onset of puberty after the follicle receives proper hormonal signal and immediately completes the MI and progress through metaphase of meiosis II (MII) where it pauses until it is fertilized and the meiosis is then completed. Thus the individual oocyte remains arrested in prophase I for 10 to 50 years, depending on the time of ovulation in reproductive life. This protracted event of oocyte growth includes three distinct error prone phases (Hassold et al., 2007). First, the prophase event in fetal ovary, at which change in usual pattern of recombination might lead to subsequent aneuploid oocyte formation. The second risk prone phase is the follicular growth during which the meiosis remains arrested and the genetic and environmental challenges get chance to accumulate in ovarian milieu. The third and the final risk phase is the maturation of oocyte which is associated with the adverse effect of advancing maternal age on protein components involved in chromosome separation system and rapidly deteriorating endocrine environments. In contrast, spermatogenesis begins at puberty and spermatogonial cells complete both MI and MII without any delay (Sherman et al. 2007).

As mentioned earlier, the overwhelming majority of Ch21 NDJ is maternal in origin among all the ethnic varieties of human population studied to date. Based on results from the US (Allen et al. 2009) and other population-based studies (Mikkelsen et al., 1995; Gomez et al., 2000), it has now been estimated that over 90% of NDJ errors leading to trisomy 21 arise in the oocyte and the majority of those occur at MI.

We carried out similar study on Indian trisomy 21 samples, particularly from eastern part of the country and obtained strong replication of those observations (Table 1). This study was started from the year 2001 and till date we included about 400 families having free trisomy21 child. Our STR(short tandem repeat)-PCR analyses estimated over 88% maternal errors with majority of cases (~77%) having NDJ events at MI. The paternal errors account for about 10 % with almost equal distribution of MI and MII NDJ events. The post zygotic mitotic error was estimated about 2%. Very concordant results were also reported for Ukraine and Russian cohorts (Machatkova et al. 2005), and Spanish cohort (Gomez et al. 2000). Little difference among these datasets that does exist is probably due to sampling variation. In this article we discuss the maternal stress factors responsible for the origin of nondisjunction.

2. Effect of advanced maternal age

The effect of 'maternal age' remains as 'black-box' for DS birth. Initially Penrose identified that advanced maternal age as risk for DS birth (Penrose 1933, 1934) and postulated that the maternal age dependent increase in birth rate of DS is in some way associated with the NDJ mechanism. But this effect is restricted only to NDJ that occur in the oocyte (Antonarakis et al., 1992; Ballesta et al., 1999; Muller et al., 2000; Sherman et al., 2005). That is, adverse effect of advanced maternal age is not evident among mothers whose offspring received an extra copy of chromosome 21 as a result of: (1) a NDJ error in spermatogenesis i.e., paternal errors (Yoon et al., 1996; Sherman et al., 2005), (2) a post zygotic mitotic error (Antonarakis et al., 1993; Sherman et al., 2005), or (3) a translocation (inherited or de novo) (Hook, 1983).

The results of earlier studies (Antonarakis et al. 1992; Ballesta et al. 1999; Muller et al. 2000), revealed that the average age of mother at the time of conception of a fetus with DS is significantly higher than that of mothers with normal euploid baby. This observation was confirmed further in the population based study in the Atlanta Down syndrome project (Allen et al. 2009) for US population and recently by us (Ghosh et al. 2010a) for Indian population. All these reports suggest that the advanced maternal age is risk factor for both the MI and MII errors and both types of error are potentially related in respect to their association with risk factors. Further, Atlanta Down syndrome project suggests (Allen et al. 2009) that maternal age specific incidence rate for live birth with free trisomy 21 may differ between MI and MII errors: the increasing risk for MII errors is shifted to the older maternal ages compared with MI errors. Interestingly, the women with MII errors are in average older than mothers with MI errors, as evident in both US (Allen et al. 2009) and Indian cohorts (Table 1). All these observations led the workers to propose several hypotheses to explain the intriguing association between advanced maternal age and an increasing chance of Ch21 nondisjunction.

Parental Origin	Meiotic Stage of Nondis-junction	Sample size	Proportion	Frequency	Maternal Age at Conception (Years+SD)	Paternal Age at Conception (Years+SD)
Maternal	Meiosis I (MI)	242	MI/(MI+MII)=242 /314	77.07%	29.91+6.12	33.95+2.04
	Meiosis II (MII)	72	MII/(MI+MII)=72 /314	22.9%	31.01+ 3.44	34.01+4.66
	Stage Unknown	17				
	Subtotal	331	Maternal/All=331 /373	88.73%		
Paternal	Meiosis I (PI)	11	PI/(PI+PII)=11/27	40.74%	24.55+3.02	31.85+5.6
	Meiosis II (PII)	16	PII/(PI+PII)=16/ 27	59.25%	26.92+4.91	33.98+4.4
	Stage Unknown	7				
	Subtotal	34	Paternal/All=34/ 314	10.82%		
Post Zygotic Mitotic Error		8	8/373	2.14%	25.66+3.26	31.76+5.21
Origin Unknown		19	19/392	4.8%		
Total Informative Cases		373				
Total Cases		392				
Control		206			24.82+3.9	32.01+4.04

Table 1. Origin of Trisomy 21 in Indian Cohort and Parental Age at conception of Trisomy Foetus

3. Biological aging hypothesis

The hypothesis was originally proposed by Brook et al (1984). The central idea of this hypothesis is that the increasing rate of meiotic errors and subsequent aneuploid birth is related to 'biological aging' of ovary not to the chronological age of women. Two different views do exist about how the biological aging is implicated for increased incidence of trisomic birth. The first view relates the suboptimal level of hormonal signal with higher rate of meiotic errors in aging ovary. The number of antral follicle at various stages of development also declines with increasing maternal age as the fact has been confirmed in several studies (Reuss et al. 1996; Gougeon 1998; Scheffer et al. 1999; Kline et al. 2004). This decline in antral follicle count, together with the accompanying decrease in total oocyte pool generates an imbalance in the hormonal environment in ovary (Warburton, 2005) which predisposes the women for aneuploid conception. Support to this postulate came from the studies on human and mouse (Freeman et al., 2000; Roberts et al. 2005). Alternate to this concept has been proposed by Warburton (1989) in her "limited oocyte pool" hypothesis which suggests a more direct effect of antral oocyte pool size on the risk of aneuploidy. Among older women available antral follicles are limited and ovary has to compromise in selecting a suboptimal or erroneous oocyte for ovulation.

The 'biological aging' can also be interpreted in term of senescence associated degradation of ovarian protein components that are implicated in chromosome separation system in oocyte (Sherman 2005). Interestingly, level of hundred of transcripts, including cell cycle genes have been reported to decrease with increased maternal age in mice and women (Hamatani et al., 2004; Steuerwald et al., 2007).

4. Genetic aging hypothesis

We proposed 'genetic aging' hypothesis (Ghosh et al. 2010b), which states that some of the mothers who have DS baby are genetically older than the mothers of same chronological age who have euploid baby (Ghosh et al. 2010b) and this genetic aging is the underlying cause of biological aging in ovary. In this analyses we estimated the telomere length (TL) of age matched controls and cases to get insight into the state of molecular aging, stratifying the mothers by stage of NDJ and their age of conception (young ,<29 years; middle ,29-35 years; and old ,>35 years). Our results showed that all three groups(M1,MII & control) have similar TL on average for younger mothers. As age increases, all groups show telomere loss, but that loss is largest in the meiosis II mother group and smallest in the euploid mother group with the meiosis I mother group in the middle(Figure 1). Our results do not support the theory that younger women who have babies with Down syndrome do so because they are '*genetically older*' than their chronological age, but we proposed that older mothers who have DS baby are "*genetically older*" than controls, who have euploid babies at the same age. This finding, however, is consistent with the previous result (Dorland et al. 1998), showing no difference in genetic age among young DS mothers and young controls.

The fact of telomere shortening among women with DS child can be explained in several ways. Apparently, the result suggests a possible functional link between telomere maintenance system and chromosome segregating apparatus at molecular level. Degradation of this possible 'molecular link' with age may affect the both system simultaneously. In this regard BubR1 is most promising candidate as mutation in this gene causes rapid senescence and high rate of aneuploidy in mouse (Baker et al., 2004) and the protein shows rapid fall with age. Alternatively, the environmental factor that induces rapid telomere loss at advanced reproductive age might simultaneously affect the chromosome separation system in oocyte. (Chen et al.,2007; Sebastián et al., 2009; Eichenlaub-Ritter et al,. 2007; Susiarjo et al., 2007).

5. Reduced meiotic recombination and its interaction with maternal age

Aside from maternal age, only single factor that has been identified unambiguously to be associated with maternal NDJ is altered pattern of meiotic recombination. The first evidence for association of reduced recombination with the events of NDJ of Ch21 was provided by Warren et al. (1987). Chiasmata are physical connections between homologous chromosomes at the site of recombination and they function to stabilize the paired homologues or tetrad at MI along with sister chromatids and centromere cohesion. It aids in proper chromosome orientation on the meiotic spindle (Carpenter 1994) and ensure their proper segregation to opposite poles. Absence of chiasma formation left the homologous pair free to drift randomly to the poles and if they move together to same pole aneuploidy results. As far as chromosome 21 NDJ is concerned, achiasmate meiosis is the major cause of reduction in recombination frequency (Lamb et al., 2005a, 2005b), although fall in double exchange frequency was reported too (Hawley et al. 1994).

In our analysis of etiology of DS birth in Indian cohort, we recorded only ~22% detectable crossover on MI nondisjoined chromosome in maternal meiosis (Ghosh et al., 2009). This observation was very consistent with the previous observation by Sherman et al. (2007), who reported 45% achiasmate meiosis associated with MI NDJ of Ch 21 in US population. Sherman and her co-workers constructed the linkage map of nondisjoined Ch21 (1994) and estimated 55% reduction in map length than the control CEPH map (39.4cM in contrast to 72.1cM). With similar approach for Indian DS population (Ghosh et al. 2010a), we scored 30.8cM map length of maternal MI nondisjoined Ch 21, which further confirmed the fact that reduced recombination due to absence of chiasma or less recombination frequency in some way increases the risk of NDJ.

In elucidation of the relationship between reduced recombination and maternal age, Sherman et al. (1994) hypothesized that the trisomy 21 conception at advanced maternal age is strongly associated with reduction in recombination frequency. The authors estimated shorter map length of Ch21 for mothers of >35 years with their linkage analysis approach. Very recently, Oliver et al. (2008) also reported a highest occurrence of non-exchange Ch21 pair among the old age (>34 years) women in compare to young (<29 yrs) and middle (29-35 yrs.), although the frequency of non-exchange tetrads remain most frequent among all the risk factors when only young mothers (<29 years) were considered. The authors proposed a model for explaining the risk of Ch21 NDJ in relation to maternal age categories. Among the young mothers risks related to aging is minimum and therefore absence of recombination becomes the predominant cause of NDJ in total risk scenario. If this remains true, then lack of recombination is an age-independent risk factor for Ch21 NDJ. This hypothesis was supported by our previous studies (Ghosh et al. 2009; 2010a) in which we estimated about 80% of younger mothers with achiasmate Ch21 who had NDJ at MI.

The highest frequency of non-exchange Ch 21 among older mothers is difficult to explain as the events of chiasma formation and recombination take place in foetal ovary. The fact led workers (Oliver et al. 2008; Ghosh et al. 2009) to speculate presence of maternal age dependent NDJ mechanism which gains support from the studies on model organisms. Mutation in the gene *nod* (no distributive disjunction) in *Drosphila* causes high frequency of NDJ of non-exchange chromosome (Knowles and Hawley, 1991) and it suggests existence of the genetic component that acts as surveillance system to ensure proper segregation of non-exchange meiotic chromosomes. Presence of such 'back-up system' is also evident in yeast in which, the gene *Mad3* performs the same function (Gillett et al. 2004). Interestingly, proteins with similar function in human have been shown to be down regulated with increasing ovarian age (Baker et al. 2004; Steuerwald et al. 2001). Thus, age-dependent down-regulation of these essential proteins may lead to the decreased ability to segregate properly the non-exchange chromosomes in aging oocyte. However, more direct evidence is needed to establish this speculation as fact.

6. Susceptible chiasma formation and its interaction with maternal age

Aside reduced recombination, unusual chiasma placement is another risk for Ch21 NDJ. Chiasma formation usually takes place at the middle of normally disjoining chromosomes (Lynn et al. 2000). This medially placed chiasma probably maintains the proper balance by counteracting the pull from opposite poles which is needed for proper segregation of chromosomes. But a chiasma close to centromere or close to telomere seems to confer instability and makes the Ch21 susceptible for random segregation and subsequent NDJ (Lamb et al. 1996; 2005a, 2005b). The increased risk of NDJ due to sub-optimally placed chiasma on the chromosome is also evident in model organisms such as *Drosophila* (Rasooly et al.1991; Moore et al. 1994; Koehler et al. 1996a), yeast (Sears et al. 1995;Krawchuk and Wahls,1999) and *Caenorhabditis elegans* (Zetka and Rose, 1995). The study of Lamb et al. (1996), suggested for the first time that a single telomeric chiasma is a risk for malsegregation of Ch21 at MI in oocyte in contrast to single pericentromeric chiasma which increases risk of MII NDJ.

Very recently, Oliver et al.(2008) and we (Ghosh et al.2009) independently conducted population based studies on US and Indian DS populations respectively to get an insight into the interaction between susceptible chiasma configuration on Ch21 in oocyte and maternal age. In doing so we used family linkage approach to detect exchange pattern on nondisjoined Ch21, using set of microsatellite markers and all the analyses were done by stratifying the participating mothers into three age groups:young (>29 yrs.), middle (29-34 yrs) and old (>34 yrs). Surprisingly, the two sets (US set and Indian set) of results were very concordant and revealed that single telomeric exchange is prevalent among younger mothers whose Ch21 nondisjoined at MI. In contrary, single centromeric chiasma is risk for MII NDJ, particularly at older age. For Indian DS sample, we recorded susceptible single chiasma within the 3.1Mb peri-telomeric and 4Mb peri-centromeric segment of 21q for MI younger and MII older categories, respectively (unpublished data). These observations led us (Oliver et al. 2008; Ghosh et al. 2009) to propose a hypothesis which states that maternal age independent risk factor is one which affects all the age groups equally and be detected in highest frequency among younger mothers for whom aging related risk factors are minimum. Alternately, age-dependent risk factors usually intensify with advancing age and so one would expect highest frequency of such factors among older age group (Figure 2). If our prediction is true, the telomeric single chiasma is maternal age independent risk, whereas, the single peri-centromeric chiasma is maternal age dependent factor.

The relationship between centromeric exchange and advancing maternal age can be interpreted in two different ways: 1) pericentromeric exchange set up a sub-optimal configuration that initiates or exacerbates the susceptibility to maternal age-related risk factors, or 2) a pericentromeric exchange protect the bivalent against age related risk factor allowing proper segregation of homologues, but not the sister chromatids at MII (Oliver et al., 2008). A chiasma very close to centromere may cause 'chromosomal entanglement' at MI, with the bivalent being unable to separate, passing intact to MII metaphase plate (Lamb et al.1996). Upon MII division, the bivalent divides reductionally, resulting in disomic gamete with identical centromeres. In this manner, proximal pericentromeric exchange, which occurred during MI, is resolved and visualized as MII error. According to an alternate model, studied in *Drosophila* (Koehler et al. 1996b), proximal chiasma lead to premature sister chromatid separation just prior to anaphase I. Resolution of chiasma requires the release of sister chromatid cohesion distal to the site of exchange (Hawley et al., 1994). Attempt to resolve chiasmata that are very near to centromere could result in premature separation of chromatids. If the sister chromatids migrate to a common pole at MI, they have 50% probability to move randomly into the same pole at MII, resulting in an apparent MII NDJ. Similar observation is evident in yeast in which centromere-proximal crossover promotes local loss of sister-chromatid cohesion (Rockmill et al., 2006). One of the members of centromeric cohesion complex *shugoshin*, when down regulated due to aging shows high frequency of MII NDJ of bivalent with peri-centromeric exchange (Marston et al. 2004). Alternatively, a pericentromeric exchange may protect the bivalent from maternal age related risk factors. The effect of degradation of centromere or sister chromatid cohesion complexes or of spindle proteins with age of oocyte may lead to premature sister chromatid separation. Perhaps the pericentromeric exchanges help to stabilize the compromised tetrad through MI. This would lead to an enrichment of MII errors among the older oocytes. Although there is no specific model system in favor of this mechanism, but some findings in model organisms can be interpreted in this way.

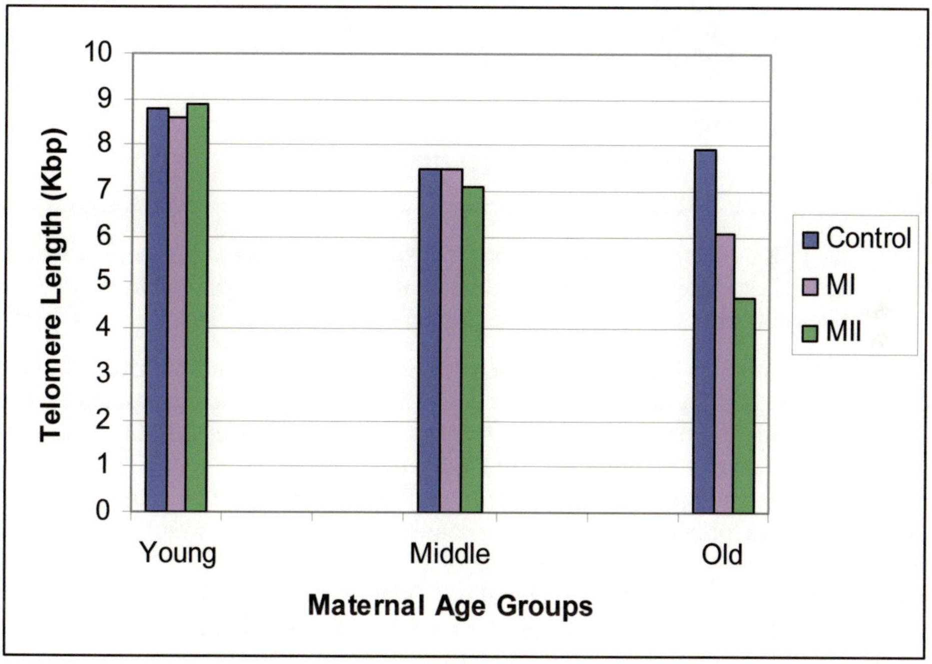

Fig. 1. Telomere length (Kbp) among control and meiotic outcome groups stratified by age categories.

A telomeric chiasma imparts its susceptibility for MI NDJ probably due to recruitment of minimal amount of sister chromatid cohesion complex remaining distal to the exchange event (Orr-Weaver, 1996). Specifically, when the exchange is too far from kinetochore, this could prevent the bi-orientation of the homologues on the meiotic spindle (Nicklas 1974; Hawley et al.1994; Koehler et al.1996b). Alternatively, the integrity of chiasma may be compromised when a minimum amount of cohesin remains to hold homologue together. Thus bivalent may act as pair of functional univalents during MI, as has been evident in human oocyte (Angell 1994, 1995).

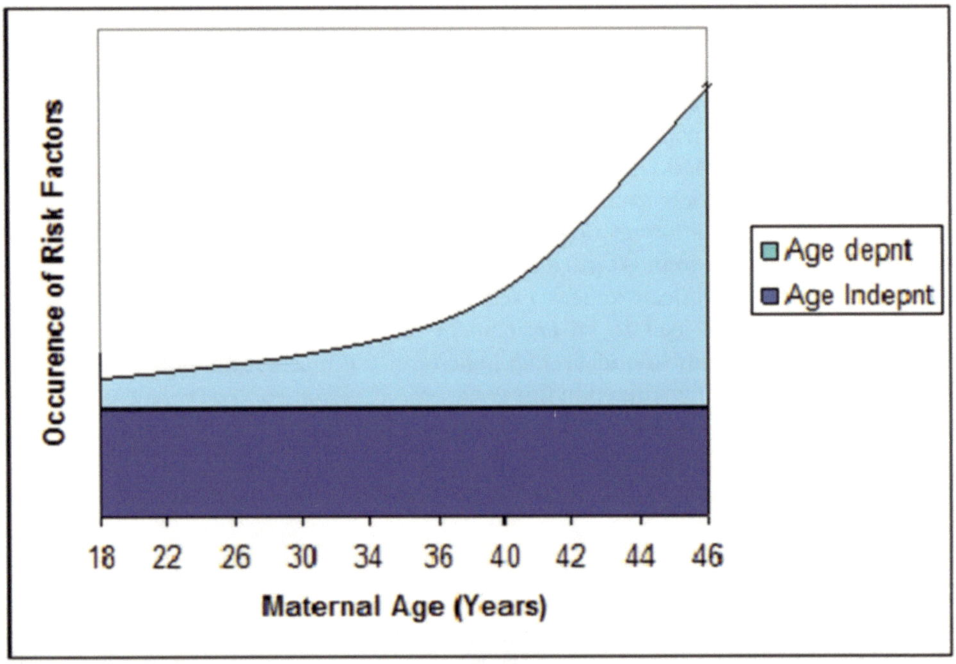

Fig. 2. Risk factor model for Down syndrome birth showing consistent presence of maternal age independent risk factors (Age Indepnt) among all the ages and gradual increased incidence of age dependent risk factors (Age Depnt) with increasing age.

Further, we evaluated the interaction between maternal age and multiple chiasmata on MI nondisjoined Ch21 and found that there is a linear increase in multiple chiasama frequency with advancing age (Ghosh et al.2010a). Interestingly, similar trend is also evident for chromosome 15, 18 and X chromosome (Robinson et al. 1998; Thomas et al. 2001; Bugge et al.1998). This finding suggests two important possibilities. The first one is that the multiple chiasmata might be protective and chromosomes with multiple recombinants probably more resistant to NDJ at least at MI because of an increase in bivalent stability. Secondly, instead of enjoying multiple recombinations some bivalents segregate improperly, particularly in older oocyte, which suggests presence of some aging associated factors that impart risk to these otherwise recombination perfect chromosomes.

7. Summary and conclusion

We have paved half of a century after the initial discovery of cause of DS, but we are still in dark regarding etiology of DS. Although advanced maternal age has been identified unambiguously as risk, its molecular relation with chromosome separation system is enigmatic. It is still elusive whether or not some women are genetically predisposed to altered meiotic recombination and subsequent chromosomal NDJ. Very recently, the gene

PRDM9 has drawn the interest. The gene controls the recombination hotspot of meiotic homologues (Parvanov et al. 2010). The variant of this gene has been reported to make the women susceptible for recurrent miscarriages, infertility and aneuploid pregnancy (Cheung et al. 2010). So PRDM9 is prospective candidate gene whose altered functional state might increase susceptibility of Ch21 NDJ. Similarly, genetic variant of any component of meiotic chromosome separation system could increase the risk for chromosome missegregation in oocyte. Intuitively, the gene BubR1 is of special interest as it is a member of centromere cohesion complex and also known for its role in cellular aging (Baker et al. 2004). In *Drosophila* hypomorphic bubR1 causes high rate of NDJ at MII due to premature sister chromatid separation and these nondisjoined chromosome exhibited centromeric exchange. All these findings suggest the possibility of BubR1 to be a 'missing link' between the molecular mechanism of cellular aging and higher incidence of chromosomal NDJ at advanced age.

The effect of environmental agents on chromosome segregation, particularly in connection with maternal age and recombination remains unexplored. As environmental aneugens have great opportunity to become accumulated within the ovarian microenvironment during protracted oocyte growth phase, their probable effects cannot be underestimated. Although epidemiologic association of some environmental agents with DS birth have been identified, their influence on meiotic recombination and aging is intriguing. The periconceptional smoking and contraceptive use have been identified as potential risk for Ch21 NDJ (Yang et al. 1999), but this observation needs further confirmation. We conducted an epidemiological study on the risk of chewing tobacco and contraceptive use among mothers having DS baby and found some association of chewing tobacco with MI NDJ and contraceptive for both MII and MI (unpublished data). Moreover, the fetal incidence of chiasma formation and recombination make us curious to the probable 'grand maternal' influence on DS birth. Presently we are in position to realize at least that the risk factors associated with DS birth is multidimensional and several mechanisms are involved for chromosome 21 NDJ in women. At this point, it is worth mentioning that the etiology of maternal Ch21 NDJ and subsequent DS birth may be similar across the human population divides irrespective of ethnic and socio-cultural differences. The future investigations should be focused to resolve all these pending issues so that we could move towards complete understanding of risk factors associated with DS birth.

8. Acknowledgements

The project was funded by University Grants Commission (UGC), New Delhi, India. We are grateful to Prof. Eleanor Feingold, Department of Human Genetics & Biostatistics, Graduate School of Public Health, University of Pittsburgh, Pittsburgh,USA for help in statistical analysis.

9. References

Allen EG, Freeman SB, Druschel C, Hobbs CA, O'Leary LA, Romitti PA, Royle MH, Torfs CP, Sherman SL (2009) Maternal age and risk for trisomy 21 assessed by the origin of chromosome nondisjunction: a report from the Atlanta and National Down Syndrome Projects.Hum Genet 125: 41-52.

Angell R (1994) Higher rates of aneuploidy in oocytes from older women. Hum Reprod 9:1199-2000.

Angell R (1995) Mechanism of chromosome nondisjunction in human oocytes.Prog Clin Biol Res 393:13-26.

Antonarakis SE (1991) Parental origin of the extra chromosome in trisomy 21 as indicated by analysis of DNA polymorphisms. Down Syndrome Collaborative Group.N Engl J Med 324: 872-876.

Antonarakis SE, Avramopoulos D, Blouin JL, Talbot CC Jr, Schinzel AA (1993) Mitotic errors in somatic cells cause trisomy 21 in about 4.5% of cases and are not associated with advanced maternal age.Nat Genet 3:146-150.

Antonarakis SE, Petersen MB, McInnis MG, Adelsberger PA, Schinzel AA, Binkert F, Pangalos C, Raoul O, Slaugenhaupt SA, Hafez M, et al.(1992) The meiotic stage of nondisjunction in trisomy 21: determination by using DNA polymorphisms. Am J Hum Genet 50:544-550.

Baker DJ, Jeganathan KB, Cameron JD, Thompson M, Juneja S, Kopecka A, Kumar R, Jenkins RB, de Groen PC, Roche P, van Deursen JM (2004) BubR1 insufficiency causes early onset of aging-associated phenotypes and infertility in mice.Nat Genet 36:744-749.

Ballesta F, Queralt R, Gomez D, Solsona E, Guitart M, Ezquerra M, Moreno J, Oliva R (1999) Parental origin and meiotic stage of non-disjunction in 139 cases of trisomy 21. Ann Genet 42:11-15.

Brook JD, Gosden RG, Chandley AC (1984) Maternal ageing and aneuploid embryos--evidence from the mouse that biological and not chronological age is the important influence. Hum Genet. 66:41-45.

Bugge M, Collins A, Petersen MB, Fisher J, Brandt C, Hertz JM, Tranebjaerg L, de Lozier-Blanchet C, Nicolaides P, Brøndum-Nielsen K, Morton N, Mikkelsen M (1998): Non-disjunction of chromosome 18. Hum Mol Genet 7: 661-669.

Carpenter AT (1994) Chiasma function. Cell 77: 957–962.

Chen JH, Hales CN, Ozanne SE (2007) DNA damage, cellular senescence and organismal ageing: causal or correlative? Nucleic Acids Res 35:7417–7428.

Cheung VG, Sherman SL, Feingold E (2010). Genetic control of hotspots. Science 327:791-792.

Dorland M, van Montfrans JM, van Kooij RJ, Lambalk CB, te Velde ER (1998) Normal telomere lengths in young mothers of children with Down's syndrome. Lancet 352: 961-962.

Eichenlaub-Ritter U, Winterscheidt U, Vogt E, Shen Y, Tinneberg HR, Sorensen R (2007) 2-Methoxyestradiol induces spindle aberrations, chromosome congression failure, and nondisjunction in mouse oocytes. Biol Reprod 76:784–793.

Freeman SB, Allen EG, Oxford-Wright CL, Tinker SW, Druschel C, Hobbs CA, O'Leary LA, Romitti PA, Royle MH, Torfs CP, Sherman SL (2007) The National Down Syndrome Project: design and implementation. Public Health Rep 122:62-72.

Freeman SB, Yang Q, Allran K, Taft LF, Sherman SL. (2000) Women with a reduced ovarian complement may have an increased risk for a child with Down syndrome. Am J Hum Genet. 66:1680-1683.

Ghosh S, Bhaumik P, Ghosh P, Dey SK (2010a) Chromosome 21 nondisjunction and Down syndrome birth in Indian cohort: analysis of incidence and etiology from family linkage data. Genet Res Cambridge 92: 189-197.

Ghosh S, Feingold E, Chakraborty S, Dey SK (2010b) Telomere length is associated with types of chromosome 21 nondisjunction: a new insight into the maternal age effect on Down Syndrome birth. Hum Genet 127: 403-409.

Ghosh S, Feingold E, Dey SK (2009) Etiology of Down Syndrome: Evidence for Consistent Association among Altered Meiotic Recombination, Nondisjunction and Maternal Age Across Populations. Am J Med Genet 149A: 1415-1420.

Gillett ES, Espelin CW, Sorger PK. (2004) Spindle checkpoint proteins and chromosome-microtubule attachment in budding yeast. J Cell Biol.164:535-546.

Gómez D, Solsona E, Guitart M, Baena N, Gabau E, Egozcue J, Caballín MR (2000) Origin of trisomy 21 in Down syndrome cases from a Spanish population registry.Ann Genet 43:23-28.

Gondos, B. et al. (1986) Initiation of oogenesis in the human fetal ovary: ultrastructural and squash preparation study. Am. J. Obstet. Gynecol.155, 189–195.

Gougeon A (1998) Ovarian follicular growth in humans: ovarian ageing and population of growing follicles. Maturitus 30:137-142.

Hamatani T, Falco G, Carter MG, Akutsu H, Stagg CA, Sharov AA, Dudekula DB, Van Buren V, Ko MS. (2004) Age-associated alteration of gene expression patterns in mouse oocytes. Hum Mol Genet. 13:2263-2278.

Hassold T, Chiu D (1985) Maternal age-specific rates of numerical chromosome abnormalities with special reference to trisomy. Hum Genet 70:11-17.

Hassold T, Hall H, Hunt P (2007) The origin of human aneuploidy: where we have been, where we are going. Hum Mol Genet 2: 203-208.

Hawley RS, Frazier JA, Rasooly R (1994) Separation anxiety: the etiology of nondisjunction in flies and people. Hum Mol Genet 3:1521-1528.

Hook EB (1983) Chromosome abnormalities and spontaneous fetal death following amniocentesis: further data and associations with maternal age.Am J Hum Genet 35:110-116.

Kline J, Kinney A, Reuss ML, Kelly A, Levin B, Ferin M, Warburton D (2004) Trisomic pregnancy and the oocyte pool.Hum Reprod 19:1633-1643.

Knowles BA, Hawley RS (1991) Genetic analysis of microtubule motor proteins in *Drosophila*: a mutation at the ncd locus is a dominant enhancer of nod. Proc Natl Acad Sci USA 88:7165-7169.

Koehler KE, Boulton CL, Collins HE, French RL, Herman KC, Lacefield SM, Madden LD, Schuetz CD, Hawley RS (1996a) Spontaneous X chromosome MI and MII nondisjunction events in Drosophila melanogaster oocytes have different recombinational histories. Nat Genet 14: 406-414.

Koehler KE, Hawley RS, Sherman S, Hassold T (1996b) Recombination and nondisjunction in humans and flies. Hum Mol Genet 5:1495-1504.

Krawchuk MD, Wahls WP (1999) Centromere mapping functions for aneuploid meiotic products: Analysis of rec8, rec10 and rec11 mutants of the fission yeast Schizosaccharomyces pombe. Genetics. 153:49-55.

Lamb NE, Freeman SB, Savage-Austin A, Pettay D, Taft L, Hersey J, Gu Y, Shen J, Saker D, May KM, Avramopoulos D, Petersen MB, Hallberg A, Mikkelsen M, Hassold TJ, Sherman SL (1996) Susceptible chiasmate configurations of chromosome 21 predispose to non-disjunction in both maternal meiosis I and meiosis II. Nat Genet 1996 14: 400-405.

Lamb NE, Sherman SL, Hassold TJ (2005a) Effect of meiotic recombination on the production of aneuploid gametes in humans. Cytogenet Genome Res 111: 250-255.

Lamb NE, Yu K, Shaffer J, Feingold E, Sherman SL (2005b) Association between maternal age and meiotic recombination for trisomy 21. Am J Hum Genet 76: 91-99.

Lejeune J, Gauthier M, Turpin R (1959) Les chromosomes humains en culture de tissues. C R Acad Sci Paris 248: 602-603.

Lynn A, Kashuk C, Petersen MB, Bailey JA, Cox DR, Antonarakis SE, Chakravarti A (2000) Patterns of meiotic recombination on the long arm of human chromosome 21. Genome Res 10:1319-1332.

Machatkova M, Brouckova M, Matejckova M, Krebsova A, Sperling K, Vorsanova S, Kutsev S, Zerova T, Arbuzova S, Krejci R, Petersen M, Macek M Sr (2005) QF-PCR examination of parental and meiotic origin of trisomy 21 in Central and Eastern Europe.J Histochem Cytochem 53: 371-373.

Marston AL, Tham WH, Shah H, Amon A (2004) A genome-wide screen identifies genes required for centromeric cohesion. Science 303: 1367–1370.

Mikkelsen M, Hallberg A, Poulsen H, Frantzen M, Hensen J, Petersen MB (1995) Epidemiology study of Down syndrome in Denmark, including family studies of chromosomes and DNA markers. Dev Brain Dysfunct 8:4-12.

Moore DP, Miyazaki WY, Tomkiel JE, Orr-Weaver TL (1994) Double or nothing: a *Drosophila* mutation affecting meiotic chromosome segregation in both females and males. Genetics 136: 953-964.

Muller F, Rebiffe M, taillandier A, Oury JF, Mornet E (2000) Parental origin of extra chromosome in prenatally diagnosed fetal trisomy 21. Hum Gent 106: 340-344.

Nicklas RB (1974) Chromosome segregation mechanisms.Genetics 78:205-213.

Oliver TR, Feingold E, Yu K, Cheung V, Tinker S, Yadav-Shah M, Masse N, Sherman SL (2008) New insights into human nondisjunction of chromosome 21 in oocytes. PLoS Genet 4:e1000033.

Orr-Weaver T (1996) Meiotic nondisjunction does the two-step. Nat Genet 14: 374-376.

Parvanov ED, Petkov PM, Paigen K. (2010) Prdm9 controls activation of mammalian recombination hotspots. Science 12:835.

Penrose LS (1933) The relative effect of paternal and maternal age in Mongolism. J Genet 27: 219-224.

Penrose LS (1934) The relative etiological importance of birth order and maternal age in Mongolism.Proc R Soc B Biol Sci 115: 431-450.

Rasooly RS, New CM, Zhang P, Hawley RS, Baker BS (1991) The lethal(1)TW-6cs mutation of *Drosophila melanogaster* is a dominant antimorphic allele of nod and is associated with a single base change in the putative ATP-binding domain. Genetics 129: 409-422.

Reuss ML, King J, Santos R, Levin B, Timor-Tritsch I (1996) Age and the ovarian follicle pool assessed with transvaginal ultrasonography. Am J Obstet Gynecol 174:624-627.

Roberts R, Iatropoulou A, Ciantar D, Stark J, Becker DL, Franks S, Hardy K (2005) Follicle-stimulating hormone affects metaphase I chromosome alignment and increases aneuploidy in mouse oocytes matured in vitro. Biol Reprod 72: 107-118.

Robinson WP, Kuchinka BD, Bernasconi F, Petersen MB, Schulze A, Brondum-Nielsen K, Christian SL, Ledbetter DH, Schinzel AA, Horsthemke B, Schuffenhauer S, Michaelis RC, Langlois S, Hassold TJ (1998) Maternal meiosis I non-disjunction of chromosome 15: dependence of the maternal age effect on level of recombination. Hum Mol Genet 7:1011-1019.

Rockmill B, Voelkel-Meiman K, Roeder GS (2006) Centromere-proximal crossovers are associated with precocious separation of sister chromatids during meiosis in *Saccharomyces cerevisiae*.Genetics 174:1745-1754.

Scheffer GJ, Broekmans FJ, Dorland M, Habbema JD, Looman CW, te Velde ER (1999) Antral follicle counts by transvaginal ultrasonography are related to age in women with proven natural fertility. Fertil Steril 72: 845-851.

Sears DD, Hegemann JH, Shero JH, Hieter P (1995) Cis-acting determinants affecting centromere function, sister-chromatid cohesion and reciprocal recombination during meiosis in *Saccharomyces cerevisiae*.Genetics 139:1159-1173.

Sebastián C, Herrero C, Serra M, Lloberas J, Blasco MA, Celada A (2009) Telomere shortening and oxidative stress in aged macrophages results in impaired STAT5a phosphorylation. J Immunol 183:2356–2364.

Sherman SL, Allen EG, Bean LH, Freeman SB (2007) Epidemiology of Down syndrome.Ment Retard Dev Disabil Res Rev 13:221-227.

Sherman SL, Freeman SB, Allen EG, Lamb NE (2005) Risk factors for nondisjunction of trisomy 21.Cytogenet Genome Res 111: 273-280.

Sherman SL, Petersen MB, Freeman SB, Hersey J, Pettay D, Taft L, Frantzen M, Mikkelsen M, Hassold TJ (1994) Non-disjunction of chromosome 21 in maternal meiosis I: evidence for a maternal age-dependent mechanism involving reduced recombination. Hum Mol Genet 3:1529-1535.

Sherman SL, Takaesu N, Freeman SB, Grantham M, Phillips C, Blackston RD, Jacobs PA, Cockwell AE , Freeman V, Uchida I et al.(1991) Trisomy 21: association between reduced recombination and nondisjunction. Am J Hum Genet 49: 608-620.

Steuerwald N, Cohen J, Herrera RJ, Sandalinas M, Brenner CA (2001) Association between spindle assembly checkpoint expression and maternal age in human oocytes.Mol Hum Reprod 7: 49-55.

Steuerwald NM, Bermúdez MG, Wells D, Munné S, Cohen J. (2007) Maternal age-related differential global expression profiles observed in human oocytes. Reprod Biomed Online14:700-708.

Susiarjo M, Hassold TJ, Freeman E, Hunt PA (2007) Bisphenol A exposure in utero disrupts early oogenesis in the mouse. PLoS Genet 3:e5.

Thomas NS, Ennis S, Sharp AJ, Durkie M, Hassold TJ, Collins AR, Jacobs PA (2001) Maternal sex chromosome non-disjunction: evidence for X chromosome-specific risk factors. Hum Mol Genet 10: 243-250

Warburton D (1989) The effect of maternal age on the frequency of trisomy: change in meiosis or in utero selection?Prog Clin Biol Res 311:165-181.

Warburton D (2005) Biological aging and the etiology of aneuploidy. Cytogenet Genome Res 111: 266-272.

Warren AC, Chakravarti A, Wong C, Slaugenhaupt SA, Halloran SL, Watkins PC, Metaxotou C, Antonarakis SE (1987) Evidence for reduced recombination on the nondisjoined chromosomes 21 in Down syndrome.Science 237: 652-654.

Yang Q, Sherman SL, Hassold TJ, Allran K, Taft L, Pettay D, Khoury MJ, Erickson JD, Freeman SB (1999) Risk factors for trisomy 21: maternal cigarette smoking and oral contraceptive use in a population-based case-control study. Genet Med 1:80-88.

Yoon PW, Freeman SB, Sherman SL, Taft LF, Gu Y, Pettay D, Flanders WD, Khoury MJ, Hassold TJ (1996) Advanced maternal age and the risk of Down syndrome characterized by the meiotic stage of chromosomal error: a population-based study. Am J Hum Genet 58: 628-633

Zetka MC, Rose AM (1995) Mutant rec-1 eliminates the meiotic pattern of crossing over in *Caenorhabditis elegans*. Genetics 141:1339-1349

3

Combinatorial Gene Effects on the Neural Progenitor Pool in Down Syndrome

Jie Lu and Volney Sheen
Beth Israel Deaconess Medical Center, Harvard Medical School
USA

1. Introduction

Down syndrome (DS) arises from triplication of genes on chromosome 21 (HSA21) and is characterized by neurological complications including cognitive dysfunction, epilepsy, and early onset Alzheimer's disease (AD). At the histological and cellular level, DS brains show prolongation in the cell cycle length of neural progenitors, increased oxidative stress, and mitochondrial dysfunction. These pathological processes likely contribute to the observed decrease in neurogenesis, increased neuronal cell death, enhanced gliosis in the cortex, and a corresponding decrease in both neuronal glutamatergic and GABAergic expression.

With recent advances in molecular biology and human genetics, many HSA21 genes have been identified, putative functions assigned to these genes and network analyses used to predict interconnecting, functional gene pathways. Interactions at this level are further complicated by gene regulatory mechanisms such as DNA methylation, histone acetylation and microRNA. In this respect, the neurological phenotypes seen in DS are not merely due to genomic imbalance from triplication of HSA21 genes, but also additive effects due to influences on associated genes within a given network or pathway and modification of gene expression due to epigenetic factors.

The development of stem cell technologies has provided the opportunity to isolate human neural progenitors (HNPs) and induced pluripotent stem cells (iPS) from patients with known neurological disorders. These reagents are also used as tools to study molecular mechanisms and pharmacological therapies in various human diseases. They provide a means by which an understanding is established for interactions between various genes causal for a human disorder, especially in contiguous gene syndromes that are difficult to faithfully replicate in animal models. We have focused on the study of DS HNPs in relation to neurological phenotypes in the early onset of DS in these individuals.

In the current review, we summarize the approaches taken, recent progress and insights gained from studies of DS during neural development, incorporating insights gained from the use of human DS neural progenitors.

2. Down syndrome phenotype and genotype during neurodevelopment

The most prominent neurological phenotypes in DS include mental retardation (MR), epilepsy, and dementia (early onset AD). Individuals with DS generally have mild to moderate MR with average intelligence quotient (IQ) among children at 50, as compared with normal children at an IQ of 100. Children with DS generally exhibit better visual motor skills (such as drawing) than auditory and linguistic skills, which typically lead to a delay in language skill development. MR can also be accompanied by behavioural issues such as attention-deficit disorder (sometimes with hyperactivity) and autistic behaviour, especially in those with severe intellectual disability. The onset of seizures tends to occur in a bimodal distribution. At early ages, individuals with DS are susceptible to infantile spasms and tonic clonic seizures with myoclonus. These epilepsies are associated with MR and likely due to early impairments in brain development. Individuals with DS in the third decade of life are more prone to developing simple partial or complex partial seizures in addition to tonic-clonic seizures. These focal epilepsies are likely associated with the increasing burden of parenchymal damage sustained from the progressive neuronal degeneration. It is estimated that 46% of Down's patients over the age of 50 have a diagnosis of epilepsy. Finally, AD is generally considered a neurodegenerative disorder that affects the elderly at 60 years of age and over. Premature AD is seen in DS in the early 40s (Arya et al., 2011; Contestabile et al., 2010; Lott and Dierssen, 2010; Menendez, 2005)

The clinical phenotypes in DS correlate with functional changes seen at the histological and cellular levels in DS brain. DS cortex shows increased simplified gyral patterning and delayed myelination (Banik et al., 1975; Cragg, 1975; Koo et al., 1992; Wisniewski, 1990; Wisniewski and Schmidt-Sidor, 1989). Neuronal loss has been seen in DS brain both during development, following differentiation and aging (Becker et al., 1991; Benda, 1947; Colon, 1972; Davidoff, 1928; Golden and Hyman, 1994; Guidi et al., 2008; Ross et al., 1984; Wisniewski et al., 1984). Histological evidence of neurofibrillary plaques and tangles can be seen in the DS brain, consistent with the premature onset of AD (Motte and Williams, 1989). Changes in dendritic branching as well as neurotransmitter levels have also been reported in the DS brain tissue and likely correlate with the behavioural and cognitive difficulties seen in these individuals (Reynolds and Warner, 1988; Ross et al., 1984). At the cellular level, DS progenitors have prolonged cell cycle lengths, thereby impairing neurogenesis (Chakrabarti et al., 2007; Contestabile et al., 2007; Guidi et al., 2008). Neuronal numbers further decline presumably through increased levels of reactive oxygen species (ROS), mitochondrial dysfunction and increased cell death in mature neurons (Busciglio et al., 2002; Guidi et al., 2008; Seidl et al., 2001). Following differentiation, neurons also show an imbalance of excitatory-inhibitory neurotransmission (Bhattacharyya et al., 2009), with reduced dendritic branching and spine density (Benavides-Piccione et al., 2004). Overall, these changes could all contribute to the MR, epilepsy and AD phenotypes seen in DS.

Various neurological features in DS have been attributed to over-expression of individual genes on HSA21, and several of these genes might contribute to a final common pathway. For example, APP has been shown to promote neuronal degeneration and oxidative stress. Similar functions have been implicated in other HSA21 genes including BACH1, SOD1, and S100B, raising a possible role in AD. Other HSA21 genes (TIAM1, SYNJ1, ITSN1, DSCR1) have been associated with synaptic dysfunction (suggestive of a pathological role in MR and epilepsy). Individual HSA21 genes with proposed neurological functions are summarized in Table 1.

3. Identification of genes and pathways responsible for AD or MR

Although HSA21 is a relatively small chromosome and single candidate genes have been shown to mimic certain DS features, the combinatorial effects of contiguous genes on

HSA21 genes	Downstream targets	Endophenotype	Exophenotype	Ref
NRIP1		Inhibit estrogen and glucocorticoid receptors		(Cavailles et al., 1995; Gardiner and Costa, 2006; Subramaniam et al., 1999; Teyssier et al., 2003)
APP	Ptch1/smo Tau RAGE Tau IL6/gp130 Notch MAP kinases	Abeta deposition, astocytosis, microgliosis, neuronal loss, hyperphosphorylation Tau, decreased proliferation, increased cell death, mitochondrial dysfunction	Dementia, learning and memory deficits	(Abramov et al., 2004; Arancio et al., 2004; Harris-Cerruti et al., 2004; Howlett and Richardson, 2009; Korbel et al., 2009; Kwak et al., 2010; Kwak et al., 2011; Mori et al., 2010; Prasher et al., 1998; Rovelet-Lecrux et al., 2006; Takuma et al., 2009; Trazzi et al.)
BACH1		Increase ROS		(Ferrando-Miguel et al., 2003; Shim et al., 2003)
TIAM1	RAC, NMDAR EphBR	Altered neurite formation, abnormal dendrite spines		(Matsuo et al., 2002; Siddiqui et al., 2008; Tolias et al., 2005; Tolias et al., 2007)
SOD1	APP	Increase ROS, mitochondrial dysfunction	Learning and memory deficits	(Furuta et al., 1995; Harris-Cerruti et al., 2004; Iannello et al., 1999; Lott et al., 2006)
SYNJ1	PtdIns(4,5)P(2)	Synaptic dysfunction, abnormal vesicle trafficking Astrogliagenesis	Learning and memory deficits	(Arai et al., 2002; Chang and Min, 2009; Herrera et al., 2009; Voronov et al., 2008)
Olig2	S100B	Increased inhibitory neurons Increased gliosis Decreased IPSC		(Chakrabarti et al.; Chen et al., 2008; Lu et al., 2002; Tatsumi et al., 2008; Zhou and Anderson, 2002)
Olig1		Increased inhibitory neurons Decreased IPSC		(Chakrabarti et al.; Zhou and Anderson, 2002)
ITSN1		Synaptic dysfunction, abnormal vesicle trafficking		(Chang and Min, 2009; Keating et al., 2006; Yu et al., 2008)
DSCR1	NFAT Calcineurin Tollip ILR1 Caspase9/3	Synaptic dysfunction; abnormal vesicle trafficking, increased neuronal susceptibility to oxidative stress, neuronal apoptosis, mitochondrial dysfunction		(Arron et al., 2006; Chang and Min, 2005; Keating et al., 2008; Lee et al., 2009; Porta et al., 2007; Sun et al.)

HSA21 genes	**Downstream targets**	**Endophenotype**	**Exophenotype**	**Ref**
SIM2	Drebrin		Learning and memory impairment, reduced exploratory behavior and social interactions, increased tolerance to pain	(Chrast et al., 2000; Ema et al., 1999; Vialard et al., 2000)
DYRK1A	NRSF/REST Calcineurin CREB NFAT Tau Notch P53 APP	↓neuroectodermal progenitor, less neuron with abnormal branched neurites, LTP deficits, hyperphosphorylation Tau and APP, premature neuronal differentiation	Learning and memory deficits, motor defects	(Altafaj et al., 2001; Arron et al., 2006; Canzonetta et al., 2008; Fernandez-Martinez et al., 2009; Guimera et al., 1999; O'Doherty et al., 2005; Olson et al., 2004b; Park et al., 2010; Park et al., 2007; Ryoo et al., 2007; Sago et al., 1998; Siarey et al., 2005; Smith et al., 1997; Woods et al., 2001; Yabut et al., 2010; Yang et al., 2001)
KCNJ6 (GIRK2)	GABAB	Imbalance of excitatory-inhibitory neuronal transmission		(Best et al., 2007; Cramer et al., 2010; Harashima et al., 2006)
ETS2	APP	Increased neuronal apoptosis, increased APP production, mitochondrial dysfunction		(Helguera et al., 2005; Wolvetang et al., 2003a; Wolvetang et al., 2003b)
PCP4	Calmodulin			(Kleerekoper and Putkey, 2009; Thomas et al., 2003; Utal et al., 1998)
DSCAM		Overexpression in Purkinje cells, cortical neurons and senile plaques		(Hattori et al., 2007; Saito et al., 2000; Yamakawa et al., 1998)
PKNOX1	FABP7			(Sanchez-Font et al., 2003)
DNMT3L	DNMT3A/3B HDAC	Transcription repression		(Deplus et al., 2002; Holz-Schietinger and Reich, 2010)
SUMO3	APP NRIP1 ELK	Inhibit glucocorticoid receptors		(Dorval et al., 2007; Gardiner, 2006; Holmstrom et al., 2003)

HSA21 genes	Downstream targets	Endophenotype	Exophenotype	Ref
S100B	RAGE AQP4 JNK GSK3ß Tau P53 ATAD3A	Increased ROS, mitochondrial dysfunction and cell death, GSK3ß and Tau hyperphosphorylation, astrocytosis and neurite proliferation	Premature neurological aging	(Esposito et al., 2008a; Esposito et al., 2008b; Gilquin et al., 2010; Lin et al., 2001; Mori et al., 2010; Reeves et al., 1994)

Table 1. HSA21 genes implicated in neurodevelopment

particular DS phenotypes are not known. Several approaches have been used to ascertain HSA21 genotype phenotype contributions: analyses of gene clusters based on their physical linkage, common function/ interactions and/or temporal-spatial distribution of expression.

3.1 Structure-based clusters

Genes that are physically linked based on their location within the same region are usually active together and often contribute to the same phenotype. Based on these structure-based clusters, comparison of full trisomy 21 and partial trisomy 21 genotypes provide some insight between contiguous genes and DS phenotypes. One such region includes APP, which is positioned between 27.25 to 27.54Mb on the long arm of HSA21. Five families with various segmental trisomies that range from 0.58 to 6.37Mb in length and contain APP were all shown to have abundant parenchymal and vascular deposits of beta amyloid without MR on brain autopsy, strongly linking APP to AD (Rovelet-Lecrux et al., 2006).

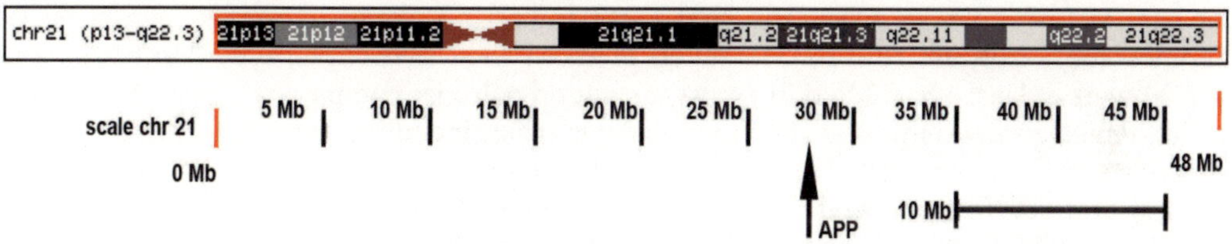

Fig. 1. APP is positioned between 27.25 to 27.54Mb on the long arm of HSA21.

Furthermore, a DS patient with duplication of the distal last 12Mb of HSA21 (a fragment that does not include APP) did not develop typical AD pathology (Prasher et al., 1998). Recently, Korbel et al. analyzed 30 patients carrying rare segmental trisomies of various regions of HSA21 and identified discrete regions between 1.8-16.3Mb in length that were likely to be involved in 8 DS CNS and non-CNS phenotypes including MR and AD (Korbel et al., 2009). They described a patient with a duplication of 18.8 Mb (28.12-telo) without APP, who did not have dementia and had no amyloid accumulation by fMRI. Conversely, several patients with segmental trisomies containing APP did show AD characteristics in the absence of severe MR, which supports the involvement of APP in AD but not MR. These authors were able to narrow down a 1.95Mb interval including APP responsible for the AD phenotype, that excludes genes located distal to 28.12 Mb on HSA21q, including BACH1 and SOD1. These genes were previously suggested to play important roles in the development of AD and MR in DS (Ferrando-Miguel et al., 2003; Lott et al., 2006).

Collectively, these studies conclude a small-segment containing APP as the basis for AD phenotype, with multiple focal regions contributing to MR.

Through segmental trisomy analyses, the primary features of DS have previously been ascribed to the Down syndrome critical region (DSCR). This interval spans about 5Mb around 21q22.12-q22.2 and contains about 33 conserved genes, including DSCR1 (35.88-35.99 Mb), SIM2 (38.07-38.13 Mb), DYRK1A (38.74-38.89), KCNJ6 (38.99-39.29Mb), ETS2 (40.18-40.2Mb), PCP4 (41.24-41.3Mb) and DSCAM (41.38-42.22Mb). The contiguous genes are thought to be sufficient to replicate the DS features including craniofacial abnormalities, short stature, joint hyperlaxity, hypotonia and mental retardation (Delabar et al., 1993; Korenberg, 1990; Korenberg, 1993; McCormick et al., 1989; Olson et al., 2004a; Rahmani et al., 1989). Further studies suggest that DSCR1 and DYRA1A cooperatively destabilize NFATC and induce DS features (Arron et al., 2006; de la Luna and Estivill, 2006). However, several genotype-phenotype correlation studies argue against this hypothesis, given that other patients with partial trisomy 21 that do not include DSCR1, DSCAM or genes within the DSCR have severe DS features including MR (Korbel et al., 2009; Lyle et al., 2009; Ronan et al., 2007).

3.2 Function-based clusters

Microarray expression profiling and sequencing of the human genome have allowed for data analyses and interconnection of functional pathways responsible for various human disorders. By comparing differentially expressed genes between normal and pathological samples, function-based clusters can be generated and attributed to certain disease pathways. We have used this approach in the study of DS human neural progenitors (HNPs) at 18 weeks gestation age (Esposito et al., 2008a). Through pairwise comparison of mRNA expression levels for approximately 54,000 probes in the HU133 plus 2.0 Affymetrix microarray, we observed that some 1900 transcripts (3.8%) were significantly different between WT and DS samples, and that these transcripts were distributed across every chromosome - not just HSA21. Moreover, of these 1900 transcripts, only 330 transcripts (0.07%) were at least 1.5 to 2 fold in excess/deficit on pairwise comparison. These transcripts could then be grouped into specific functional networks, including gene clusters involved in cell cycle (proliferation), cell compromise (cell death, oxidative stress), cell signalling (stress kinases) and cell function and maintenance (differentiation and survival). For example, HSA21 genes such as S100B and amyloid precursor protein (APP) were constitutively over-expressed in DS HNPs along with various stress related kinases and the water channel aquaporin 4 (AQP4). These dysregulated genes comprised a cell signaling functional cluster, whereby HSA21 associated S100B and APP led to increased ROS formation, activation of stress response kinases, and compensatory AQP4 expression. siRNA inhibition of AQP4 resulted in elevated levels of ROS following S100B exposure whereas loss of AQP4 expression led to increased programmed cell death. Results from these studies support the hypothesis that HSA21 gene overdose lead to profound disruption of the entire transcriptome, but presumably in fairly specific functional groups (FitzPatrick et al., 2002; Saran et al., 2003; Tang et al., 2004).

Using a similar strategy, Bhattacharyya et al. compared the differential expression of genes in DS versus WT HNPs at 13 weeks gestation age. Within these earlier aged progenitors, they observed similar functional clusters involved in cell death, cell cycle/ proliferation, and cell fate/ neuronal development. These studies focused on impairments in interneuron neurogenesis, perhaps related to increased expression of gliocentric genes such as Olig1, Olig2, OMG and COUP-TF1/NR2F1 and downregulation of the interneuron related genes DLX1, DLX2 and DLX5.

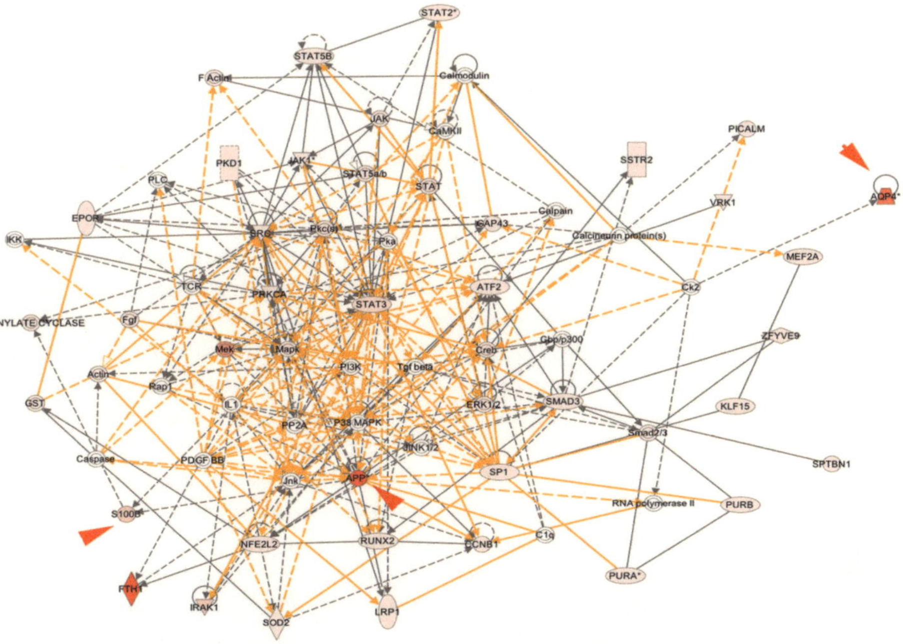

Fig. 2. Constitutively overexpressed genes on HSA21 (S100B & APP) and AQP4 (shown by red arrows) are predicted to form tight interrelationships within known cell signaling pathways shown in the networks pooled out from many differentially expressed genes in DS HNPs with microarray.

In another report, Canzonetta used differential expression analyses following microarray profiling of normal and trsisomy 21 mouse ES cells and pooled the differentially expressed genes into endodermal, mesodermal or ectodermal subgroups. They found reduced expression of stem cell genes controlling pluripotency such as Nanog and Sox2; increased expression of endodermal genes such as Gata4, Gata6 and Foxa2; increased expression of mesodermal genes such as Snail1 and Pitx2 and reduced expression of neuroectodermal genes, such as Nestin, Tubb3, Map2 in trisomy 21 ES cells (Canzonetta et al., 2008). More pervasively, they observed a decrease in Nrsf/Rest, a key regulator of neuronal differentiation and pluripotency. Quantitative linkage analysis (QTL) mapped the REST level change to a 3Mb region of HSA21 containing DYRK1A, suggesting that dysregulation of this HSA21 gene was an early regulator of various embryonic lineages.

3.3 Temporal-spatial mapping-based clusters

Although structure and function cluster approaches provide correlation between DS genotype-phenotypes, temporal and spatial distribution of gene expression further refines the contribution of individual HSA21 genes in DS neural development and later maturation. Previous reports analyzing human trisomy 21 tissue or cells have shown that overexpression of different chromosome 21 genes is cell type and developmental time specific (Ait Yahya-Graison et al., 2007; Chung et al., 2005; Giannone et al., 2004; Gross et al., 2002; Li et al., 2006; Lubec and Sohn, 2003; Mao et al., 2005; Mao et al., 2003; Rozovski et al., 2007). For example, by RNA whole-mount in situ hybridization, gene expression maps of

HSA21 orthologues in various aged embryonic or newborn mouse brain have been reported (Gitton et al., 2002; Reymond et al., 2002). Of the 158 orthologous genes examined in postnatal day 2 mouse brain, 41% were expressed in new cortex, 25% in hippocampus and 25% in cerebellum. The transcripts expressed in neocortex represent a pool of candidate genes for MR of DS, and include DSCAM, SYNJ1 and TIAM1. These genes are implicated in synaptic function, axonal guidance, cell migration and neurite outgrowth (Leeuwen et al., 1997; Saito et al., 2000; Yamakawa et al., 1998).

While several studies have used human cortical progenitors to identify changes in expression profiling, the findings of gene expression levels vary between studies. The temporal-spatial variations in DS HNPs may account for these differences. For example, the REST/NRSF transcription factor was previously reported to be selectively repressed in the DS HNPs (Bahn et al., 2002). These changes were not seen in our studies or those of others (Bhattacharyya et al., 2009; Esposito et al., 2008a). However, this discrepancy could be due to the fact that the gestational ages of the euploid and DS fetal tissues used in these differential expression studies were not the same. Similarly, our observations of increased S100B and aquaporin 4 levels in 19 week gestational age DS HNPs were not appreciated in 13 week gestational age HNPs. This difference would be consistent with the previous notion that HNPs mimic normal developmental patterns such that later generated or propagated HNPs generate fewer neurons than HNPs harvested at an earlier age. Given that S100B and AQP4 are associated with more gliocentric phenotypes, upregulation of these genes would be expected in later gestational aged HNPs. Similar differences appear to exist with other HSA21 genes such as Olig1/2 and DNMT3L (unpublished observations).

4. Characterization of endophenotypes for AD or MR

Endophenotypes are pathological changes observed at the histological, cellular or molecular levels, which provide an association between candidate genes and the clinical symptoms. Clinical neurological symptoms of DS include early onset AD, mental retardation and seizures. Histological changes such as increased cell death, gliosis, demyelination, loss in neuronal numbers, and gyral simplification are thought to contribute to AD and/or MR in DS brain. At the cellular level, DS cells show impairments in mitochondrial function, increased levels of oxidative stress, and changes in proliferative rates. An imbalance in excitatory-inhibitory neurotransmission, expression changes of genes that affect cell fate/differentiation, proliferation/cell cycle and cell injury have been observed at the molecular level.

4.1 Mitochondrial dysfunction and apoptosis

Oxidative stress is increased in DS brain and the imbalance of reactive oxygen species (ROS) metabolism may be the key component giving rise to DS pathogenesis- namely neuronal degeneration (Brooksbank and Balazs, 1984; Busciglio and Yankner, 1995). The mitochondrial respiratory system is the primary source of ROS, and dysregulation of the redox states may induce sequential apoptosis. Several lines of evidence implicate multiple HSA21 genes in mitochondrial dysfunction and DS/AD neuropathology. APP is a membrane protein associated with neuronal survival and overexpression of APP and its products Abeta has been attributed to neurodegeneration in DS and AD (Conti et al., 2010; Isacson et al., 2002; Salehi et al., 2006). APP and Abeta are located in mitochondria (Devi and Anandatheerthavarada, 2010; Manczak et al., 2006). Abeta peptides induce mitochondrial dysfunction and oxidative stress in astrocytes leading to cell death in neurons (Abramov et al., 2004). Impairments in mitochondrial function in astrocytes also alter metabolism and secretion of neuroprotective APP and increase neuronal vulnerability (Busciglio et al., 2002). Mitochondrial dysfunction, however, does not require aberrant APP and Abeta processing specifically. The Ts1Cje DS mouse model, whose partial trisomy 16 does not include the APP gene, also exhibits diminished mitochondrial activity (Shukkur et al., 2006). These mice show decreased mitochondrial membrane potential and ATP production, increased ROS, and increased GSK3ß and JNK/SAPK activities. GSK3ß preserves mitochondrial function, and inhibits Ca(2+)-induced mitochondrial permeability (Mio et al., 2009). In addition to GSK3ß, several other genes within the Ts1Cje trisomic segment are thought to be involved in mitochondrial function. DSCR1 has been reported to be located in the mitochondria and to play a critical role in mitochondrial function (Chang and Min, 2005). DYRK1A can phosphorylate tau and APP (Park et al., 2007; Woods et al., 2001), and the transcription factor ETS-2 increases APP production and promotes the activation of a mitochondrial death pathway in DS neurons (Helguera et al., 2005; Wolvetang et al., 2003a; Wolvetang et al., 2003b). S100B is another HSA21 gene that can increase ROS, it is a calcium binding protein that affects calcium-dependent signals, targeting mitochondrial proteins such as p53 and ATPase ATAD3A, thereby assisting the cytoplasmic processing of proteins for proper folding and subcellular localization. S100B overexpression can also lead to p53 inactivation (Donato, 2003; Gilquin et al., 2010; Leclerc et al., 2010; Lin et al., 2001; Mihara et al., 2003). Finally, similar mechanisms involving mitochondrial dysfunction have been proposed with other HSA21 genes including SOD1 and BATCH1 (Arbuzova et al., 2002; Ferrando-Miguel et al., 2003; Furuta et al., 1995; Harris-Cerruti et al., 2004; Iannello et al., 1999; Lott et al., 2006; Shim et al., 2003). The added, combinatorial effects of these various HSA21 genes in oxidative stress, apoptosis in neurons and neuronal progenitors are not known.

While mitochondrial dysfunction, oxidative stress, and subsequent apoptosis have been well appreciated in neurons, only recently changes have been reported in DS HNPs. We have shown that upregulation of glial-associated proteins such as S100B lead to tau and GSK3ß hyperphosphorylation, suggesting loss of mitochondrial function (Esposito et al., 2008a; Esposito et al., 2008b). HNPs over-express the HSA21-localized S100B, leading to increased ROS formation such as hydrogen peroxide and nitric oxide, activation of stress response kinase pathways (JNK/STAT), and the upregulation of the glial-associated water channel AQP4 (Esposito et al., 2008a). This same functional network also predicts an added contribution through HSA21 localized APP. Both APP and S100B are upregulated in DS HNPs, they reciprocally enhance the expression of one another, have an additive effect on increasing hydrogen peroxide, decreasing mitochondrial membrane potential and increasing apoptosis (unpublished data). The co-localization of APP and S100B within the same HNPs along VZ of cortex may make progenitors even more vulnerable to oxidative stress, which is supported by the fact that increased progenitor cell death is seen at nano or pico level of S100B or Abeta stimulation (unpublished observations). These same doses are neuroprotective in more mature neurons (Lambert et al., 1998; Van Eldik and Wainwright, 2003; Yankner and Lu, 2009). The additive effects from S100B and APP may depend upon their common activation through the extracellular RAGE receptor which has been shown to regulate intracellular mitochondrial function (Devi and Anandatheerthavarada, 2010; Donato, 2003; Leclerc et al., 2010; Manczak et al., 2006). The *in vitro* observations from DS HNPs are consistent with *in vivo* observations in polytransgenic mice. S100B/APP double transgenic (Tg2576/APP-huS100B) mice display augmented reactive astrocytosis and microgliosis, increased levels of pro-inflammatory cytokines and enhanced apoptosis (Mori et al., 2010). The double transgenic (mutant APP (mAPP)/RAGE) mice demonstrate increased activation of stress pathways (phosphorylation of p38 and JNK) and altered expression of markers of synaptic plasticity (MAP kinases), leading to early abnormalities in spatial learning/memory (Arancio et al., 2004).

4.2 Gliosis and inflammatory changes

Increased astrocytes and gliosis have previously been reported in DS brain (Guidi et al., 2008). Altered redox states and mitochondrial compromise leading to cell death are thought to promote these inflammatory changes in mature DS brain (Griffin et al., 1989). In DS the increase in the glial marker S100B could be explained, in part, by a gene dosage effect and in part by reactive gliosis (Selinfreund et al., 1991).

A shift in the DS progenitor pool may contribute to the neuronal reduction and increase in glial cells within the mature trisomy 21 brain. Some studies have suggested impairments in interneuron neurogenesis within the DS HNP pool, possibly due to over-expression of the transcription factor COUP-TF1/NR2F1 (Bhattacharyya et al., 2009). Increased levels of COUP-TF1/NR2F1 cause increases in the generation of earlier born neurons and depletion of later born interneurons. Alternatively, other reports suggest that HSA21 associated DYRK1A causes a skewed ratio of primitive endoderm at the expense of neuroectodermal progenitors, leading to a reduction in neurogenesis (Canzonetta et al., 2008). Mensah also reported an inhibition of neuroectodermal differentiation in a teratoma model transplanted with mouse ES cells injected with HSA21 (Mensah et al., 2007). Our prior studies of DS HNPs had demonstrated a constitutive increase in the glial and HSA21 associated S100B protein, which in turn, enhanced expression of another glial-associated protein, the water channel AQP4. Aquaporins can partially mitigate damage due to ROS, such that glial progenitors are more resistant to oxidative damage (Esposito et al., 2008a). In this setting endogenous overexpression of a glial-associated gene S100B might drive gliogenic progenitors, while the inflammatory changes from oxidative stressors would further promote a gliocentric progenitor pool. Other candidate genes such as HSA21-localized Olig1 and Olig2 are basic helix-loop-helix (bHLH) transcription factors essential for development of oligodendrocytes (Jakovcevski and Zecevic, 2005; Lu et al., 2002; Takebayashi et al., 2002; Zhou and Anderson, 2002) or astrocytes (Cai et al., 2007; Marshall et al., 2005; Ono et al., 2008); and SYNJ1 could increase astrogliosis (Herrera et al., 2009). The number of Olig1/Olig2(+) progenitors increases in the injured CNS (Arnett et al., 2004), and Olig2(+) cells preferentially differentiate into GFAP-expressing astrocytes, the main contributors to glial scars which further secrete S100B (Chen et al., 2008; Tatsumi et al., 2008). S100B also contributes to oligodendrocyte progenitor cells (OPC) differentiation in response to demyelinating insults (Deloulme et al., 2004). In addition to transcription factors, epigenetic regulation can also control the cell fate changes within progenitors. One possible candidate gene in DS is HSA21 associated DNMT3L. DNMT3L is a DNA methyltransferase like gene playing a role in DNA methylation by activating DNMT3A or DNMT3B (Jia et al., 2007; Ooi et al., 2007; Suetake et al., 2004). It also represses transcription by recruiting histone deacetylase (HDAC) (Aapola et al., 2002; Deplus et al., 2002). Hypomethylation in neural progenitors leads to precocious astroglial differentiation and perturbed neuronal maturation in DNMT1 or DNMT3A knockout mice (Fan et al., 2005; Hutnick et al., 2009), whereas HDAC activation increases oligodendrocytes differentiation (Hsieh et al., 2004; Liu et al.,

2009; Liu and Casaccia, 2010; Shen et al., 2005; Ye et al., 2009). Again the combinatorial effects from these various HSA21 genes associated with cell fate changes are not known.

4.3 Prolonged cell cycle and reduced proliferation

Proliferation changes during development have been thought to contribute to the decreased neuronal numbers and reduced cortical volume in DS brains. Recent studies demonstrated impairments in proliferation within both hippocampus and neocortical germinal matrix of 17 weeks to 21 weeks gestation age fetal DS brains (Contestabile et al., 2007; Guidi et al., 2008). The DS progenitor cell cycle is prolonged with more cells remaining in G2 phase, thereby causing a reduction in neurogenesis and presumptive increase in astrocytosis. Similar endophenotypes are also found in animal models, which show a reduced progenitor pool and neurogenesis in ventricular zone or dentate gyrus (Contestabile et al., 2009; Haydar et al., 2000; Lorenzi and Reeves, 2006; Moldrich et al., 2009). The molecular mechanisms behind G2 phase prolongation are not known although many genes on HSA21 can cause proliferation changes. Overexpression of APP would antagonistically compete with the APP-BP1, which is required for the cell cycle progression from G1 to S phase. This change would lead to a predicted slowing in proliferation but at the G1 to S phase (Joo et al., 2010). Overexpression of S100B could promote p53 nuclear accumulation and inhibit proliferation (Scotto et al., 1999). Olig2 overexpression has been shown to increase CDK inhibitor p27, leading to decreased proliferation (Tabu et al., 2006). Presumably, various HSA21 genes may directly act in a combinatorial fashion to affect progenitor proliferation.
Studies from human DS HNPs raise another potential explanation for altered progenitor proliferative rates. Consistent with previous reports, we have also found reduced proliferation in HNPs, localized along the ventricular zone of DS cortex, and within DS HNPs cultured *in vitro*. However, characterization of these progenitors have shown that these progenitors, while retaining neural progenitor markers, are more gliocentric in their expression profile. Some preliminary studies suggest that the DS HNPs have reduced voltage gated, outward rectifying potassium channel activity, which correlated to decreased proliferation. Increased potassium channel activity has been correlated with increased proliferation, whereas decreased channel activity coincides with oligodendrocyte differentiation (Chittajallu et al., 2002). Taken in this context, changes in progenitor cell fates (due to such HSA21 genes as S100B, APP, and Olig2) may in part explain the reduction in cell proliferation.

4.4 Imbalance of excitatory-inhibitory neurotransmission

The balance of neurotransmission is important for maintaining normal physiology and behavior. Imbalance of excitatory-inhibitory neurotransmission could contribute to the MR phenotypes seen in DS. Prior studies have shown decreased excitatory and increased inhibitory activities in DS neurons or Trisomy 16 mice. The excitatory neurotransmitter glutamate and inhibitory neurotransmitter GABA are both decreased in DS fetal brain (Reynolds and Warner, 1988; Risser et al., 1997; Smigielska-Kuzia et al., 2010; Whittle et al., 2007). Ts65Dn mice show increased inhibitory synapses and decreased excitatory synapses in the hippocampus (Belichenko et al., 2009; Belichenko et al., 2004; Kurt et al., 2000; Perez-Cremades et al., 2010). Excessive GABA inhibition also alters LTP in the hippocampus (Costa and Grybko, 2005; Kleschevnikov et al., 2004; Siarey et al., 1997). Likewise, Ts1Cje mice show a shortened long term potentiation and an increase in long term depression, as well as a decrease in the evoked field excitatory postsynaptic potentials- all consistent with impairments in short and long term plasticity (Siarey et al., 2005).

Various HSA21 genes could theoretically affect synaptic function and thereby alter memory and learning. TINM1, SYNJ1 and ITSN1 are thought to play some role in synaptic plasticity, KCNJ6, KCNJ15, KCNE1 and KCNE2 would alter channel activity, whereas NRIP1, ETS2, PCP4, DSCR1, DYRK1A, S100B and APP have some role in affecting neurotransmitter receptors or intracellular signaling. Another more closely scrutinized HSA21 gene GIRK2 (KCNJ6), an inwardly rectifying K channel, could contribute to synaptic inhibition. GIRK2 channels are overexpressed in Ts65Dn hippocampus and frontal cortex (Harashima et al., 2006). The overexpression leads to a significant increase in GABAB-mediated GIRK current in primary cultured hippocampal neurons, and likely affects the balance between excitatory and inhibitory neuronal transmission (Best et al., 2007). Pharmacological treatment of the trisomy 16 mice with GABAA antagonists at non-epileptic doses causes a persistent post-drug recovery of cognition and LTP (Fernandez et al., 2007). Interestingly, treatment of these same mice with the uncompetitive NMDAR antagonist memantine rescues the performance deficits on a fear-conditioning test (Costa et al., 2008). Memantine mimics calcineurin action and the HSA21 DSCR1 gene inhibits calcineurin activity. This raises the hypothesis that DSCR1 overexpression produces a pathological increase in NMDAR activity.

Earlier developmental changes in DS HNPs could also contribute to the imbalance of excitatory and inhibitory neurotransmission. Alterations in cell fate through genes such as Olig1 and Olig2 could lead to an abnormal ratio or distribution of excitatory and inhibitory neurons. Overexpression of HSA21 located Olig1 and Olig2 have been shown to increase GABAergic interneuron neurogenesis in Ts65Dn mice, and the dysregulation of excitatory-inhibitory imbalance could be rescued by knocking down the extra copy of these two genes (Chakrabarti et al., 2010). This phenotype contrasts with our observations and those from other groups, who have observed a reduction of interneurons in DS HNPs at the expense of increasing oligodendrocytes (Bhattacharyya et al., 2009). We see a shift from neuronal to gliocentric progenitors with overexpression of S100B (Esposito et al., 2008a) and APP (unpublished observations), which would potentially further compromise the interneuron population. This decline in interneuron neuronal production is consistent with the loss in GABA-ergic interneurons, as opposed to total neuronal numbers, reported in the DS cortex, further reiterating differences between the mouse and human disorders (Golden and Hyman, 1994; Ross et al., 1984; Weitzdoerfer et al., 2001).

5. Combinatorial gene effects in DS HNPs contribute to the DS phenotype

HSA21 associated genes which are implicated in cell death and oxidative stress could contribute to the later endophenotypes seen in DS. To identify functional modules of gene expression and interacting partners relevant to DS HNPs, we had applied network-based analyses through the Ingenuity Pathways Knowledge Base (IPA) (Calvano et al., 2005). Among 1902 genes that were significantly different on pairwise comparison between WT-DS expression profiling of HNPs, 334 genes were shown to interact within 46 functional networks (Esposito et al., 2008a). The top four interactive networks incorporated 93 dysregulated genes involved in cell cycle, cell death, oxidative stress and several canonical signal transduction pathways. These findings would suggest that genes involved in these primary functional clusters might later contribute to the observed DS endophenotypes.

To understand the role of HSA21 genes in progenitor cell death and changes in redox state, we first focused on HSA21 genes APP and S100B. These molecules were included in one of the top functional clusters and were associated with other cell signaling molecules, including JAK/STAT and MAPK, which have been implicated in the stress response pathway, inflammation and potentially gliosis. Using this potential pathway, we found that upregulation of S100B activated the JAK/STAT MAPK pathway through the RAGE receptor. RAGE receptor activation induced mitochondrial disruption and oxidative stress. Activation of this pathway enhanced progenitor cell death and likely gliosis, as suggested by increased expression of glial associated water channel AQP4 (Esposito et al., 2008a). We have also been able to observe a S100B-mediated induction of tau protein hyperphosphorylation via Dickopff-1 up-regulation and disruption of the Wnt pathway, suggesting a shared common final pathway with APP (Esposito et al., 2008b).

Although APP and S100B have previously been implicated in oxidative stress and cell death, constitutive over-expression of these and other HSA21 genes would also predict upregulation of inflammatory responses (astrocytosis), leading to a skewed gliocentric progenitor phenotype. The ongoing cell death and inflammation from APP and S100B promote reactive astrocytosis and astrocytes secrete S100B, causing further cell injury and death (Li et al., 2011). This same mechanism of injury in the mature brain could also take place within the progenitor population during development. Additionally, the transcription factors Olig1/2 increase oligodendroglial progenitor numbers and would likely augment any gliocentric shift. Similarly, the HSA21 DNA methylthansferase like DNMT3L gene recruits HDACs, which compete with beta catenin to regulate TCF4 dependent transcriptional inhibition of neuronal progenitor proliferation and activation of oligoprogenitor phenotypes (Aapola et al., 2002; Deplus et al., 2002; Liu et al., 2009; Ye et al., 2009).

A gliocentric shift in the progenitor pool could alter rates of proliferation and create an imbalance in excitatory-inhibitory transmission. Gliocentric progenitors would be predicted to demonstrate reduced voltage gated, outward rectifying potassium channel activity, and consequent slower rates of proliferation. Moreover, the ongoing neural progenitor cell death from oxidative stress enhances gliocentric progenitor characteristics at the expense of neuronal progenitor phenotypes. This shift becomes more prominent later in cortical development when the cyclical and synergistic roles played by such inflammatory mediators such as S100B and APP become more pronounced. Under this paradigm, the loss in neuronogenic progenitors would manifest later in development and thereby affect interneuron production.

These observations raise a hypothetical paradigm whereby several specific HSA21-localized genes promote a deleterious, cyclical pathway involving ROS, hypersecretion of S100B, APP overproduction and proliferation of gliocentric progenitors. A gliocentric shift in the progenitor pool would provide a potential explanation for the predominant endophenotypes seen in the DS brain.

6. Pharmacological approach using DS HNPs

From a translational standpoint, human neurally-derived reagents will be useful to identify pathological mechanisms and address the efficacy of pharmacotherapeutics. Given that DS is a contiguous gene syndrome, multiple genes on HSA21 will interact, share substrates, and/or influence the same processes or pathways relevant to neural function. Our ongoing work demonstrates that some genes such as S100B and APP are over-expressed from development into adulthood and would therefore have potentially cumulative effects over time. In this respect, treatment directed toward correcting aberrant pathways regulated by these genes may require early and ongoing management to achieve efficacy. Other genes which might also contribute to gliocentric phenotypes and which reside on HSA21 such as Olig1/2 appear to be more temporally restricted (personal observations, Lu and Sheen) and therefore might be more amenable to a finite pharmacological approach. It remains to be seen to what extent the observations made from various treatment modalities for trisomy mouse models and/or DS HNPs are faithfully replicated in actual individuals with DS. That said, the use of DS HNPs would provide another measure of validation for pharmocotherapies devised in treatment of these disorders.

7. Conclusion

DS is a contiguous gene syndrome giving rise to MR, dementia, and seizures. These clinical outcomes are mirrored by endophenotypes including mitochondrial dysfunction, oxidative stress, cell death, gliosis, inflammation, prolonged cell cycle, reduction in proliferation and imbalances in excitatory and inhibitory neurotransmission. While these characteristics have largely been observed in neurons in the mature brain, function based cluster analyses of pair-wise comparisons between normal and DS human neural progenitors suggest that similar changes are ongoing during development. Moreover, these endophenotypes likely arise from the integration of various genetic and epigenetic factors on chromosome 21 such as APP, S100B, Olig1/2 and DNMT3L. The ongoing disruption of mitochondrial redux states and inflammation promote early gliocentric phenotypes in the progenitor pool, which would alter progenitor proliferative rates and contribute to a decline in interneuron production. Overall, early developmental changes in the progenitor population could promote many of the deleterious changes seen later in the mature DS brain.

8. Acknowledgment

This work was supported by grants to V.L.S from NINDS 1R01NS063997, NICHD 1R21HD054347, and the Harvard Neurodiscovery Center. V.L.S. is a Doris Duke Clinical Scientist Development Award recipient and Alzheimer's Association New Investigator. C.J.C. is an Investigator at the Howard Hughes Medical Institute and thanks the NIH (GM 79465) for research support.

9. References

Aapola, U., Liiv, I., and Peterson, P. (2002). Imprinting regulator DNMT3L is a transcriptional repressor associated with histone deacetylase activity. Nucleic Acids Res *30*, 3602-3608.

Abramov, A. Y., Canevari, L., and Duchen, M. R. (2004). Beta-amyloid peptides induce mitochondrial dysfunction and oxidative stress in astrocytes and death of neurons through activation of NADPH oxidase. J Neurosci *24*, 565-575.

Ait Yahya-Graison, E., Aubert, J., Dauphinot, L., Rivals, I., Prieur, M., Golfier, G., Rossier, J., Personnaz, L., Creau, N., Blehaut, H., *et al.* (2007). Classification of human chromosome 21 gene-expression variations in Down syndrome: impact on disease phenotypes. Am J Hum Genet *81*, 475-491.

Altafaj, X., Dierssen, M., Baamonde, C., Marti, E., Visa, J., Guimera, J., Oset, M., Gonzalez, J. R., Florez, J., Fillat, C., and Estivill, X. (2001). Neurodevelopmental delay, motor abnormalities and cognitive deficits in transgenic mice overexpressing Dyrk1A (minibrain), a murine model of Down's syndrome. Hum Mol Genet *10*, 1915-1923.

Arai, Y., Ijuin, T., Takenawa, T., Becker, L. E., and Takashima, S. (2002). Excessive expression of synaptojanin in brains with Down syndrome. Brain Dev *24*, 67-72.

Arancio, O., Zhang, H. P., Chen, X., Lin, C., Trinchese, F., Puzzo, D., Liu, S., Hegde, A., Yan, S. F., Stern, A., *et al.* (2004). RAGE potentiates Abeta-induced perturbation of neuronal function in transgenic mice. Embo J *23*, 4096-4105.

Arbuzova, S., Hutchin, T., and Cuckle, H. (2002). Mitochondrial dysfunction and Down's syndrome. Bioessays *24*, 681-684.

Arnett, H. A., Fancy, S. P., Alberta, J. A., Zhao, C., Plant, S. R., Kaing, S., Raine, C. S., Rowitch, D. H., Franklin, R. J., and Stiles, C. D. (2004). bHLH transcription factor Olig1 is required to repair demyelinated lesions in the CNS. Science *306*, 2111-2115.

Arron, J. R., Winslow, M. M., Polleri, A., Chang, C. P., Wu, H., Gao, X., Neilson, J. R., Chen, L., Heit, J. J., Kim, S. K., *et al.* (2006). NFAT dysregulation by increased dosage of DSCR1 and DYRK1A on chromosome 21. Nature *441*, 595-600.

Arya, R., Kabra, M., and Gulati, S. (2011). Epilepsy in children with Down syndrome. Epileptic Disord *13*, 1-7.

Bahn, S., Mimmack, M., Ryan, M., Caldwell, M. A., Jauniaux, E., Starkey, M., Svendsen, C. N., and Emson, P. (2002). Neuronal target genes of the neuron-restrictive silencer factor in neurospheres derived from fetuses with Down's syndrome: a gene expression study. Lancet *359*, 310-315.

Banik, N. L., Davison, A. N., Palo, J., and Savolainen, H. (1975). Biochemical studies on myelin isolated from the brains of patients with Down's syndrome. Brain *98*, 213-218.

Becker, L., Mito, T., Takashima, S., and Onodera, K. (1991). Growth and development of the brain in Down syndrome. Prog Clin Biol Res *373*, 133-152.

Belichenko, P. V., Kleschevnikov, A. M., Masliah, E., Wu, C., Takimoto-Kimura, R., Salehi, A., and Mobley, W. C. (2009). Excitatory-inhibitory relationship in the fascia dentata in the Ts65Dn mouse model of Down syndrome. J Comp Neurol *512*, 453-466.

Belichenko, P. V., Masliah, E., Kleschevnikov, A. M., Villar, A. J., Epstein, C. J., Salehi, A., and Mobley, W. C. (2004). Synaptic structural abnormalities in the Ts65Dn mouse model of Down Syndrome. J Comp Neurol *480*, 281-298.

Benavides-Piccione, R., Ballesteros-Yanez, I., de Lagran, M. M., Elston, G., Estivill, X., Fillat, C., Defelipe, J., and Dierssen, M. (2004). On dendrites in Down syndrome and DS murine models: a spiny way to learn. Prog Neurobiol *74*, 111-126.

Benda, C. E. (1947). Neuropsychiatric aspects of mental deficiency; a clinicopathologic study based on 200 autopsies. N C Med J *8*, 72-82.

Best, T. K., Siarey, R. J., and Galdzicki, Z. (2007). Ts65Dn, a mouse model of Down syndrome, exhibits increased GABAB-induced potassium current. J Neurophysiol *97*, 892-900.

Bhattacharyya, A., McMillan, E., Chen, S. I., Wallace, K., and Svendsen, C. N. (2009). A critical period in cortical interneuron neurogenesis in down syndrome revealed by human neural progenitor cells. Dev Neurosci *31*, 497-510.

Brooksbank, B. W., and Balazs, R. (1984). Superoxide dismutase, glutathione peroxidase and lipoperoxidation in Down's syndrome fetal brain. Brain Res *318*, 37-44.

Busciglio, J., Pelsman, A., Wong, C., Pigino, G., Yuan, M., Mori, H., and Yankner, B. A. (2002). Altered metabolism of the amyloid beta precursor protein is associated with mitochondrial dysfunction in Down's syndrome. Neuron *33*, 677-688.

Busciglio, J., and Yankner, B. A. (1995). Apoptosis and increased generation of reactive oxygen species in Down's syndrome neurons in vitro. Nature *378*, 776-779.

Cai, J., Chen, Y., Cai, W. H., Hurlock, E. C., Wu, H., Kernie, S. G., Parada, L. F., and Lu, Q. R. (2007). A crucial role for Olig2 in white matter astrocyte development. Development *134*, 1887-1899.

Calvano, S. E., Xiao, W., Richards, D. R., Felciano, R. M., Baker, H. V., Cho, R. J., Chen, R. O., Brownstein, B. H., Cobb, J. P., Tschoeke, S. K., *et al.* (2005). A network-based analysis of systemic inflammation in humans. Nature *437*, 1032-1037.

Canzonetta, C., Mulligan, C., Deutsch, S., Ruf, S., O'Doherty, A., Lyle, R., Borel, C., Lin-Marq, N., Delom, F., Groet, J., *et al.* (2008). DYRK1A-dosage imbalance perturbs NRSF/REST levels, deregulating pluripotency and embryonic stem cell fate in Down syndrome. Am J Hum Genet *83*, 388-400.

Cavailles, V., Dauvois, S., L'Horset, F., Lopez, G., Hoare, S., Kushner, P. J., and Parker, M. G. (1995). Nuclear factor RIP140 modulates transcriptional activation by the estrogen receptor. Embo J *14*, 3741-3751.

Chakrabarti, L., Best, T. K., Cramer, N. P., Carney, R. S., Isaac, J. T., Galdzicki, Z., and Haydar, T. F. Olig1 and Olig2 triplication causes developmental brain defects in Down syndrome. Nat Neurosci *13*, 927-934.

Chakrabarti, L., Best, T. K., Cramer, N. P., Carney, R. S., Isaac, J. T., Galdzicki, Z., and Haydar, T. F. (2010). Olig1 and Olig2 triplication causes developmental brain defects in Down syndrome. Nat Neurosci *13*, 927-934.

Chakrabarti, L., Galdzicki, Z., and Haydar, T. F. (2007). Defects in embryonic neurogenesis and initial synapse formation in the forebrain of the Ts65Dn mouse model of Down syndrome. J Neurosci *27*, 11483-11495.

Chang, K. T., and Min, K. T. (2005). Drosophila melanogaster homolog of Down syndrome critical region 1 is critical for mitochondrial function. Nat Neurosci *8*, 1577-1585.

Chang, K. T., and Min, K. T. (2009). Upregulation of three Drosophila homologs of human chromosome 21 genes alters synaptic function: implications for Down syndrome. Proc Natl Acad Sci U S A *106*, 17117-17122.

Chen, Y., Miles, D. K., Hoang, T., Shi, J., Hurlock, E., Kernie, S. G., and Lu, Q. R. (2008). The basic helix-loop-helix transcription factor olig2 is critical for reactive astrocyte proliferation after cortical injury. J Neurosci *28*, 10983-10989.

Chittajallu, R., Chen, Y., Wang, H., Yuan, X., Ghiani, C. A., Heckman, T., McBain, C. J., and Gallo, V. (2002). Regulation of Kv1 subunit expression in oligodendrocyte progenitor cells and their role in G1/S phase progression of the cell cycle. Proc Natl Acad Sci U S A *99*, 2350-2355.

Chrast, R., Scott, H. S., Madani, R., Huber, L., Wolfer, D. P., Prinz, M., Aguzzi, A., Lipp, H. P., and Antonarakis, S. E. (2000). Mice trisomic for a bacterial artificial chromosome with the single-minded 2 gene (Sim2) show phenotypes similar to some of those present in the partial trisomy 16 mouse models of Down syndrome. Hum Mol Genet *9*, 1853-1864.

Chung, I. H., Lee, S. H., Lee, K. W., Park, S. H., Cha, K. Y., Kim, N. S., Yoo, H. S., Kim, Y. S., and Lee, S. (2005). Gene expression analysis of cultured amniotic fluid cell with Down syndrome by DNA microarray. J Korean Med Sci *20*, 82-87.

Colon, E. J. (1972). The elderly brain. A quantitative analysis in the cerebral cortex of two cases. Psychiatr Neurol Neurochir *75*, 261-270.

Contestabile, A., Benfenati, F., and Gasparini, L. (2010). Communication breaks-Down: from neurodevelopment defects to cognitive disabilities in Down syndrome. Prog Neurobiol *91*, 1-22.

Contestabile, A., Fila, T., Cappellini, A., Bartesaghi, R., and Ciani, E. (2009). Widespread impairment of cell proliferation in the neonate Ts65Dn mouse, a model for Down syndrome. Cell Prolif *42*, 171-181.

Contestabile, A., Fila, T., Ceccarelli, C., Bonasoni, P., Bonapace, L., Santini, D., Bartesaghi, R., and Ciani, E. (2007). Cell cycle alteration and decreased cell proliferation in the hippocampal dentate gyrus and in the neocortical germinal matrix of fetuses with Down syndrome and in Ts65Dn mice. Hippocampus *17*, 665-678.

Conti, E., Galimberti, G., Piazza, F., Raggi, M. E., and Ferrarese, C. (2010). Increased soluble APPalpha, Abeta 1-42, and anti-Abeta 1-42 antibodies in plasma from down syndrome patients. Alzheimer Dis Assoc Disord *24*, 96-100.

Costa, A. C., and Grybko, M. J. (2005). Deficits in hippocampal CA1 LTP induced by TBS but not HFS in the Ts65Dn mouse: a model of Down syndrome. Neurosci Lett *382*, 317-322.

Costa, A. C., Scott-McKean, J. J., and Stasko, M. R. (2008). Acute injections of the NMDA receptor antagonist memantine rescue performance deficits of the Ts65Dn mouse model of Down syndrome on a fear conditioning test. Neuropsychopharmacology *33*, 1624-1632.

Cragg, B. G. (1975). The density of synapses and neurons in normal, mentally defective ageing human brains. Brain *98*, 81-90.

Cramer, N. P., Best, T. K., Stoffel, M., Siarey, R. J., and Galdzicki, Z. (2010). GABAB-GIRK2-mediated signaling in Down syndrome. Adv Pharmacol *58*, 397-426.

Davidoff, L. M. (1928). Staining Fibrillary Neuroglia in Formalin-Fixed Material. Am J Pathol *4*, 493-496.1.

de la Luna, S., and Estivill, X. (2006). Cooperation to amplify gene-dosage-imbalance effects. Trends Mol Med *12*, 451-454.

Delabar, J. M., Theophile, D., Rahmani, Z., Chettouh, Z., Blouin, J. L., Prieur, M., Noel, B., and Sinet, P. M. (1993). Molecular mapping of twenty-four features of Down syndrome on chromosome 21. Eur J Hum Genet *1*, 114-124.

Deloulme, J. C., Raponi, E., Gentil, B. J., Bertacchi, N., Marks, A., Labourdette, G., and Baudier, J. (2004). Nuclear expression of S100B in oligodendrocyte progenitor cells correlates with differentiation toward the oligodendroglial lineage and modulates oligodendrocytes maturation. Mol Cell Neurosci *27*, 453-465.

Deplus, R., Brenner, C., Burgers, W. A., Putmans, P., Kouzarides, T., de Launoit, Y., and Fuks, F. (2002). Dnmt3L is a transcriptional repressor that recruits histone deacetylase. Nucleic Acids Res *30*, 3831-3838.

Devi, L., and Anandatheerthavarada, H. K. (2010). Mitochondrial trafficking of APP and alpha synuclein: Relevance to mitochondrial dysfunction in Alzheimer's and Parkinson's diseases. Biochim Biophys Acta *1802*, 11-19.

Donato, R. (2003). Intracellular and extracellular roles of S100 proteins. Microsc Res Tech *60*, 540-551.

Dorval, V., Mazzella, M. J., Mathews, P. M., Hay, R. T., and Fraser, P. E. (2007). Modulation of Abeta generation by small ubiquitin-like modifiers does not require conjugation to target proteins. Biochem J *404*, 309-316.

Ema, M., Ikegami, S., Hosoya, T., Mimura, J., Ohtani, H., Nakao, K., Inokuchi, K., Katsuki, M., and Fujii-Kuriyama, Y. (1999). Mild impairment of learning and memory in mice overexpressing the mSim2 gene located on chromosome 16: an animal model of Down's syndrome. Hum Mol Genet *8*, 1409-1415.

Esposito, G., Imitola, J., Lu, J., De Filippis, D., Scuderi, C., Ganesh, V. S., Folkerth, R., Hecht, J., Shin, S., Iuvone, T., *et al.* (2008a). Genomic and functional profiling of human Down syndrome neural progenitors implicates S100B and aquaporin 4 in cell injury. Hum Mol Genet *17*, 440-457.

Esposito, G., Scuderi, C., Lu, J., Savani, C., De Filippis, D., Iuvone, T., Steardo, L., Jr., Sheen, V., and Steardo, L. (2008b). S100B induces tau protein hyperphosphorylation via Dickopff-1 up-regulation and disrupts the Wnt pathway in human neural stem cells. J Cell Mol Med *12*, 914-927.

Fan, G., Martinowich, K., Chin, M. H., He, F., Fouse, S. D., Hutnick, L., Hattori, D., Ge, W., Shen, Y., Wu, H., *et al.* (2005). DNA methylation controls the timing of astrogliogenesis through regulation of JAK-STAT signaling. Development *132*, 3345-3356.

Fernandez-Martinez, J., Vela, E. M., Tora-Ponsioen, M., Ocana, O. H., Nieto, M. A., and Galceran, J. (2009). Attenuation of Notch signalling by the Down-syndrome-associated kinase DYRK1A. J Cell Sci *122*, 1574-1583.

Fernandez, F., Morishita, W., Zuniga, E., Nguyen, J., Blank, M., Malenka, R. C., and Garner, C. C. (2007). Pharmacotherapy for cognitive impairment in a mouse model of Down syndrome. Nat Neurosci *10*, 411-413.

Ferrando-Miguel, R., Cheon, M. S., Yang, J. W., and Lubec, G. (2003). Overexpression of transcription factor BACH1 in fetal Down syndrome brain. J Neural Transm Suppl, 193-205.

FitzPatrick, D. R., Ramsay, J., McGill, N. I., Shade, M., Carothers, A. D., and Hastie, N. D. (2002). Transcriptome analysis of human autosomal trisomy. Hum Mol Genet *11*, 3249-3256.

Furuta, A., Price, D. L., Pardo, C. A., Troncoso, J. C., Xu, Z. S., Taniguchi, N., and Martin, L. J. (1995). Localization of superoxide dismutases in Alzheimer's disease and Down's syndrome neocortex and hippocampus. Am J Pathol *146*, 357-367.

Gardiner, K. (2006). Transcriptional dysregulation in Down syndrome: predictions for altered protein complex stoichiometries and post-translational modifications, and consequences for learning/behavior genes ELK, CREB, and the estrogen and glucocorticoid receptors. Behav Genet *36*, 439-453.

Gardiner, K., and Costa, A. C. (2006). The proteins of human chromosome 21. Am J Med Genet C Semin Med Genet *142C*, 196-205.

Giannone, S., Strippoli, P., Vitale, L., Casadei, R., Canaider, S., Lenzi, L., D'Addabbo, P., Frabetti, F., Facchin, F., Farina, A., *et al.* (2004). Gene expression profile analysis in human T lymphocytes from patients with Down Syndrome. Ann Hum Genet *68*, 546-554.

Gilquin, B., Cannon, B. R., Hubstenberger, A., Moulouel, B., Falk, E., Merle, N., Assard, N., Kieffer, S., Rousseau, D., Wilder, P. T., *et al.* (2010). The calcium-dependent interaction between S100B and the mitochondrial AAA ATPase ATAD3A and the role of this complex in the cytoplasmic processing of ATAD3A. Mol Cell Biol *30,* 2724-2736.

Gitton, Y., Dahmane, N., Baik, S., Ruiz i Altaba, A., Neidhardt, L., Scholze, M., Herrmann, B. G., Kahlem, P., Benkahla, A., Schrinner, S., *et al.* (2002). A gene expression map of human chromosome 21 orthologues in the mouse. Nature *420,* 586-590.

Golden, J. A., and Hyman, B. T. (1994). Development of the superior temporal neocortex is anomalous in trisomy 21. J Neuropathol Exp Neurol *53,* 513-520.

Griffin, W. S., Stanley, L. C., Ling, C., White, L., MacLeod, V., Perrot, L. J., White, C. L., 3rd, and Araoz, C. (1989). Brain interleukin 1 and S-100 immunoreactivity are elevated in Down syndrome and Alzheimer disease. Proc Natl Acad Sci U S A *86,* 7611-7615.

Gross, S. J., Ferreira, J. C., Morrow, B., Dar, P., Funke, B., Khabele, D., and Merkatz, I. (2002). Gene expression profile of trisomy 21 placentas: a potential approach for designing noninvasive techniques of prenatal diagnosis. Am J Obstet Gynecol *187,* 457-462.

Guidi, S., Bonasoni, P., Ceccarelli, C., Santini, D., Gualtieri, F., Ciani, E., and Bartesaghi, R. (2008). Neurogenesis impairment and increased cell death reduce total neuron number in the hippocampal region of fetuses with Down syndrome. Brain Pathol *18,* 180-197.

Guimera, J., Casas, C., Estivill, X., and Pritchard, M. (1999). Human minibrain homologue (MNBH/DYRK1): characterization, alternative splicing, differential tissue expression, and overexpression in Down syndrome. Genomics *57,* 407-418.

Harashima, C., Jacobowitz, D. M., Witta, J., Borke, R. C., Best, T. K., Siarey, R. J., and Galdzicki, Z. (2006). Abnormal expression of the G-protein-activated inwardly rectifying potassium channel 2 (GIRK2) in hippocampus, frontal cortex, and substantia nigra of Ts65Dn mouse: a model of Down syndrome. J Comp Neurol *494,* 815-833.

Harris-Cerruti, C., Kamsler, A., Kaplan, B., Lamb, B., Segal, M., and Groner, Y. (2004). Functional and morphological alterations in compound transgenic mice overexpressing Cu/Zn superoxide dismutase and amyloid precursor protein [correction]. Eur J Neurosci *19,* 1174-1190.

Hattori, D., Demir, E., Kim, H. W., Viragh, E., Zipursky, S. L., and Dickson, B. J. (2007). Dscam diversity is essential for neuronal wiring and self-recognition. Nature *449,* 223-227.

Haydar, T. F., Wang, F., Schwartz, M. L., and Rakic, P. (2000). Differential modulation of proliferation in the neocortical ventricular and subventricular zones. J Neurosci *20,* 5764-5774.

Helguera, P., Pelsman, A., Pigino, G., Wolvetang, E., Head, E., and Busciglio, J. (2005). ets-2 promotes the activation of a mitochondrial death pathway in Down's syndrome neurons. J Neurosci *25,* 2295-2303.

Herrera, F., Chen, Q., Fischer, W. H., Maher, P., and Schubert, D. R. (2009). Synaptojanin-1 plays a key role in astrogliogenesis: possible relevance for Down's syndrome. Cell Death Differ *16,* 910-920.

Holmstrom, S., Van Antwerp, M. E., and Iniguez-Lluhi, J. A. (2003). Direct and distinguishable inhibitory roles for SUMO isoforms in the control of transcriptional synergy. Proc Natl Acad Sci U S A *100*, 15758-15763.

Holz-Schietinger, C., and Reich, N. O. (2010). The inherent processivity of the human de novo methyltransferase 3A (DNMT3A) is enhanced by DNMT3L. J Biol Chem *285*, 29091-29100.

Howlett, D. R., and Richardson, J. C. (2009). The pathology of APP transgenic mice: a model of Alzheimer's disease or simply overexpression of APP? Histol Histopathol *24*, 83-100.

Hsieh, J., Nakashima, K., Kuwabara, T., Mejia, E., and Gage, F. H. (2004). Histone deacetylase inhibition-mediated neuronal differentiation of multipotent adult neural progenitor cells. Proc Natl Acad Sci U S A *101*, 16659-16664.

Hutnick, L. K., Golshani, P., Namihira, M., Xue, Z., Matynia, A., Yang, X. W., Silva, A. J., Schweizer, F. E., and Fan, G. (2009). DNA hypomethylation restricted to the murine forebrain induces cortical degeneration and impairs postnatal neuronal maturation. Hum Mol Genet *18*, 2875-2888.

Iannello, R. C., Crack, P. J., de Haan, J. B., and Kola, I. (1999). Oxidative stress and neural dysfunction in Down syndrome. J Neural Transm Suppl *57*, 257-267.

Isacson, O., Seo, H., Lin, L., Albeck, D., and Granholm, A. C. (2002). Alzheimer's disease and Down's syndrome: roles of APP, trophic factors and ACh. Trends Neurosci *25*, 79-84.

Jakovcevski, I., and Zecevic, N. (2005). Olig transcription factors are expressed in oligodendrocyte and neuronal cells in human fetal CNS. J Neurosci *25*, 10064-10073.

Jia, D., Jurkowska, R. Z., Zhang, X., Jeltsch, A., and Cheng, X. (2007). Structure of Dnmt3a bound to Dnmt3L suggests a model for de novo DNA methylation. Nature *449*, 248-251.

Joo, Y., Ha, S., Hong, B. H., Kim, J., Chang, K. A., Liew, H., Kim, S., Sun, W., Kim, J. H., Chong, Y. H., *et al.* (2010). Amyloid precursor protein binding protein-1 modulates cell cycle progression in fetal neural stem cells. PLoS One *5*, e14203.

Keating, D. J., Chen, C., and Pritchard, M. A. (2006). Alzheimer's disease and endocytic dysfunction: clues from the Down syndrome-related proteins, DSCR1 and ITSN1. Ageing Res Rev *5*, 388-401.

Keating, D. J., Dubach, D., Zanin, M. P., Yu, Y., Martin, K., Zhao, Y. F., Chen, C., Porta, S., Arbones, M. L., Mittaz, L., and Pritchard, M. A. (2008). DSCR1/RCAN1 regulates vesicle exocytosis and fusion pore kinetics: implications for Down syndrome and Alzheimer's disease. Hum Mol Genet *17*, 1020-1030.

Kleerekoper, Q. K., and Putkey, J. A. (2009). PEP-19, an intrinsically disordered regulator of calmodulin signaling. J Biol Chem *284*, 7455-7464.

Kleschevnikov, A. M., Belichenko, P. V., Villar, A. J., Epstein, C. J., Malenka, R. C., and Mobley, W. C. (2004). Hippocampal long-term potentiation suppressed by increased inhibition in the Ts65Dn mouse, a genetic model of Down syndrome. J Neurosci *24*, 8153-8160.

Koo, B. K., Blaser, S., Harwood-Nash, D., Becker, L. E., and Murphy, E. G. (1992). Magnetic resonance imaging evaluation of delayed myelination in Down syndrome: a case report and review of the literature. J Child Neurol *7*, 417-421.

Korbel, J. O., Tirosh-Wagner, T., Urban, A. E., Chen, X. N., Kasowski, M., Dai, L., Grubert, F., Erdman, C., Gao, M. C., Lange, K., *et al.* (2009). The genetic architecture of Down syndrome phenotypes revealed by high-resolution analysis of human segmental trisomies. Proc Natl Acad Sci U S A *106*, 12031-12036.

Korenberg, J. R. (1990). Molecular mapping of the Down syndrome phenotype. Prog Clin Biol Res *360*, 105-115.

Korenberg, J. R. (1993). Toward a molecular understanding of Down syndrome. Prog Clin Biol Res *384*, 87-115.

Kurt, M. A., Davies, D. C., Kidd, M., Dierssen, M., and Florez, J. (2000). Synaptic deficit in the temporal cortex of partial trisomy 16 (Ts65Dn) mice. Brain Res *858*, 191-197.

Kwak, Y. D., Dantuma, E., Merchant, S., Bushnev, S., and Sugaya, K. (2010). Amyloid-beta precursor protein induces glial differentiation of neural progenitor cells by activation of the IL-6/gp130 signaling pathway. Neurotox Res *18*, 328-338.

Kwak, Y. D., Marutle, A., Dantuma, E., Merchant, S., Bushnev, S., and Sugaya, K. (2011). Involvement of notch signaling pathway in amyloid precursor protein induced glial differentiation. Eur J Pharmacol *650*, 18-27.

Lambert, M. P., Barlow, A. K., Chromy, B. A., Edwards, C., Freed, R., Liosatos, M., Morgan, T. E., Rozovsky, I., Trommer, B., Viola, K. L., *et al.* (1998). Diffusible, nonfibrillar ligands derived from Abeta1-42 are potent central nervous system neurotoxins. Proc Natl Acad Sci U S A *95*, 6448-6453.

Leclerc, E., Sturchler, E., and Vetter, S. W. (2010). The S100B/RAGE Axis in Alzheimer's Disease. Cardiovasc Psychiatry Neurol *2010*, 539581.

Lee, J. Y., Lee, H. J., Lee, E. J., Jang, S. H., Kim, H., Yoon, J. H., and Chung, K. C. (2009). Down syndrome candidate region-1 protein interacts with Tollip and positively modulates interleukin-1 receptor-mediated signaling. Biochim Biophys Acta *1790*, 1673-1680.

Leeuwen, F. N., Kain, H. E., Kammen, R. A., Michiels, F., Kranenburg, O. W., and Collard, J. G. (1997). The guanine nucleotide exchange factor Tiam1 affects neuronal morphology; opposing roles for the small GTPases Rac and Rho. J Cell Biol *139*, 797-807.

Li, C., Zhao, R., Gao, K., Wei, Z., Yin, M. Y., Lau, L. T., Chui, D., and Hoi Yu, A. C. (2011). Astrocytes: implications for neuroinflammatory pathogenesis of Alzheimer's disease. Curr Alzheimer Res *8*, 67-80.

Li, C. M., Guo, M., Salas, M., Schupf, N., Silverman, W., Zigman, W. B., Husain, S., Warburton, D., Thaker, H., and Tycko, B. (2006). Cell type-specific over-expression of chromosome 21 genes in fibroblasts and fetal hearts with trisomy 21. BMC Med Genet *7*, 24.

Lin, J., Blake, M., Tang, C., Zimmer, D., Rustandi, R. R., Weber, D. J., and Carrier, F. (2001). Inhibition of p53 transcriptional activity by the S100B calcium-binding protein. J Biol Chem *276*, 35037-35041.

Liu, H., Hu, Q., D'Ercole A, J., and Ye, P. (2009). Histone deacetylase 11 regulates oligodendrocyte-specific gene expression and cell development in OL-1 oligodendroglia cells. Glia *57*, 1-12.

Liu, J., and Casaccia, P. (2010). Epigenetic regulation of oligodendrocyte identity. Trends Neurosci *33*, 193-201.

Lorenzi, H. A., and Reeves, R. H. (2006). Hippocampal hypocellularity in the Ts65Dn mouse originates early in development. Brain Res *1104*, 153-159.

Lott, I. T., and Dierssen, M. (2010). Cognitive deficits and associated neurological complications in individuals with Down's syndrome. Lancet Neurol *9*, 623-633.

Lott, I. T., Head, E., Doran, E., and Busciglio, J. (2006). Beta-amyloid, oxidative stress and down syndrome. Curr Alzheimer Res *3*, 521-528.

Lu, Q. R., Sun, T., Zhu, Z., Ma, N., Garcia, M., Stiles, C. D., and Rowitch, D. H. (2002). Common developmental requirement for Olig function indicates a motor neuron/oligodendrocyte connection. Cell *109*, 75-86.

Lubec, G., and Sohn, S. Y. (2003). RNA microarray analysis of channels and transporters in normal and fetal Down syndrome (trisomy 21) brain. J Neural Transm Suppl, 215-224.

Lyle, R., Bena, F., Gagos, S., Gehrig, C., Lopez, G., Schinzel, A., Lespinasse, J., Bottani, A., Dahoun, S., Taine, L., *et al.* (2009). Genotype-phenotype correlations in Down syndrome identified by array CGH in 30 cases of partial trisomy and partial monosomy chromosome 21. Eur J Hum Genet *17*, 454-466.

Manczak, M., Anekonda, T. S., Henson, E., Park, B. S., Quinn, J., and Reddy, P. H. (2006). Mitochondria are a direct site of A beta accumulation in Alzheimer's disease neurons: implications for free radical generation and oxidative damage in disease progression. Hum Mol Genet *15*, 1437-1449.

Mao, R., Wang, X., Spitznagel, E. L., Jr., Frelin, L. P., Ting, J. C., Ding, H., Kim, J. W., Ruczinski, I., Downey, T. J., and Pevsner, J. (2005). Primary and secondary transcriptional effects in the developing human Down syndrome brain and heart. Genome Biol *6*, R107.

Mao, R., Zielke, C. L., Zielke, H. R., and Pevsner, J. (2003). Global up-regulation of chromosome 21 gene expression in the developing Down syndrome brain. Genomics *81*, 457-467.

Marshall, C. A., Novitch, B. G., and Goldman, J. E. (2005). Olig2 directs astrocyte and oligodendrocyte formation in postnatal subventricular zone cells. J Neurosci *25*, 7289-7298.

Matsuo, N., Hoshino, M., Yoshizawa, M., and Nabeshima, Y. (2002). Characterization of STEF, a guanine nucleotide exchange factor for Rac1, required for neurite growth. J Biol Chem *277*, 2860-2868.

McCormick, M. K., Schinzel, A., Petersen, M. B., Stetten, G., Driscoll, D. J., Cantu, E. S., Tranebjaerg, L., Mikkelsen, M., Watkins, P. C., and Antonarakis, S. E. (1989). Molecular genetic approach to the characterization of the "Down syndrome region" of chromosome 21. Genomics *5*, 325-331.

Menendez, M. (2005). Down syndrome, Alzheimer's disease and seizures. Brain Dev *27*, 246-252.

Mensah, A., Mulligan, C., Linehan, J., Ruf, S., O'Doherty, A., Grygalewicz, B., Shipley, J., Groet, J., Tybulewicz, V., Fisher, E., *et al.* (2007). An additional human chromosome 21 causes suppression of neural fate of pluripotent mouse embryonic stem cells in a teratoma model. BMC Dev Biol *7*, 131.

Mihara, M., Erster, S., Zaika, A., Petrenko, O., Chittenden, T., Pancoska, P., and Moll, U. M. (2003). p53 has a direct apoptogenic role at the mitochondria. Mol Cell *11*, 577-590.

Mio, Y., Shim, Y. H., Richards, E., Bosnjak, Z. J., Pagel, P. S., and Bienengraeber, M. (2009). Xenon preconditioning: the role of prosurvival signaling, mitochondrial permeability transition and bioenergetics in rats. Anesth Analg *108*, 858-866.

Moldrich, R. X., Dauphinot, L., Laffaire, J., Vitalis, T., Herault, Y., Beart, P. M., Rossier, J., Vivien, D., Gehrig, C., Antonarakis, S. E., *et al.* (2009). Proliferation deficits and gene expression dysregulation in Down's syndrome (Ts1Cje) neural progenitor cells cultured from neurospheres. J Neurosci Res *87*, 3143-3152.

Mori, T., Koyama, N., Arendash, G. W., Horikoshi-Sakuraba, Y., Tan, J., and Town, T. (2010). Overexpression of human S100B exacerbates cerebral amyloidosis and gliosis in the Tg2576 mouse model of Alzheimer's disease. Glia *58*, 300-314.

Motte, J., and Williams, R. S. (1989). Age-related changes in the density and morphology of plaques and neurofibrillary tangles in Down syndrome brain. Acta Neuropathol *77*, 535-546.

O'Doherty, A., Ruf, S., Mulligan, C., Hildreth, V., Errington, M. L., Cooke, S., Sesay, A., Modino, S., Vanes, L., Hernandez, D., *et al.* (2005). An aneuploid mouse strain carrying human chromosome 21 with Down syndrome phenotypes. Science *309*, 2033-2037.

Olson, L. E., Richtsmeier, J. T., Leszl, J., and Reeves, R. H. (2004a). A chromosome 21 critical region does not cause specific Down syndrome phenotypes. Science *306*, 687-690.

Olson, L. E., Roper, R. J., Baxter, L. L., Carlson, E. J., Epstein, C. J., and Reeves, R. H. (2004b). Down syndrome mouse models Ts65Dn, Ts1Cje, and Ms1Cje/Ts65Dn exhibit variable severity of cerebellar phenotypes. Dev Dyn *230*, 581-589.

Ono, K., Takebayashi, H., Ikeda, K., Furusho, M., Nishizawa, T., Watanabe, K., and Ikenaka, K. (2008). Regional- and temporal-dependent changes in the differentiation of Olig2 progenitors in the forebrain, and the impact on astrocyte development in the dorsal pallium. Dev Biol *320*, 456-468.

Ooi, S. K., Qiu, C., Bernstein, E., Li, K., Jia, D., Yang, Z., Erdjument-Bromage, H., Tempst, P., Lin, S. P., Allis, C. D., *et al.* (2007). DNMT3L connects unmethylated lysine 4 of histone H3 to de novo methylation of DNA. Nature *448*, 714-717.

Park, J., Oh, Y., Yoo, L., Jung, M. S., Song, W. J., Lee, S. H., Seo, H., and Chung, K. C. (2010). Dyrk1A phosphorylates p53 and inhibits proliferation of embryonic neuronal cells. J Biol Chem *285*, 31895-31906.

Park, J., Yang, E. J., Yoon, J. H., and Chung, K. C. (2007). Dyrk1A overexpression in immortalized hippocampal cells produces the neuropathological features of Down syndrome. Mol Cell Neurosci *36*, 270-279.

Perez-Cremades, D., Hernandez, S., Blasco-Ibanez, J. M., Crespo, C., Nacher, J., and Varea, E. (2010). Alteration of inhibitory circuits in the somatosensory cortex of Ts65Dn mice, a model for Down's syndrome. J Neural Transm *117*, 445-455.

Porta, S., Serra, S. A., Huch, M., Valverde, M. A., Llorens, F., Estivill, X., Arbones, M. L., and Marti, E. (2007). RCAN1 (DSCR1) increases neuronal susceptibility to oxidative stress: a potential pathogenic process in neurodegeneration. Hum Mol Genet *16*, 1039-1050.

Prasher, V. P., Farrer, M. J., Kessling, A. M., Fisher, E. M., West, R. J., Barber, P. C., and Butler, A. C. (1998). Molecular mapping of Alzheimer-type dementia in Down's syndrome. Ann Neurol *43*, 380-383.

Rahmani, Z., Blouin, J. L., Creau-Goldberg, N., Watkins, P. C., Mattei, J. F., Poissonnier, M., Prieur, M., Chettouh, Z., Nicole, A., Aurias, A., and et al. (1989). Critical role of the D21S55 region on chromosome 21 in the pathogenesis of Down syndrome. Proc Natl Acad Sci U S A *86*, 5958-5962.

Reeves, R. H., Yao, J., Crowley, M. R., Buck, S., Zhang, X., Yarowsky, P., Gearhart, J. D., and Hilt, D. C. (1994). Astrocytosis and axonal proliferation in the hippocampus of S100b transgenic mice. Proc Natl Acad Sci U S A *91*, 5359-5363.

Reymond, A., Marigo, V., Yaylaoglu, M. B., Leoni, A., Ucla, C., Scamuffa, N., Caccioppoli, C., Dermitzakis, E. T., Lyle, R., Banfi, S., *et al.* (2002). Human chromosome 21 gene expression atlas in the mouse. Nature *420*, 582-586.

Reynolds, G. P., and Warner, C. E. (1988). Amino acid neurotransmitter deficits in adult Down's syndrome brain tissue. Neurosci Lett *94*, 224-227.

Risser, D., Lubec, G., Cairns, N., and Herrera-Marschitz, M. (1997). Excitatory amino acids and monoamines in parahippocampal gyrus and frontal cortical pole of adults with Down syndrome. Life Sci *60*, 1231-1237.

Ronan, A., Fagan, K., Christie, L., Conroy, J., Nowak, N. J., and Turner, G. (2007). Familial 4.3 Mb duplication of 21q22 sheds new light on the Down syndrome critical region. J Med Genet *44*, 448-451.

Ross, M. H., Galaburda, A. M., and Kemper, T. L. (1984). Down's syndrome: is there a decreased population of neurons? Neurology *34*, 909-916.

Rovelet-Lecrux, A., Hannequin, D., Raux, G., Le Meur, N., Laquerriere, A., Vital, A., Dumanchin, C., Feuillette, S., Brice, A., Vercelletto, M., *et al.* (2006). APP locus duplication causes autosomal dominant early-onset Alzheimer disease with cerebral amyloid angiopathy. Nat Genet *38*, 24-26.

Rozovski, U., Jonish-Grossman, A., Bar-Shira, A., Ochshorn, Y., Goldstein, M., and Yaron, Y. (2007). Genome-wide expression analysis of cultured trophoblast with trisomy 21 karyotype. Hum Reprod *22*, 2538-2545.

Ryoo, S. R., Jeong, H. K., Radnaabazar, C., Yoo, J. J., Cho, H. J., Lee, H. W., Kim, I. S., Cheon, Y. H., Ahn, Y. S., Chung, S. H., and Song, W. J. (2007). DYRK1A-mediated hyperphosphorylation of Tau. A functional link between Down syndrome and Alzheimer disease. J Biol Chem *282*, 34850-34857.

Sago, H., Carlson, E. J., Smith, D. J., Kilbridge, J., Rubin, E. M., Mobley, W. C., Epstein, C. J., and Huang, T. T. (1998). Ts1Cje, a partial trisomy 16 mouse model for Down syndrome, exhibits learning and behavioral abnormalities. Proc Natl Acad Sci U S A *95*, 6256-6261.

Saito, Y., Oka, A., Mizuguchi, M., Motonaga, K., Mori, Y., Becker, L. E., Arima, K., Miyauchi, J., and Takashima, S. (2000). The developmental and aging changes of Down's syndrome cell adhesion molecule expression in normal and Down's syndrome brains. Acta Neuropathol *100*, 654-664.

Salehi, A., Delcroix, J. D., Belichenko, P. V., Zhan, K., Wu, C., Valletta, J. S., Takimoto-Kimura, R., Kleschevnikov, A. M., Sambamurti, K., Chung, P. P., *et al.* (2006). Increased App expression in a mouse model of Down's syndrome disrupts NGF transport and causes cholinergic neuron degeneration. Neuron *51*, 29-42.

Sanchez-Font, M. F., Bosch-Comas, A., Gonzalez-Duarte, R., and Marfany, G. (2003). Overexpression of FABP7 in Down syndrome fetal brains is associated with PKNOX1 gene-dosage imbalance. Nucleic Acids Res *31*, 2769-2777.

Saran, N. G., Pletcher, M. T., Natale, J. E., Cheng, Y., and Reeves, R. H. (2003). Global disruption of the cerebellar transcriptome in a Down syndrome mouse model. Hum Mol Genet *12*, 2013-2019.

Scotto, C., Delphin, C., Deloulme, J. C., and Baudier, J. (1999). Concerted regulation of wild-type p53 nuclear accumulation and activation by S100B and calcium-dependent protein kinase C. Mol Cell Biol *19*, 7168-7180.

Seidl, R., Bidmon, B., Bajo, M., Yoo, P. C., Cairns, N., LaCasse, E. C., and Lubec, G. (2001). Evidence for apoptosis in the fetal Down syndrome brain. J Child Neurol *16*, 438-442.

Selinfreund, R. H., Barger, S. W., Pledger, W. J., and Van Eldik, L. J. (1991). Neurotrophic protein S100 beta stimulates glial cell proliferation. Proc Natl Acad Sci U S A *88*, 3554-3558.

Shen, S., Li, J., and Casaccia-Bonnefil, P. (2005). Histone modifications affect timing of oligodendrocyte progenitor differentiation in the developing rat brain. J Cell Biol *169*, 577-589.

Shim, K. S., Ferrando-Miguel, R., and Lubec, G. (2003). Aberrant protein expression of transcription factors BACH1 and ERG, both encoded on chromosome 21, in brains of patients with Down syndrome and Alzheimer's disease. J Neural Transm Suppl, 39-49.

Shukkur, E. A., Shimohata, A., Akagi, T., Yu, W., Yamaguchi, M., Murayama, M., Chui, D., Takeuchi, T., Amano, K., Subramhanya, K. H., *et al.* (2006). Mitochondrial dysfunction and tau hyperphosphorylation in Ts1Cje, a mouse model for Down syndrome. Hum Mol Genet *15*, 2752-2762.

Siarey, R. J., Stoll, J., Rapoport, S. I., and Galdzicki, Z. (1997). Altered long-term potentiation in the young and old Ts65Dn mouse, a model for Down Syndrome. Neuropharmacology *36*, 1549-1554.

Siarey, R. J., Villar, A. J., Epstein, C. J., and Galdzicki, Z. (2005). Abnormal synaptic plasticity in the Ts1Cje segmental trisomy 16 mouse model of Down syndrome. Neuropharmacology *49*, 122-128.

Siddiqui, A., Lacroix, T., Stasko, M. R., Scott-McKean, J. J., Costa, A. C., and Gardiner, K. J. (2008). Molecular responses of the Ts65Dn and Ts1Cje mouse models of Down syndrome to MK-801. Genes Brain Behav *7*, 810-820.

Smigielska-Kuzia, J., Bockowski, L., Sobaniec, W., Kulak, W., and Sendrowski, K. (2010). Amino acid metabolic processes in the temporal lobes assessed by proton magnetic resonance spectroscopy (1H MRS) in children with Down syndrome. Pharmacol Rep *62*, 1070-1077.

Smith, D. J., Stevens, M. E., Sudanagunta, S. P., Bronson, R. T., Makhinson, M., Watabe, A. M., O'Dell, T. J., Fung, J., Weier, H. U., Cheng, J. F., and Rubin, E. M. (1997). Functional screening of 2 Mb of human chromosome 21q22.2 in transgenic mice implicates minibrain in learning defects associated with Down syndrome. Nat Genet *16*, 28-36.

Subramaniam, N., Treuter, E., and Okret, S. (1999). Receptor interacting protein RIP140 inhibits both positive and negative gene regulation by glucocorticoids. J Biol Chem *274*, 18121-18127.

Suetake, I., Shinozaki, F., Miyagawa, J., Takeshima, H., and Tajima, S. (2004). DNMT3L stimulates the DNA methylation activity of Dnmt3a and Dnmt3b through a direct interaction. J Biol Chem *279*, 27816-27823.

Sun, X., Wu, Y., Chen, B., Zhang, Z., Zhou, W., Tong, Y., Yuan, J., Xia, K., Gronemeyer, H., Flavell, R. A., and Song, W. (2011). Regulator of calcineurin 1 (RCAN1) facilitates neuronal apoptosis through caspase 3 activation. J Biol Chem *286*, 9049-9062.

Tabu, K., Ohnishi, A., Sunden, Y., Suzuki, T., Tsuda, M., Tanaka, S., Sakai, T., Nagashima, K., and Sawa, H. (2006). A novel function of OLIG2 to suppress human glial tumor cell growth via p27Kip1 transactivation. J Cell Sci *119*, 1433-1441.

Takebayashi, H., Ohtsuki, T., Uchida, T., Kawamoto, S., Okubo, K., Ikenaka, K., Takeichi, M., Chisaka, O., and Nabeshima, Y. (2002). Non-overlapping expression of Olig3 and Olig2 in the embryonic neural tube. Mech Dev *113*, 169-174.

Takuma, K., Fang, F., Zhang, W., Yan, S., Fukuzaki, E., Du, H., Sosunov, A., McKhann, G., Funatsu, Y., Nakamichi, N., *et al.* (2009). RAGE-mediated signaling contributes to intraneuronal transport of amyloid-beta and neuronal dysfunction. Proc Natl Acad Sci U S A *106*, 20021-20026.

Tang, Y., Schapiro, M. B., Franz, D. N., Patterson, B. J., Hickey, F. J., Schorry, E. K., Hopkin, R. J., Wylie, M., Narayan, T., Glauser, T. A., *et al.* (2004). Blood expression profiles for tuberous sclerosis complex 2, neurofibromatosis type 1, and Down's syndrome. Ann Neurol *56*, 808-814.

Tatsumi, K., Takebayashi, H., Manabe, T., Tanaka, K. F., Makinodan, M., Yamauchi, T., Makinodan, E., Matsuyoshi, H., Okuda, H., Ikenaka, K., and Wanaka, A. (2008). Genetic fate mapping of Olig2 progenitors in the injured adult cerebral cortex reveals preferential differentiation into astrocytes. J Neurosci Res *86*, 3494-3502.

Teyssier, C., Belguise, K., Galtier, F., Cavailles, V., and Chalbos, D. (2003). Receptor-interacting protein 140 binds c-Jun and inhibits estradiol-induced activator protein-1 activity by reversing glucocorticoid receptor-interacting protein 1 effect. Mol Endocrinol *17*, 287-299.

Thomas, S., Thiery, E., Aflalo, R., Vayssettes, C., Verney, C., Berthuy, I., and Creau, N. (2003). PCP4 is highly expressed in ectoderm and particularly in neuroectoderm derivatives during mouse embryogenesis. Gene Expr Patterns *3*, 93-97.

Tolias, K. F., Bikoff, J. B., Burette, A., Paradis, S., Harrar, D., Tavazoie, S., Weinberg, R. J., and Greenberg, M. E. (2005). The Rac1-GEF Tiam1 couples the NMDA receptor to the activity-dependent development of dendritic arbors and spines. Neuron *45*, 525-538.

Tolias, K. F., Bikoff, J. B., Kane, C. G., Tolias, C. S., Hu, L., and Greenberg, M. E. (2007). The Rac1 guanine nucleotide exchange factor Tiam1 mediates EphB receptor-dependent dendritic spine development. Proc Natl Acad Sci U S A *104*, 7265-7270.

Trazzi, S., Mitrugno, V. M., Valli, E., Fuchs, C., Rizzi, S., Guidi, S., Perini, G., Bartesaghi, R., and Ciani, E. (2011). APP-dependent up-regulation of Ptch1 underlies proliferation impairment of neural precursors in Down syndrome. Hum Mol Genet *20*, 1560-1573.

Utal, A. K., Stopka, A. L., Roy, M., and Coleman, P. D. (1998). PEP-19 immunohistochemistry defines the basal ganglia and associated structures in the adult human brain, and is dramatically reduced in Huntington's disease. Neuroscience *86*, 1055-1063.

Van Eldik, L. J., and Wainwright, M. S. (2003). The Janus face of glial-derived S100B: beneficial and detrimental functions in the brain. Restor Neurol Neurosci *21*, 97-108.

Vialard, F., Toyama, K., Vernoux, S., Carlson, E. J., Epstein, C. J., Sinet, P. M., and Rahmani, Z. (2000). Overexpression of mSim2 gene in the zona limitans of the diencephalon of segmental trisomy 16 Ts1Cje fetuses, a mouse model for trisomy 21: a novel whole-mount based RNA hybridization study. Brain Res Dev Brain Res *121*, 73-78.

Voronov, S. V., Frere, S. G., Giovedi, S., Pollina, E. A., Borel, C., Zhang, H., Schmidt, C., Akeson, E. C., Wenk, M. R., Cimasoni, L., *et al.* (2008). Synaptojanin 1-linked phosphoinositide dyshomeostasis and cognitive deficits in mouse models of Down's syndrome. Proc Natl Acad Sci U S A *105*, 9415-9420.

Weitzdoerfer, R., Dierssen, M., Fountoulakis, M., and Lubec, G. (2001). Fetal life in Down syndrome starts with normal neuronal density but impaired dendritic spines and synaptosomal structure. J Neural Transm Suppl, 59-70.

Whittle, N., Sartori, S. B., Dierssen, M., Lubec, G., and Singewald, N. (2007). Fetal Down syndrome brains exhibit aberrant levels of neurotransmitters critical for normal brain development. Pediatrics *120*, e1465-1471.

Wisniewski, K. E. (1990). Down syndrome children often have brain with maturation delay, retardation of growth, and cortical dysgenesis. Am J Med Genet Suppl *7*, 274-281.

Wisniewski, K. E., Laure-Kamionowska, M., and Wisniewski, H. M. (1984). Evidence of arrest of neurogenesis and synaptogenesis in brains of patients with Down's syndrome. N Engl J Med *311*, 1187-1188.

Wisniewski, K. E., and Schmidt-Sidor, B. (1989). Postnatal delay of myelin formation in brains from Down syndrome infants and children. Clin Neuropathol *8*, 55-62.

Wolvetang, E. J., Wilson, T. J., Sanij, E., Busciglio, J., Hatzistavrou, T., Seth, A., Hertzog, P. J., and Kola, I. (2003a). ETS2 overexpression in transgenic models and in Down syndrome predisposes to apoptosis via the p53 pathway. Hum Mol Genet *12*, 247-255.

Wolvetang, E. W., Bradfield, O. M., Tymms, M., Zavarsek, S., Hatzistavrou, T., Kola, I., and Hertzog, P. J. (2003b). The chromosome 21 transcription factor ETS2 transactivates the beta-APP promoter: implications for Down syndrome. Biochim Biophys Acta *1628*, 105-110.

Woods, Y. L., Rena, G., Morrice, N., Barthel, A., Becker, W., Guo, S., Unterman, T. G., and Cohen, P. (2001). The kinase DYRK1A phosphorylates the transcription factor FKHR at Ser329 in vitro, a novel in vivo phosphorylation site. Biochem J *355*, 597-607.

Yabut, O., Domogauer, J., and D'Arcangelo, G. (2010). Dyrk1A overexpression inhibits proliferation and induces premature neuronal differentiation of neural progenitor cells. J Neurosci *30*, 4004-4014.

Yamakawa, K., Huot, Y. K., Haendelt, M. A., Hubert, R., Chen, X. N., Lyons, G. E., and Korenberg, J. R. (1998). DSCAM: a novel member of the immunoglobulin superfamily maps in a Down syndrome region and is involved in the development of the nervous system. Hum Mol Genet *7*, 227-237.

Yang, E. J., Ahn, Y. S., and Chung, K. C. (2001). Protein kinase Dyrk1 activates cAMP response element-binding protein during neuronal differentiation in hippocampal progenitor cells. J Biol Chem *276*, 39819-39824.

Yankner, B. A., and Lu, T. (2009). Amyloid beta-protein toxicity and the pathogenesis of Alzheimer disease. J Biol Chem *284*, 4755-4759.

Ye, F., Chen, Y., Hoang, T., Montgomery, R. L., Zhao, X. H., Bu, H., Hu, T., Taketo, M. M., van Es, J. H., Clevers, H., *et al.* (2009). HDAC1 and HDAC2 regulate oligodendrocyte differentiation by disrupting the beta-catenin-TCF interaction. Nat Neurosci *12*, 829-838.

Yu, Y., Chu, P. Y., Bowser, D. N., Keating, D. J., Dubach, D., Harper, I., Tkalcevic, J., Finkelstein, D. I., and Pritchard, M. A. (2008). Mice deficient for the chromosome 21 ortholog Itsn1 exhibit vesicle-trafficking abnormalities. Hum Mol Genet *17*, 3281-3290.

Zhou, Q., and Anderson, D. J. (2002). The bHLH transcription factors OLIG2 and OLIG1 couple neuronal and glial subtype specification. Cell *109*, 61-73.

4

Down Syndrome: A Complex and Interactive Genetic Disorder

Samantha L. Deitz, Joshua D. Blazek, Jeffrey P. Solzak and Randall J. Roper
Indiana University-Purdue University Indianapolis
United States of America

1. Introduction

1.1 Trisomy 21 causes phenotypes associated with Down syndrome

Down syndrome (DS) occurs in approximately 1 out of 700 live births and most commonly results from three copies of human chromosome 21 (Hsa21) (Christianson, 2006). DS is a multifaceted disorder with over 80 clinically defined phenotypes including those affecting the central nervous system, heart, gastrointestinal tract, skeleton and immune system (Epstein, 2001; Van Cleve and Cohen, 2006). Phenotypes associated with individuals with DS vary in both incidence and severity, leading to a vast array of phenotypic combinations among those with Trisomy 21 (Ts21) (Deutsch et al., 2005; Epstein, 2001; Van Cleve et al., 2006; Van Cleve and Cohen, 2006). For example, cognitive impairment, hypotonia and craniofacial features are universal phenotypes, whereas cardiac abnormalities only affect approximately half of individuals with DS. Individual phenotypes similar to those seen in DS have been documented in individuals without Ts21, but a general higher incidence and severity of these phenotypes in individuals with DS suggests that trisomy plays an important role in initiating or modifying these features (Epstein, 2001; Roper and Reeves, 2006). Although it has been suggested that common mechanisms may be involved in similar phenotypes seen in individuals with and without Ts21, common pathophysiology must be proven for each individual phenotype.

A chromosomal basis for DS was postulated as early as 1932 (Patterson and Costa, 2005). After Jerome Lejeune established that DS was caused by an extra Hsa21, he studied the metabolic pathways associated with Ts21 phenotypes in an attempt to cure DS (Neri and Opitz, 2009). Alternate causes of DS, including translocations and mosaicism of extra material from Hsa21, were established shortly after the chromosomal basis of DS had been discovered (Patterson and Costa, 2005). These early genetic findings set the stage for current paradigms and research surrounding the gene-phenotype relationships in DS.

Although ~95% of the incidence of DS is due to trisomy of the entire Hsa21, DS also results from extra genetic material from Hsa21 translocated to other chromosomes. Additionally, some individuals with DS phenotypes have Ts21 in only a portion of their cells (mosaicism). Differences in genetic and cellular composition of the trisomy may lead to the observed differences in DS phenotypic incidence and severity. Genotypic and phenotypic variations have also been used to hypothesize about trisomic genes or chromosomal regions that may cause or significantly alter DS phenotypes. Such genotype-phenotype correlations are important in defining the etiology of traits associated with DS as well as suggesting possible therapeutic mechanisms to overcome deficits seen in individuals with DS.

1.2 Hypotheses regarding genotype-phenotype correlation in DS

Early investigations into the genotype-phenotype relationship drew upon information from individuals with partial Ts21. By examining these individuals, determining the extra chromosomal material and corresponding phenotypes, an early causal hypothesis linked DS to trisomy of the distal end of Hsa21 (Patterson and Costa, 2005). A reductionist variation of this hypothesis later stated that individual phenotypes and features could be mapped to specific regions of the genome, and the addition of these regions with their respective phenotypes would cause the multitude of traits associated with DS (Neri and Opitz, 2009). Others had a more global or genomic view of the genotype-phenotype relationship and hypothesized that DS phenotypes were due to a general genomic imbalance initiated by Ts21. Many new ideas have extended or combined previous hypotheses as well as proposed novel views about the correlation between genes and phenotypes in DS, especially with an increased ability to precisely define the genotypes and phenotypes associated with DS. Yet, the exact mechanisms of how the triplication of genes on Hsa21, the smallest and least gene dense of the autosomes, causes one of the myriad phenotypes associated with DS have still largely not been established. One or more of the hypothesized mechanisms may be correct for a single phenotype associated with DS, yet it is unlikely that a single overriding mechanism would describe the etiology of all Ts21 phenotypes (Epstein, 2001).

1.2.1 Gene dosage imbalance hypothesis

The "gene dosage imbalance" hypothesis suggests that an increased dosage or copy number of genes on Hsa21 would lead to an increase in gene expression and protein product in the individual (Antonarakis et al., 2004; Epstein, 2001; Pritchard and Kola, 1999). In essence, overexpression of the products of dosage sensitive genes on Hsa21 would lead to DS phenotypes. This hypothesis has been extended to include the possibility that specific genes or subsets of genes may control specific DS phenotypes (Patterson, 2007). Most studies have concluded that three copies of Hsa21 genes leads to an average 50% higher expression of trisomic genes as compared to euploid (normal chromosomal complement) individuals (Gardiner et al., 2010). As additional high throughput analyses are performed, however it is becoming increasingly clear that the gene expression changes may be specific to a group of genes in a particular tissue at a precise developmental or mature stage. Additionally, some trisomic gene expression changes may overlap with normal expression of these genes in the euploid chromosomal component (Ait Yahya-Graison et al., 2007; Prandini et al., 2007; Wiseman et al., 2009).

1.2.2 Amplified developmental instability hypothesis

The "amplified developmental instability" hypothesis states that a non-specific dosage of a number of trisomic genes leads to a genetic imbalance that causes a large impact on the expression and regulation of many genes throughout the genome (Pritchard and Kola, 1999; Shapiro, 1983). This disruption in genetic homeostasis or more generalized change in gene expression throughout the genome would affect signaling pathways and lead to phenotypes associated with DS. Therefore, it has been hypothesized that traits in individuals with DS are not caused by the altered expression of a particular gene, but rather the general changes in expression throughout the genome caused by trisomy that lead to DS traits (Patterson, 2009). An additional premise of this hypothesis is that the larger the number of trisomic genes, the higher the incidence and severity of DS phenotypes due to increased genetic instability. An extension of this hypothesis is that some phenotypic changes associated with

DS may not be attributable to specific genetic changes but rather to changes in the expression of the entire chromosomal domain (Gardiner et al., 2010).

1.2.3 Critical region(s) hypothesis

Phenotypic analyses conducted on individuals with partial trisomy for Hsa21 led to a hypothesis that only one or a few small chromosomal regions, termed "Down syndrome critical regions" (DSCR), contain genes responsible for the majority of DS phenotypes (Delabar et al., 1993; Korenberg et al., 1990). It has been suggested that DS (including many of the major, most well defined phenotypes) was caused by one specific DSCR (Epstein, 2001). Even before the identification of specific genes on Hsa21, a region of 1.6-2.5 Mb on Hsa21was thought to be responsible and sufficient to cause most DS phenotypes (Dahmane et al., 1998; Ohira et al., 1996). The sequencing of Hsa21 proved to be an important factor in the progression of DS research (Hattori et al., 2000) and led to further insight into genotype-phenotype correlations associated with DS and precise characterizations of DSCR regions (Patterson, 2009). A region of 3.8-6.5 Mb on 21q21.22 containing approximately 30 genes has been traditionally identified as the DSCR, although recent studies have demonstrated that this DSCR is not sufficient for all major DS phenotypes, though its inclusive genes may be relevant for some individual phenotypes (Delabar et al., 1993; Lyle et al., 2009). A current hypothesis states that certain chromosomal regions may contain a significant gene or genes necessary for the development or maintenance of specific but not all DS phenotypes (Korbel et al., 2009; Lyle et al., 2009; Olson et al., 2007).

1.2.4 Other genetic, epigenetic and environmental considerations

The hypotheses of how genetic mechanisms control DS phenotypes are not mutually exclusive, may include a combination of different mechanisms and may be unique for each particular phenotype. It is now believed that contributions to phenotypes associated with DS are likely to come from a number of genes. Variability in genomes may also come from allelic heterogeneity or other differences in the genetic architecture (Antonarakis et al., 2004). There may be genes that have a larger effect on certain phenotypes (Epstein, 2001; Patterson, 2009), or genetic contributions may be additive, subtractive, or epistatic (Gardiner et al., 2010). Recently it has been shown that epigenetic modifications and allelic differences also play a significant role in the development of these phenotypes, not just the simple presence of the chromosomal imbalance (Belichenko et al., 2009; Elton et al., 2010). Other factors including environmental influences and stochastic events also add to the differential manifestation of phenotypes.

1.2.5 Dosage compensation

Extra copies of genes may be found as a result of a number of duplication events, yet many of the resultant trisomies may be difficult to detect or have subtle phenotypes. Though there may be an extra copy of a gene, and even alterations in gene expression with the resultant protein product, dosage imbalance for a specific gene may have no effect on a phenotype. Such genes have been "dosage compensated" by some mechanism (Antonarakis et al., 2004). Gene expression experiments of cells with Ts21 have shown that a high percentage of three copy genes may undergo dosage compensation (Ait Yahya-Graison et al., 2007). This compensation could be accomplished by gene regulatory networks or negative feedback loops. Dosage compensation may be tissue or time dependent and may play an important role in the development and progression of DS phenotypes.

1.3 Mouse models of DS to understand genotype-phenotype correlation

In addition to being valuable tools for better understanding Ts21 and DS phenotypes, DS mouse models have also been utilized as predictive models of novel DS phenotypes (Baxter et al., 2000). Mice provide access to all tissues at all developmental stages, the ability to understand genetic and cellular mechanisms caused by trisomy, and a resource to understand potential treatments for phenotypes. Genes found on Hsa21 are highly conserved in order and homology on three different mouse chromosomes: mouse chromosome (Mmu)16, 17, and 10. Several DS mouse models have been created with segmental trisomy for different regions of the distal portion Mmu16, that contains nearly half the gene homologs found on Hsa21 (Hattori et al., 2000; Pletcher et al., 2001). The Ts65Dn mouse is the most commonly used DS model with segmental trisomy for the distal portion of Mmu16. Three copies of the region between *Mrpl39* and *Znf295* spanning 13.6 Mb on Mmu16 and containing over 100 Hsa21 gene homologs results in several DS-like phenotypes (Reeves et al., 1995). The Ts1Cje mouse contains segmental trisomy for approximately 78% (*Sod1-Znf295* excluding *Sod1*) of the triplicated genes in the Ts65Dn model (Olson et al., 2004b; Sago et al., 1998). Both Ts65Dn and Ts1Cje mice contain three copies of the putative DSCR region and exhibit a significant amount of phenotypic similarity to humans with DS. The Ts1Rhr/Ms1Rhr mouse models were created by generating a 3.9 Mb reciprocal duplication/deletion containing 33 genes (*Cbr1-Orf9*) homologous to those found in the most commonly defined human DSCR (Olson et al., 2004a). The transchromosomal Tc1 mouse model of DS has a copy of Hsa21 in its cells, though there are some deletions of Hsa21 regions and significant mosaicism in this model (O'Doherty et al., 2005). The Ts1Yey model contains the entire region of Hsa21 homology on Mmu16 from *D930038D03Rik-Znf295* duplicated on one Mmu16 and results in trisomy for this region in the mouse model (Li et al., 2007) (See Table 1).

More recently, mouse models of DS have been made that contain small regions of homology from chromosomes other than Mmu16. The Ts1Yah model contains a duplication of Mmu17 from *Abcg1-U2af1* with homology to Hsa21 (Pereira et al., 2009). The Ts2Yey model has a duplication of the entire region of Mmu10 homologous to Hsa21 (*Prmt2-Pdxk*). The Ts3Yey mouse has a duplication of the entire Mmu17 chromosomal region that corresponds to Hsa21 (*Abcg1-Rrp1b*) (Yu et al., 2010). Mice containing entire regions of homology to Hsa21 are being generated to examine DS phenotypes. Mouse models of DS may exhibit certain DS-like phenotypes with differing severity, but phenotypes may not be conserved across models, thus adding to the usefulness of the models for understanding the genotype-phenotype relationships associated with DS.

1.4 Using modern genetic and genomic tools to understand genotype-phenotype correlation in DS

Because DS and its resultant phenotypes are caused by trisomy, the gene-phenotype correlation (the genes responsible for the cellular or developmental changes) is of great importance in understanding DS. DS may be viewed as a chromosomal disorder due to three copies of Hsa21, a genetic disorder resulting from the altered expression of trisomic genes, or a disorder that results from alterations in gene expression and pathways

Common Name	Genetic triplication	Number of triplicated genes
Ts65Dn	Ts(17^{16})65Dn	104 (Mmu 16)
Ts1Rhr	Dp(16*Cbr1-Orf9*)1Rhr	33 (Mmu 16)
Ts1Cje	Ts(12^{16}C-tel)1Cje	81 (Mmu16)
Tc1	Tc(Hsa21)1TybEmcf	131 (~92% of Hsa 21)
Ts1Yey	*Dp(16 D930038D03Rik-Znf295)1Yey*	Mmu 16
Ts2Yey	*Dp(10Prmt2-Pdxk)2Yey*	Mmu 10
Ts3Yey	*Dp(17Abcg1-Rrp1b)3Yey*	Mmu 17

Table 1. Common DS mouse models with defined trisomic regions.

throughout the entire genome. Several studies have documented differential gene expression in tissues originating from varying spatial and developmental environments in attempts to determine genetic mechanisms affecting DS phenotypes (Conti et al., 2007; Lintas et al., 2010; Lyle et al., 2004; Moldrich et al., 2007). High throughput analysis utilizing tools such as microarray analysis, qPCR (quantitative polymerase chain reaction) and SAGE (serial analysis of gene expression) not only allow for a better understanding of gene expression aberrations in a spatiotemporal sense, but also permit for a better understanding of gene interactions within the context of natural physiological conditions. Though disparities exist between tissues and developmental time points, such analyses have provided insight into genes that appear to be critical to the development of specific DS phenotypes. New genetic information, coupled with precisely defined cellular and molecular phenotypes, (often using mouse models), has allowed the testing of multiple hypotheses concerning the gene-phenotype relationship. Functional groupings of dysregulated genes may add additional mechanistic insight into the origin of DS phenotypes, and such groupings may transcend both time and tissue type. The intersection of genetic and functional information may lead to new insights into the gene-phenotype relationship and the mechanisms leading to the development of DS phenotypes. With increasing ability to assess large scale gene expression, the importance of both trisomic and non-trisomic genes and genetic pathways utilizing gene products from the entire genome has been investigated. Instead of a simple notion of trisomy for Hsa21 causing a disorder or trisomic expression of specific genes on Hsa21 causing a disorder, current technologies and techniques now suggest that DS, with its myriad phenotypes, is a complex disorder with many interactions on genetic and mechanistic levels.

2. Trisomic and non-trisomic genes

2.1 The importance of trisomic and non-trisomic genes

Numerous gene expression studies have been performed on an assortment of tissues from individuals with DS as well as mouse models of DS (Tables 2 and 3). Although these assays vary widely in technique and scope, they have generally focused on the altered expression of trisomic genes. A strict interpretation of the gene dosage hypothesis suggests that all trisomic genes theoretically exhibit a 1.5 fold upregulation in every tissue and cell when compared to normal subjects, and nearly all studies use this expected fold change as a standard for expression analysis (Giannone et al., 2004; Mao et al., 2003). Interestingly, in studies that have analyzed both trisomic and disomic (non-trisomic) gene expression in trisomic compared to normal individuals, a significant number of non-trisomic genes have been found to be dysregulated in association with DS phenotypes (Table 4) (Lockstone et al., 2007; Rozovski et al., 2007; Slonim et al., 2009).

Study	Strain	Age	Tissue	Platform
Chrast et al. 2000	Ts65Dn	Adult	Brain	SAGE
Saran et al. 2003	Ts65Dn	3-4 months	Cerebellum	Microarray
Amano et al. 2004	Ts1Cje	Postnatal 0	Brain	Microarray
Lyle et al. 2004	Ts65Dn	Adult	Brain, Heart, Kidney, Liver, Lung, Muscle	qPCR
Dauphinot et al. 2005	Ts1Cje	Postnatal 0, 15, 30	Cerebellum	Microarray
Kahlem et al 2007	Ts65Dn	3-4 months	Lung, Skeletal Muscle, Midbrain, Cerebellum, Cortex, Testis, Liver, Heart, Kidney	Microarray
Sultan et al. 2007	Ts65Dn	13-26 weeks	Cerebellum, Midbrain, Cortex	qPCR
Laffaire et al. 2009	Ts1Cje	Postnatal 0, 3, 7, 10	Cerebellum, Granule Cell Layer	Microarray
Moldrich et al. 2009	Ts1Cje	E14	Neural Progenitor Cells	Microarray
Hewitt et al. 2010	Ts1Cje	Adult	Neural Stem Cells	Microarray, qPCR

Table 2. Features of gene expression assays performed in mice.

Study	Age	Tissue	Platform
Gross et al. 2002	Gest. 16-24 weeks	Placenta	Microarray
FitzPatrick et al. 2002	Fetal	Amniocytes	Microarray, qPCR
Mao et al. 2003	Gest. 17-21 weeks	Cerebral cortex, astrocytes	Microarray
Giannone et al. 2004	Adult	T lymphocytes	Microarray
Tang et al. 2004	Adult	Blood	Microarray
Chung et al. 2005	Fetal	Amniocytes	Microarray
Deutsch et al. 2005	Adult	Lymphoblastoids	qPCR
Mao et al. 2005	Fetal	Cerebellum, heart	Microarray
Li et al. 2006	Gest. 15-23 weeks	Heart, fibroblasts	Microarray, qPCR
Ait Yahya-Graison et al. 2007	Adult	Lymphoblasts	Microarray
Altug-Teber et al. 2007	Fetal	Amniocytes, Chorionic Villus Cells	Microarray
Conti et al. 2007	Gest. 18-22 weeks	Heart	Microarray
Lockstone et al. 2007	47-76 years	Brain	Microarray
Prandini et al. 2007	25 years	Lymphoblasts, Fibroblasts	qPCR
Rozovski et al. 2007	Fetal	Placenta	Microarray, qPCR
Chou et al. 2008	Gest. 16-21 weeks	Amniocytes	Microarray
Esposito et al. 2008	Gest. 19-21 weeks	Frontal cortex	Microarray
Sommer et al. 2008	1-4 years	Lymphocytes	SAGE, qPCR
Slonim et al. 2009	Fetal	Aminocytes	Microarray

Table 3. Features of gene expression assays from human derived tissues.

The number and variety of genes found to be dysregulated in response to trisomy seems to vary greatly in a spatiotemporal dependent manner, and provide evidence against the idea of a specific 1.5 fold dysregulation of trisomic genes in all tissue types (Mao et al., 2005; Potier et al., 2006; Sultan et al., 2007). Additionally, much of the variation in both trisomic and disomic gene expression in subjects with trisomy overlaps with the variation observed among normal individuals, which may limit the number of trisomic genes found to be differentially expressed (Prandini et al., 2007), and contribute to the variable phenotypes associated with DS (Chou et al., 2008). We therefore hypothesize that both trisomic and non-trisomic genes are important for the origin and development of DS phenotypes.

2.2 Gene expression studies in humans and mouse models of DS

2.2.1 Altered expression of trisomic genes and the gene dosage hypothesis

The gene dosage hypothesis and the proposed 1.5 fold increase in all trisomic gene expression have motivated much of the gene expression research of DS phenotypes. Assessment of gene expression in human fetal brain tissue and astrocyte cell lines taken at 17-20 weeks gestation revealed a general upregulation of trisomic gene expression, and seemed to agree with the 1.5 fold change hypothesis (Mao et al., 2003). Analysis of brain tissue isolated from 13-16 week old Ts65Dn mice also identified a global upregulation of trisomic genes in the cerebellum, cortex, and midbrain, and the average fold changes of trisomic gene expression were 1.44, 1.37, and 1.39, respectively, in Ts65Dn mice (Sultan et al., 2007).

Yet, other studies suggest the global upregulation of trisomic genes in agreement with the gene-dosage hypothesis is likely not occurring in DS. Many studies indicate that not all trisomic genes are dysregulated in all trisomic tissues. Furthermore, several studies on trisomic tissues have demonstrated expression levels significantly different from the expected 1.5 fold increase, indicating that having three copies of a gene does not necessarily confer a 1.5 fold upregulation. For example, expression analysis of 99 genes in 6 different tissues (brain, heart, lung, kidney, liver, and muscle) in P30 and 11 month old Ts65Dn mice revealed that 37% of the trisomic genes were expressed at a 1.5 fold increase, 45% were <1.5 increase, 18% >1.5 increase, and 9% were not significantly different from normal mice (Lyle et al., 2004). Additionally, only 15% and 29% of tested trisomic genes were found to be overexpressed in DS fetal hearts and cultured fibroblasts, respectively (Li et al., 2006). Of 134 differentially expressed genes assessed in lymphoblastoid cell lines (LCLs), 58/134 had overexpression greater than 1, (1.25-2.27), and 86/134 exhibited fold changes significantly different from 1.5 (9 were greater than 1.5 fold (1.64-2.27) and 77 were less than 1.5 (0.74-1.4)) (Ait Yahya-Graison et al., 2007). Of 117 trisomic genes in LCLs and 114 trisomic genes in fibroblasts, only 39% and 62% respectively were found to have significant expression differences from euploid cells (Prandini et al., 2007). Based on these data, four classes of genes in trisomic tissues have been suggested: those that exhibit expression significantly different from 1 but not different from 1.5 fold, amplified genes (expression significantly greater than 1.5 fold), compensated genes (expression significantly less than 1.5 fold), and the genes with expression differences not different from 1 or 1.5 fold (Ait Yahya-Graison et al., 2007; Prandini et al., 2007). These extensive studies indicate that a global 1.5 fold upregulation of all trisomic genes in DS tissues is unlikely and suggest that mechanisms in addition to trisomy are also affecting gene regulation. Although the expression levels of some trisomic genes fit within the theoretical 50% upregulation, trisomic genes in several tissues at different time points exhibit expression levels much different from the expected 1.5 fold increase.

Study	Trisomic Genes	Disomic Genes	# Significant Trisomic Genes	# Significant Disomic Genes	# Genes Examined
Gross et al. 2002	*C21ORF3*	*KRT8, ALDH7, KISS1*	2	5	8976
FitzPatrick et al. 2002	*N/A*	*IGFBP3, RGS5, IGFBP5*	39	1934	8020
Mao et al. 2003	*DSCR2, SOD1*	N/A	Global upregulation	N/A	~15,000
Giannone et al. 2004	*SOD1,CSTB*	*HLA-DRB3, GABRG2, ACAT2*	2	15	334
Tang et al. 2004	*DSCR2, CSTB*	*FHL1, ALOX12, RGS10*	~20%	6%	~12,000
Chung et al. 2005	*COL6A1, PRSS7*	*AKT, CASP5, JUN*	2	8	102
Deutsch et al. 2005	*APP*	N/A	25	7	41
Mao et al. 2005	*SOD1, SON, DSCR3*	*ADAMTS1*	26	14	~12,500
Li et al. 2006	*SH3BGR, MX1, GART*	*IFI27*	17	41	~10,000
Ait Yahya-Graison et al. 2007	*SAMSN1, DYRK1A SNF1LK, MX1*	N/A	29%	N/A	359
Altug-Teber et al. 2007	*DSCR1*	N/A	16	N/A	~12,500
Conti et al. 2007	*DSCR1, DYRK1A*	*NFATc*	32	441	~6300
Lockstone et al. 2007	*APP, RCAN, BACE2*	*APOE, NOTCH2*	40 (25%)	4.4% dysregulated	~12,500
Prandini et al. 2007	*GABAPA, PFKL, U2AF1*		39%, 62%	N/A	123, 132
Rozovski et al. 2007	*APP*	*LOX, MEST, MAT2A*	41 overexpressed	709 overexpressed	~12,500
Chou et al. 2008	N/A	N/A	~1.28 fold	17 with high variation	~18,000
Esposito et al. 2008	*APP, S100B*	*AQP4*	~1.5 fold in DSCR	Modest pathway-specific changes	~12,500
Sommer et al. 2008	*N/A*	*2M, CD74, CD52*	7	~250	N/A
Slonim et al. 2009	*CLIC6, ITGB2, RUNX1*	N/A	5	409	~12,500
Chrast et al. 2000	*Ifnar2, Ifngr2, Cbr*	N/A	3	330	N/A
Saran et al. 2003	N/A	N/A	~1.45 fold average	~1.1 fold average	~12,500
Amano et al. 2004	N/A	N/A	~1.5 fold average	~1.0 fold average	~11,300
Lyle et al. 2004	*Adamts1, Mx1*	N/A	~1.5 fold average	N/A	99
Dauphinot et al. 2005	*Dscr3, Hmgp14, Donson*	*HoxA5, Dlx1*	~1.5 fold average	~1.0 fold average	~12,500
Kahlem et al 2007	*Bace2, App, Mx1*	N/A	~1.5 fold average	N/A	136
Sultan et al. 2007	*Bace2, Kcne2, App, Cbr1*	N/A	~1.5 fold average	N/A	50
Laffaire et al. 2009	*Olig1, Dscam, Girk2, Son*	N/A	11-13 in cerebellum 23 in GCL	372-1164 in cerebellum 9 in GCL	~15,600
Moldrich et al. 2009	*Olig1, Olig2, Dscam, Dscr3*	*Sox21, Calcoco1*	29 of 54	1847	~25,000
Hewitt et al. 2010	*Itsn1*	*Mcm7, Brca2,Prim1*	~1.5 fold average	6.5% of probes	~14,000

Table 4. Significant trisomic and disomic genes highlighted by gene expression studies. Common genes of interest were selected from studies that stated more than three genes. N/A= not applicable or available.

2.2.2 Altered expression of non-trisomic genes

While many gene expression studies have focused on expression levels of genes in three copies, increasingly the expression of non-trisomic genes has also been analyzed. Two early microarray studies using amniotic fluid and placenta found extreme variation associated with the genes on Hsa21, however both of these studies showed that disomic genes also contained high variation in expression in trisomic tissue (Chung et al., 2005; Deutsch et al., 2005). It was observed that two-copy genes were downregulated implying that Ts21 was affecting genes on other chromosomes (Chung et al., 2005). An additional microarray analysis on cells derived from DS fetal placenta found 750 genes were overexpressed with the majority located on chromosomes other than 21, implicating non-trisomic genes as significant contributors to DS phenotypes (Rozovski et al., 2007). Adult human DS brains exhibited 400 differentially expressed genes when compared to normal individuals and approximately 350 of these were not found on Hsa21 (Lockstone et al., 2007). Expression analyses conducted on uncultured DS amniotic fluid cells identified a total of 414 dysregulated genes with only five located on Hsa21 (Slonim et al., 2009). Two recent analyses of cells from developing Ts1Cje brains have also indicated a large number of dysregulated non-trisomic genes in addition to significantly dysregulated trisomic genes (Laffaire et al., 2009; Moldrich et al., 2009). Additionally, 6.5% of all disomic genes were found to be dysregulated in the primary neural progenitor cells isolated from the brains of adult DS mice (Hewitt et al., 2010). Based on these findings, it has been suggested that trisomy causes a disruption in gene regulation throughout the entire genome and not just of the genes in three copies. Despite these findings, the phenotypic effects of altered disomic gene expression in DS is highly debated and not well understood (Lyle et al., 2004; Mao et al., 2005; Saran et al., 2003).

2.3 Measuring gene regulation with tissue and age specificity

The most tissue-specific developmental microarray research in mouse models of DS has focused on the developing cerebellum, which continues to develop after birth. Extensive microarray analyses of the hypocellular cerebellum in adult and early postnatal trisomic mice have revealed dysregulation of both trisomic and non-trisomic genes. For example, microarray analyses were performed on the entire cerebellum during postnatal days 0, 15, and 30 (P0, P15, P30) in the Ts1Cje model of DS. Though genes present in three copies had an average relative expression of about 1.5 fold, only five (P0), nine (P15), and seven (P30) three copy genes of the 63 trisomic genes tested were expressed at levels >2 or <1.2. Additionally, 406 of 8250 two copy (non-trisomic) genes examined had ratios comparing trisomic and euploid expression that were significantly different from 1 (Dauphinot et al., 2005). Three trisomic genes were dysregulated at all developmental time points. Interestingly, changes in development influenced gene expression differences between stages more than between trisomy and euploid animals (Dauphinot et al., 2005; Potier et al., 2006). As these studies showed, gene expression can vary greatly in one tissue from early in development to adulthood. Because individual genes are shown to have variation in expression throughout development, certain genes may be relevant to a particular phenotype at one time point and unrelated at another.

2.4 Gene expression variation in response to Trisomy 21

In addition to the importance of understanding the temporal and spatial relationships associated with trisomic gene expression, variation in gene expression of both disomic and trisomic genes may contribute to DS phenotypes. Expression studies conducted on fibroblasts and LCLs identified large gene expression variation between cell lines as well as between individual genes (Ait Yahya-Graison et al., 2007; Deutsch et al., 2005; Prandini et al., 2007). It was suggested that high levels of gene expression variation could explain why the majority of Hsa21 genes were not significantly upregulated and the variability in DS phenotypes. The latter is explained by the level of overlap between gene expression in trisomic and euploid individuals. Genes with distinct expression profiles may be candidates for the constant features of DS, whereas the genes that exhibit overlapping expression profiles may be responsible for the variable DS phenotypes (Prandini et al., 2007).

Studies conducted in Ts65Dn mice also exhibited differing levels of variable gene expression. Sultan et al. showed that 31 out of 33 trisomic genes were upregulated in the Ts65Dn brain. Of these 31 genes, 24 genes exhibited a small amount of variation (coefficient of variation of <0.2) and seven genes exhibited high variation. These authors suggested that the level of variation in gene expression indicated how tightly the genes were being regulated in the brain tissue of Ts65Dn animals.

Understanding gene expression variation in trisomic tissues is a key component in the study of DS gene-phenotype relationships. This expression variation may influence the results of microarray and qPCR studies and lead to the false identification/exclusion of candidate genes for specific phenotypes. Additionally the phenotypic variability observed in individuals with DS may be attributed to trisomic gene expression variation in different tissues, and it is likely that the level of variation within an individual gene is directly related to how tightly that particular gene is regulated. Further research is needed to identify the exact role expression variation plays in the development of DS phenotypes.

2.5 Summary

Gene expression assays in DS are an essential tool for understanding the mechanisms behind Ts21. While the gene dosage hypothesis may be applicable to specific genes with spatiotemporal specific expression, gene expression analyses suggest that not all trisomic genes are dysregulated at a 1.5 fold ratio, the expression of some trisomic genes is similar to euploid, and variation in gene expression plays a significant role in influencing phenotypic development. Differences in developmental stages as well as particular tissue types may contribute to some of the variable findings across studies. Additionally, the level of gene expression variation differs between individuals of the same genotype, adding to the complexity of understanding expression analyses. Though trisomic genes are important and are the likely initiators of DS phenotypes, disomic genes are also dysregulated suggesting that both trisomic and disomic genes can influence the DS phenotype.

3. Complex genotype-phenotype relationships

Characterization of certain DS phenotypes along with the genetic analysis of individuals with partial trisomies led to a hypothesis of the "Down syndrome critical or chromosomal region" (DSCR) believed to contain the genes necessary for the development of the most common phenotypes observed in individuals with DS (Delabar et al., 1993; Korenberg et al., 1990). The sequencing of Hsa21 and mapping of specific genes in the putative DSCR further defined the genetic content of the region and allowed for a more detailed trisomic gene-phenotype correlation. More recent analyses of critical regions using mouse models of DS as well as samples from individuals with partial trisomies have questioned the validity of the original DSCR hypothesis of a single region or gene important for most of the common DS traits (Korbel et al., 2009; Lyle et al., 2009; Olson et al., 2004a). Current data suggest a single critical region or critical gene is not sufficient to cause multiple characteristic DS phenotypes. Rather, specific genes within susceptibility regions may play important roles in the establishment and maintenance of specific, but not all, DS phenotypes.

3.1 Origins of the Down syndrome critical region hypothesis

The DSCR was originally hypothesized based on the assessment of a family with partial Hsa21 trisomy and the variable expression of several of the characteristic physical features of DS. A "critical region" within 21q22 was believed to be responsible for several DS phenotypes including craniofacial abnormalities, congenital heart defects of the endocardial cushions, clinodactyly of the fifth finger and mental retardation (Niebuhr, 1974). Soon after the DSCR hypothesis, genetic analyses of the Hsa21 DNA revealed several gene-rich segments located within 21q22 and placed further emphasis on this region as critical to the development of DS phenotypes (Brahe et al., 1990).

The hypothesis of a DSCR shifted the focus of many in the DS research community toward understanding how these genomic regions could correlate with the development of DS phenotypes. Regions linked to congenital heart defects (CHD), duodenal stenosis and craniofacial abnormalities in individuals with DS were identified through further analyses (Korenberg et al., 1992). An analysis of ten patients with partial trisomy for different segments of Hsa21 led to the mapping of 24 DS phenotypes to six chromosomal regions. Of these 24 phenotypes, 13 were mapped to 21g22.2 - proximal 21q22.3 region and six were linked to the *D21S55-MX1* region (Delabar et al., 1993). CHD was not included in the phenotypes associated with the D21S55-*MX1* region, and a later assessment of 19 individuals led to the mapping of CHD to a region outside of the D21S55-*MX1* region on 21q22.3 including *DSCAM,* a gene known to be involved in cell adhesion and expressed in the heart during development (Barlow et al., 2001a). A similar experiment comparing gene overlap regions with the phenotypic traits of 16 individuals with partial Ts21 along with the phenotypic variability observed in DS led to the hypothesis that factors in addition to trisomic genes both within and outside the DSCR likely contribute to most DS phenotypes, as opposed to a single critical region (Korenberg et al., 1994). Several additional genetic aspects including allelic heterogeneity, epistatic interactions, imprinting effects, uncharacterized epigenetic modifications and environmental events as well as the general variability observed in non-affected individuals were also suggested to have an impact on phenotypic variability (Korenberg et al., 1994).

The DSCR hypothesis, derived from analyses of the shortest region of overlap in individuals with partial Ts21, paved the way for the establishment of gene-phenotype relationships associated with DS. However, the high variability in phenotypic expression caused by an array of trisomic genetic consequences severely restricts the resolution of the gene-phenotype relationships associated with DS. The sequencing of Hsa21 as well as the development of several mouse models of DS provided further insight into the DSCR hypothesis.

3.2 Disproving the DSCR with mouse models

Unlike the analyses of partial trisomy in humans, comparisons of DS mouse models with differing segmental aneuploidies (both on their own and crossed between each other) has allowed for a systematic and meticulous analysis of the relationship between certain chromosomal regions and DS phenotypes. The Ts1Rhr/Ms1Rhr mouse model was created by generating a 3.9 Mb reciprocal duplication/deletion containing 33 genes (*Cbr1-Orf9*) homologous to those found in the most commonly recognized putative human DSCR (Olson et al., 2004a). Human DS-like phenotypes documented in Ts65Dn and Ts1Cje mice, which contain larger segmental trisomies, and the creation of Ts1Rhr and Ms1Rhr mice, established a system suitable to test the DSCR hypothesis in mice. Ts65Dn mice are smaller in size with shorter femurs and exhibit craniofacial abnormalities including smaller skulls and mandible bones, as well as brachycephaly when compared to euploid littermates—defects also found in humans with DS and previously attributed to the DSCR (Delabar et al., 1993; Richtsmeier et al., 2000). Analysis of Ts1Rhr mice revealed significant increases in overall size, length of femur, and mandible size when compared to euploid littermates and an absence of brachycephaly, indicating major differences between Ts1Rhr and Ts65Dn or Ts1Cje phenotypes (Olson et al., 2004a). Mice generated from a cross between Ts65Dn and Ms1Rhr mice (removing triplication of the DSCR in the Ts65Dn mouse) exhibited craniofacial phenotypes similar to those observed in Ts65Dn mice (Olson et al., 2004a). Comparison of the craniofacial phenotypes observed in Ts1Rhr and Ts65Dn/Ms1Rhr mice indicated that the DSCR is not sufficient to produce these phenotypes in DS mouse models, but may still contribute in the genetic context of the phenotypes observed in Ts65Dn mice through genetic interactions.

In addition to the studies conducted on craniofacial skeletal abnormalities, DS-associated brain phenotypes have also been compared in DS mouse models. Ts65Dn mice exhibit a similar sized brain and hippocampus but smaller cerebellum and reductions in granule and Purkinje cell density when compared to euploid littermates (Baxter et al., 2000). Ts1Cje and Ms1Cje/Ts65Dn mice exhibit similar but less severe defects to those observed in Ts65Dn mice (Olson et al., 2004b). Analysis of Ts1Rhr mice revealed a similar sized brain and hippocampus when compared to euploid littermates, analogous to what was observed in Ts65Dn and Ts1Cje mouse models. The cerebellum of Ts1Rhr mice exhibited a small but significant reduction in size compared to euploid mice, but no differences were found in granule or Purkinje cell density, suggesting that trisomy for the DSCR is not sufficient to produce some brain phenotypes associated with DS (Olson et al., 2007).

Furthermore, studies have shown that Ts65Dn mice exhibit impairment of hippocampal function similar to that observed in individuals with DS (Holtzman et al., 1996; Reeves et al., 1995). Based on the DSCR hypothesis, genes within this region control the cognitive impairment phenotype associated with DS. If this were true, Ts1Rhr mice should exhibit similar deficits to Ts65Dn mice in hippocampal function. In contrast to Ts65Dn mice, Ts1Rhr exhibited normal hippocampal function in the Morris water maze test and normal induction of long term potentiation (LTP) in the CA1 suggesting the DSCR is not sufficient to cause the cognitive impairment associated with DS (Aldridge et al., 2007; Olson et al., 2007). Interestingly, when three copies of the DSCR were reduced to two, Ts65Dn/Ms1Rhr mice performed similarly to euploid animals in the water maze test suggesting that although the DSCR is not sufficient on its own to cause cognitive impairment, it is necessary for the phenotype to occur (Olson et al., 2007).

It is important to note that there are background differences between Ts65Dn, Ts1Cje, Ms1Rhr, and Ts1Rhr mice utilized in the studies described above. Inbreeding strategies for Ts65Dn and Ms1Rhr mice have not been successful, and these mice are maintained on an ~50% B6 and 50% C3H advanced intercross genetic background. The majority of studies previously documented in Ts1Rhr mice used a mixed background of approximately 50% B6, 25% 129 and 25% C3H (except for the Morris water maze and LTP study where Ts1Rhr were on a B6 background) and it is possible that background differences may cloud direct comparisons between these mouse models. Behavioral and neurophysiologic phenotypes were assessed in Ts1Rhr mice maintained on a ~50% B6 and 50% C3H background to mimic the same genetic background as Ts65Dn mice. In contrast to what was observed in Ts1Rhr mice on other backgrounds, these mice exhibited several (20 of 48) similar neurologic phenotypes as Ts65Dn mice suggesting that the DSCR may be sufficient to confer some characteristic DS cognitive and brain abnormalities (Belichenko et al., 2009). The differences in neurological phenotypes in Ts1Rhr mice on different genetic backgrounds suggest the importance of understanding the complex genetic interactions associated with DS. Although evidence in mouse models implies that there is no single region critical to the majority of DS phenotypes, it is apparent that a gene or genes within this region are important in certain phenotypes and these phenotypes may be dependent on genetic background. Either allelic differences associated with trisomic genes or other two-copy genes in the genome may be responsible for the differences observed between trisomies with different genetic backgrounds.

3.3 New views on the DSCR and additional analyses in humans

Advancements in DNA technology as well as additional individuals identified with partial trisomy have led to more information on the hypothesized DSCR and gene-phenotype relationships in individuals with DS. A genotype-phenotype correlation analysis conducted on 30 individuals with either partial trisomy or partial monosomy for Hsa21 using array comparative genome hybridization found that four individuals with partial trisomy for the proximal portion of Hsa21 (not including the putative DSCR) exhibited several DS phenotypes (Lyle et al., 2009). Additionally, it was shown that there are multiple regions necessary to produce the cognitive impairment and hypotonia associated with DS, as well as a region previously identified as a candidate for CHD (*D21S3-PFKL*) (Barlow et al., 2001a). These new results suggest that the concept of one chromosomal region important for the majority of DS phenotypes does not exist due to multiple genetic regions critical for DS phenotypes. Due to the identification of multiple regions contributing to the same phenotypes, these regions may be more aptly termed "susceptibility" regions and may correspond to one or a limited number of phenotypes (Lyle et al., 2009). Individuals with triplication of these genes are more likely to exhibit the DS phenotypes associated with these regions.

High-resolution genetic mapping to determine gene involvement of eight specific DS phenotypes using 30 individuals with segmental trisomy for Hsa21 also concluded that specific genetic regions may be important for certain DS phenotypes. Genomic analysis revealed that the interaction of *DYRK1A* and *RCAN1*, thought to be involved in many DS phenotypes (Arron et al., 2006), were not essential in the development of CHD and mental retardation because individuals without trisomy for these genes exhibited severe abnormalities (Korbel et al., 2009). Additionally, several DS phenotypes, including transient myeloproliferative disorder, AMKL, and cognitive impairment, require triplication of multiple Hsa21 regions and genes (Korbel et al., 2009). A combination of data from this work and that in mouse models led to the specification of a CHD-causing region smaller than but included in a previously defined region for CHD (Barlow et al., 2001a). The newly defined region contains only 10 genes including *DSCAM*, a cell adhesion molecule highly expressed in the developing heart, also believed to contribute to the high levels of Hirschprung disease associated with DS (Korbel et al., 2009; Korbel et al., 2007).

Additional evidence against the synergy of *DYRK1A* and *RCAN1* in causing craniofacial and cardiac abnormalities associated with DS (Arron et al., 2006; Richtsmeier et al., 2000) came from a family with a 4.3 Mb duplication of chromosome 21q22 (including *DYRK1A* but not *RCAN1* or *DSCAM*). Individuals with the duplication presented with severe DS-like craniofacial abnormalities, but other malformations including cardiac defects were not observed. Based on these observations, the authors suggested two distinct regions important for these DS phenotypes with the distal region containing the genes including *DYRK1A* associated with craniofacial abnormalities and the proximal region (including *RCAN1* and *DSCAM*) associated with cardiac abnormalities (Ronan et al., 2007).

Interestingly, studies of individuals without DS provide evidence against the theory of only these distal and proximal specific regions associated with DS phenotypes. A patient with Silver-Russell syndrome, which has little similarity with DS, and his healthy father displayed a 0.46 Mb duplication of 21q22 including the *RCAN1* gene. No DS-associated phenotypes were documented in either individual suggesting that *RCAN1* alone is not sufficient to produce DS phenotypes (Eggermann et al., 2010). Furthermore, a child with a non-mosaic ring chromosome 21 duplication containing most of the long arm of Hsa21 including the hypothesized DSCR was found to have several characteristic DS phenotypes including cardiac and gastrointestinal defects but lacked the usual facial features associated with DS (Crombez et al., 2005).

Taken together, these studies provide evidence against the original DSCR hypothesis. It has been shown that genes and regions of genes located both within and outside of the hypothesized DSCR are critical to the initiation and severity of specific DS phenotypes. Studies conducted on humans with DS, DS mouse models, and other transgenic models have uncovered that several genes found within the putative DSCR are known to have a major effect on DS phenotypes. Thus, although the DSCR concept as traditionally defined does not seem to be correct, there are critical genes within this region that have a major impact on specific DS phenotypes.

3.4 Individual genes associated with the DSCR

Although it is evident the DSCR does not contribute to all of the phenotypes associated with DS, because the DSCR has been heavily studied, several genes found within this region have been implicated as candidate genes for individual DS phenotypes. The most extensively studied genes found within this region are Regulator of calcineurin1 (*RCAN1/DSCR1*) and dual specificity tyrosine-phosphorylation kinase 1a (*DYRK1A*), which are hypothesized to play important roles in several developmental pathways, including CNS, craniofacial skeletal and cardiac (Arron et al., 2006; Park et al., 2009; Richtsmeier et al., 2000). *DYRK1A* and *RCAN1* are both involved in the regulation of NFAT, a critical transcription factor necessary for the processes of vertebrate development and organogenesis (Graef et al., 2001). Transgenic *Nfatc* mutant mice exhibit several characteristics similar to DS mouse models as well as humans with DS including cognitive impairment and craniofacial and cardiac abnormalities. Mice with overexpression of *Dyrk1a* and *Rcan1* exhibited similar phenotypes to *Nfatc* mutants, suggesting that these genes are likely playing a part in the development of DS phenotypes (Arron et al., 2006).

In addition to *DYRK1A* and *RCAN1*, Down syndrome cell adhesion molecule (*DSCAM*) has been suggested to play a critical role in the developing brain and has also been identified as a candidate gene for the increased levels of CHD observed in DS individuals (Alves-Sampaio et al., 2010; Barlow et al., 2001a; Barlow et al., 2002). DSCAM is a critical factor in neural differentiation, axon guidance, and the establishment of neural networks and it has been suggested that the disruption of these processes contributes to the DS neurocognitive phenotype (Agarwala et al., 2001; Barlow et al., 2001b; Yamakawa et al., 1998). A recent study found that *Dscam* was overexpressed in hippocampal neurons of the Ts1Cje mouse model. Overexpression of *Dscam* impaired dendritic branching leading to an inhibitory effect on synaptogenesis and neurite outgrowth, further implicating the role of *Dscam* in the development of the DS brain phenotype (Alves-Sampaio et al., 2010).

Also found within the DSCR, *ETS2* is a transcription factor known to be involved in the regulation of cellular proliferation, differentiation, transformation and apoptosis (Seth and Watson, 2005). Extensive studies on *Ets2* in transgenic and DS mouse models have revealed that the gene may play a role in the neuronal, tumor suppressive, and craniofacial phenotypes associated with DS (Hill et al., 2009; Sussan et al., 2008; Wolvetang et al., 2003). Additionally, *KCNJ6/GIRK2* overexpression in the hippocampus of Ts65Dn mice has been shown to cause an abnormal balance between inhibitory and excitatory synapses, implicating the gene in the DS-brain phenotype (Best et al., 2007). Additionally, this overexpression was also implicated in the reduced cerebellar size and alterations in granule cell neuron differentiation observed in the weaver mouse (Patil et al., 1995).

3.5 Gene(s)-phenotype relationships

The establishment of a specific phenotype requires the successful coordination of a number of genetic interactions. In many human disorders a single gene or gene network is responsible for causing the associated phenotypes. However, evidence from both humans and mouse models of DS suggests that specific DS phenotypes are influenced by genetic aberrations in multiple genes as opposed to a single gene. The most glaring case of multiple genes affecting a phenotype comes from the study of cognitive impairment through the analysis of human and mouse DS brains. *DYRK1A, RCAN1,* and *DSCAM* have all been shown to regulate the stages of neuronal cell maturation (proliferation, differentiation, and apoptosis) in the developing brain (Agarwala et al., 2001; Barlow et al., 2001b; Park et al., 2010; Sun et al., 2011). Triplication of *Olig1, Olig2,* and *Kcnj6,* leads to significant changes in the ratio of inhibitory to excitatory neurons in the Ts65Dn forebrain (Best et al., 2007; Chakrabarti et al., 2010) and *DSCAM* regulates dendritic branching and neuronal network establishment (Alves-Sampaio et al., 2010), suggesting that increased inhibitory activity and the inability to form neuronal networks are also contributing to the cognitive impairment phenotype. In addition to cognitive impairment, an AD-like phenotype is apparent in most adult individuals with DS. Dysregulation of *DYRK1A, RCAN1,* and/or *Ets2* lead to an increase in the number of neurofibrillary tangles and β-amyloid plaques in the brains of humans and mice (Ermak et al., 2001; Ryoo et al., 2008; Sun et al., 2011), respectively, indicating that multiple genes are contributing to the DS-AD phenotype.

3.6 Summary

Based on thorough analyses of studies on humans and DS mouse models, it is evident that there is not a single critical region of genes sufficient to cause all DS phenotypes. Alternatively, it is likely that there are multiple critical regions or critical genes contributing to a respective phenotype or group of phenotypes associated with DS (Lyle et al., 2009). Although studies conducted regarding the DSCR have provided a wealth of evidence refuting the idea, it is important to understand that several genes within this region have been identified as key contributors to more specific DS phenotypes. Furthermore, both non-trisomic genes and trisomic genes located outside of the hypothesized DSCR have also been implicated in the development of specific DS phenotypes and in some cases may be linked with DSCR associated genes. It is evident that DS phenotypes are influenced by a multitude of complex genetic interactions and it seems likely that multiple genes and gene networks will be involved in the development of most DS phenotypes. Important genes or regions of genes contributing to specific DS phenotypes should be defined as susceptibility genes or regions, as opposed to defining a single Down syndrome critical region or single gene-phenotype relationship (Lyle et al., 2009).

4. Functional analysis of genes

4.1 Introduction

Although hypotheses have been developed concerning cellular and developmental mechanisms relating to DS phenotypes, no conclusive evidence exists for a single mechanism likely responsible for the majority of DS phenotypes. Instead, multiple common mechanisms may be responsible for individual phenotypes in specific tissues or at precise developmental stages and groups of genes with related functions may also be dysregulated in DS pathology. Functional databases provide the foundation for elucidating gene-phenotype relationships by clustering dysregulated genes with common functions. These clusters identify potential cellular, developmental and biological functions, as well as the number of genes in each cluster and significance of those categories. Depending on the functional annotation tool, relevant pathways, molecules for potential pharmacological interventions or insight into genetic mechanisms may be suggested. The use of functional databases extends the value of high throughput arrays and tests hypotheses that specific groups of genes with related function may be dysregulated in DS. Rather than a simple dosage increase of Hsa21 genes, it has been hypothesized that trisomy has a more global dysregulational effect on the genome, though developmental changes and tissue type do maintain a significant role (Altug-Teber et al., 2007; Dauphinot et al., 2005; Sommer et al., 2008). We hypothesize that the interaction between trisomic and disomic genes have a significant effect on the way DS phenotypes arise, manifest and progress.

Several studies have documented differential gene expression in unique spatial and developmental environments to determine mechanisms affecting DS phenotypes (Conti et al., 2007; Lyle et al., 2004; Moldrich et al., 2007). Other studies often concentrate on the cellular or developmental mechanisms as a causative factor of DS phenotypes (Chakrabarti et al., 2007; Contestabile et al., 2009; Cooper et al., 2001; Roper et al., 2006; Roper et al., 2009). High throughput analyses are important for investigating gene-phenotype relationships in analyses of various tissue and cell types from individuals with DS, mouse models of DS, and cell lines previously derived from individuals with DS or engineered to contain this extra genetic material. We hypothesize that a single generalized pathway or mechanism does not underlie the phenotypes of DS, but rather several pathways and mechanisms contribute to the phenotypes of DS, though some functional groups may cluster together in certain tissues or within phenotypes. Assessment of the gene-phenotype relationships in high throughput meta-analysis provides novel information regarding the importance of developmental processes in the DS pathophysiology.

4.2 Previously established functional analyses

Studies of DS have utilized high throughput analysis on several tissues including cultured DS neural progenitor cells and tissue samples from DS amniocytes, hearts, cerebra and cerebella and cultured Ts1Cje neural progenitor cells (NPCs). Though differences are present between developmental time points and tissues, genes involved with cellular cycling, cell adhesion, signal transduction, DNA and RNA metabolism and binding, gene expression regulation and transcription, mitochondrial function and oxidative phosphorylation, kinase activity, and ECM production and maintenance were the most highly dysregulated and common categories observed, as well as maintain the ability to transcend time and tissue differences (Table 5). More specifically, certain cell types of representative models of DS or from individuals with DS share multiple common annotation results. We suggest a similar phenomenon may regulate multiple DS phenotypes in which dysregulated mechanisms affect the same tissue in order to produce a phenotype (Figure 1).

4.2.1 Cell cycle alterations contribute to neurological phenotypes

NPCs display altered gene expression related to cell cycling, proliferation, signaling, transcription and metabolism of chromosomal material. It is well established that deficits in proliferation and mitotic activity of specific cellular populations in the DS brain exist, including areas of the cerebellum and multiple areas of the cerebrum (Baxter et al., 2000; Chakrabarti et al., 2007; Gardiner et al., 2010; Roper et al., 2006). Additionally, impairment of proliferation in the cerebellum of fetuses with DS has also been reported (Guidi et al., 2010) as well as in the Ts65Dn neonate peripheral tissues and fibroblasts, suggesting a general deficit in proliferation as a mechanism for multiple DS abnormalities (Contestabile et al., 2009). Individuals born with DS have reduced brain weights coupled with a smaller, dysmorphic skull and multiple cellular abnormalities within the brain including reduction in the number of neurons in the cerebral cortex as well as cellular deficiencies in multiple other structures (Aylward et al., 1997; Fink et al., 1975; Wisniewski, 1990). Therefore, these phenotypic deficits may be caused by a similar mechanism. However, downregulation of genes with proliferation-promoting function or upregulation of genes involved in the arrest of proliferation could equally, if not synergistically, contribute to the general proliferation deficit hypothesized to occur in several DS phenotypes. Overexpression of *Dyrk1a* in mouse NPCs was recently found to inhibit proliferation and stimulate precocious neuronal differentiation (Park et al., 2010; Yabut et al., 2010). *DYRK1A* has previously been implicated in the physiopathology of the cognitive impairment observed in individuals with DS (Altafaj et al., 2001; Smith et al., 1997) and is overexpressed approximately 1.5 fold in the DS and Ts65Dn brain (Dowjat et al., 2007; Guimera et al., 1999), suggesting upregulation of *DYRK1A* in concert with other Hsa21 and disomic genes in the DS brain may lead to deficits that underlie both cognitive phenotypes and other cellular phenotypes of DS.

4.2.2 Changes in cell adhesion contribute to DS phenotypes

In addition to brain, other tissues appear to be affected by alterations in cell homeostasis. Because cell cycling, cell adhesion, signal transduction, and ECM production all display dysregulation in DS fetal amniocytes, heart, cerebra and cerebella, one cannot conclude that a simple deficit in proliferation, such as that observed in DS skin fibroblasts (Kimura et al., 2005), is sufficient to result in the DS phenotypes observed. While the DS brain is reduced in size overall, it is also dysmorphic, pointing to both a decrease in proliferation, but perhaps also altered cell cycling, changes in the migratory pattern of progenitor cells and even the decreased founder population of these cells due to decreases in neurogenesis, implicating a complex interaction of mechanisms in the DS neurological phenotype (Bhattacharyya et al., 2009; Guidi et al., 2010).

Study	Tissue	Time point	Analysis Tool	RNA/DNA metabolism	Cell cycling	Cell adhesion	Cell fate	Transcription	Oxidative phosphorylation	Mitochondria	Cell Proliferation	Apoptosis	Regulation of gene expression	RNA/DNA binding	Signal Transduction	Cytoskeleton organization	Monovalent cation transport	Collagen	Integral to plasma membrane	Other annotations of interest
(Mao et al., 2005)	DS cerebrum		G					+		+				+			+			Monovalent cation transport
(Mao et al., 2005)	DS cerebellum		G	+										+						Nerve impulses
(Mao et al., 2005)	DS astrocytes		G	+		+												+	+	
(Mao et al., 2005)	DS heart		G	+						+							+		+	Cell-cell signalling
(Conti et al., 2007)	DS heart	18-22 wks	G			22			9	48								8		ATP synthesis, ECM, phosphate transport
(Lockstone et al., 2007)	DS dorsolateral prefrontal cortex		O		16	3	3	5			9	7	6			6				Immune system, Notch and tyrosine signalling, cell migration, endocytosis
(Rozovski et al., 2007)	DS trophoblasts	Fetal	N	4					6											Ubiquitine cycle, purine biosynthesis
(Chou et al., 2008)	DS amniocytes	16-22 wks	G			+		+							+					
(Esposito et al., 2008)	DS NPCs	19-21 wks	I		25								20		25					Molecular transport
(Sommer et al., 2008)	DS lymphocytes	1-4 yrs	D	12	5				14							12				Protein synthesis, kinase binding, antigen presentation
(Bhattacharyya et al., 2009)	DS NPCs		G		131		131				131	81								Neurogenesis
(Moldrich et al., 2009)	Ts1Cje NPCs	E14.5	G				75													Development, homeostasis

Table 5. Published functional analysis data for phenotypes of DS. Functional annotations were selected by lowest p-values for the categories established by the investigators and of specific interest to the authors. Studies are listed by tissue type and annotations are listed by most common to least common categories horizontally. Analysis tool abbreviations: G: GeneOntology (www.geneontology.org), I: Ingenuity Pathway Analysis (www.ingenuity.com), O: OntoExpress (vortex.cs.wayne.edu/projects.htm), N: NetAffex (www.affymetrix.com/analysis/index.affx), D: DAVID (david.abcc.ncifcrf.gov).

In addition, approximately 50% of newborns with DS display a congenital heart defect, most of which involve septal and canal defects (Pediatrics, 2001). Previous studies have established a link between DS atrioventricular septal defects (AVSDs) and the importance of collagen VI in developing endocardial cushions (Baptista et al., 2000; Davies et al., 1995). Characterization of the involvement of collagen VI in cardiac development was later established when investigators observed altered collagen VI expression in AV endocardial cushions in the DS heart (Gittenberger-de Groot et al., 2003). Interestingly, genes encoding collagen VI are found on Hsa21 and its role as an extracellular matrix (ECM) component makes its presence ubiquitous throughout the body (Aumailley et al., 1991). A similar idea has recently been proposed in which atrioventricular canal (AVC) defects, which comprise the majority of congenital heart defects observed in DS, are a result of increased cell adhesion. Deficits in cell adhesion may lead to decreased cell migration to the ventricular canal because of changes in the ECM, leading to alterations in epithelial-mesenchymal transformations (Delom et al., 2009). Using a transchromosomic model of DS, investigators found both decreased cell migration and an increased affinity for adhesion to collagen VI (Delom et al., 2009). Importantly, differences in Hsa21 genes or groups of genes causing aberrations in both cellular properties may act in concert to lead to the development of AVC defects. It is therefore plausible that cell adhesion complexes coupled with ECM component alterations significantly contribute to congenital heart abnormalities in DS.

In addition to congenital heart defects, individuals with DS are at an increased risk for dermatological disorders such as atopic dermatitis, causing susceptibility toward opportunistic infections (Madan et al., 2006). Studies utilizing DS skin fibroblasts have shown that these cells display an increased adhesion to collagen VI, likely leading to aberrant migration of these cells to target areas of the body (Jongewaard et al., 2002). This decreased migration would leave a smaller population of cells to make up an epidermal barrier and thus would compromise the integrity of the skin. Dysregulation of genes involved in cell adhesion may also lead to changes in junctional complexes that are found to be altered in functional analyses, and these changes may contribute to atypical migration of the cells with which they interact.

4.2.3 Changes in DNA and RNA metabolism may lead to transcription and translation dysregulation

Genes involved with the metabolism and expression of nucleic acids are highly dysregulated in multiple DS tissue types (brain, heart, trophoblasts) and time points in multiple functional analyses. The observed dysregulation of the genome due to the presence of the extra chromosomal material and its interaction with the rest of the genome is likely directed by multiple types of regulation. It may be that fewer transcripts are formed given a higher rate of metabolism of genetic material. The reduced transcripts directing cellular proliferation, migration or an anti-apoptotic state could lead to the smaller or altered structures observed in DS.

In particular, changes in metabolism of genetic transcripts have been documented in the expression of multiple genes in both DS-related and unrelated tissues. Several studies sampling multiple DS-derived tissues have described the transcriptional alterations of Hsa21 genes, including two genes involved in nucleic acid metabolism: GART (purine metabolism) and ZNF294 (transcriptional regulation) (Lintas et al., 2010). DNA and RNA binding and metabolism may also be related to transcription factor activity, dysregulating genes downstream of these alterations. Alterations of transcription factors such as NFAT, as a result of dysregulation of *DYRK1A* and *DSCR1*, have the potential to lead to DS developmental phenotypes (Arron et al., 2006). The dysregulation of NFAT may initiate a cascade of events affecting multiple downstream targets. Many of these genes may also be involved with cell cycling and maintenance as well as DNA and RNA binding and metabolism. Such studies, however, remain to be performed.

4.2.4 Mitochondrial changes penetrate neurological and metabolic phenotypes

The high incidence of mitochondria-related dysregulation in DS hearts, lymphocytes, and trophoblasts coupled with the increased prevalence of biomarkers of reactive oxygen species (ROS) in individuals with DS (Jovanovic et al., 1998) is an interesting and well-studied paradigm. Mitochondrial impairment in fetal hearts suggested by the downregulation of genes from five mitochondrial complexes, as well as the cerebellum and other brain regions, platelets, astrocytes and cultured fibroblasts suggests pervasive impairment of mitochondria in individuals with DS (Arbuzova et al., 2002; Busciglio et al., 2002; Conti et al., 2007; Kim et al., 2001; Kim et al., 2000; Prince et al., 1994). Interestingly, this mitochondrial impairment may affect other DS pathophysiology. Dysregulation of the mitochondria has the ability to cause alterations in ATP synthesis, electron transport, monovalent cation transporter activity, oxidative phosphorylation, and general changes in physical components (Conti et al., 2007) (all found as dysregulated functional groups in Table 5). Furthermore, changes in membrane potential caused by this dysregulation may lead to increased mitochondrial susceptibility to other insults, leading to a constant feedback in the balance of genetic regulation (Roat et al., 2007). Two genes in particular located on Hsa21, *SOD1* and *BACH1*, have been implicated the generation of ROS due to elevated H_2O_2 levels and decreased transcriptional activity, respectively. Elevated levels of *SOD1* have been implicated in deposition of β amyloid and *BACH1* downregulation has been proposed as a contributing mechanism to the development of Alzheimer disease neuropathology (Percy et al., 1990; Shim et al., 2003). High levels of oxidative stress in the brains of individuals with DS may indicate that dysregulation of normal processes in the mitochondria lead to anomalies including Alzheimer pathology (de Haan et al., 1997; Lockstone et al., 2007). A disproportionate number of ROS, caused by mitochondrial and other changes, combined with altered metabolism and feedback mechanisms suggest the complexity of the interacting mechanisms involved in DS phenotypes affecting the brain, heart and skin (Busciglio and Yankner, 1995; Li et al., 2006; Sinha, 2005).

4.3 DAVID analysis of trisomic genes in humans with DS and DS mouse models

DS mouse models have the ability to predict phenotypes not previously observed in individuals with DS (Baxter et al., 2000; Pennington et al., 2003). We hypothesized that by analyzing the genes trisomic genes on Hsa21 as well as their homologs in two DS mouse models, we would observe common mechanisms as found by functional analysis of altered gene expression. Using DAVID (http://david.abcc.ncifcrf.gov/) we analyzed trisomic genes from Hsa21 and the Ts1Rhr and Ts65Dn mouse models (http://chr21.molgen.mpg.de/HSA21db.html). Functional annotations were obtained using the protocol described by Huang et al. 2009.

Our analyses of Hsa21 genes revealed dysregulation of functional annotations including keratin, intermediate filament/cytoskeleton digestion, protein dimerization, interferon receptor activity, cytokine receptor activity, multiple junctions, cell adhesion, ionic channels and ECM (Table 6). Analysis of the genes triplicated in Ts65Dn mice revealed dysregulation of genes involved in ion transport, voltage-gated channels, ionic channels, monovalent inorganic cation transport, tight junctions, calcium dependent cell-cell adhesion, regulation of transcription, DNA binding, behavior, neuron development, neuron differentiation and synaptic transmission and cell-cell signaling. Analysis of genes in three copies from the Ts1Rhr mouse model identified functions integral to binding and related to regulation of transcription factor activity, transcription and DNA binding as the most enriched categories with the lowest p-values.

As predicted, some, but not all functional groups found in previous analyses were also seen in our DAVID analysis. Data compiled using DAVID analysis of Hsa21 and two DS mouse models provide insight into what mechanisms appear to be generally dysregulated when trisomy for these regions occurs. Ts65Dn mice display many similarities to individuals with DS with regard to general brain, behavior, stature, heart and craniofacial phenotypes. Interestingly, a high level of overlap in functional categories also exists between the two analyses. For example, our analysis of Hsa21 and Ts65Dn revealed dysregulation of genes involved in cell adhesion, tight junctions and ionic transport. Ts65Dn mice replicate some of the heart defects observed in DS, and aberrant cell adhesion and migration have been implicated in these defects (Delom et al., 2009; Moore, 2006; Williams et al., 2008). Ts1Rhr and Ts65Dn triplicated genes led to functional hits in transcription, transcription factor activity, and RNA/DNA binding. While Ts1Rhr and Ts65Dn mice display some similar phenotypes, Ts1Rhr mice exhibit a number of phenotypes contrary to those seen in DS. It is noteworthy, though, that though these functional groups are dysregulated, they may be regulated in a manner divergent from one another, such as higher levels of transcription and RNA/DNA binding in Ts1Rhr than Ts65Dn, leading to the exaggerated phenotypes which Ts1Rhr mice display. Interestingly, no functional groups overlapped between the Hsa21 and Ts1Rhr analyses and this result provides additional evidence for the different phenotypes observed between humans with DS and this mouse model. Clearly, the involvement of other trisomic genes as well as disomic genes plays an important role in the identification of functional categories. Given that our analyses only included trisomic genes, it seems plausible that significant overlap between the past and current studies was not found.

Study	RNA/DNA binding	Cell adhesion	Transcription	Transcription factor activity	Tight Junctions	Ionic transport	Voltage-gated channel	Cell junctions	Cell signaling	Apical Junction Complex	Intermediate Filaments	Protein dimerization activity	ECM	
Hsa21 Genes		13			6	8		7		6	27	11	6	Keratin, digestion, interferon receptor activity, cytokine receptor activity
Ts65Dn mouse model	7	4	7	6	5	8	5		3					Behavior, neuron development, neuron differentiation, synaptic transmission
Ts1Rhr mouse model	3		4	3										Integral to membrane

Table 6. DAVID analysis of trisomic genes from Hsa21 and Ts65Dn and Ts1Rhr mice. Functional annotations are listed in columns by most common dysregulated annotations, then by highest to lowest enrichment score and smallest to largest p-value in succession for each category.

4.4 Summary

Functional analyses of genetic information for DS have the potential to revolutionize our understanding about the gene-phenotype relationships in DS (Ait Yahya-Graison et al., 2007; Gardiner, 2010). Our meta-analysis of current functional analyses has indicated that cell cycling, maintenance, function, and adhesion, as well as DNA and RNA metabolism and binding and mitochondrial function are leading common mechanisms underlying DS phenotypes. The combination of multiple genes to produce specific disorder-related phenotypes appears to be a common theme in DS phenotypes. Groups of genes may act in concert to produce one or more phenotypes, or contribute a key factor in the development or maintenance of a phenotype. In many cases, functional groups and mechanisms overlap between tissues of different origins, but no general mechanism appears to be ubiquitously dysregulated amongst the tissues studied (Figure 1).

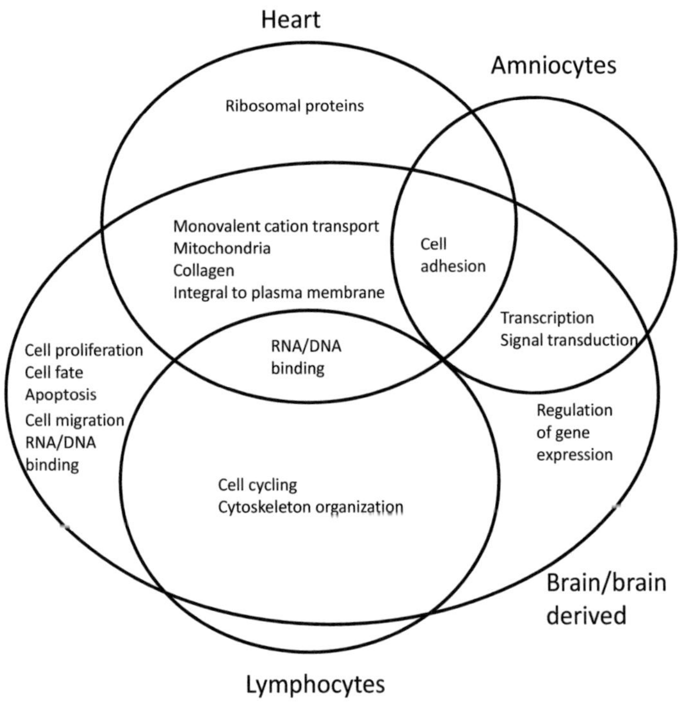

Fig. 1. Overlap of dysregulated functional groups occurs between multiple tissues, but no single mechanism appears to be dysregulated among all tissues studied.

5. Conclusions

Although the initial genetic insult is known and the phenotypes related to DS have been characterized, the relationship between genes and phenotypes has not been well distinguished for most DS phenotypes. Though phenotypes associated with DS must be caused by Ts21, high throughput gene expression analyses demonstrate the dysregulation of both trisomic and non-trisomic genes in tissues that are important for traits associated with Ts21. Hypotheses concerning critical regions and genes, thought to be important in most of the major phenotypes associated with DS, have been disproved. Instead, it is postulated that a region of Hsa21 may be critical for a specific phenotype and a genomic region may contain a gene that is important (but not exclusive) for the causation of the trait. Moreover, there may be singular genes that are important in many, but not all, phenotypes associated with DS. Functional analyses of differentially expressed genes and genes in three copies may be used to further understand the relationships between genes and phenotypes. A number of differentially expressed genes may be tied into a mechanism and there may be mechanisms that are critical to a number of phenotypes. Thus, more accurate genotyping, large scale gene expression meta-analysis and functional mechanism investigations are helping to define gene-phenotype relationships in this complex and interactive disorder.

6. Acknowledgement

The laboratory of RJR is supported by the National Institutes of Health (NIH) Grant DE021034 . Samantha L. Deitz and Joshua D. Blazek contributed equally to this work.

7. References

Agarwala, K. L., Ganesh, S., Suzuki, T., Akagi, T., Kaneko, K., Amano, K., Tsutsumi, Y., Yamaguchi, K., Hashikawa, T., Yamakawa, K., 2001. Dscam is associated with axonal and dendritic features of neuronal cells. J Neurosci Res. 66, 337-46.

Ait Yahya-Graison, E., Aubert, J., Dauphinot, L., Rivals, I., Prieur, M., Golfier, G., Rossier, J., Personnaz, L., Creau, N., Blehaut, H., Robin, S., Delabar, J. M., Potier, M. C., 2007. Classification of human chromosome 21 gene-expression variations in Down syndrome: impact on disease phenotypes. Am J Hum Genet. 81, 475-91.

Aldridge, K., Reeves, R. H., Olson, L. E., Richtsmeier, J. T., 2007. Differential effects of trisomy on brain shape and volume in related aneuploid mouse models. Am J Med Genet A. 143A, 1060-70.

Altafaj, X., Dierssen, M., Baamonde, C., Marti, E., Visa, J., Guimera, J., Oset, M., Gonzalez, J. R., Florez, J., Fillat, C., Estivill, X., 2001. Neurodevelopmental delay, motor abnormalities and cognitive deficits in transgenic mice overexpressing Dyrk1A (minibrain), a murine model of Down's syndrome. Hum Mol Genet. 10, 1915-23.

Altug-Teber, O., Bonin, M., Walter, M., Mau-Holzmann, U. A., Dufke, A., Stappert, H., Tekesin, I., Heilbronner, H., Nieselt, K., Riess, O., 2007. Specific transcriptional changes in human fetuses with autosomal trisomies. Cytogenet Genome Res. 119, 171-84.

Alves-Sampaio, A., Troca-Marin, J. A., Montesinos, M. L., 2010. NMDA-mediated regulation of DSCAM dendritic local translation is lost in a mouse model of Down's syndrome. J Neurosci. 30, 13537-48.

Amano, K., Sago, H., Uchikawa, C., Suzuki, T., Kotliarova, S.E., Nukina, N., Epstein, C.J., Yamakawa, K., 2004. Dosage-dependent over-expression of genes in the trisomic region of Ts1Cje mouse model for Down syndrome. Hum Mol Genet 13, 1333-1340.

Antonarakis, S. E., Lyle, R., Dermitzakis, E. T., Reymond, A., Deutsch, S., 2004. Chromosome 21 and down syndrome: from genomics to pathophysiology. Nat Rev Genet. 5, 725-38.

Arbuzova, S., Hutchin, T., Cuckle, H., 2002. Mitochondrial dysfunction and Down's syndrome. Bioessays. 24, 681-4.

Arron, J. R., Winslow, M. M., Polleri, A., Chang, C. P., Wu, H., Gao, X., Neilson, J. R., Chen, L., Heit, J. J., Kim, S. K., Yamasaki, N., Miyakawa, T., Francke, U., Graef, I. A., Crabtree, G. R., 2006. NFAT dysregulation by increased dosage of DSCR1 and DYRK1A on chromosome 21. Nature. 441, 595-600.

Aumailley, M., Specks, U., Timpl, R., 1991. Cell adhesion to type-VI collagen. Biochem Soc Trans. 19, 843-7.

Aylward, E. H., Habbak, R., Warren, A. C., Pulsifer, M. B., Barta, P. E., Jerram, M., Pearlson, G. D., 1997. Cerebellar volume in adults with Down syndrome. Arch Neurol. 54, 209-12.

Baptista, M. J., Fairbrother, U. L., Howard, C. M., Farrer, M. J., Davies, G. E., Trikka, D., Maratou, K., Redington, A., Greve, G., Njolstad, P. R., Kessling, A. M., 2000. Heterotrisomy, a significant contributing factor to ventricular septal defect associated with Down syndrome? Hum Genet. 107, 476-82.

Barlow, G. M., Chen, X. N., Shi, Z. Y., Lyons, G. E., Kurnit, D. M., Celle, L., Spinner, N. B., Zackai, E., Pettenati, M. J., Van Riper, A. J., Vekemans, M. J., Mjaatvedt, C. H., Korenberg, J. R., 2001a. Down syndrome congenital heart disease: a narrowed region and a candidate gene. Genet Med. 3, 91-101.

Barlow, G. M., Lyons, G. E., Richardson, J. A., Sarnat, H. B., Korenberg, J. R., 2002. DSCAM: an endogenous promoter drives expression in the developing CNS and neural crest. Biochem Biophys Res Commun. 299, 1-6.

Barlow, G. M., Micales, B., Lyons, G. E., Korenberg, J. R., 2001b. Down syndrome cell adhesion molecule is conserved in mouse and highly expressed in the adult mouse brain. Cytogenet Cell Genet. 94, 155-62.

Baxter, L. L., Moran, T. H., Richtsmeier, J. T., Troncoso, J., Reeves, R. H., 2000. Discovery and genetic localization of Down syndrome cerebellar phenotypes using the Ts65Dn mouse. Hum Mol Genet. 9, 195-202.

Belichenko, N. P., Belichenko, P. V., Kleschevnikov, A. M., Salehi, A., Reeves, R. H., Mobley, W. C., 2009. The "Down syndrome critical region" is sufficient in the mouse model to confer behavioral, neurophysiological, and synaptic phenotypes characteristic of Down syndrome. J Neurosci. 29, 5938-48.

Best, T. K., Siarey, R. J., Galdzicki, Z., 2007. Ts65Dn, a mouse model of Down syndrome, exhibits increased GABAB-induced potassium current. J Neurophysiol. 97, 892-900.

Bhattacharyya, A., McMillan, E., Chen, S. I., Wallace, K., Svendsen, C. N., 2009. A critical period in cortical interneuron neurogenesis in down syndrome revealed by human neural progenitor cells. Dev Neurosci. 31, 497-510.

Brahe, C., Tassone, F., Millington-Ward, A., Serra, A., Gardiner, K., 1990. Potential gene sequence isolation and regional mapping in human chromosome 21. Am J Med Genet Suppl. 7, 120-4.

Busciglio, J., Pelsman, A., Wong, C., Pigino, G., Yuan, M., Mori, H., Yankner, B. A., 2002. Altered metabolism of the amyloid beta precursor protein is associated with mitochondrial dysfunction in Down's syndrome. Neuron. 33, 677-88.

Busciglio, J., Yankner, B. A., 1995. Apoptosis and increased generation of reactive oxygen species in Down's syndrome neurons in vitro. Nature. 378, 776-9.

Chakrabarti, L., Best, T. K., Cramer, N. P., Carney, R. S., Isaac, J. T., Galdzicki, Z., Haydar, T. F., 2010. Olig1 and Olig2 triplication causes developmental brain defects in Down syndrome. Nat Neurosci. 13, 927-34.

Chakrabarti, L., Galdzicki, Z., Haydar, T. F., 2007. Defects in embryonic neurogenesis and initial synapse formation in the forebrain of the Ts65Dn mouse model of Down syndrome. J Neurosci. 27, 11483-95.

Chou, C. Y., Liu, L. Y., Chen, C. Y., Tsai, C. H., Hwa, H. L., Chang, L. Y., Lin, Y. S., Hsieh, F. J., 2008. Gene expression variation increase in trisomy 21 tissues. Mamm Genome. 19, 398-405.

Chrast, R., Scott, H.S., Papasavvas, M.P., Rossier, C., Antonarakis, E.S., Barras, C., Davisson, M.T., Schmidt, C., Estivill, X., Dierssen, M., Pritchard, M., Antonarakis, S.E., 2000. The mouse brain transcriptome by SAGE: differences in gene expression between P30 brains of the partial trisomy 16 mouse model of Down syndrome (Ts65Dn) and normals. Genome Res 10, 2006-2021.

Christianson, A., C.P. Howson and B. Modell, March of Dimes Global Report on Birth Defects: The Hidden Toll of Dying and Disabled Children., 2006, pp. pp. 1-98. March of Dimes Birth Defect Foundation, White Plains, NY.

Chung, I. H., Lee, S. H., Lee, K. W., Park, S. H., Cha, K. Y., Kim, N. S., Yoo, H. S., Kim, Y. S., Lee, S., 2005. Gene expression analysis of cultured amniotic fluid cell with Down syndrome by DNA microarray. J Korean Med Sci. 20, 82-7.

Contestabile, A., Fila, T., Cappellini, A., Bartesaghi, R., Ciani, E., 2009. Widespread impairment of cell proliferation in the neonate Ts65Dn mouse, a model for Down syndrome. Cell Prolif. 42, 171-81.

Conti, A., Fabbrini, F., D'Agostino, P., Negri, R., Greco, D., Genesio, R., D'Armiento, M., Olla, C., Paladini, D., Zannini, M., Nitsch, L., 2007. Altered expression of mitochondrial and extracellular matrix genes in the heart of human fetuses with chromosome 21 trisomy. BMC Genomics. 8, 268.

Cooper, J. D., Salehi, A., Delcroix, J. D., Howe, C. L., Belichenko, P. V., Chua-Couzens, J., Kilbridge, J. F., Carlson, E. J., Epstein, C. J., Mobley, W. C., 2001. Failed retrograde transport of NGF in a mouse model of Down's syndrome: reversal of cholinergic neurodegenerative phenotypes following NGF infusion. Proc Natl Acad Sci U S A. 98, 10439-44.

Crombez, E. A., Dipple, K. M., Schimmenti, L. A., Rao, N., 2005. Duplication of the Down syndrome critical region does not predict facial phenotype in a baby with a ring chromosome 21. Clin Dysmorphol. 14, 183-7.

Dahmane, N., Ghezala, G. A., Gosset, P., Chamoun, Z., Dufresne-Zacharia, M. C., Lopes, C., Rabatel, N., Gassanova-Maugenre, S., Chettouh, Z., Abramowski, V., Fayet, E., Yaspo, M. L., Korn, B., Blouin, J. L., Lehrach, H., Poutska, A., Antonarakis, S. E., Sinet, P. M., Creau, N., Delabar, J. M., 1998. Transcriptional map of the 2.5-Mb CBR-ERG region of chromosome 21 involved in Down syndrome. Genomics. 48, 12-23.

Dauphinot, L., Lyle, R., Rivals, I., Dang, M. T., Moldrich, R. X., Golfier, G., Ettwiller, L., Toyama, K., Rossier, J., Personnaz, L., Antonarakis, S. E., Epstein, C. J., Sinet, P. M., Potier, M. C., 2005. The cerebellar transcriptome during postnatal development of the Ts1Cje mouse, a segmental trisomy model for Down syndrome. Hum Mol Genet. 14, 373-84.

Davies, G. E., Howard, C. M., Farrer, M. J., Coleman, M. M., Bennett, L. B., Cullen, L. M., Wyse, R. K., Burn, J., Williamson, R., Kessling, A. M., 1995. Genetic variation in the COL6A1 region is associated with congenital heart defects in trisomy 21 (Down's syndrome). Ann Hum Genet. 59, 253-69.

de Haan, J. B., Wolvetang, E. J., Cristiano, F., Iannello, R., Bladier, C., Kelner, M. J., Kola, I., 1997. Reactive oxygen species and their contribution to pathology in Down syndrome. Adv Pharmacol. 38, 379-402.

Delabar, J. M., Theophile, D., Rahmani, Z., Chettouh, Z., Blouin, J. L., Prieur, M., Noel, B., Sinet, P. M., 1993. Molecular mapping of twenty-four features of Down syndrome on chromosome 21. Eur J Hum Genet. 1, 114-24.

Delom, F., Burt, E., Hoischen, A., Veltman, J., Groet, J., Cotter, F. E., Nizetic, D., 2009. Transchromosomic cell model of Down syndrome shows aberrant migration, adhesion and proteome response to extracellular matrix. Proteome Sci. 7, 31.

Deutsch, S., Lyle, R., Dermitzakis, E. T., Attar, H., Subrahmanyan, L., Gehrig, C., Parand, L., Gagnebin, M., Rougemont, J., Jongeneel, C. V., Antonarakis, S. E., 2005. Gene expression variation and expression quantitative trait mapping of human chromosome 21 genes. Hum Mol Genet. 14, 3741-9.

Dowjat, W. K., Adayev, T., Kuchna, I., Nowicki, K., Palminiello, S., Hwang, Y. W., Wegiel, J., 2007. Trisomy-driven overexpression of DYRK1A kinase in the brain of subjects with Down syndrome. Neurosci Lett. 413, 77-81.

Eggermann, T., Schonherr, N., Spengler, S., Jager, S., Denecke, B., Binder, G., Baudis, M., 2010. Identification of a 21q22 duplication in a Silver-Russell syndrome patient further narrows down the Down syndrome critical region. Am J Med Genet A. 152A, 356-9.

Elton, T. S., Sansom, S. E., Martin, M. M., 2010. Trisomy-21 gene dosage over-expression of miRNAs results in the haploinsufficiency of specific target proteins. RNA Biol. 7, 35-42.

Epstein, C. J., Down Syndrome (Trisomy 21). In: C. R. Scriver, A. L. Beaudet, W. S. Sly, D. Valle, Eds.), The Metabolic & Molecular Bases of Inherited Disease. McGraw-Hill, New York, 2001, pp. 1223-1256.

Ermak, G., Morgan, T. E., Davies, K. J., 2001. Chronic overexpression of the calcineurin inhibitory gene DSCR1 (Adapt78) is associated with Alzheimer's disease. J Biol Chem. 276, 38787-94.

Esposito, G., Imitola, J., Lu, J., De Filippis, D., Scuderi, C., Ganesh, V. S., Folkerth, R., Hecht, J., Shin, S., Iuvone, T., Chesnut, J., Steardo, L., Sheen, V., 2008. Genomic and functional profiling of human Down syndrome neural progenitors implicates S100B and aquaporin 4 in cell injury. Hum Mol Genet. 17, 440-57.

Fink, G. B., Madaus, W. K., Walker, G. F., 1975. A quantitative study of the face in Down's syndrome. Am J Orthod. 67, 540-53.

FitzPatrick, D.R., Ramsay, J., McGill, N.I., Shade, M., Carothers, A.D., Hastie, N.D., 2002. Transcriptome analysis of human autosomal trisomy. Hum Mol Genet 11, 3249-3256.

Gardiner, K., Herault, Y., Lott, I. T., Antonarakis, S. E., Reeves, R. H., Dierssen, M., 2010. Down syndrome: from understanding the neurobiology to therapy. J Neurosci. 30, 14943-5.

Gardiner, K. J., 2010. Molecular basis of pharmacotherapies for cognition in Down syndrome. Trends Pharmacol Sci. 31, 66-73.

Giannone, S., Strippoli, P., Vitale, L., Casadei, R., Canaider, S., Lenzi, L., D'Addabbo, P., Frabetti, F., Facchin, F., Farina, A., Carinci, P., Zannotti, M., 2004. Gene expression profile analysis in human T lymphocytes from patients with Down Syndrome. Ann Hum Genet. 68, 546-54.

Gittenberger-de Groot, A. C., Bartram, U., Oosthoek, P. W., Bartelings, M. M., Hogers, B., Poelmann, R. E., Jongewaard, I. N., Klewer, S. E., 2003. Collagen type VI expression during cardiac development and in human fetuses with trisomy 21. Anat Rec A Discov Mol Cell Evol Biol. 275, 1109-16.

Graef, I. A., Chen, F., Crabtree, G. R., 2001. NFAT signaling in vertebrate development. Curr Opin Genet Dev. 11, 505-12.

Gross, S.J., Ferreira, J.C., Morrow, B., Dar, P., Funke, B., Khabele, D., Merkatz, I., 2002. Gene expression profile of trisomy 21 placentas: a potential approach for designing noninvasive techniques of prenatal diagnosis. Am J Obstet Gynecol 187, 457-462.

Guidi, S., Ciani, E., Bonasoni, P., Santini, D., Bartesaghi, R., 2010. Widespread Proliferation Impairment and Hypocellularity in the Cerebellum of Fetuses with Down Syndrome. Brain Pathol.

Guimera, J., Casas, C., Estivill, X., Pritchard, M., 1999. Human minibrain homologue (MNBH/DYRK1): characterization, alternative splicing, differential tissue expression, and overexpression in Down syndrome. Genomics. 57, 407-18.

Hattori, M., Fujiyama, A., Taylor, T. D., Watanabe, H., Yada, T., Park, H. S., Toyoda, A., Ishii, K., Totoki, Y., Choi, D. K., Groner, Y., Soeda, E., Ohki, M., Takagi, T., Sakaki, Y., Taudien, S., Blechschmidt, K., Polley, A., Menzel, U., Delabar, J., Kumpf, K., Lehmann, R., Patterson, D., Reichwald, K., Rump, A., Schillhabel, M., Schudy, A., Zimmermann, W., Rosenthal, A., Kudoh, J., Schibuya, K., Kawasaki, K., Asakawa, S., Shintani, A., Sasaki, T., Nagamine, K., Mitsuyama, S., Antonarakis, S. E., Minoshima, S., Shimizu, N., Nordsiek, G., Hornischer, K., Brant, P., Scharfe, M., Schon, O., Desario, A., Reichelt, J., Kauer, G., Blocker, H., Ramser, J., Beck, A., Klages, S., Hennig, S., Riesselmann, L., Dagand, E., Haaf, T., Wehrmeyer, S., Borzym, K., Gardiner, K., Nizetic, D., Francis, F., Lehrach, H., Reinhardt, R., Yaspo, M. L., 2000. The DNA sequence of human chromosome 21. Nature. 405, 311-9.

Hewitt, C. A., Ling, K. H., Merson, T. D., Simpson, K. M., Ritchie, M. E., King, S. L., Pritchard, M. A., Smyth, G. K., Thomas, T., Scott, H. S., Voss, A. K., 2010. Gene network disruptions and neurogenesis defects in the adult Ts1Cje mouse model of Down syndrome. PLoS One. 5, e11561.

Hill, C. A., Sussan, T. E., Reeves, R. H., Richtsmeier, J. T., 2009. Complex contributions of Ets2 to craniofacial and thymus phenotypes of trisomic "Down syndrome" mice. Am J Med Genet A. 149A, 2158-65.

Holtzman, D. M., Santucci, D., Kilbridge, J., Chua-Couzens, J., Fontana, D. J., Daniels, S. E., Johnson, R. M., Chen, K., Sun, Y., Carlson, E., Alleva, E., Epstein, C. J., Mobley, W. C., 1996. Developmental abnormalities and age-related neurodegeneration in a mouse model of Down syndrome. Proc Natl Acad Sci U S A. 93, 13333-8.

Jongewaard, I. N., Lauer, R. M., Behrendt, D. A., Patil, S., Klewer, S. E., 2002. Beta 1 integrin activation mediates adhesive differences between trisomy 21 and non-trisomic fibroblasts on type VI collagen. Am J Med Genet. 109, 298-305.

Jovanovic, S. V., Clements, D., MacLeod, K., 1998. Biomarkers of oxidative stress are significantly elevated in Down syndrome. Free Radic Biol Med. 25, 1044-8.

Kahlem, P., Sultan, M., Herwig, R., Steinfath, M., Balzereit, D., Eppens, B., Saran, N.G., Pletcher, M.T., South, S.T., Stetten, G., Lehrach, H., Reeves, R.H., Yaspo, M.L., 2004. Transcript level alterations reflect gene dosage effects across multiple tissues in a mouse model of down syndrome. Genome Res 14, 1258-1267.

Kim, S. H., Vlkolinsky, R., Cairns, N., Fountoulakis, M., Lubec, G., 2001. The reduction of NADH ubiquinone oxidoreductase 24- and 75-kDa subunits in brains of patients with Down syndrome and Alzheimer's disease. Life Sci. 68, 2741-50.

Kim, S. H., Vlkolinsky, R., Cairns, N., Lubec, G., 2000. Decreased levels of complex III core protein 1 and complex V beta chain in brains from patients with Alzheimer's disease and Down syndrome. Cell Mol Life Sci. 57, 1810-6.

Kimura, M., Cao, X., Skurnick, J., Cody, M., Soteropoulos, P., Aviv, A., 2005. Proliferation dynamics in cultured skin fibroblasts from Down syndrome subjects. Free Radic Biol Med. 39, 374-80.

Korbel, J. O., Tirosh-Wagner, T., Urban, A. E., Chen, X. N., Kasowski, M., Dai, L., Grubert, F., Erdman, C., Gao, M. C., Lange, K., Sobel, E. M., Barlow, G. M., Aylsworth, A. S., Carpenter, N. J., Clark, R. D., Cohen, M. Y., Doran, E., Falik-Zaccai, T., Lewin, S. O., Lott, I. T., McGillivray, B. C., Moeschler, J. B., Pettenati, M. J., Pueschel, S. M., Rao, K. W., Shaffer, L. G., Shohat, M., Van Riper, A. J., Warburton, D., Weissman, S., Gerstein, M. B., Snyder, M., Korenberg, J. R., 2009. The genetic architecture of Down syndrome phenotypes revealed by high-resolution analysis of human segmental trisomies. Proc Natl Acad Sci U S A. 106, 12031-6.

Korbel, J. O., Urban, A. E., Grubert, F., Du, J., Royce, T. E., Starr, P., Zhong, G., Emanuel, B. S., Weissman, S. M., Snyder, M., Gerstein, M. B., 2007. Systematic prediction and validation of breakpoints associated with copy-number variants in the human genome. Proc Natl Acad Sci U S A. 104, 10110-5.

Korenberg, J. R., Bradley, C., Disteche, C. M., 1992. Down syndrome: molecular mapping of the congenital heart disease and duodenal stenosis. Am J Hum Genet. 50, 294-302.

Korenberg, J. R., Chen, X. N., Schipper, R., Sun, Z., Gonsky, R., Gerwehr, S., Carpenter, N., Daumer, C., Dignan, P., Disteche, C., et al., 1994. Down syndrome phenotypes: the consequences of chromosomal imbalance. Proc Natl Acad Sci U S A. 91, 4997-5001.

Korenberg, J. R., Kawashima, H., Pulst, S. M., Ikeuchi, T., Ogasawara, N., Yamamoto, K., Schonberg, S. A., West, R., Allen, L., Magenis, E., et al., 1990. Molecular definition of a region of chromosome 21 that causes features of the Down syndrome phenotype. Am J Hum Genet. 47, 236-46.

Laffaire, J., Rivals, I., Dauphinot, L., Pasteau, F., Wehrle, R., Larrat, B., Vitalis, T., Moldrich, R.X., Rossier, J., Sinkus, R., Herault, Y., Dusart, I., Potier, M.C., 2009. Gene expression signature of cerebellar hypoplasia in a mouse model of Down syndrome during postnatal development. BMC Genomics 10, 138.

Li, C. M., Guo, M., Salas, M., Schupf, N., Silverman, W., Zigman, W. B., Husain, S., Warburton, D., Thaker, H., Tycko, B., 2006. Cell type-specific over-expression of chromosome 21 genes in fibroblasts and fetal hearts with trisomy 21. BMC Med Genet. 7, 24.

Li, Z., Yu, T., Morishima, M., Pao, A., Laduca, J., Conroy, J., Nowak, N., Matsui, S., Shiraishi, I., Yu, Y. E., 2007. Duplication of the entire 22.9 Mb human chromosome 21 syntenic region on mouse chromosome 16 causes cardiovascular and gastrointestinal abnormalities. Hum Mol Genet. 16, 1359-66.

Lintas, C., Sacco, R., Persico, A. M., 2010. Genome-wide expression studies in Autism spectrum disorder, Rett syndrome, and Down syndrome. Neurobiol Dis.

Lockstone, H. E., Harris, L. W., Swatton, J. E., Wayland, M. T., Holland, A. J., Bahn, S., 2007. Gene expression profiling in the adult Down syndrome brain. Genomics. 90, 647-60.

Lyle, R., Bena, F., Gagos, S., Gehrig, C., Lopez, G., Schinzel, A., Lespinasse, J., Bottani, A., Dahoun, S., Taine, L., Doco-Fenzy, M., Cornillet-Lefebvre, P., Pelet, A., Lyonnet, S., Toutain, A., Colleaux, L., Horst, J., Kennerknecht, I., Wakamatsu, N., Descartes, M., Franklin, J. C., Florentin-Arar, L., Kitsiou, S., Ait Yahya-Graison, E., Costantine, M., Sinet, P. M., Delabar, J. M., Antonarakis, S. E., 2009. Genotype-phenotype correlations in Down syndrome identified by array CGH in 30 cases of partial trisomy and partial monosomy chromosome 21. Eur J Hum Genet. 17, 454-66.

Lyle, R., Gehrig, C., Neergaard-Henrichsen, C., Deutsch, S., Antonarakis, S. E., 2004. Gene expression from the aneuploid chromosome in a trisomy mouse model of down syndrome. Genome Res. 14, 1268-74.

Madan, V., Williams, J., Lear, J. T., 2006. Dermatological manifestations of Down's syndrome. Clin Exp Dermatol. 31, 623-9.

Mao, R., Wang, X., Spitznagel, E. L., Jr., Frelin, L. P., Ting, J. C., Ding, H., Kim, J. W., Ruczinski, I., Downey, T. J., Pevsner, J., 2005. Primary and secondary transcriptional effects in the developing human Down syndrome brain and heart. Genome Biol. 6, R107.

Mao, R., Zielke, C. L., Zielke, H. R., Pevsner, J., 2003. Global up-regulation of chromosome 21 gene expression in the developing Down syndrome brain. Genomics. 81, 457-67.

Moldrich, R. X., Dauphinot, L., Laffaire, J., Rossier, J., Potier, M. C., 2007. Down syndrome gene dosage imbalance on cerebellum development. Prog Neurobiol. 82, 87-94.

Moldrich, R. X., Dauphinot, L., Laffaire, J., Vitalis, T., Herault, Y., Beart, P. M., Rossier, J., Vivien, D., Gehrig, C., Antonarakis, S. E., Lyle, R., Potier, M. C., 2009. Proliferation deficits and gene expression dysregulation in Down's syndrome (Ts1Cje) neural progenitor cells cultured from neurospheres. J Neurosci Res. 87, 3143-52.

Moore, C. S., 2006. Postnatal lethality and cardiac anomalies in the Ts65Dn Down syndrome mouse model. Mamm Genome. 17, 1005-12.

Neri, G., Opitz, J. M., 2009. Down syndrome: comments and reflections on the 50th anniversary of Lejeune's discovery. Am J Med Genet A. 149A, 2647-54.

Niebuhr, E., 1974. Down's syndrome. The possibility of a pathogenetic segment on chromosome no. 21. Humangenetik. 21, 99-101.

O'Doherty, A., Ruf, S., Mulligan, C., Hildreth, V., Errington, M. L., Cooke, S., Sesay, A., Modino, S., Vanes, L., Hernandez, D., Linehan, J. M., Sharpe, P. T., Brandner, S., Bliss, T. V., Henderson, D. J., Nizetic, D., Tybulewicz, V. L., Fisher, E. M., 2005. An aneuploid mouse strain carrying human chromosome 21 with Down syndrome phenotypes. Science. 309, 2033-7.

Ohira, M., Ichikawa, H., Suzuki, E., Iwaki, M., Suzuki, K., Saito-Ohara, F., Ikeuchi, T., Chumakov, I., Tanahashi, H., Tashiro, K., Sakaki, Y., 1996. A 1.6-Mb P1-based physical map of the Down syndrome region on chromosome 21. Genomics. 33, 65-74.

Olson, L. E., Richtsmeier, J. T., Leszl, J., Reeves, R. H., 2004a. A chromosome 21 critical region does not cause specific Down syndrome phenotypes. Science. 306, 687-90.

Olson, L. E., Roper, R. J., Baxter, L. L., Carlson, E. J., Epstein, C. J., Reeves, R. H., 2004b. Down syndrome mouse models Ts65Dn, Ts1Cje, and Ms1Cje/Ts65Dn exhibit variable severity of cerebellar phenotypes. Dev Dyn. 230, 581-9.

Olson, L. E., Roper, R. J., Sengstaken, C. L., Peterson, E. A., Aquino, V., Galdzicki, Z., Siarey, R., Pletnikov, M., Moran, T. H., Reeves, R. H., 2007. Trisomy for the Down syndrome 'critical region' is necessary but not sufficient for brain phenotypes of trisomic mice. Hum Mol Genet. 16, 774-82.

Park, J., Oh, Y., Chung, K. C., 2009. Two key genes closely implicated with the neuropathological characteristics in Down syndrome: DYRK1A and RCAN1. BMB Rep. 42, 6-15.

Park, J., Oh, Y., Yoo, L., Jung, M. S., Song, W. J., Lee, S. H., Seo, H., Chung, K. C., 2010. Dyrk1A phosphorylates p53 and inhibits proliferation of embryonic neuronal cells. J Biol Chem. 285, 31895-906.

Patil, N., Cox, D. R., Bhat, D., Faham, M., Myers, R. M., Peterson, A. S., 1995. A potassium channel mutation in weaver mice implicates membrane excitability in granule cell differentiation. Nat Genet. 11, 126-9.

Patterson, D., 2007. Genetic mechanisms involved in the phenotype of Down syndrome. Ment Retard Dev Disabil Res Rev. 13, 199-206.

Patterson, D., 2009. Molecular genetic analysis of Down syndrome. Hum Genet. 126, 195-214.

Patterson, D., Costa, A. C., 2005. Down syndrome and genetics - a case of linked histories. Nat Rev Genet. 6, 137-47.

Pediatrics, A. A. o., 2001. Health Supervision for Children with Down Syndrome. Pediatrics. 107, 8.

Pennington, B. F., Moon, J., Edgin, J., Stedron, J., Nadel, L., 2003. The neuropsychology of Down syndrome: evidence for hippocampal dysfunction. Child Dev. 74, 75-93.

Percy, M. E., Dalton, A. J., Markovic, V. D., McLachlan, D. R., Hummel, J. T., Rusk, A. C., Andrews, D. F., 1990. Red cell superoxide dismutase, glutathione peroxidase and catalase in Down syndrome patients with and without manifestations of Alzheimer disease. Am J Med Genet. 35, 459-67.

Pereira, P. L., Magnol, L., Sahun, I., Brault, V., Duchon, A., Prandini, P., Gruart, A., Bizot, J. C., Chadefaux-Vekemans, B., Deutsch, S., Trovero, F., Delgado-Garcia, J. M., Antonarakis, S. E., Dierssen, M., Herault, Y., 2009. A new mouse model for the trisomy of the Abcg1-U2af1 region reveals the complexity of the combinatorial genetic code of down syndrome. Hum Mol Genet. 18, 4756-69.

Pletcher, M. T., Wiltshire, T., Cabin, D. E., Villanueva, M., Reeves, R. H., 2001. Use of comparative physical and sequence mapping to annotate mouse chromosome 16 and human chromosome 21. Genomics. 74, 45-54.

Potier, M. C., Rivals, I., Mercier, G., Ettwiller, L., Moldrich, R. X., Laffaire, J., Personnaz, L., Rossier, J., Dauphinot, L., 2006. Transcriptional disruptions in Down syndrome: a case study in the Ts1Cje mouse cerebellum during post-natal development. J Neurochem. 97 Suppl 1, 104-9.

Prandini, P., Deutsch, S., Lyle, R., Gagnebin, M., Delucinge Vivier, C., Delorenzi, M., Gehrig, C., Descombes, P., Sherman, S., Dagna Bricarelli, F., Baldo, C., Novelli, A., Dallapiccola, B., Antonarakis, S. E., 2007. Natural gene-expression variation in Down syndrome modulates the outcome of gene-dosage imbalance. Am J Hum Genet. 81, 252-63.

Prince, J., Jia, S., Bave, U., Anneren, G., Oreland, L., 1994. Mitochondrial enzyme deficiencies in Down's syndrome. J Neural Transm Park Dis Dement Sect. 8, 171-81.

Pritchard, M. A., Kola, I., 1999. The "gene dosage effect" hypothesis versus the "amplified developmental instability" hypothesis in Down syndrome. J Neural Transm Suppl. 57, 293-303.

Reeves, R. H., Irving, N. G., Moran, T. H., Wohn, A., Kitt, C., Sisodia, S. S., Schmidt, C., Bronson, R. T., Davisson, M. T., 1995. A mouse model for Down syndrome exhibits learning and behaviour deficits. Nat Genet. 11, 177-84.

Richtsmeier, J. T., Baxter, L. L., Reeves, R. H., 2000. Parallels of craniofacial maldevelopment in Down syndrome and Ts65Dn mice. Dev Dyn. 217, 137-45.

Roat, E., Prada, N., Ferraresi, R., Giovenzana, C., Nasi, M., Troiano, L., Pinti, M., Nemes, E., Lugli, E., Biagioni, O., Mariotti, M., Ciacci, L., Consolo, U., Balli, F., Cossarizza, A., 2007. Mitochondrial alterations and tendency to apoptosis in peripheral blood cells from children with Down syndrome. FEBS Lett. 581, 521-5.

Ronan, A., Fagan, K., Christie, L., Conroy, J., Nowak, N. J., Turner, G., 2007. Familial 4.3 Mb duplication of 21q22 sheds new light on the Down syndrome critical region. J Med Genet. 44, 448-51.

Roper, R. J., Baxter, L. L., Saran, N. G., Klinedinst, D. K., Beachy, P. A., Reeves, R. H., 2006. Defective cerebellar response to mitogenic Hedgehog signaling in Down [corrected] syndrome mice. Proc Natl Acad Sci U S A. 103, 1452-6.

Roper, R. J., Reeves, R. H., 2006. Understanding the basis for Down syndrome phenotypes. PLoS Genet. 2, e50.

Roper, R. J., VanHorn, J. F., Cain, C. C., Reeves, R. H., 2009. A neural crest deficit in Down syndrome mice is associated with deficient mitotic response to Sonic hedgehog. Mech Dev. 126, 212-9.

Rozovski, U., Jonish-Grossman, A., Bar-Shira, A., Ochshorn, Y., Goldstein, M., Yaron, Y., 2007. Genome-wide expression analysis of cultured trophoblast with trisomy 21 karyotype. Hum Reprod. 22, 2538-45.

Ryoo, S. R., Cho, H. J., Lee, H. W., Jeong, H. K., Radnaabazar, C., Kim, Y. S., Kim, M. J., Son, M. Y., Seo, H., Chung, S. H., Song, W. J., 2008. Dual-specificity tyrosine(Y)-phosphorylation regulated kinase 1A-mediated phosphorylation of amyloid precursor protein: evidence for a functional link between Down syndrome and Alzheimer's disease. J Neurochem. 104, 1333-44.

Sago, H., Carlson, E. J., Smith, D. J., Kilbridge, J., Rubin, E. M., Mobley, W. C., Epstein, C. J., Huang, T. T., 1998. Ts1Cje, a partial trisomy 16 mouse model for Down syndrome, exhibits learning and behavioral abnormalities. Proc Natl Acad Sci U S A. 95, 6256-61.

Saran, N. G., Pletcher, M. T., Natale, J. E., Cheng, Y., Reeves, R. H., 2003. Global disruption of the cerebellar transcriptome in a Down syndrome mouse model. Hum Mol Genet. 12, 2013-9.

Seth, A., Watson, D. K., 2005. ETS transcription factors and their emerging roles in human cancer. Eur J Cancer. 41, 2462-78.

Shapiro, B. L., 1983. Down syndrome--a disruption of homeostasis. Am J Med Genet. 14, 241-69.

Shim, K. S., Ferrando-Miguel, R., Lubec, G., 2003. Aberrant protein expression of transcription factors BACH1 and ERG, both encoded on chromosome 21, in brains of patients with Down syndrome and Alzheimer's disease. J Neural Transm Suppl. 39-49.

Sinha, S., 2005. Anti-oxidant gene expression imbalance, aging and Down syndrome. Life Sci. 76, 1407-26.

Slonim, D. K., Koide, K., Johnson, K. L., Tantravahi, U., Cowan, J. M., Jarrah, Z., Bianchi, D. W., 2009. Functional genomic analysis of amniotic fluid cell-free mRNA suggests that oxidative stress is significant in Down syndrome fetuses. Proc Natl Acad Sci U S A. 106, 9425-9.

Smith, D. J., Stevens, M. E., Sudanagunta, S. P., Bronson, R. T., Makhinson, M., Watabe, A. M., O'Dell, T. J., Fung, J., Weier, H. U., Cheng, J. F., Rubin, E. M., 1997. Functional screening of 2 Mb of human chromosome 21q22.2 in transgenic mice implicates minibrain in learning defects associated with Down syndrome. Nat Genet. 16, 28-36.

Sommer, C. A., Pavarino-Bertelli, E. C., Goloni-Bertollo, E. M., Henrique-Silva, F., 2008. Identification of dysregulated genes in lymphocytes from children with Down syndrome. Genome. 51, 19-29.

Sultan, M., Piccini, I., Balzereit, D., Herwig, R., Saran, N. G., Lehrach, H., Reeves, R. H., Yaspo, M. L., 2007. Gene expression variation in Down's syndrome mice allows prioritization of candidate genes. Genome Biol. 8, R91.

Sun, X., Wu, Y., Chen, B., Zhang, Z., Zhou, W., Tong, Y., Yuan, J., Xia, K., Gronemeyer, H., Flavell, R. A., Song, W., 2011. Regulator of calcineurin 1 (RCAN1) facilitates neuronal apoptosis through caspase 3 activation. J Biol Chem.

Sussan, T. E., Yang, A., Li, F., Ostrowski, M. C., Reeves, R. H., 2008. Trisomy represses Apc(Min)-mediated tumours in mouse models of Down's syndrome. Nature. 451, 73-5.

Tang, Y., Schapiro, M.B., Franz, D.N., Patterson, B.J., Hickey, F.J., Schorry, E.K., Hopkin, R.J., Wylie, M., Narayan, T., Glauser, T.A., Gilbert, D.L., Hershey, A.D., Sharp, F.R., 2004. Blood expression profiles for tuberous sclerosis complex 2, neurofibromatosis type 1, and Down's syndrome. Ann Neurol 56, 808-814.

Van Cleve, S. N., Cannon, S., Cohen, W. I., 2006. Part II: Clinical Practice Guidelines for adolescents and young adults with Down Syndrome: 12 to 21 Years. J Pediatr Health Care. 20, 198-205.

Van Cleve, S. N., Cohen, W. I., 2006. Part I: clinical practice guidelines for children with Down syndrome from birth to 12 years. J Pediatr Health Care. 20, 47-54.

Williams, A. D., Mjaatvedt, C. H., Moore, C. S., 2008. Characterization of the cardiac phenotype in neonatal Ts65Dn mice. Dev Dyn. 237, 426-35.

Wiseman, F. K., Alford, K. A., Tybulewicz, V. L., Fisher, E. M., 2009. Down syndrome--recent progress and future prospects. Hum Mol Genet. 18, R75-83.

Wisniewski, K. E., 1990. Down syndrome children often have brain with maturation delay, retardation of growth, and cortical dysgenesis. Am J Med Genet Suppl. 7, 274-81.

Wolvetang, E. J., Bradfield, O. M., Hatzistavrou, T., Crack, P. J., Busciglio, J., Kola, I., Hertzog, P. J., 2003. Overexpression of the chromosome 21 transcription factor Ets2 induces neuronal apoptosis. Neurobiol Dis. 14, 349-56.

Yabut, O., Domogauer, J., D'Arcangelo, G., 2010. Dyrk1A overexpression inhibits proliferation and induces premature neuronal differentiation of neural progenitor cells. J Neurosci. 30, 4004-14.

Yamakawa, K., Huot, Y. K., Haendelt, M. A., Hubert, R., Chen, X. N., Lyons, G. E., Korenberg, J. R., 1998. DSCAM: a novel member of the immunoglobulin superfamily maps in a Down syndrome region and is involved in the development of the nervous system. Hum Mol Genet. 7, 227-37.

Yu, T., Li, Z., Jia, Z., Clapcote, S. J., Liu, C., Li, S., Asrar, S., Pao, A., Chen, R., Fan, N., Carattini-Rivera, S., Bechard, A. R., Spring, S., Henkelman, R. M., Stoica, G., Matsui, S., Nowak, N. J., Roder, J. C., Chen, C., Bradley, A., Yu, Y. E., 2010. A mouse model of Down syndrome trisomic for all human chromosome 21 syntenic regions. Hum Mol Genet. 19, 2780-91.

5

Abnormal Folate Metabolism and Maternal Risk for Down Syndrome

Érika Cristina Pavarino[1], Bruna Lancia Zampieri[2], Joice Matos Biselli[2] and Eny Maria Goloni Bertollo[1]

[1]*Faculdade de Medicina de São José do Rio Preto – FAMERP, Unidade de Pesquisa em Genética e Biologia Molecular - UPGEM, Equipe Ding-Down;*

[2]*Faculdade de Medicina de São José do Rio Preto – FAMERP, Unidade de Pesquisa em Genética e Biologia Molecular - UPGEM,*

Brazil

1. Introduction

Down syndrome (DS) or trisomy 21 (MIM 190685) is the most common genetic disorder with a prevalence of 1 in 660 live births (Jones, 2006). DS is the leading cause of genetically-defined intellectual disability (Contestabile et al., 2010) and its phenotype is complex and variable among individuals, who may present with a combination of dysmorphic features (Ahmed et al., 2005; Pavarino-Bertelli et al., 2009), congenital heart disease (Abbag, 2006), neurological abnormalities such as early manifestations of Alzheimer's disease (Lott & Head, 2005), immunological impairments (Ram & Chinen, 2011), elevated risk of specific types of leukemia (Hasle et al., 2000), and other clinical complications (Venail et al., 2004).

Trisomy 21 can be caused by three types of chromosomal abnormalities: free trisomy, translocation, or mosaicism. Mosaicism accounts for the minority of DS cases (about 1%) and is characterized by some cells containing 46 chromosomes and others, 47 chromosomes. Translocations are attributed to 3-4% of the cases, with Robertsonian translocation involving chromosomes 14 and 21 being the most common type. Finally, free trisomy occurs in about 95% of cases (Ahmed et al., 2005; J.M. Biselli et al., 2008b) and is characterized by the presence of three complete copies of chromosome 21.

Free trisomy, the main chromosomal abnormality leading to DS, is caused by the failure of normal chromosome 21 segregation during meiosis (meiotic nondisjunction) (Hassold & Hunt, 2000). The parental origin of the extra chromosome 21 is maternal in about 80% of cases (Jyothy et al., 2001), and most (about 77%) occur during the first maternal meiotic division in the maturing oocyte, before conception (Antonarakis et al., 1992).

2. Meiosis and chromosomal segregation

Faithful transmission of a genome from one generation to another depends on the mechanism of cell division in which each pair of replicated chromosomes is separated and equally distributed to mother and daughter cells. Meiosis generates haploid gametes through a specialized cell division process that consists of one round of DNA replication followed by two cell divisions. The first division, meiosis I (MI), involves the segregation of homologous chromosomes from each other, whereas meiosis II (MII) involves the segregation of the sister chromatids (Hassold & Hunt, 2000).

Timing of chromosome attachment and loss of cohesion is essential to faithful chromosome segregation. During MI, the cohesion between sister chromatid arms assures physical attachment by the chiasmata of homologous chromosomes, ensuring their alignment on the meiosis-I spindle, and maintains them at the site of recombination. Chiasmata are resolved at anaphase I by the loss of cohesion between the arms of sister chromatids in the homologous chromosomes; the chromosomes then segregate to opposite poles of the cell. Cohesion, however, must be maintained at centromeres between sister chromatids beyond meiosis I to prevent premature chromatid separation (predivision) and ensure proper attachment of the sister chromatids to opposite spindle poles in meiosis II (Barbero, 2011; Sakuno & Watanabe, 2009; Vogt et al., 2008).

The centromeric cohesion during meiosis I results from the attachment of kinetochores of sister chromatids to only one spindle pole (Sakuno & Watanabe, 2009). Kinetochores are situated on opposite sides of the centromeric heterochromatin at the centromeres of each sister chromatid and they capture and stabilize microtubules for the formation of kinetochore fibers, only then they are capable of chromosome bi-orientation during the metaphase and chromosome segregation during the anaphase of meiosis (Vogt et al., 2008).

During cell division, several chromosomal mal-segregation mechanisms can occur. Classical nondisjunction is due to the failure to resolve chiasmata between homologous chromosomes, whereby both homologues segregate together. In addition, premature resolution of chiasmata or the failure to establish a chiasma between a pair of homologues results in the independent segregation of homologues at MI, which leads to an error if both segregate to the same pole of the MI spindle. A MI error can also involve the segregation of sister chromatids, rather than homologous chromosomes, whereby the premature separation of sister chromatids at MI can result in the segregation of a whole chromosome and a single chromatid to one of the poles. At MII, errors result from the failure of sister chromatid separation (Hassold & Hunt, 2000).

3. The origin of maternal chromosome 21 nondisjunction

The molecular mechanisms involved in meiotic nondisjunction leading to trisomy 21 are still poorly understood and the only well-established risk factor for DS is advanced maternal age at conception (35 years or older) (Allen et al., 2009; Jyothy et al., 2001; Lamb et al., 2005). Studies have suggested many explanations for the maternal age-associated increase in aneuploidy. One model attributes the effect of advanced maternal age to the uterine environment, indicating that there might be an age-related decline in the ability to recognize and then abort trisomic fetuses (Aymé & Lippman-Hand, 1982; Stein et al., 1986). However, the observation that the advanced maternal age effect is restricted to chromosome 21 nondisjunction of maternal origin, but not associated with cases resulting from sperm or post-zygotic mitotic errors, suggests that the uterus is the source of the age effect (Allen et al., 2009).

On the other hand, Zheng & Byers (1993) proposed that age-dependent trisomy 21 results primarily from a mechanism that favors maturation and utilization of euploid oocytes over the pre-existing aneuploid products of mitotic (premeiotic) nondisjunction at an early stage of the reproductive lifespan. In addition, decreased expression of checkpoint proteins in aging oocytes (Vogt et al., 2008) and failure to effectively replace cohesion proteins that are lost from chromosomes during aging (Chiang et al., 2010) also are pointed out as risk factors for predisposing oocytes to errors in chromosome segregation.

A link between altered recombination and maternal age-related nondisjunction has been described. It was observed that recombination is reduced among nondisjoined chromosomes 21 at MI, and this reduction seems to be age-related (Sherman et al., 1994). Lamb et al. (1996) proposed that at least two "hits" are required for chromosome 21 nondisjuntion: (1) the establishment in the fetal ovary of a susceptible pattern of meiotic recombination, and (2) the abnormal processing of susceptible chromosomes in the adult ovary. The second "hit" would involve degradation of a meiotic process (e.g., a spindle component, a sister chromatid cohesion protein, a meiotic motor protein, a checkpoint control protein) that increases the risk of improper segregation for these susceptible bivalents (Hassold & Sherman, 2000). Further studies have shown susceptible patterns of chromosome 21 meiotic recombination, including pericentromeric and telomeric exchanges, described as maternal risk factors for DS even in young DS mothers (Gosh et al., 2009; Lamb et al., 2005).

Besides advanced maternal age, the age of the maternal grandmother at the time of birth of the mother has also been pointed out as a risk factor for the occurrence of DS. At an advanced age, the grandmother's reproductive system may fail to make the essential proteins needed for proper meiotic segregation in the germ cells of her daughter, leading to nondisjunction of chromosome 21 during the embryogenesis of DS child's mother when she was in the grandmother's womb (Malini & Ramachandra, 2006). However, more recent studies failed to support the suggestion that advanced age of the DS grandmother is responsible for meiotic disturbances in her daughter (Allen et al., 2009; Kovaleva et al., 2010).

Although the risk of bearing a child with DS increases substantially with increasing maternal age, many DS children are born to mothers aged less than 35 years-old, suggesting other risk factors influencing DS etiology. In 1999, James et al. produced the first evidence that the occurrence of DS independent of maternal age is associated with DNA hypomethylation due to impairments in folate metabolism.

4. Folate metabolism

Folate represents an essential nutrition component in the human diet, and is involved in many metabolic pathways, mainly the folate metabolism, i.e., a single-carbon transfer from one molecule to another through a series of interconnected biochemical reactions. Folate is a generic term for a family of compounds present in most foods, e.g., legumes, leafy greens, some fruits, vegetables (e.g., spinach, broccoli, asparagus, and lettuce), liver, milk, and dairy products (Lin & Young, 2000). Humans, as all mammals, are unable to synthesize folate, thus its ingestion, either from normal diet or nutritional supplements, is very important. After intestinal absorption, natural folate, known as polyglutamate, requires reduction into monoglutamate by conjugases in the small intestine before it can be absorbed. On the other hand, in its synthetic form, folic acid exists as monoglutamate and does not need to be reduced for release into the blood and cellular uptake (Bailey & Gregory, 1999; Hall & Solehdin, 1998). Another disadvantage of natural food folate is its poor stability especially under typical cooking conditions, which can substantially reduce the vitamin content before it is even ingested, a significant additional factor limiting the ability of natural food folates to enhance folate status (McNulty & Pentieva, 2004; McNulty & Scott, 2008).

Folate metabolism is a complex metabolic pathway that involves multiple enzymes and water-soluble B vitamins such as folate, vitamin B_6 and vitamin B_{12}, that play key roles as enzyme cofactors or substrates in this metabolism. It includes two main cycles: purine and pyrimidine synthesis, necessary for synthesis and repair of DNA, and DNA methylation, an epigenetic process that acts on the control associated with gene expression and genomic stability essential for normal cellular methylation reactions (Figure 1).

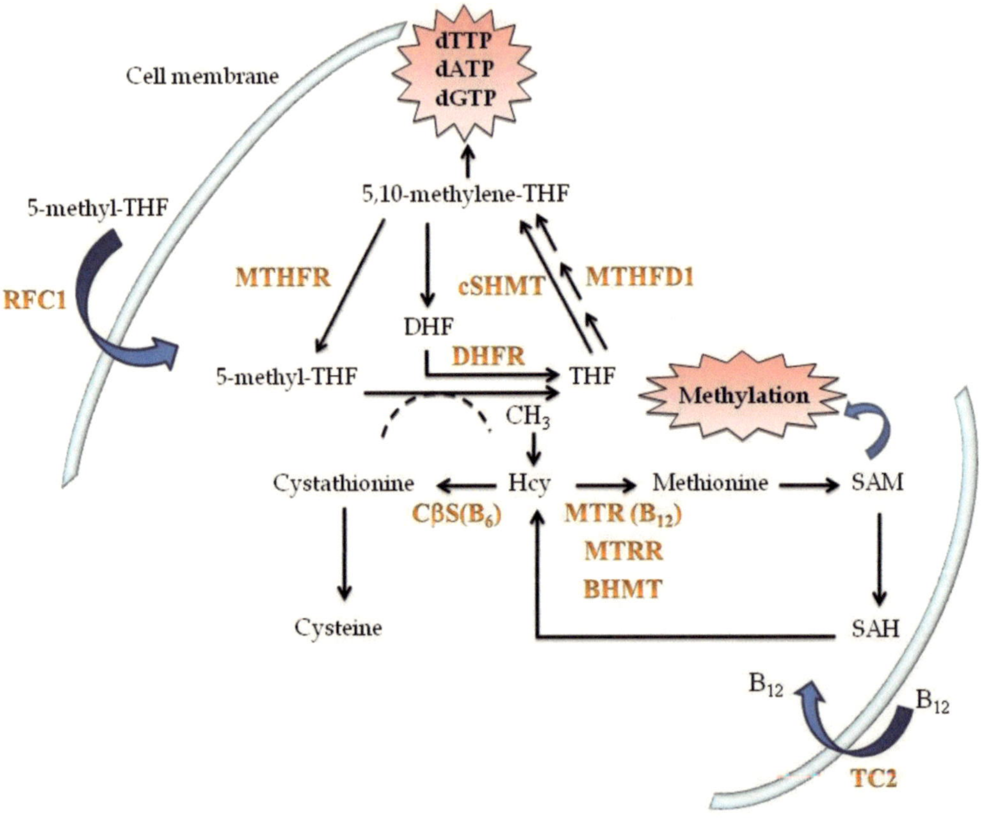

Fig. 1. Folate metabolism. BHMT = Betaine-homocysteine methyltransferase; B_6 = vitamin B6; B_{12} = vitamin B12; CβS = Cystathionine β- synthase; CH_3 = Methyl; dATP = Deoxyadenosine 5′-triphosphate; dGTP = Deoxyguanosine 5′-triphosphate; dTTP = Deoxythymidine 5′-triphosphate; DHF = Dihydrofolate; DHFR = Dihydrofolate reductase; Hcy = Homocysteine; MTHFD1 = Methylenetetrahydrofolate dehydrogenase 1; MTHFR = Methylenetetrahydrofolate reductase; MTR = Methionine synthase; MTRR = Methionine synthase reductase; RFC1 = Reduced folate carrier 1; SAH = S-adenosylhomocysteine; SAM = S- adenosylmethionine; cSHMT= Serine hydroxymethyltransferase; TC2 = Transcobalamin 2; THF = Tetrahydrofolate.

Folate requires several transport systems to enter the cells and the one best characterized is the reduced folate carrier (RFC1), an enzyme located on intestinal cell membranes that carries out the transport of 5-methyltetrahydrofolate (5-methyl-THF) to the interior of a variety of cells, representing an important determinant of folate concentration in the interior of cells (Nguyen et al., 1997). In addition to the folate transport system, several genes and their respective enzymes play important roles in folate metabolism. The *Dihydrofolate reductase* (*DHFR*) gene encodes an enzyme that catalyzes the conversion of dihydrofolate

(DHF) into tetrahydrofolate (THF) (Stanisiawska-Sachadyn et al., 2008), which is then converted into the corresponding 10-formyl, 5,10-methenyl, and 5,10-methylene derivatives by Methylenetetrahydrofolate dehydrogenase 1 (MTHFD1), a trifunctional nicotinamide adenine dinucleotide phosphate-dependent cytoplasmic enzyme. The donor cofactors for *de novo* purine and pyrimidine biosynthesis and, thus, the biosynthesis of DNA (Hum, 1988) are 10-formyl-THF and 5,10-methylene-THF. By an alternative route, THF is converted into 5,10-methylene-THF and glycine by the cytosolic form of the enzyme Serine hydroxymethyltransferase (cSHMT) (Steck et al., 2008).

Methylenetetrahydrofolate reductase (MTHFR) is responsible for the conversion of 5,10-methylene-THF to 5-methyl-THF, the main circulating form of folate that donates methyl groups for homocysteine (Hcy) remethylation into methionine. This latter reaction is catalyzed by the enzyme Methionine synthase (MTR), which requires vitamin B_{12} or cobalamin (Cbl) as a cofactor, and results in the formation of S-adenosylmethionine (SAM), the primary methyl (CH_3) donor for DNA methylation reactions (Finkelstein & Martin, 2000). SAM is demethylated to form S-adenosylhomocysteine (SAH) and then hydrolyzed to form adenine and Hcy. The DNA methyltransferase (DNMTs) enzymes catalyze the transfer of the methyl group, obtained from conversion of SAM into SAH, to position 5′ of cytosine residues located mainly in dinucleotide cytosine-guanine (CpG) (Bestor, 2000; DeAngelis et al., 2008).

Methionine synthase reductase (MTRR), an enzyme codified by the *MTRR* gene, is responsible for the maintenance of the active form of the enzyme MTR. During remethylation of Hcy to methionine, a reaction catalyzed by MTR, methylcob(III)alamine acts as a methyl donor. In this reaction, the transfer of a methyl group from methylcob(III)alamine results in the formation of highly reactive cob(I)alamine, which is oxidized into cob(II)alamine, resulting in MTR inactivation (Yamada et al., 2006). In this inactivation process, a complex is formed between the enzymes MTR and MTRR, and derivative electrons from the oxidation of nicotinamide adenine dinucleotide phosphate (NADPH), catalyzed by MTR, are transferred to the inactive form of MTR. This process favors the transfer of methyl from the SAM to the MTR enzyme, resulting in methylcob(III)alamine, thus reestablishing MTR activity (Leclerc et al., 1999; Olteanu et al., 2001, 2002).

Betaine-homocysteine methyltransferase (BHMT) catalyses the conversion of Hcy to methionine by an alternative pathway of remethylation using the amino acid bethaine as methyl donor. When the Hcy folate-dependent remethylation catalyzed by the MTR enzyme is impaired by genetics or environmental factors, the BHMT enzyme plays an important role maintaining the homeostasis of Hcy (Pajares & Pérez-Salab, 2006).

In the transsulfuration cycle, Hcy is converted into cystathionine by Cystathionine β-synthase (CβS), a vitamin B_6-dependent enzyme, and then into cysteine (Kraus et al., 1998). Under normal physical conditions, all Hcy is remethylated into methionine or catalyzed into cystathionine. The increase of Hcy concentration represents impairment in folate metabolism and thus in methylation reactions (Fenech, 2002).

Besides the enzymes that act directly on folate metabolism, cobalamin-transporting proteins also play an important role in this metabolic pathway, since the MTR enzyme is cobalamin-dependent. The enzyme Transcobalamin 2 (TC2) is synthesized in the intestinal villi and binds itself to Cbl in the interstitial fluid. This formed complex goes into the intestinal villi microcirculation and then reaches the systemic circulation. This circulation distributes the vitamin to all tissues where specific receptors on cell membranes bind and internalize the TC2-Cbl complex by endocytosis (Quadros et al., 1999; Seetharam & Li, 2000).

5. Folate metabolism, genomic stability, and maternal risk for chromosome 21 nondisjunction

Based on evidence that stable centromeric DNA chromatin may depend on the epigenetic inheritance of specific centromeric methylation patterns and on the binding of specific methyl-sensitive proteins to maintain the higher order DNA architecture necessary for kinetochore assembly (Karpen & Allshire, 1997), James et al. (1999) hypothesized that pericentromeric hypomethylation, resulting from impaired folate metabolism secondary to polymorphism of the *MTHFR* gene, could impair chromosomal segregation and increase the risk for chromosome 21 nondisjunction in young mothers. They observed that the risk of having a child with DS was 2.6-fold higher in mothers with 677 C→T substitution in one or both alleles of the *MTHFR* gene than in mothers without the 677 C→T substitution. In addition, DS mothers displayed a significant increase in plasma Hcy concentrations and lymphocyte methotrexate cytotoxicity, consistent with abnormal folate and methyl metabolism.

As described above, the MTHFR enzyme plays an important role in regulating DNA methylation through the reduction of 5,10-methylene-THF to 5-methyl-THF (Figure 1). The 677 C→T polymorphism is known to decrease the affinity of the enzyme for the flavin-adenine-dinucleotide (FAD) cofactor, decreasing enzyme activity (Guenther et al., 1999; Yamada et al., 2001). The *MTHFR* 677 CT genotype seems to reduce enzyme activity by about 35% and the homozygous TT genotype by 70% (Frosst et al., 1995). Since the study by James et al. (1999), polymorphisms in the *MTHFR* gene are the most frequently investigated in attempt to clarify the role of folate and methyl metabolism in the maternal risk for DS (Martínez-Frías et al., 2008). Several studies have associated the MTHFR 677C→T polymorphism and the risk of bearing a child with DS (da Silva et al., 2005; Meguid et al., 2008; Sadiq et al., 2011; Wang et al., 2008) as well as with increasing plasma Hcy concentration (P.M. Biselli et al., 2007; da Silva et al., 2005; Narayanan et al., 2004; Ulvik et al., 2007).

Another common polymorphism in the *MTHFR* gene, the substitution of alanine for cytosine at the 1298 position, was already associated with DS risk and increased plasma Hcy concentration (Martínez-Frías et al., 2006; Meguid et al., 2008; Narayanan et al., 2004, Rai et al., 2006; Scala et al., 2006; Weisberg et al., 2001). This polymorphism proved to have an impact on enzyme activity resulting in an even more pronounced decrease in its activity in homozygous 1298 CC compared to the heterozygous individuals (van der Putt et al., 1998).

In addition to the *MTHFR* gene, other genetic polymorphisms involved in the folate pathway seem to modulate the maternal risk for bearing a child with DS (Bosco et al., 2003; J.M. Biselli et al., 2008a; Meguid et al., 2008; Pozzi et al., 2009; Sadiq et al., 2011; Scala et al., 2006; Wang et al., 2008) as well as the concentrations of metabolites involved in the folate pathway (Ananth et al. 2007; Barbosa et al., 2008; Cheng et al., 2010; Devos et al., 2008). The *MTR* 2756 A→G polymorphism has been associated with increased maternal risk for DS in the presence of AG or GG genotypes, as well as when combined with polymorphisms *MTRR* 66 A→G (*MTR* 2756AG/*MTRR* 66AG) (Bosco et al., 2003) and *MTHFR* 677 C→T (*MTHFR* 677TT/*MTR* 2756AA). In addition, the allele *MTR* 2756 G proved to be more frequent, both in homozygosis and heterozygosis, in DS mothers as compared to mothers of individuals without the syndrome (Pozzi et al., 2009). Concerning its influence on Hcy concentrations, studies have shown conflicting results, since some have associated the *MTR* 2756 A allele to increased Hcy concentration (Fredriksen et al., 2007; Harmon et al., 1999), while others found the same association, but with the polymorphic 2756 G alelle (Feix et al., 2001; Fillon-Emery et al., 2004).

As to the *MTRR* 66 A→G polymorphism, some studies have supported an independent role for this polymorphism in the maternal risk for DS in the presence of the homozygous *MTRR* 66 GG genotype (Hobbs et al., 2000; Pozzi et al., 2009; Wang et al., 2008). Most of the studies have associated this polymorphism with the risk of DS and increased Hcy concentration when combined to other polymorphisms, such as *MTHFR* 677 C→T (Hobbs et al., 2000; Martínez-Frías et al., 2006; O'Leary et al, 2002; Yang et al., 2008). Additionally, a steady state kinetic analysis showed a significantly decreased affinity of *MTRR* for *MTR* accompanying substitution 66 A→G, revealing a significant difference in the relative efficacies of the MTRR enzyme (Olteanu et al., 2002). However, several studies have failed to find association between DS risk and the *MTRR* 66 A→G polymorphism, whether alone or combined with other genetic variants (Coppedè et al., 2009; Chango et al., 2005; Scala et al., 2006).

The *RFC1* gene is polymorphic at nucleotide 80 (A→G), and investigation of the impact of this polymorphism on protein function have demonstrated a difference in its affinity for subtracts and/or efficiency in transport in comparison with the wild type enzyme (Whetstine et al., 2001). Few studies have evaluated the influence of the *RFC1* 80 A→G polymorphism on DS risk (J.M. Biselli, 2008a, 2008c; Chango et al., 2005; Coppedè et al., 2006). Some studies have found no association between this polymorphism and DS (Chango et al. 2005; Fintelman-Rodrigues et al., 2009); however, Coppedè et al. (2006) and J.M. Biselli et al. (2008a) suggest a role for this polymorphism when combined with other polymorphisms in genes involved in folate metabolism. Supporting this hypothesis, the combined *RFC1* 80 GG/*MTHFR* 677 TT genotype has been associated with increased Hcy concentration and the *RFC1* 80 AA/*MTHFR* 677 CT combined genotype with higher plasma folate concentration (Chango et al., 2000).

A common polymorphism in the *CβS* gene, 68-base pair (bp) insertion at nucleotide position 844 (844ins68), is also investigated in the risk for DS, but there is no evidence that this variant plays an independent role on this risk (da Silva et al., 2005; Chango et al., 2005; Scala et al., 2006). The *CβS* 844ins68 polymorphism has been associated with reduction of Hcy concentration in the presence of the insertion (Tsai et al., 1996; Tsai et al., 1999; Tsai et al., 2000), and it is believed that this insertion is related to increased enzyme activity (Tsai et al., 1996, Tsai et al., 1999). This variant is always found to be associated in *cis* with an additional polymorphism in the *CβS* gene, a thymine-to-cytosine transition at nucleotide position 833, which causes a threonine-to-isoleucine amino acid substitution, and is reported, together with *CβS* 844ins68, as a 833 T→C/844ins68 *in cis* double mutation (Pepe et al., 1999; Vyletal et al., 2007). Da Silva et al., (2005) observed that the 844ins68 polymorphism, in association with other polymorphisms of the folate pathway, is related to increased risk for DS. Concerning its influence on folate metabolite concentrations, such as folate, Hcy, and vitamin B_{12}, the *CβS* 844ins68 polymorphism showed no significant association with any of the biochemical variables involved in folate metabolism (Bowron et al., 2005; Kumar et al., 2010; Summers et al., 2008).

The *MTHFD1* gene presents a functional polymorphism, a guanine-to-adenine substitution at position 1958 (1958 G→A), that has been shown to reduce the activity and stability of the variant enzyme (Christensen et al., 2008). There are only two studies to date on the influence of this polymorphism on maternal risk for DS. Scala et al. (2006) showed an association of the *MTHFD1* 1958 AA genotype with DS risk, but only when combined with the *RFC1* 80

GG genotype; however, more recently, Neagos et al. (2010) failed to find association. Thus, further investigations are necessary to clarify the role of *MTHFD*1 1958 G→A in the chromosome 21 nondisjunction.

Johnson et al. (2004) described a 19-base pair (bp) deletion polymorphism in intron-1 of the *DHFR* gene and hypothesized that this polymorphism could be functional since the deletion removes a possible transcription factor binding site that affects gene regulation. A study with mothers of individuals with spina bifida showed that the expression of the messenger ribonucleic acid (mRNA) from the *DHFR* gene was 50% higher in the presence of del/del genotype than in the ins/ins genotype (Parle-McDermott et al., 2007). This polymorphism has been associated with the modulation of metabolites' concentrations involved in the folate pathway. Gellekink et al. (2007) reported association between the del/del genotype and reduction of plasma Hcy concentration, but found no association between this genotype and concentrations of serum and erythrocyte folate. Another study found no effect on Hcy concentration, but found increased plasma and erythrocyte folate levels in del/del individuals (Stanislawska-Sachadyn et al., 2008). The results of the only study that investigated the 19-bp deletion polymorphism of *DHFR* gene in DS mothers did not support an association between this variant and the maternal risk for DS. In addition, the polymorphism was not associated with variations in serum folate and plasma Hcy and methylmalonic acid (MMA) concentrations in the study population (Mendes et al., 2010).

The *TC2* gene, which codifies a transporting protein required for the cellular uptake of vitamin B_{12} (Seetharam &Li, 2000), is polymorphic at nucleotide position 776 (C→G). There is evidence that the presence of the *TC2* 776 CC genotype may be more efficient in delivering vitamin B_{12} to tissues, resulting in enhanced B_{12} functional status (Miller et al., 2002; Namour et al., 1998). In other studies, the presence of the *TC2* 776 GG genotype was shown to affect negatively the serum concentration of the TC2 protein-vitamin B_{12} complex (von Castel-Dunwoody et al., 2005) and was associated with low concentrations of SAM in childbearing-age women (Barbosa et al., 2008). Considering that SAM is the major methyl donor for DNA methylation reactions, it was hypothesized that the variant *TC2* 776 C→G could influence the maternal risk for DS by modifying the DNA methylation pattern. This polymorphism has only been investigated in DS risk by two groups to date (J.M. Biselli et al., 2008c; Fintelman-Rodrigues et al., 2009), but no association has been found.

The conflicting results shown by literature have raised the suggestion that the presence of individual polymorphisms in genes involved in folate metabolism might not increase the risk of having a child with DS, although the effect of combined risk genotypes might modify their individual effect and increase DS risk (J.M., Biselli et al., 2008a; Brandalize et al., 2010; Coppedè et al., 2006; Coppedè et al., 2009; da Silva et al., 2005; Martínez-Frías, et al., 2006; Scala et al., 2006; Wang et al., 2008). Moreover, there is evidence that the significance of genetic polymorphisms seems to depend on interactions with nutritional factors (Papoutsakis et al., 2010; Stover & Caudill, 2008).

6. Folate metabolism, genomic stability, and genetic polymorphisms

Both *in vitro* and *in vivo* studies have shown that DNA methylation is an important mechanism for the maintenance of genomic stability. Literature provides several examples that genome-wide DNA hypomethylation enhances the occurrence of aneuploidy and chromosomal rearrangements (Herrera et al., 2008), loss of heterozygosity (Matsuzaki et al., 2005), and chromosome malsegregation (Fenech et al., 2011). Folate and vitamin B_{12} are among the most important minerals and vitamins required for DNA maintenance and prevention of DNA damage that could be induced by inadequate intake of these antimutagenic vitamins (Fenech, 2002). In human cells, folate deficiency is associated with DNA hypomethylation (Chang et al., 2011; Linhart et al., 2009), DNA instability (strand breakage, uracil misincorporation) (Linhart et al., 2009; Williams & Jacobson, 2010), aneuploidy of chromosomes 17 and 21 (Beetstra et al., 2005; Wang et al., 2004), apoptosis (Li et al., 2003), and necrosis (Beetstra et al., 2005). Low vitamin B_{12} status is also associated with DNA hypomethylation (Brunaud et al., 2003) and genetic instability (Andreassi et al., 2003; Botto et al., 2003).

There is increasing evidence of association between polymorphisms in folate and Hcy metabolizing genes and levels of chromosome damage. The *MTHFR* 677 C→T polymorphism is associated with diminished levels of 5-methylcytosine and DNA hypomethylation (Chen et al., 2010; Friso et al., 2002; Paz et al., 2002), micronucleus formation (Andreassi et al., 2003; Botto et al., 2003), and microsatellite instability (Naghibalhossaini et al., 2010) in the presence of the variant T allele. The homozygous variant genotype of another polymorphism of the *MTHFR* gene, 1298 A→C, was more frequent in patients with Turner syndrome (de Oliveira et al., 2008), and a higher frequency of the C allele was observed in spontaneous abortions with fetal chromosomal aneuploidy as compared to those with normal fetal karyotypes (Kim et al., 2011), suggesting its involvement in the origin of chromosomal imbalances. The *MTR* 2756 A→G polymorphism was associated with reduced number of hypermethylated CpG islands of suppressor tumor genes and with higher micronucleus rates in the presence of the *MTRR* 66 GG variant genotype (Botto et al., 2003; Paz et al., 2002; Zijno et al., 2003).

The polymorphism *RFC1* 80 A→G has been associated with reduced percentage of 5-methylcytosine in the DNA of mothers of children with autism in the presence of homozygous and heterozygous genotypes for the G allele as compared to AA genotype (James et al., 2010); however, the presence of the A allele was recently associated with increased oxidative DNA damage, while the *cSHMT* 1420 C→T polymorphism was associated with reduced oxidative DNA damage (CC>CT>TT) (Mohammad et al., 2011).

Moreover, Piskac-Collier et al. (2011) recently demonstrated that lymphocytes from lung cancer patients showed a considerably increased frequency of cytogenetic damage in the presence of *MTHFR* 677 C→T, *MTHFR* 1298 A→C, and *cSHMT* 435 C→T allelic variants, suggesting that interactions between genetic polymorphisms may also have a significant impact on genetic instability.

7. Predisposition to chromosome malsegregation in young DS mothers and its association with folate-metabolizing gene polymorphisms

Studies with women who have a DS child at a young age have suggested that they present genetic predispositions to chromosome malsegregation in both somatic and germ line cells. Migliore et al. (2006) observed increased frequency of binucleated-micronucleated lymphocytes in women who had a DS child before 35 years of age, and fluorescence in situ hybridization analysis revealed that micronuclei were mainly originating from chromosomal malsegregation events, including chromosome 21 malsegregation. Further studies from their group confirmed increased chromosome damage in blood cells of young DS mothers and showed a significant correlation between micronucleated cells and both

MTHFR 677C→T and 1298A→C polymorphisms. The mean frequency of binucleated-micronucleated cells increased significantly with the increasing number of *MTHFR* 677 T alleles, and *MTHFR* 1298 AA women have significantly higher binucleated-micronucleated cells frequency than do *MTHFR* 1298 AC + CC carriers (Coppedè et al., 2007; Coppedè, 2009). In addition, mothers who had a DS child at a young age showed increased frequency (of about 5-fold) of Alzheimer's disease (AD) (Schupf, et al., 2001). A unifying hypothesis trying to relate DS, trisomy 21, and AD has proposed that trisomy 21 mosaicism at the germ cell level or in brain cells could account for the familial aggregation of AD and DS (Potter, 1991). Together, these results suggest that young DS mothers are more prone to chromosome malsegregation, which could be true both for somatic (peripheral blood lymphocytes, brain) and for germ cells and, importantly, folate-metabolizing gene polymorphisms seem to play an important role on this susceptibility to aneuploidy.

8. Folate supplementation and DS prevention

Two important emerging areas of nutrition science are nutrigenomics, which refers to the effect of diet on DNA stability, and nutrigenetics, which refers to the impact of genetic differences between individuals on their response to a specific dietary pattern, functional food, or supplement for a specific health outcome. On these terms, two premises are important: (a) inappropriate nutrient supply can cause considerable levels of genome mutation and alter the expression of genes required for genome maintenance, and (b) common genetic polymorphisms may alter the activity of genes that affect the bioavailability of micronutrients and/or the affinity for micronutrient cofactors in key enzymes involved in DNA metabolism or repair, resulting in a lower or higher reaction rate (Bull & Fenech, 2008; Fenech, 2005).

As mentioned before, the folate-dependent biosynthesis of nucleotide precursors for DNA synthesis and genome methylation is dependent on the availability of many vitamins, including B_{12}, B_6, niacin, riboflavin, and minerals (zinc, cobalt), and is subject to regulation by other nutrients, such as iron and vitamin A, not directly involved in DNA or SAM biosynthesis (Stover, & Caudill 2008). Therefore, impairments in one-carbon metabolism, and the SAM cycle in particular, induced by nutritional deficiencies and/or genetic polymorphisms that encode folate-dependent enzymes, alter genome methylation patterns and gene expression levels (Stover, 2004; Stover, & Caudill 2008).

Since 1992, supplementation with 0.4 mg/daily of folic acid is recommended for women of childbearing age for the prevention of neural tube defects (Centers for Disease Control, 1992). Barkai et al. (2003) observed that families at risk for neural tube defects present with a higher frequency of DS cases and vice-versa, suggesting that both disorders are influenced by the same folate-related risk factors. However, two issues ought to be considered in the prevention of DS by folic acid: the dose and the timing of folic acid intake (Scala et al., 2006). It has been proposed that genomic instability is reduced at plasma folate concentrations above 34 nmol/L and Hcy concentrations below 7.5 μmol/L; these concentrations can only be reached with the ingestion of more than 0.4 mg/day of folic acid (Fenech, 2002). A report of a decreased occurrence of DS offspring in mothers supplemented with high doses of folic acid (6 mg/day) (Czeizel & Puho, 2005) supports the hypothesis of an involvement of folate in the etiology of DS. Concerning the timing of folate intake, it should be remembered that maternal MI errors in the primary oocyte may occur in a process that begins during fetal life and ends at the time of ovulation, whereas MII errors occur at the time of fertilization (Yoon et al., 1996). Therefore, it is likely that only MII errors would be immediately affected by folic acid intake in adult women (Ray et al., 2003).

9. Conclusion

Currently available literature suggests that abnormal folate metabolism is associated with increased maternal risk for DS, with a complex interaction between genetic polymorphisms, environmental factors (i.e., nutritional factors), and epigenetic processes. However, given the complexity of the folate pathway, these complex interactions cannot be easily understood and none of the polymorphisms studied so far can be used in genetic counseling to predict the maternal risk for having a DS child (Coppedè et al., 2009). However, nutrigenetics and nutrigenomics are promising areas for evaluating the possibility of DS prevention with folic acid supplementation associated with susceptible genotypes. Thus, further large-scale studies are necessary to better understand the complex association between chromosomal 21 nondisjunction and folate metabolism.

10. References

Abbag, F.I. (2006). Congenital heart diseases and other major anomalies in patients with Down syndrome. Saudi Medical Journal, Vol.27, No.2, (February 2006), pp. 219-222, ISSN 0379-5284

Ahmed, I.; Ghafoor, T.; Samore, N.A. & Chattha, M.N. (2005). Down syndrome: clinical and cytogenetic analysis. Journal of the College of Physicians and Surgeons - Pakistan: JCPSP, Vol.15, No.7, (July 2005), pp. 426-429, ISSN 1022-386X

Allen, E.G.; Freeman, S.B.; Druschel, C.; Hobbs, C.A.; O'Leary, L.A.; Romitti, P.A.; Royle, M.H.; Torfs, C.P. & Sherman, S.L. (2009). Maternal age and risk for trisomy 21 assessed by the origin of chromosome nondisjunction: a report from the Atlanta and National Down Syndrome Projects. Human Genetics, Vol.125, No.1, (February 2009), pp. 41-52, ISSN 0340-6717

Ananth, C.V.; Elsasser D.A.; Kinzler, W.L.; Peltier, M.R.; Getahun, D.; Leclerc, D.; Rozen, R.R. & New Jersey Placental Abruption Study Investigators. (2007). Polymorphisms in methionine synthase reductase and betaine-homocysteine S-methyltransferase genes: Risk of placental abruption. Molecular Genetics and Metabolism, Vol.91, No.1, (May 2007), pp. 104–110, ISSN 1096-7192

Andreassi, M.G.; Botto, N.; Cocci, F.; Battaglia, D.; Antonioli, E.; Masetti, S.; Manfredi, S.; Colombo, M.G.; Biagini, A. & Clerico, A. (2003). Methylenetetrahydrofolate reductase gene C677T polymorphism, homocysteine, vitamin B12, and DNA damage in coronary artery disease. Human Genetics, Vol.112, No.2, (February 2003), pp. 171-177, ISSN 0340-6717

Antonarakis, S.E.; Petersen, M.B.; McInnis, M.G.; Adelsberger, P.A.; Schinzel, A.A.; Binkert, F.; Pangalos, C.; Raoul, O.; Slaugenhaupt, S.A.; Hafez, M.; Cohen, M.M.; Roulson, D.; Schwartz, S.; Mikkelsen, M.; Tranebjaerg, L.; Greenberg, F.; Hoar, D.I.; Rudd, N.L.; Warren, A.C.; Metaxotou, C.; Bartsocas, C. & Chakravarti, A. (1992). The meiotic stage of nondisjunction in trisomy 21: determination by using DNA polymorphisms. American Journal of Human Genetics, Vol.50, No.3, (March 1992), pp. 544-550, ISSN 0340-6717

Aymé, S. & Lippman-Hand, A. (1982). Maternal-age effect in aneuploidy: does altered embryonic selection play a role? American Journal of Human Genetics, Vol.34, No.4, (July 1982), pp. 558-565, ISSN 0002-9297

Bailey, L.B. & Gregory, J.F. (1999). Folate metabolism and requirements. The Journal of Nutrition, Vol.129, No.4, (April 1999), pp. 779-782, ISSN 0022-3166

Barbero, J.L. (2011). Chromatid Cohesion Control and Aneuploidy. Cytogenetic and Genome Research, (January 2011), Epub ahead of print, ISSN 1424-8581

Barbosa, P.R.; Stabler, S.P.; Trentin, R.; Carvalho, F.R.; Luchessi, A.D.; Hirata, R.D.; Hirata, M.H.; Allen, R.H. & Guerra-Shinohara, E.M. (2008). Evaluation of nutritional and genetic determinants of total homocysteine, methylmalonic acid and S-adenosylmethionine/S-adenosylhomocysteine values in Brazilian childbearing-age women. Clinica Chimica Acta; International Journal of Clinical Chemistry, Vol.388, No.1-2, (February 2008), pp. 139–147, ISSN 0009-8981

Barkai, G.; Arbuzova, S.; Berkenstadt, M.; Heifetz, S. & Cuckle H. (2003). Frequency of Down's syndrome and neural-tube defects in the same family. Lancet, Vol.361, No.9366, (April 2003), pp. 1331-1335, ISSN 0140-6736

Beetstra, S.; Thomas, P.; Salisbury, C.; Turner, J. & Fenech, M. (2005). Folic acid deficiency increases chromosomal instability, chromosome 21 aneuploidy and sensitivity to radiation-induced micronuclei. Mutation Research, Vol.578, No.1-2, (October 2005), pp. 317–326, ISSN 0027-5107

Bestor, T.H. (2000). The DNA methyltransferases of mammals. Human Molecular Genetics, Vol.9, No.16, (October 2000), pp. 2395–2402, ISSN 0964-6906

Biselli, P.M.; Sanches de Alvarenga, M.P.; Abbud-Filho, M.; Ferreira-Baptista, M.A.; Galbiatti, A.L.; Goto, M.T.; Cardoso, M.A.; Eberlin, M.N.; Haddad, R.; Goloni-Bertoll,o E.M. & Pavarino-Bertelli E.C. (2007). Effect of folate, vitamin B6, and vitamin B12 intake and MTHFR C677T polymorphism on homocysteine concentrations of renal transplant recipients. Transplantation proceedings, Vol.39, No.10, (December 2007), pp. 3163-3165, ISSN 0041-1345

Biselli, J.M.; Goloni-Bertollo, E.M.; Zampieri, B.L.; Haddad, R.; Eberlin, M.N. & Pavarino-Bertelli EC. (2008a). Genetic polymorphisms involved in folate metabolism and elevated concentrations of plasma homocysteine: maternal risk factors for Down syndrome in Brazil. Genetics and Molecular Research, Vol. 7, No.1, (January 2008), pp. 33-42, ISSN 1676-5680

Biselli, J.M.; Goloni-Bertollo, E. M.; Ruiz, M.T.; & Pavarino-Bertelli, E.C. (2008b). Cytogenetic profile of Down syndrome cases seen by a general genetics outpatient service in Brazil. Down's syndrome, research and practice, Vol.12, No.3, (February 2008), ISSN 0968-7912

Biselli, J.M.; Brumati, D.; Frigeri, V.F.; Zampieri, B.L.; Goloni-Bertollo, E.M. & Pavarino-Bertelli, E.C. (2008c). A80G polymorphism of reduced folate carrier 1 (RFC1) and C776G polymorphism of transcobalamin 2 (TC2) genes in Down's syndrome etiology. Sao Paulo Medical Journal, Vol.126, No.6, (November 2008), pp. 329-332, ISSN 1516-3180

Bosco, P.; Guéant-Rodriguez, R.M.; Anello, G.; Barone, C.; Namour, F.; Caraci, F.; Romano, A.; Romano, C. & Guéant, J.L. (2003). Methionine synthase (MTR) 2756 (A→G) polymorphism, double heterozygosity Methionine synthase 2756AG / Methionine synthase reductase (MTRR 66AG) and elevated homocysteinemia are three risk factors for having a child with Down syndrome. American Journal of Medical Genetics Part A, Vol.121, No.3, (September 2003), pp. 219-224, ISSN 1552-4825

Botto, N.; Andreassi, M.G.; Manfredi, S.; Masetti, S.; Cocci, F.; Colombo, M.G.; Storti, S.; Rizza, A. & Biagini, A. (2003). Genetic polymorphisms in folate and homocysteine metabolism as risk factors for DNA damage. European Journal of Human Genetics, Vol.11. No.9, (September 2003), pp. 671-678, ISSN 1018-4813

Bowron, A.; Scott, J. & Stansbie, D. (2005). The influence of genetic and environmental factors on plasma homocysteine concentrations in a population at high risk for coronary artery disease. Annals of Clinical Biochemistry, Vol.42, No.Pt6, (November 2005), pp. 459–462, ISSN 0004-5632

Brandalize, A.P.; Bandinelli, E.; dos Santos, P.A. & Schüler-Faccini, L. (2010). Maternal gene polymorphisms involved in folate metabolism as risk factors for Down syndrome offspring in Southern Brazil. Disease Markers, Vol.29, No.2, pp. 95-101, ISSN 0278-0240

Brunaud, L.; Alberto, J.M.; Ayav, A.; Gérard, P.; Namour, F.; Antunes, L.; Braun, M.; Bronowicki. J.P.; Bresler, L. & Guéant, J.L. (2003). Vitamin B12 is a strong determinant of low methionine synthase activity and DNA hypomethylation in gastrectomized rats. Digestion, Vol.68, No.2-3, (November 2003), pp. 133-40, ISSN 0012-2823

Bull, C. & Fenech, M. (2008). Genome-health nutrigenomics and nutrigenetics: nutritional requirements or 'nutriomes' for chromosomal stability and telomere maintenance at the individual level. The Proceedings of Nutrition Society, Vol.67, No.2, (May 2008), pp. 146-156, ISSN 0029-6651

Centers for Disease Control. (1992). Recommendations for the use of folic acid to reduce the number of cases of spina bifida and other neural tube defects. MMWR. Recommendations and reports: Morbidity and mortality weekly report. Recommendations and reports / Centers for Disease Control, Vol.41, No. RR-14, (September 1992), pp. 1-7, ISSN 1057-5987

Chang, H.; Zhang, T.; Zhang, Z.; Bao, R.; Fu, C.; Wang, Z.; Bao, Y.; Li, Y.; Wu, L.; Zheng, X. & Wu, J. (2011). Tissue-specific distribution of aberrant DNA methylation associated with maternal low-folate status in human neural tube defects. The Journal of Nutritional Biochemistry, (February 2011), Epub ahead of print, ISSN 0955-2863

Chango, A.; Fillon-Emery, N.; de Courcy, G.P.; Lambert, D.; Pfister, M.; Rosenblatt, D.S. & Nicolas, J.P. (2000). A polymorphism (80G->A) in the Reduced folate carrier gene and its associations with folate status and homocysteinemia. Molecular Genetics and Metabolism, Vol.70, No.4, (August 2000), pp. 310-315, ISSN 1096-7192

Chango, A.; Fillon-Emery, N.; Mircher, C.; Bléhaut, H.; Lambert, D.; Herbeth, B.; James, S.J.; Réthoré, M.O. & Nicolas, J.P. (2005). No association between common polymorphisms in genes of folate/homocysteine metabolism and the risk of Down syndrome among French mothers. The British Journal of Nutrition, Vol.95, No.2, (August 2005), pp. 166-169, ISSN 0007-1145

Chen, X.; Guo, J.; Lei, Y.; Zou, J.; Lu, X.;, Bao, Y.; Wu, L.; Wu, J.; Zheng, X.; Shen, Y.; Wu, B.L. & Zhang, T. (2010). Global DNA hypomethylation is associated with NTD-affected pregnancy: A case-control study. Birth Defects Research. Part A, Clinical and Molecular Teratology, Vol.88, No.7, (July 2010), pp. 575-581, ISSN 1542-0760

Cheng, D.M.; Jiang, Y.G.; Huang, C.Y.; Kong, H.Y.; Pang, W. & Yang, H.P. (2010). Polymorphism of MTHFR C677T, serum vitamin levels and cognition in subjects with hyperhomocysteinemia in China. Nutritional Neuroscience, Vol.13, No.4, (August 2010), pp. 175-182, ISSN 1028-415X

Chiang, T.; Duncan, F.E.; Schindler, K.; Schultz, R.M. & Lampson, M.A. (2010). Evidence that weakened centromere cohesion is a leading cause of age-related aneuploidy in oocytes. Current Biology: CB, Vol.20, No.17, (September 2010), pp.1522-1528, ISSN 0960-9822

Christensen, K.E.; Rohlicek, C.V.; Andelfinger, G.U.; Michaud, J.; Bigras, J.L.; Richter, A.; Mackenzie, R.E. & Rozen, R. (2008). The MTHFD1 p.Arg653Gln variant alters enzyme function and increases risk for congenital heart defects. Human Mutation, Vol.30, No.2, (February 2008), pp. 212-220, ISSN 1098-1004

Contestabile, A.; Benfenati, F. & Gasparini, L. (2010). Communication breaks-Down: from neurodevelopment defects to cognitive disabilities in Down syndrome. Progress in Neurobiology, Vol.91, No.1, (May 2010), pp. 1-22, ISSN 0301-0082

Coppedè, F.; Marini, G.; Bargagna, S.; Stuppia, L.; Minichilli, F.; Fontana, I.; Colognato, R.; Astrea, G.; Palka, G. & Migliore, L. (2006). Folate gene polymorphisms and the risk of Down syndrome pregnancies in young Italian women. American Journal of Medical Genetics Part A, Vol.140, No.10, (May 2006), pp. 1083-1091, ISSN 1552-4825

Coppedè, F.; Colognato, R.; Bonelli, A.; Astrea, G.; Bargagna, S.; Siciliano, G. & Migliore. L. (2007). Polymorphisms in folate and homocysteine metabolizing genes and chromosome damage in mothers of Down syndrome children. American Journal of Medical Genetics. Part A, Vol.143A, No.17, (September 2007), pp. 2006-2015, ISSN 1552-4825

Coppedè, F.; Migheli, F.; Bargagna, S.; Siciliano, G.; Antonucci ,I.; Stuppia, L.; Palka, G. & Migliore, L. (2009). Association of maternal polymorphisms in folate metabolizing genes with chromosome damageand risk of Down syndrome offspring. Neuroscience Letters, Vol.449, No.1, (January 2009), pp. 15-19, ISSN 0304-3940

Coppedè, F. (2009). The complex relationship between folate/homocysteine metabolism and risk of Down syndrome. Mutation Research, Vol.682, No.1, (July-August 2009), pp. 54-70, ISSN 0027-5107

Czeizel, A.E. & Puhó, E. (2005). Maternal use of nutritional supplements during the first month of pregnancy and decreased risk of Down's syndrome: case-control study. Nutrition, Vol.21, No.6, (June 2005), pp.698-704, ISSN 0899-9007

da Silva, L.R.; Vergani, N.; Galdieri, Lde.C.; Ribeiro Porto, M.P.; Longhitanom, S.B.; Brunoni, D.; D'Almeida, V. & Alvarez Perez AB. (2005). Relationship between polymorphisms in genes involved in homocysteine metabolism and maternal risk for Down syndrome in Brazil. American Journal of Medical Genetics Part A, Vol.135, No. 3, (June 2005), pp. 263–267, ISSN 1552-4825

De Oliveira, K.C.; Bianco, B.B.; Verreschi, I.T.; Guedes, A.D.; Galera, B.B.; Galera, M.F.; Barbosa, C.P. & Lipay, M.V. (2008). Prevalence of the polymorphism MTHFR A1298C and not MTHFR C677T is related to chromosomal aneuploidy in Brazilian Turner Syndrome patients. Arquivos Brasileiros de Endocrinologia e Metabologia, Vol.52, No.8, (November 2008), pp. 1374–1381, ISSN 0004-2730

DeAngelis, J.T.; Farrington, W.J. & Tollefsbol, T.O. (2008). An overview of epigenetic assays. Molecular Biotechnology, Vol.38, No.2, (February 2008), pp. 179-183, ISSN 1073-6085

DeVos, L.; Chanson, A.; Liu, Z.; Ciappio, E.D.; Parnell, L.D.; Mason, J.B.; Tucker, K.L. & Crott, J.W. (2008). Associations between single nucleotide polymorphisms in folate uptake and metabolizing genes with blood folate, homocysteine, and DNA uracil concentrations. American Journal of Clinical Nutrition, Vol.88, No.4, (October 2008), pp. 1149-1158, ISSN 0002-9165

Feix, A.; Fritsche-Polanz, R.; Kletzmayr, J.; Vychytil, A.; Horl, W.H.; Sunder-Plassmann, G. & Födinger, M. (2001). Increased prevalence of combined MTR and MTHFR genotypes among individuals with severely elevated total homocysteine plasma levels. American journal of kidney diseases: the official journal of the National Kidney Foundation, Vol.38, No.5, (November 2001), pp. 956-964, ISSN 0272-6386

Fenech, M. (2002). Micronutrients and genomic stability: a new paradigm for recommended dietary allowances (RDAs). Food and chemical toxicology: an international journal published for the British Industrial Biological Research Association, Vol.40, No.8, (August 2002), pp. 1113-1117, ISSN 0278-6915

Fenech, M.; Baghurst, P.; Luderer, W.; Turner, J.; Record, S.; Ceppi, M. & Bonassi, S. (2005). Low intake of calcium, folate, nicotinic acid, vitamin E, retinol, b-carotene and high intake of pantothenic acid, biotin and riboflavin are significantly associated with increased genome instability - results from a dietary intake and micronucleus index survey in South Australia. Carcinogenesis, Vol. 26, No.5, (May 2005), pp. 991–999, ISSN 0143-3334

Fenech, M.; Kirsch-Volders, M.; Natarajan, A.T.; Surralles, J.; Crott, J.W.; Parry, J.; Norppa, H.; Eastmond, D.A.; Tucker, J.D. & Thomas P. (2011). Molecular mechanisms of micronucleus, nucleoplasmic bridge and nuclear bud formation in mammalian and human cells. Mutagenesis, Vol.26, No.1, (January 2011), pp. 125-132, ISSN 0267-8357

Fillon-Emery, N.; Chango, A.; Mircher, C.; Barbé, F.; Bléhaut, H.; Herbeth, B.; Rosenblatt, D.S.; Réthoré, M.O.; Lambert, D. & Nicolas, J.P. (2004). Homocysteine concentrations in adults with trisomy 21: effect of B vitamins and genetic polymorphisms. The American Journal of Clinical Nutrition,Vol.80, No.6, (December 2004), pp. 1551–1557, ISSN 0002-9165

Finkelstein, J.D. & Martin, J.J. (2000). Homocysteine. The International Journal of Biochemistry & Cell Biology, Vol.32, No.4, (April 2000), pp. 385-389, ISSN 1357-2725

Fintelman-Rodrigues, N.; Corrêa, J.C.; Santos, J.M.; Pimentel, M.M. & Santos-Rebouças, C.B. (2009). Investigation of CBS, MTR, RFC-1 and TC polymorphisms as maternal risk factors for Down syndrome. Disease Markers,Vol.26, No.4, pp. 155-161, ISSN 0278-0240

Fredriksen, A.; Meyer, K.; Ueland, P.M.; Vollset, S.E.; Grotmol, T. & Schneede, J. (2007). Large-scale population-based metabolic phenotyping of thirteen genetic polymorphisms related to one-carbon metabolism. Human Mutation,Vol.28, No.9, (September 2007), pp. 856–865, ISSN 1098-1004

Friso, S.; Choi, S.W.; Girelli, D.; Mason, J.B.; Dolnikowski, G.G.; Bagley, P.J.; Olivieri, O.; Jacques, P.F.; Rosenberg, I.H.; Corrocher, R. & Selhub, J. (2002). A common mutation in the 5,10-methylenetetrahydrofolate reductase gene affects genomic DNA methylation through an interaction with folate status. Proceedings of the National Academy of Sciences of the United States of America, Vol.99, No.8, (April 2002), pp. 5606-5611, ISSN 0027-8424

Frosst, P.; Blom, H.J.; Milos, R.; Goyette, P.; Sheppard, C.A.; Matthews, R.G.; Boers, G.J.H.; den Heijer, M.; Kluijtmans, L.A.J.; van den Heuve, L.P. & Rozen, R. (1995). A candidate genetic risk factor for vascular disease: a common mutation in Methylenetetrahydrofolate reductase. Nature Genetics,Vol.10,No.1, (May 1995), pp. 111-113, ISSN 1061-4036

Gellekink, H.; Blom, H.J.; van der Linden, I.J. & den Heijer, M. (2007). Molecular genetic analysis of the human dihydrofolate reductase gene: relation with plasma total homocysteine, serum and red blood cell folate levels. European Journal of Human Genetics: EJHG,Vol.15, No.1, (January 2007), pp. 103-109, ISSN 1018-4813

Ghosh, S.; Feingold, E. & Dey, S.K. (2009). Etiology of Down syndrome: Evidence for consistent association among altered meiotic recombination, nondisjunction, and maternal age across populations. American Journal of Medical Genetics Part A, Vol.149A, No.7, (July 2009), pp. 1415-1420, ISSN 1552-4825

Guenther, B.D.F.; Sheppard, C.A.; Tran, P.; Rozen, R.; Matthews, R.G. & Ludwig, M.L. (1999). The structure and properties of methylenetetrahydrofolate reductase from Escherichia coli suggest how folate ameliorates human hyperhomocysteinemia. Nature Structural and Molecular Biology, Vol.6, No.4, (April 1999), pp. 359-365, ISSN 1072-8368

Hall, J. & Solehdin, F. (1998). Folic acid for the prevention of congenital anomalies. European Journal of Pediatrics,Vol.157, No.6, (June 1998), pp. 445-450, ISSN 0340-6199

Harmon, D.L.; Shields, D.C.; Woodside, J.V.; McMaster, D.; Yarnell, J.W.G.; Young, I.S.; Peng, K.; Shane, B.; Evans, A.E. & Whitehead, A.S. (1999). Methionine synthase D919G polymorphism is a significant but modest determinant of circulating homocysteine concentrations. Genetic Epidemiology, Vol.17, No.4, (November 1999),pp. 298–309, ISSN 0741-0395

Hasle, H.; Clemmensen, I.H. & Mikkelsen, M. (2000). Risks of leukaemia and solid tumours in individuals with Down's syndrome. Lancet, Vol.355, No.9199, (January 2000), pp. 165-169, ISSN 0140-6736

Hassold, T. & Sherman, S. (2000). Down syndrome: genetic recombination and the origin of the extra chromosome 21. Clinical Genetics, Vol.57, No.2, (February 2000), pp. 95–100, ISSN 0009-9163

Hassold, T. & Hunt, P. (2001). To err (meiotically) is human: the genesis of human aneuploidy. Nature Reviews. Genetics, Vol.2, No.4, (April 2001), pp. 280-291, ISSN 1471-0056

Herrera, L.A.; Prada, D.; Andonegui, M.A. & Dueñas-González, A. (2008). The epigenetic origin of aneuploidy. Current Genomics, Vol.9, No.1, (March 2008), pp. 43-50, ISSN 1389-2029

Hobbs, C.A.; Cleves, M.A.; Lauer, R.M.; Burns, T.L. & James, S.J. (2002). Preferential transmission of the MTHFR 677 T allele to infants with Down syndrome: implications for a survival advantage. American Journal of Medical Genetics, Vol.113, No.1, (November 2002), pp. 9-14, ISSN 1552-4825

Hum, D.W.; Bell, A.W.; Rozen, R. & MacKenzie, R.E. (1988). Primary structure of a human trifunctional enzyme. Isolation of a cDNA encoding methylenetetrahydrofolate dehydrogenase-methenyltetrahydrofolate cyclohydrolase-formyltetrahydrofolate synthetase. The Journal of Biological Chemistry, Vol.263, No.31, (November 1988), pp. 15946–15950, ISSN 0021-9258

James, S.J.; Melnyk, S.; Jernigan, S.; Pavliv, O.; Trusty, T.; Lehman, S.; Seidel, L.; Gaylor, D.W. & Cleves, M.A. (2010). A functional polymorphism in the reduced folate carrier gene and DNA hypomethylation in mothers of children with autism. American Journal of Medical Genetics. Part B, Neuropsychiatric genetics : the official publication of the International Society of Psychiatric Genetics, Vol. 153B, No. 6, (September 2010), pp. 1209-1220, ISSN 1552-4841

Johnson, W.G.; Stenroos, E.S.; Spychala, J.R.; Chatkupt, S.; Ming, S.X. & Buyske, S. (2004). New 19 bp deletion polymorphism in intron-1 of dihydrofolate reductase (DHFR): a risk factor for spina bifida acting in mothers during pregnancy? American Journal of Medical Genetics Part A, Vol.124, No.4, (February 2004), pp.339-345, ISSN 1552-4825

Jones, K.L. (2006). Smith's recognizable patterns of human malformation (6th edition), Elsevier Saunders, ISBN 0-7216-0615-6, Philadelphia.

Jyothy, A.; Kumar, K.S.; Mallikarjuna. G.N.; Babu Rao, V.; Uma Devi, B.; Sujatha M. & Reddy, P.P. (2001). Parental age and the origin of extra chromosome 21 in Down syndrome. Journal of Human Genetics, Vol.46, No.6, pp. 347-350, ISSN1434-5161

Karpen, G.H. & Allshire, R.C. (1997). The case for epigenetic effects on centromere identity and function. Trends in Genetics: TIG, Vol.13, No.12, (December 1997), pp. 489-496, ISSN 0168-9525

Kim, S.Y.; Park, S.Y.; Choi, J.W.; Kim, D.J.; Lee, S.Y.; Lim, J.H.; Han, J.Y.; Ryu, H.M. & Kim, M.H. (2011). Association between MTHFR 1298A>C polymorphism and spontaneous abortion with fetal chromosomal aneuploidy. American Journal of Reproductive Immunology (New York, N.Y.: 1989), (March 2011), Epub ahead of print, ISSN 1046- 7408

Kovaleva, N.V.; Tahmasebi-Hesari, M. & Verlinskaia, D.K. (2010). Grandmaternal age in children with Down syndrome in St. Petersburg. Tsitologiia i Genetika, Vol.44, No.5, (September-October 2010), pp. 47-53, ISSN 0564-3783

Kraus, J.P. (1998). Biochemistry and molecular genetics of cystathionine beta-synthase deficiency. European Journal of Pediatrics,Vol.157, No.Suppl 2, (April 1998),pp. S50-S53, ISSN 0340-6199

Kumar, J.; Garg, G.; Karthikeyan, G. & Sengupta, S. (2010). Cystathionine beta-synthase 844Ins68 polymorphism is not associated with the levels of homocysteine and cysteine in an Indian population. Biomarkers: biochemical indicators of exposure, response, and susceptibility to chemicals, Vol.15, No.3, (May 2010),pp. 283-287, ISSN 1354-750X

Lamb, N.E.; Freeman, S.B.; Savage-Austin, A.; Pettay, D.; Taft, L.; Hersey, J.; Gu, Y.; Shen, J.; Saker, D.; May, K.M.; Avramopoulos, D.; Petersen, M.B.; Hallberg, A.; Mikkelsen, M.; Hassold, T.J. & Sherman, S.L. (1996). Susceptible chiasmate configurations of chromosome 21 predispose to non-disjunction in both maternal meiosis I and meiosis II. Nature Genetics, Vol.14, No.4, (December 1996), pp. 400-405, ISSN 1061-4036

Lamb, N.E.; Yu, K.; Shaffer, J.; Feingold, E. & Sherman SL. (2005). Association between maternal age and meiotic recombination for trisomy 21. American Journal of Human Genetics, Vol.76, No.1, (January 2005), pp. 91-99, ISSN 0002-9297

Leclerc, D.; Odièvre, M.; Wu, Q.; Wilson, A.; Huizenga, J.J.; Rozen, R.; Scherer, S.W. & Gravel, R.A. (1999). Molecular cloning, expression and physical mapping of the human methionine synthase reductase gene. Gene, Vol.240, No.1, (November 1999),pp. 75-88, ISSN 0378-1119

Li, G.M.; Presnell SR & Gu L. (2003). Folate deficiency, mismatch repair-dependent apoptosis, and human disease. The Journal of Nutritional Biochemistry, Vol.14, No.10, (October 2003), pp. 568-75, ISSN 0955-2863

Lin, M.Y. & Young, C.M. (2000). Folate levels in cultures of lactic acid bacteria. International dairy journal / published in association with the International Dairy Federation., Vol.10, pp. 409–414, ISSN 0958-6946

Linhart, H.G.; Troen, A.; Bell, G.W.; Cantu, E.; Chao, W.H.; Moran, E.; Steine, E.; He, T. & Jaenisch, R. (2009). Folate deficiency induces genomic uracil misincorporation and hypomethylation but does not increase DNA point mutations. Gastroenterology, Vol.136, No.1, (January 2009), pp. 227-235.e3, ISSN 0016-5085

Lott, I.T. & Head, E. (2005). Alzheimer disease and Down syndrome: factors in pathogenesis. Neurobiology of Aging, Vol.26, No.3, pp. 383-389, ISSN 197-4580

Malini, S.S. & Ramachandra, N.B. (2006). Influence of advanced age of maternal grandmothers on Down syndrome. BMC Medical Genetics, Vol.14, (January 2006), pp. 7-4, ISSN 1471-2350

Martínez-Frías, M.L.; Pérez, B.; Desviat, L.R.; Castro, M.; Leal, F.; Rodríguez, L.; Mansilla, E.; Martínez-Fernández, M.L.; Bermejo, E.; Rodríguez-Pinilla, E.; Prieto, D.; Ugarte, M & ECEMC Working Group. (2006). Maternal polymorphisms 677C-T and 1298A-C of MTHFR, and 66A-G MTRR genes: is there any relationship between polymorphisms of the folate pathway, maternal homocysteine levels, and the risk for having a child with Down syndrome? American Journal of Medical Genetics. Part A,Vol.140, No.9, (May 2006), pp. 987-997, ISSN 1552-4825

Martínez-Frías, M.L. (2008). The biochemical structure and function of methylenetetrahydrofolate reductase provide the rationale to interpret the epidemiological results on the risk for infants with Down syndrome. American Journal of Medical Genetics Part A, Vol.146, No.11, (June 2008), pp.1477-1482, ISSN 1552-4825

Matsuzaki, K.; Deng, G.; Tanaka, H.; Kakar, S.; Miura, S. & Kim, Y.S. (2005). The relationship between global methylation level, loss of heterozygosity, and microsatellite instability in sporadic colorectal cancer. Clinical Cancer Research: an official journal of the American Association for Cancer Research, Vol.15, No.11, (December 2005), pp. 8564-8569, ISSN 1078-0432

McNulty, H. & Pentieva, K. (2004). Folate bioavailability. The Proceedings of the Nutrional Society, Vol.63, No.4, (November 2004), pp. 529–536, ISSN 1475-2719.

McNulty, H. & Scott, J.M. (2008). Intake and status of folate and related B-vitamins: considerations and challenges in achieving optimal status. The British Journal of Nutrition, Vol.99, No.Suppl 3, (June 2008), pp. S48-54, ISSN 0007-1145

Meguid, N.A.; Dardir, A.A.; Khass, M.; Hossieny, L.E.; Ezzat, A. & El Awady, M.K. (2008). MTHFR genetic polymorphism as a risk factor in Egyptian mothers with Down syndrome children. Disease Markers, Vol. 24, No.1, pp. 19-26, ISSN 0278-0240

Mendes, C.C.; Biselli, J.M.; Zampieri, B.L.; Goloni-Bertollo, E.M.; Eberlin, M.N.; Haddad, R.; Riccio, M.F.; Vannucchi, H.; Carvalho, V.M. & Pavarino-Bertelli, E.C. (2010). 19-base pair deletion polymorphism of the dihydrofolate reductase (DHFR) gene: maternal risk of Down syndrome and folate metabolism. Sao Paulo Medical Journal,Vol.128, No.4, (July 2010), pp. 215-218, ISSN 1516-3180

Migliore, L.; Boni, G.; Bernardini, R.; Trippi, F.; Colognato, R.; Fontana, I.; Coppedè, F. & Sbrana, I. (2006). Susceptibility to chromosome malsegregation in lymphocytes of women who had a Down syndrome child in young age. Neurobiology of Aging, Vol.27, No.5, (May 2006), pp. 710-716, ISSN 197-4580

Miller, J.W.; Ramos, M.I.; Garrod, M.G.; Flynn, M.A. & Green, R. (2002). Transcobalamin II 775G>C polymorphism and indices of vitamin B12 status in healthy older adults. Blood, Vol.100, No.2, pp. 718-720, ISSN 0006-4971

Mohammad, N.S.; Yedluri, R.; Addepalli, P.; Gottumukkala, S.R.; Digumarti, R.R. & Kutala, V.K. (2011). Aberrations in one-carbon metabolism induce oxidative DNA damage in sporadic breast cancer. Molecular and Cellular Biochemistry, Vol.349, No.1-2, (March 2011), pp. 159-167, ISSN 0300-8177

Naghibalhossaini, F.; Mokarram, P.; Khalili, I.; Vasei, M.; Hosseini, S.V.; Ashktorab, H.; Rasti, M. & Abdollahi, K. (2010). MTHFR C677T and A1298C variant genotypes and the risk of microsatellite instability among Iranian colorectal cancer patients. Cancer Genetics and Cytogenetics, Vol.197, No.2, (March 2010), pp. 142-51, ISSN 0165-4608

Namour, F.; Guy, M.; Aimone-Gastin, I.; de Nonancourt, M.; Mrabet, N. & Guéant, J.L. (1998). Isoelectrofocusing phenotype and relative concentration of transcobalamin II isoproteins related to the codon 259 Arg/Pro polymorphism. Biochemical and Biophysical Research Communications, Vol.251, No.3, (October 1999), pp. 769-774, ISSN 0006-291X

Narayanan, S.; McConnell, J.; Little, J.; Sharp, L.; Piyathilake, C.J.; Powers, H.; Basten, G. & Duthie, S.J. (2004). Associations between two common variants C677T and A1298C in the methylenetetrahydrofolate reductase gene and measures of folate metabolism and DNA stability (strand breaks, misincorporated uracil, and DNA methylation status) in human lymphocytes in vivo. Cancer epidemiology, biomarkers & prevention : a publication of the American Association for Cancer Research, cosponsored by the American Society of Preventive Oncology, Vol.13, No.9, (September 2004), pp.1436-1443, ISSN 055-9965

Nguyen, T.T.; Dyer, D.L.; Dunning, D.D.; Rubin, S.A.; Grant, K.E. & Said, H.M. (1997). Human intestinal folate transport: cloning, expression, and distribution of complementary RNA. Gastroenterology, Vol.112, No.3, (March 1997), pp. 783-791, ISSN 0016-5085

O'Leary, V.B.; Parle-McDermott, A.; Molloy, A.M.; Kirke, P.N.; Johnson, Z.; Conley, M.; Scott, J.M. & Mills, J.L. (2002). MTRR and MTHFR polymorphism: link to Down syndrome? American Journal of Medical Genetics, Vol.107, No.2, (January 2002) pp. 151-155, ISSN 0148-7299

Olteanu, H. & Banerjee, R. (2001). Human methionine synthase reductase, a soluble P-450 reductase-like dual flavoprotein, is sufficient for NADPH-dependent methionine synthase activation. The Journal of Biological Chemistry, Vol.276, No.38, (September 2001), pp. 35558-35563, ISSN 21-9258

Olteanu, H.; Munson, T. & Banerjee, R. (2002). Differences in the efficiency of reductive activation of methionine synthase and exogenous electron acceptors between the common polymorphic variants of human methionine synthase reductase. Biochemistry, Vol.41, No.45, (November 2002), pp. 13378–13385, ISSN 0006-2960

Pajares, M.A. & Pérez-Sala, D. (2006). Betaine homocysteine S-methyltransferase: just a regulator of homocysteine metabolism? Cellular and molecular life sciences : CMLS, Vol.63, No.23, (December 2006), pp. 2792-2803, ISSN 1420-682X

Papoutsakis, C.; Manios, Y.; Magkos, F.; Papaconstantinou, E.; Schulpis, K.H.; Zampelas, A.; Matalas, A.L. & Yiannakouris, N. (2010). Effect of the methylenetetrahydrofolate reductase (MTHFR 677C>T) polymorphism on plasma homocysteine concentrations in healthy children is influenced by consumption of folate-fortified foods. Nutrition (Burbank, Los Angeles County, Calif.), Vol.26, No.10, (October 2010), pp. 969-974, ISSN 0899-9007

Parle-McDermott, A.; Pangilinan, F.; Mills, J.L.; Kirke, P.N.; Gibney, E.R.; Troendle, J.; O'Leary, V.B.; Molloy, A.M.; Conley, M.; Scott, J.M. & Brody, L.C. (2007). The 19-bp deletion polymorphism in intron-1 of dihydrofolate reductase (DHFR) may decrease rather than increase risk for spina bifida in the Irish population. American Journal of Medical Genetics. Part A,Vol.143, No.11, (June 2007), pp. 1174-1180, ISSN 1552-4825

Pavarino-Bertelli, E.C.; Biselli, J.M.; Bonfim, D. & Goloni-Bertollo, E.M. (2009). Clinical profile of children with Down syndrome treated in a genetics outpatient service in the southeast of Brazil. Revista da Associação Médica Brasileira (1992), Vol.55, No.5, (September-October 2009), pp. 547-552, ISSN 0104-4230

Paz, M.F.; Ávila, S.; Fraga, M.F.; Pollan, M.; Capella, G.; Peinado, M.A.; Sanchez-Cespedes, M.; Herman, J.G. & Esteller, M. (2002). Germ-line variants in methyl-group metabolism genes and susceptibility to DNA methylation in normal tissues and human primary tumors. Cancer Research, Vol.62, No.15, (August 2002), pp. 4519-4524, ISSN 0008-5472

Pepe, G.; Vanegas, O.C.; Rickards, O.; Giusti, B.; Comeglio, P.; Brunelli, T; Marcucci, R.; Prisco, D.; Gensini, G.F. & Abbate, R. (1999). World distribution of the T833C/844INS68 CBS in cis double mutation: a reliable anthropological marker. Human Genetics, Vol. 104, No.2, (February 1999), pp. 126-129, ISSN 0340-6717

Piskac-Collier, A.L.; Monroy, C.; Lopez, M.S.; Cortes, A.; Etzel, C.J.; Greisinger, A.J.; Spitz, M.R. & El-Zein, R.A. (2011). Variants in folate pathway genes as modulators of genetic instability and lung cancer risk. Genes, Chromosomes & Cancer, Vol.50, No.1, (January 2011), pp. 1-12, ISSN 1045-2257

Potter, H. (1991). Review and hypothesis: Alzheimer disease and Down syndrome--chromosome 21 nondisjunction may underlie both disorders. American Journal of Human Genetics, Vol.48, No.6, (June 1991), pp. 1192–1200, ISSN 0002-9297

Pozzi, E.; Vergani, P.; Dalprà, L.; Combi, R.; Silvestri, D.; Crosti, F.; Dell, O. M. & Valsecchi, M.G. (2009). Maternal polymorphisms for methyltetrahydrofolate reductase and methionine synthetase reductase and risk of children with Down syndrome.

American Journal of Obstetrics and Gynecology, Vol.200, No.6, (June 2009), pp. 636.e1-6, ISSN 0002-9378

Quadros, E.V.; Regec, A.L.; Khan, K.M.; Quadros, E. & Rothenberg, S.P. (1999). Transcobalamin II synthesized in the intestinal villi facilitates transfer of cobalamin to the portal blood. The American Journal of Physiology, Vol.277, No.1 Pt 1, (July 1999), pp. G161-166, ISSN 0002-9513

Rai, A.K.; Singh, S.; Mehta, S.; Kumar, A.; Pandey, L.K. & Raman, R. (2006). MTHFR C677T and A1298C polymorphisms are risk factors for Down's syndrome in Indian mothers. Journal of Human Genetics,Vol.51, No.4, (February 2006), pp. 278-283, ISSN 4-5161

Ram, G. & Chinen, J. (2011). Infections and immunodeficiency in Down syndrome. Clinical and Experimental Immunology, Vol.164, No.1 (April 2011), pp. 9-16, ISSN 0009-9104

Ray, J.G.; Meier, C.; Vermeulen, M.J.; Cole, D.E.C. & Wyatt, P.R. (2003). Prevalence of trissomy 21 following folic acid food fortification. American Journal of Medical Genetics. Part A, Vol.120, No.3, (July 2003), pp. 309-313, ISSN 1552-4825

Sadiq, M.F.; Al-Refai, E.A.; Al-Nasser, A.; Khassawneh, M. & Al-Batayneh, Q. (2011). Methylenetetrahydrofolate Reductase Polymorphisms C677T and A1298C as Maternal Risk Factors for Down Syndrome in Jordan. Genetic Testing and Molecular Biomarkers,Vol.15, No.1-2, (January-February 2011), pp. 51-57, ISSN 1945-0265

Sakuno, T. & Watanabe, Y. (2009). Studies of meiosis disclose distinct roles of cohesion in the core centromere and pericentromeric regions. Chromosome Research: an international journal on the molecular, supramolecular and evolutionary aspects of chromosome biology, Vol.17, No.2, pp. 239-249, ISSN 0967-3849

Scala, I.; Granese, B.; Sellitto, M.; Salomè, S.; Sammartino, A.; Pepe, A.; Mastroiacovo, P.; Sebastio, G. & Andria, G. (2006). Analysis of seven maternal polymorphisms of genes involved in homocysteine/folate metabolism and risk of Down syndrome offspring. Genetics in medicine : official journal of the American College of Medical Genetics, Vol.8, No.7, (July 2006), pp. 409-416, ISSN 1098-3600

Schupf, N.; Kapell, D.; Nightingale, B.; Lee, J.H.; Mohlenhoff, J.; Bewley, S.; Ottman, R. & Mayeux, R. (2001). Specificity of the fivefold increase in AD in mothers of adults with Down syndrome. Neurology, Vol.57, No.6, (September 2001), pp. 979-984, ISSN 0028-3878

Seetharam B, & Li N. (2000). Transcobalamin II and its cell surface receptor. Vitamins and Hormones, Vol.59, pp. 337-66, ISSN 0083-6729

Sherman, S,L.; Petersen, M.B.; Freeman, S.B.; Hersey, J.; Pettay, D.; Taft, L.; Frantzen, M.; Mikkelsen, M. & Hassold, T.J. (1994). Non-disjunction of chromosome 21 in maternal meiosis I: evidence for a maternal age-dependent mechanism involving reduced recombination. Human Molecular Genetics, Vol.3, No.9, (September 1994), pp. 1529-1535, ISSN 0964-6906

Stanisiawska-Sachadyn, A.; Brown, K.S.; Mitchell, L.E.; Woodside, J.V.; Young, I.S.; Scott, J.M.; Murray, L.; Boreham, C.A.; McNulty, H.; Strain, J.J. & Whitehead, A.S. (2008). An insertion/deletion polymorphism of the Dihydrofolate reductase (DHFR) gene is associated with serum and red blood cell folate concentrations in women. Human Genetics, Vol.123, No.3, (April 2008), pp. 289-295, ISSN 0340-6717

Steck, S.E.; Keku, T.; Butler, L.M.; Galanko, J.; Massa, B.; Millikan, R.C. & Sandler, R.S. (2008). Polymorphisms in Methionine synthase, Methionine synthase reductase and Serine hydroxymethyltransferase, folate and alcohol intake, and colon cancer risk. Journal of Nutrigenetics and Nutrigenomics, 2008,Vol.1, No.4, (June 2008), pp. 196–204, ISSN 1661-6499

Stein, Z.; Stein, W. & Susser, M. (1986). Attrition of trisomies as a maternal screening device. An explanation of the association of trisomy 21 with maternal age. Lancet, Vol.1, No.8487, (April 1986), pp. 944-947, ISSN 0140-6736

Stover, P.J. & Caudill, M.A. (2008). Genetic and epigenetic contributions to human nutrition and health: managing genome-diet interactions. Journal of The American Dietetic Association, Vol.108, No.9, (September 2008), pp. 1480-1487, ISSN 0002-8223

Stover, P.J. (2004). Physiology of folate and vitamin B12 in health and disease. Nutrition Reviews,Vol.62, No.6Pt 2, (June 2004), pp. S3-S12, discussion S13, ISSN 0029-6643

Summers, C.M.; Hammons, A.L.; Mitchell, L.E.; Woodside, J.V.; Yarnell, J.W.G.; Young, I.S.; Evans, A. & Whitehead, A.S. (2008). Influence of the cystathionine b-synthase 844ins68 and methylenetetrahydrofolate reductase 677C4T polymorphisms on folate and homocysteine concentrations. European Journal of Human Genetics: EJHG,Vol.16, No.8, (August 2008), pp.1010-1013, ISSN 1018-4813

Tsai, M.Y.; Bignell, M.; Schwichtenberg, K. & Hanson, N.Q. (1996). High prevalence of a mutation in the cystathionine-b-synthase gene. American Journal of Human Genetics, Vol.59, No.5, (October 1996), pp. 1262–1267, ISSN 0002-9297

Tsai, M.Y.; Welge, B.C.; Hanson, N.Q.; Bignell, M.K.; Vessey, J.; Schwichtenberg, K.; Yang, F.; Bullemer, F.E.; Rasmussen, R. & Graham, K.J. (1999). Genetic causes of mild hyperhomocysteinemia in patients with premature occlusive coronary artery diseases. Atherosclerosis, Vol.143, No.1, (March 1999), pp. 63-170, ISSN 0021-9150

Tsai, M.Y.; Bignell, M.; Yang, F.; Welge, B.G.; Graham, K.J. & Hanson, N.Q. (2000). Polygenic influence on plasma homocysteine: association of two revalent mutations, the 844ins68 of cystathionine b-synthase and A2756G of methionine synthase, with lowered plasma homocysteine levels. Atherosclerosis, Vol.149, No.1, (March 2000), pp. 131–137, ISSN 0021-9150

Ulvik, A.; Ueland, P.M.; Fredriksen, A.; Meyer, K.; Vollset, S.E.; Hoff, G. & Schneede, J. (2007). Functional inference of the Methylenetetrahydrofolate reductase 677 C > T and 1298A > C polymorphisms from a large-scale epidemiological study. Human Genetics, Vol.121, No.1, (March 2007), pp. 57-64, ISSN 0340-6717

van der Put, N.M.; Gabreëls, F.; Stevens, E.M.; Smeitink, J.A.; Trijbels, F.J.; Eskes, T.K.; van den Heuvel, L.P. & Blom HJ. (1998). A second common mutation in the methylenetetrahydrofolate reductase gene: an additional risk factor for neural-tube defects? American Journal of Human Genetics, Vol.62, No.5, (May 1998), pp. 1044-1051, ISSN 0002-9297

Venail, F.; Gardiner, Q.; & Mondain, M. (2004). ENT and speech disorders in children with Down's syndrome: an overview of pathophysiology, clinical features, treatments, and current management. Clinical Pediatrics (Phila), Vol.43, No.9, (November-December 2004), pp. 783-791, ISSN 0009-9228

Vogt, E.; Kirsch-Volders, M.; Parry, J.; & Eichenlaub-Ritter, U. (2008). Spindle formation, chromosome segregation and the spindle checkpoint in mammalian oocytes and susceptibility to meiotic error. Mutation Research, Vol. 651, No.1-2, (March 2008), pp. 14-29, ISSN 0027-5107

von Castel-Dunwoody, K.M.; Kauwell, G.P.; Shelnutt, K.P.; Vaughn, J.D.; Griffin, E.R.; Maneval, D.R.; Theriaque, D.W. & Bailey, L.B. (2005). Transcobalamin 776C->G polymorphism negatively affects vitamin B-12 metabolism. American Journal of Clinical Nutrition,Vol.81, No.6, (June 2005), pp. 1436-1441, ISSN 0002-9165

Vyletal, P.; Sokolová, J.; Cooper, D.N.; Kraus, J.P.; Krawczak, M.; Pepe, G.; Rickards, O.; Koch, H.G.; Linnebank, M.; Kluijtmans, L.A.; Blom, H.J.; Boers, G.H.; Gaustadnes, M.; Skovby, F.; Wilcken, B.; Wilcken, D.E.; Andria, G.; Sebastio, G.; Naughten, E.R.; Yap, S.; Ohura, T.; Pronicka, E.; Laszlo, A. & Kozich, V. (2007). Diversity of cystathionine beta-synthase haplotypes bearing the most common homocystinuria mutation c.833T>C: a possible role for gene conversion. Human Mutation., Vol.28, No.3, (March 2007), pp. 255-264, ISSN 1059-7794

Wang, X.; Thomas, P.; Xue, J. & Fenech, M. (2004). Folate deficiency induces aneuploidy in human lymphocytes in vitro-evidence using cytokinesis-blocked cells and probes specific for chromosomes 17 and 21. Mutation Research, Vol.551, No.1-2, (July 2004), pp. 167-180, ISSN 0027-5107

Wang, S.S.; Qiao, F.Y.; Feng, L. & Lv, J.J. (2008) Polymorphisms in genes involved in folate metabolism as maternal risk factors for Down syndrome in China. Journal of Zhejiang University. Science. B, Vol.9, No.2, (February 2008), pp. 93-99, ISSN 1673-1581

Weisberg, I.S.; Jacques, P.F.; Selhub, J.; Bostom, A.G.; Chen, Z.; Ellison, C.; Eckfeldt, J.H. & Rozen, R. (2001). The 1298A→C polymorphism in methylenetetrahydrofolate reductase (MTHFR): in vitro expression and association with Homocysteine. Atherosclerosis, Vol.156, No.2, (June 2001), pp. 409-415, ISSN 0021-9150

Whetstine, J.R.; Gifford, A.J.; Witt, T.; Liu, X.Y.; Flatley, R.M.; Norris, M.; Haber, M.; Taub, J.W.; Ravindranath, Y. & Matherly, L.H. (2001). Single nucleotide polymorphisms in the human reduced folate carrier: characterization of a high-frequency G/A variant at position 80 and transport properties of the His(27) and Arg(27) carriers. Clinical cancer research : an official journal of the American Association for Cancer Research, Vol. 7, No. 11, (November 2001), pp. 3416-3422, ISSN 1078-0432

Williams, J.D. & Jacobson, M.K. (2010). Photobiological implications of folate depletion and repletion in cultured human keratinocytes. Journal of photochemistry and photobiology. B, Biology, Vol.99, No.1, (April 2010), pp. 49-61, ISSN 1011-1344

Yamada, K.; Chen, Z.; Rozen, R. & Matthews, R.G. (2001). Effects of common polymorphisms on the properties of recombinant human methylenetetrahydrofolate reductase. Proceedings of the National Academy of Sciences of the United States of America, Vol.98, No.26, (December 2001), pp. 14853-14858, ISSN 0027-8424

Yamada, K.; Gravel, R.A.; Toraya, T. & Matthews, R.G. (2006). Human methionine synthase reductase is a molecular chaperone for human methionine synthase. Proceedings of the National Academy of Science of the United States of America, Vol.103, No.25, (June 2006), pp. 9476-9481, ISSN 0027-8424

Yang, Q.H.; Botto, L.D.; Gallagher, M.; Friedman, J.M.; Sanders, C.L.; Koontz, D.; Nikolova, S.; Erickson, J.D. & Steinberg, K. (2008). Prevalence and effects of gene-gene and gene-nutrient interactions on serum folate and serum total homocysteine concentrations in the United States: findings from the third National Health and Nutrition Examination Survey DNA Bank. American Journal of Clinical Nutrition, Vol.88, No.1, (July 2008), pp. 232–246, ISSN 0002-9165

Yoon, P.W.; Freeman, S.B.; Sherman, S.L.; Taft, L.F.; Gu, Y.; Pettay, D.; Flanders, W.D.; Khoury, M.J. & Hassold, T.J. (1996). Advanced maternal age and the risk of Down syndrome characterized by the meiotic stage of chromosomal error: A population-based study. American Journal of Human Genetics, Vol.58, No.3, (March 19960, pp. 628–633, ISSN 0002-9297

Zheng, C.J. Byers, B. (1993). Oocyte selection: a new model for the maternal-age dependence of Down syndrome. Human Genetics, Vol.90, No.1-2, (September-October 1993), pp. 1-6, ISSN 0340-6717

Zijno, A.; Andreoli, C.; Leopardi, P.; Marcon, F.; Rossi, S.; Caiola, S.; Verdina, A.; Galati, R.; Cafolla, A. & Crebelli, R. (2003). Folate status, metabolic genotype, and biomarkers of genotoxicity in healthy subjects. Carcinogenesis, Vol.24, No.6, (June 2003), pp. 1097-1103, ISSN 0143-3334

6

Down Syndrome Expressed Protein; DSCR-1 Deters Cancer and Septic Inflammation

Takashi Minami
RCAST, The University of Tokyo
Japan

1. Introduction

Down syndrome is the most common genetic cause of mental retardation in humans, occurring in one out of 700 live births. Epidemiological studies suggest that although individuals with Down syndrome have an increased risk of infant cardiovascular malformation, muscle hypotonia, lymphatic edema, and leukemia, noteworthy they have a considerably reduced incidence of most solid tumor, atherosclerosis, and pathological angiogenesis-mediated diabetic retinopathy and kidney dysfunction.

Such data indicate that one or more of the 231 trisomic genes on chromosome 21 are responsible for protecting these individuals against cancer and vascular disease. We and others recently have identified the candidate genes are Down syndrome critical region (DSCR)-1, and A disintegrin and metalloproteinase with thrombospondin motifs (ADAMTS)-1. In primary cultured endothelial cells, vascular endothelial cell growth factor (VEGF) resulted in rapid and profound upregulation of both genes, which in turn negatively feeds back to attenuate VEGF-mediated signaling and following the endothelial cell activation. In genome-wide screening, important regulatory transcription factor for many pathological features of Down syndrome, NFAT, bound more than 10,000 independent regions in VEGF-treated activated endothelial cells. Down syndrome trisomy model mice or endothelium-specific modest DSCR-1 increases in mice resulted in significant suppression of the vascular density in matrigel-plugs, inflammatory leukocyte infiltration, and tumor growth. In contrast, DSCR-1 null mice demonstrated markedly decreased vascular integrity and increased susceptibility to tumor metastasis. In a mouse model of endotoxemia, DSCR-1 null mice showed greater morbidity and mortality compared with wild-type littermate. Conversely, adenovirus-mediated overexpression of DSCR-1 resulted in marked attenuation of lipopolysaccharide (LPS) or VEGF-mediated inflammation. Collectively, these data provide that Down syndrome overexpressed protein; DSCR-1 serves to dampen the host response to infection and the tumor growth. The molecular research for Down syndrome with patients or model mice unexpectedly provide us a great hint for therapeutic targets in solid tumor and vasculopathic disease against all individuals.

2. Down Syndrome Critical Region (DSCR)-1 expression in activated endothelium

2.1 Foundation of the DSCR-1 from endothelial cell research

The endothelium is highly malleable cell layer, constantly responding to changes within the extracellular environment and responding in ways that are usually beneficial, but at times harmful to the organism. Several mediators, including growth factors (e.g. vascular endothelial growth factor, VEGF), inflammatory cytokines (e.g. tumor necrosis factor-α, TNF-α), and thrombosis mediator (e.g. thrombin), activate gene transcription in endothelial cells, resulting in changes in hemostatic balance, increased leukocyte adhesion, loss of barrier function, increased permeability, migration, proliferation and successive angiogenesis (Minami and Aird, 2005). The tight control of these processes is essential for homeostasis - endothelial cell activation, if excessive, sustained or spatially and temporally misplaced, may result in vasculopathic disease. Indeed, different extra-cellular mediators engage the endothelium in ways that differ from one signal to the next. A major important point is to survey the temporal and spatial dynamics of endothelial cell activation. Using DNA microarrays, I carried out a global survey of mRNA in human umbilical vein endothelial cells (HUVEC) treated in the VEGF, thrombin, or TNF-α. Clustering analyses of the data revealed a far closer relationship between VEGF and thrombin, than between other pairings (Fig. 1A). Of the various transcripts that were responsive both to VEGF and thrombin, DSCR-1 was the most highly induced at the earliest time point (1 h). Compared with VEGF and thrombin, TNF-α treatment of HUVEC resulted in far less induction of DSCR-1 (3.2-fold at 1 h) (not shown). The rest of the VEGF-mediated induced gene was early growth response (Egr)-3, nerve growth factor inducible (NGFI)-Bβ, cyclooxigenase (COX)-2, and ADAMTS-1 (**Fig. 1B**).

2.2 Molecular information of the DSCR-1

The DSCR-1 gene consists of 7 exons, of which exons 1-4 can be alternatively spliced, resulting in a number of different mRNA isoforms, each of which exhibit different expression patterns. In adult, there are two major isoforms, DSCR-1 long variant (DSCR-1L) and DSCR-1 short variant (DSCR-1s), expressed in organs (Fuentes et al., 1997). DSCR-1L, encoded by exons 1, 5, 6, and 7, is highly expressed in brain. Exon 1 was originally thought to encode a 29 amino acid region, but later studies revealed a start site further upstream, resulting in a larger 84 amino acid region (Genesca et al., 2003). In contrast, DSCR-1s is encoded by exons 4-7 and is under the control of a different promoter located in intron 3 (intergenic promoter) (**Fig. 1C**). Each promoter contains different regulatory transcriptional subunits. For example, DSCR-1s is mainly regulated by the calcineurin-NFAT pathway, which is highly induced by angiogenic and inflammatory stimuli in endothelial cells (Minami et al., 2004; Minami et al., 2006).

While, the DSCR-1L isoform is under the control of a Notch and Hes-1-dependent pathway (Mammucari et al., 2005) or TEF-1 dependent pathway (Liu et al., 2008). DSCR-1s inhibits calcineurin phosphatase activity, and the C-terminal 57 residues are sufficient for this activity. DSCR-1s strongly inhibits the calcineurin mediated NFAT signaling via two ways; its ability to disrupt binding of calcineurin to NFAT, and to disrupt calcineurin enzymatic activities (**Fig. 1D**).

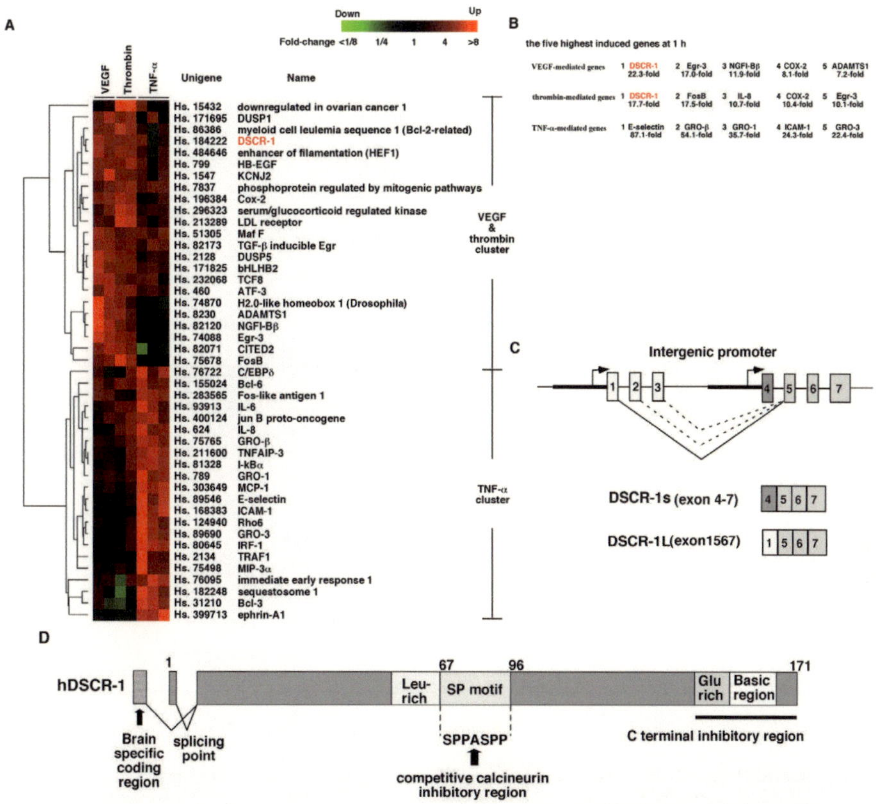

Fig. 1. VEGF / thrombin-mediated DSCR-1 induction *A*, heat map representation of induced genes in HUVEC. *B*, Top 5 genes induced via VEGF, thrombin, or TNF-α. *C*, major two variants of DSCR-1. *D*, structure information of DSCR-1

2.3 DSCR-1 expression in cultured cells

VEGF or thrombin induces the DSCR-1s expression in endothelial cells, through the coordinate binding of NFATc and GATA to closely positioned NFAT and GATA motifs in the intergenic promoter (Minami et al., 2004). VEGF/thrombin induces NFATc nuclear localization, and overexpression of the nuclear NFATc1 greatly induces the targeted DSCR-1s expression (Hesser et al., 2004; Minami et al., 2004; Minami et al., 2006). In addition, endothelial cells from the Down syndrome model mice (Ts65Dn) increased DSCR-1 mRNA by 1.7-2.0 fold (Baek et al., 2009). NFATc is an important factor for regulating the vertebrate development (Graef et al., 2001). In endothelial cells, NFATc1, c2, and c3 are expressed (Minami et al., 2009). To survey the NFATc1 binding in genome-widely, we carried out the chromatin immunoprecipitation using the antibody against NFATc1 following the comprehensive sequencing (ChIP-seq) in endothelial cells. We found totally 10,938 regions (*P* value >20) were identified as NFATc1 enrichment area from the ChIP-seq. DSCR-1 revealed the profound NFATc1 binding after the VEGF treatment within the proximal DSCR-1s promoter (**Fig. 2**). The area overlapped with positive signals from acetylated histone H4 (transcriptional active chromatin) and tri-methylated lysine of histone H3 (H3K4me3; active promoter marking) (**Fig. 2**).

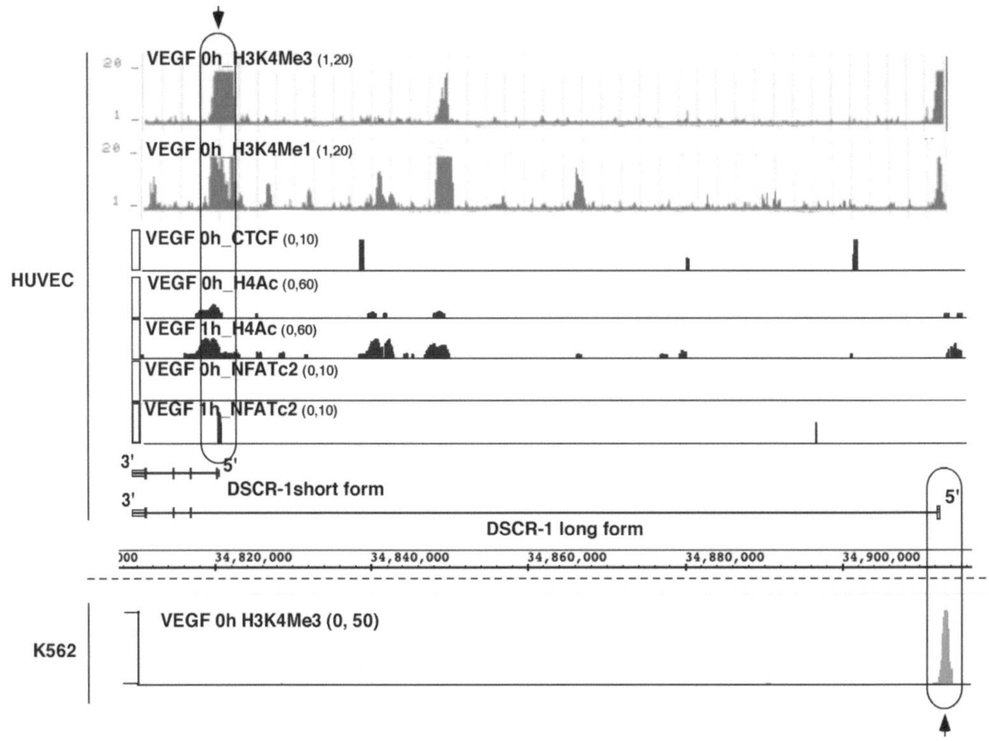

Fig. 2. Epigenetic information of the DSCR-1 locus Arrow indicates the significant enrichment from the ChIP-seq results

In contrast, erythroid lineage cells isolated from leukemia; K562 indicated the H3K4me3 positive signals within the proximal DSCR-1L promoter region, but not proximal DSCR-1s promoter region (**Fig. 2**). DSCR-1L reported the proceeding the pathological function in neurons (Cook et al., 2005). Moreover, Down syndrome patients have an increased risk of leukemia (Lott, 1982). Collectively, DSCR-1s and DSCR-1L obtained separate transcriptional machinery. VEGF mediated NFATc activation selectively transactivates the DSCR-1s via the profound binding within the promoter.

2.4 Characterization of the NFAT dependent genes overexpressed in Down syndrome

Besides DSCR-1, other genes encoded in chromosome 21 also reported as a candidate for pathogenesis on the Down syndrome. By using the combination of several NFATc knockout mice, dysfunction of NFAT was shown as a key point for the onset of Down syndrome (Arron et al., 2006). Around 1.5-fold increasing of both DSCR-1 and DYRK1A caused complete NFAT dysfunction. Thus, we test whether many Down syndrome genes obtain the NFATc1 binding on the each proximal promoter, by using the whole-genome NFATc1 ChIP-seq data (**Table 1**). Interestingly, DYRK1A obtained positive NFATc1 binding. VEGF inducible ADAMTS-1 (see **Fig. 1B**) also showed the NFATc1 positive binding. Ets family, Ets2, ERG, and GABPα, were highly expressed in endothelial cells, which was shown the regulation for the endothelial cell-specific expression or-essential function. All of them have a possibility as a NFATc1 direct target downstream gene.

	Gene	Description	NFATc1 bound	Bound peak area
From Nature (Reynolds et al.2010)				
	ADAMTS1	A disintegrin and metalloproteinase with thrombospondin motifs, type 1	+	5'UTR
	ERG	v-ets erythroblastosis virus E26 oncogene homolog	+	+5367 & 5th intron
	Ets2	v-ets erythroblastosis virus E26 oncogene homolog 2	+	+55
	JAM2	junction adhesion molecule 2	-	
	PTTG1IP	pituitary tumor-transforming 1 interacting protein	+	+883
From Lancet (Roizen and Patterson, 2003)				
Energy and reactive oxygen species metabolism				
	BTG3	B-cell translocation gene 3	+, weak	1st intron
	MRPL39	mitochondrial ribosomal protein L39	+, weak	1st exon
	ATP5J	ATP synthase, H+ transporting, subunit F6	+, weak	1st exon
	GABPA	GA binding protein transcription factor, alpha	+, weak	+80
	BACH1	BTB and CNC homology 1, basic leucine zipper transcription factor 1	+, weak	1st intron
	SOD1	superoxide dismutase 1	+	5'UTR
	CRYZL1	crystallin, zeta-like 1	+, weak	1st Exon & +520
	ATP5O	ATP synthase, H+ transporting, O subunit	+	5'UTR
	MRPS6	mitochondrial ribosomal protein S6	+, weak	5'-UTR
	DSCR-1	Down syndrome critical region gene 1	+	Indicated in Fig. 2
	CBR1	carbonyl reductase 1	+, weak	1st exon
	CBR3	carbonyl reductase 3	+	1st exon
	SH3BGR	SH3 domain binding glutamic acid-rich protein	+	5'UTR
	NDUFV3	NADH dehydrogenase flavoprotein 3, 10kDa	+	+139
	SNF1LK	salt-inducible kinase 1	-	
	C21orf2	chromosome 21 open reading frame 2	+, weak	+140
Brain development, neuronal loss, and Alzheimer's type neuropathology				
	SIM2	single-minded homolog 2	-	
	DYRK1A	dual-specificity tyrosine-phosphorylation regulated kinase 1A	+	+1680

	GART	phosphoribosylglycinamide formyltransferase	+	+513 & 5'-UTR
	PCP4	Purkinje cell protein 4	-	
	DSCAM	Down syndrome cell adhesion molecule	-	
	GRIK1	glutamate receptor, ionotropic, kainate 1	-	
	APP	amyloid beta (A4) precursor protein	+, weak	1st intron
	S100B	S100 Ca-binding protein B	-	
Folate methyl group metabolism				
	N6AMT1	N-6 adenine-specific DNA methyltransferase 1	+, weak	1st exon
	CBS	cystathionine-beta-synthase	-	
	DNMT3L	DNA methyltransferase 3-like	-	
	SLC19A1	Solute carrier family 19 , member 1	-	
	FTCD	formiminotransferase cyclodeaminase	-	
	HRMT1L1 (PRMT2)	Protein arginine methyltransferase 2	+	5'UTR

Table 1. Candidate genes for Down syndrome, where NFATc1 occupancy on the promoter. 'Weak 'means P value < 20

2.5 DSCR-1 expression in organ

Increased DSCR-1 expression was observed in human fetal Down syndrome kidney versus age-matched control kidney (**Fig. 3A**). To determine whether the DSCR-1s promoter region directed inducible expression *in vivo*, the -1664/+83 DSCR-1s promoter was coupled to the *lacZ* reporter gene and targeted the resulting transgenic cassette (DSCR-1-*lacZ*) to the *Hprt* locus of mice using homologous recombination. The *Hprt*-locus *in vivo* promoter analysis system has been previously shown to be beneficial in controlling and avoiding the undesirable and undetectable effects of copy number and integration site on promoter activity (Cvetkovic et al., 2000; Ryan and Sigmund, 2003). We have used this system successfully to show the vascular bed specific expression patterns of endothelial cell specific promoters, Flt-1, vWF, ROBO4, and Tie-2 (Minami et al., 2002; Minami et al., 2003; Okada et al., 2007). At embryonic day 11, whole-mount *lacZ* staining revealed widespread expression of the transgene in the vasculature. In cryosections, strong staining was observed in the dorsal aorta, intersomitic vessels, carotid arteries, caudal veins, the primary head vein branch, and the endocardium (**Fig. 3B**). *LacZ* colocalized with endothelial PECAM-1 (**Fig. 3B**). However, after the embryonic day 14, profound DSCR-1s promoter activation in vascular endothelium was markedly downregulated correlated with the decline of embryonic VEGF levels after the critical steps for angiogenesis and vascular remodeling. In adult mice, DSCR-1s-*lacZ* activity was detected in only a subset of endothelial cells in the brain, heart, lung and kidney. Expression was also observed in occasional neurons, vascular smooth muscle cells, cardiomyocytes, and renal epithelial cells. In contrast, DSCR-1s-*lacZ* activity was undetectable in the liver, spleen, thigh skeletal muscle, and thymus. These findings suggest that the DSCR-1s promoter, though widely expressed in the endothelium of embryonic days 11, is downregulated in the later stages of development and in adults.

Subsequently, to determine whether the DSCR-1s promoter confers response to inflammatory or angiogenic stimuli *in vivo*, DSCR-1-*lac*Z mice were systemically administrated VEGF or LPS. In whole mount preparations, the X-gal reaction product was detectable in the brain and heart of untreated mice and was further upregulated by VEGF and LPS. In contrast, *lac*Z staining was not observed in skeletal muscle, liver, and spleen vasculature even after the stimulus (data not shown).

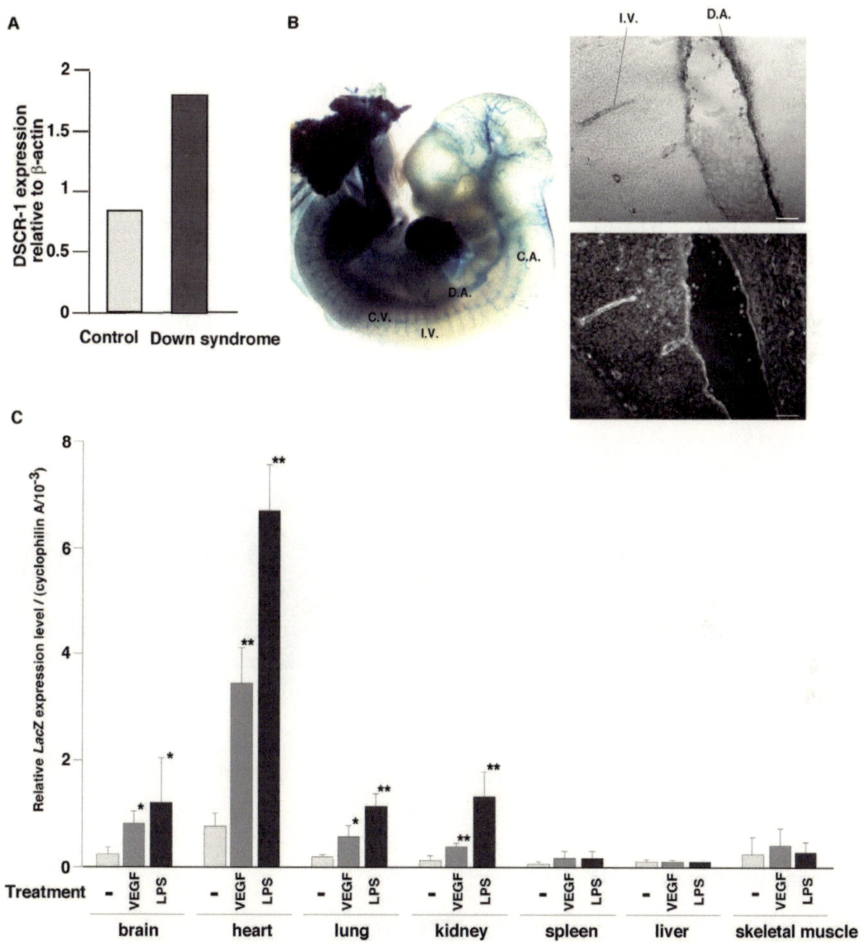

Fig. 3. DSCR-1 promoter activation *in vivo A,* highly DSCR-1 expression in kidney from Down syndrome individuals. *B, left,* whole-mount *lac*Z staining of embryonic day 11 Hprt-targeted embryos. C.A., carotid artery; D.A., dorsal aorta; I.V., intersomite vessel. *Right,* serial tissue sections from Hprt-targeted embryo. *lac*Z (*up*) and PECAM-1 (*down*) immunostainings were shown. *C,* real-time PCR quantification of *lac*Z epression in various organs. *P<0.04, **P<0.01 compared mock treatment in each organ.

Real-time PCR analysis was used to quantify changes in transgene expression. Under basal conditions, *lac*Z mRNA expression was highest in the heart, followed by the brain, lung, and kidney (**Fig. 3C**). Expression in skeletal muscle, the spleen and liver was below the level of detection. VEGF and LPS resulted in significant induction of *lac*Z transcripts in the heart, brain, lung, and kidney, but not in spleen, liver or skeletal muscle (**Fig. 3C**). LPS-mediated induction of the endogenous DSCR-1s gene was similarly restricted to the heart (25.3-fold), brain (7.0-fold), lung (10.3-fold), and kidney (9.3-fold) (not shown). Agonist treatment failed to alter DSCR-1L transcript levels. Thus, VEGF and LPS promote vascular bed-specific expression of both the DSCR-1s promoter and the endogenous DSCR-1s gene.

2.6 DSCR-1 expression in tumor

Solid tumors produce a variety of pro-angiogenic molecules and inflammatory cytokines, which have important paracrine effects on surrounding endothelial cells. To investigated whether the DSCR-1s transgene is activated in tumor blood vessels, B16-F1 melanoma and Lewis lung carcinoma (LLC) cells were implanted subcutaneously into the flank of DSCR-1s-*lacZ Hprt* mice. When tumors reached ≈2.5 cm^3 in volume, the xenografts were harvested, sectioned and stained for *lacZ*. As shown in **Fig. 4A**, there was widespread reporter gene activity within both B16-F1 melanoma and LLC tumor neovessels. In double immunofluorescence studies, *lacZ* co-localized with endothelial PECAM-1 (**Fig. 4B**). Consistent with these findings, endogenous DSCR-1 also co-localized with PECAM-1 in tumor vessels of both B16-F1 melanoma and LLC xenografts (not shown).

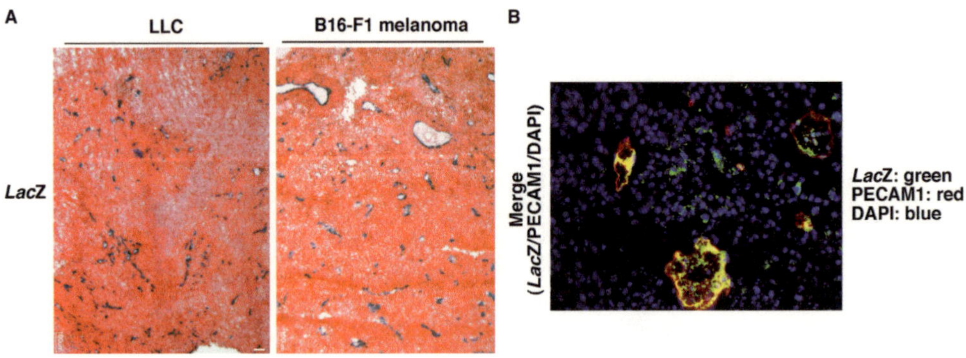

Fig. 4. DSCR-1s promoter activation in tumor vasculature. *A*, *lacZ* stainings were performed of LLC and B16-F1 melanoma xenografts. *B*, merged image of immunofluorescence staining with antibodies against *lacZ*, PECAM-1 or DAPI.

3. Biological function of DSCR-1

3.1 DSCR-1 inhibits nuclear localization of NFATc

Adenovirus mediated overexpression of DSCR-1, but not control, inhibited VEGF mediated nuclear localization of NFATc1 and NFATc2 (Minami et al., 2004). DYRK1A is another potential NFAT regulators, which encodes a nuclear serine/threonine kinase that primes substrates for phsphorylation by Glycogen synthase kinase (GSK) 3(Gwack et al., 2006). GSK3 phosphorylates NFATc proteins in the nucleus, resulting in their inactivation and export (Beals et al., 1997). DYRK1A is expressed at elevated levels in some human Down syndrome fetal tissues (Arron et al., 2006). In neuronal cells, DYRK1A inhibits FGF8-mediated induction of NFAT activity. Moreover, it has been shown that a 1.5-fold increase in the dosage of DSCR-1 and DYRK1A, both of which lie within the critical region of human chromosome 21, cooperatively destabilized the calcineurin-NFAT regulatory circuit (Fig. 5), leading to many of the features of Down syndrome (Arron et al., 2006).

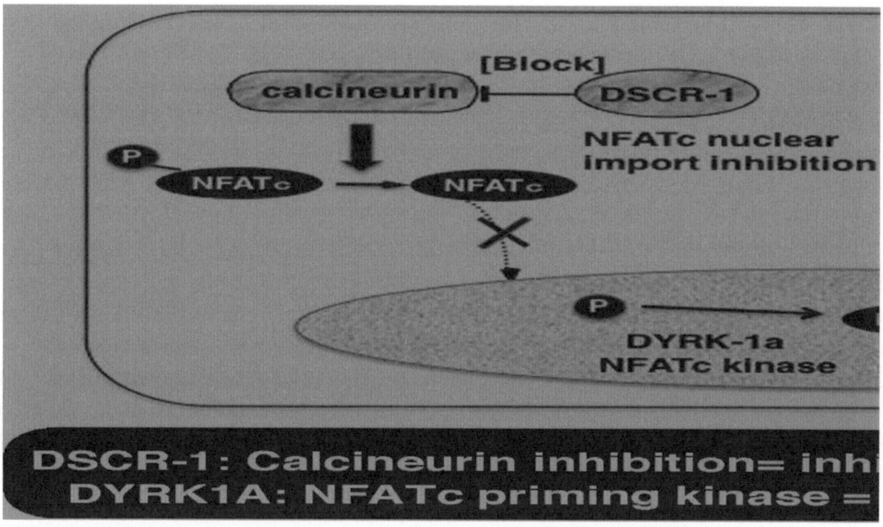

Fig. 5. schematic model of NFAT inhibition with DSCR-1 and DYRK1A.

3.2 DSCR-1s auto-inhibits the VEGF-mediated vascular activation

VEGF is an endothelial cell specific mitogen, and chemotactic agent, which is involved in wound repair, angiogenesis of ischemic tissue, tumor growth, microvascular permeability, hemostasis and endothelial cell survival (Isner and Losordo, 1999). DSCR-1 overexpression inhibits VEGF-mediated vessel growth, and monocyte cell adhesion (Minami et al., 2006). DSCR-1 overexpression did not lead in increased apoptosis (Minami et al., 2009). Taken together, these findings suggest that DSCR-1 constitutive expression lead the endothelial cells to quiescent status form the VEGF-mediated activated status.

3.3 DSCR-1s attenuates septic inflammation

As shown above, DSCR-1s attenuates VEGF-mediated activation of cultured endothelial cells. These data led us to hypothesize that VEGF- and LPS-inducible expression of DSCR-1s in mice may serve as a negative feedback inhibitor of endothelial activation *in vivo*. To test this hypothesis, I examined the effect of DSCR-1 deficiency or overexpression on endotoxemia phenotype. The generation of DSCR-1$^{-/-}$ mice, which carry a targeted deletion of both DSCR-1s and DSCR-1L. To overexpress DSCR-1s, I have chosen an adenoviral delivery system in which the endothelial-specific Flt-1 promoter is coupled to DSCR-1s cassette (Ad-Flt1-DSCR-1s). *In vivo* delivery of Ad-Flt1-DSCR-1s results in overexpression of DSCR-1s in the intact endothelium of mice. Endotoxemia in mice is associated with a reduction in heart rate, blood pressure, and body temperature, and an increase in circulating interleukin (IL)-6 levels. This effect was accentuated in DSCR-1$^{-/-}$ mice, and attenuated in DSCR-1s overexpressing animals. Recently, Yano et.al. reported that endotoxemia in mice is associated with increased circulating levels of VEGF (Yano et al., 2006). Further, VEGF plays a pathogenic role in sepsis (Yano et al., 2008). Interestingly, resting levels of plasma VEGF were 5.0-fold higher in DSCR-1$^{-/-}$ mice compared with wild-type littermates (**Fig. 6A**), which is a parallel correlation with the report that lower VEGF expression in stem cell culture derived from amniotic fluid in Down Syndrome (Salvolini et al., 2010). In response to septic treatment, DSCR-1$^{-/-}$ mice demonstrated super-induction of circulating VEGF levels (2.2-

fold higher vs. wild-type mice). Ad-Flt1-DSCR-1s-injected mice had no change in resting VEGF levels. However, in response to endotoxemia, DSCR-1s-overexpressing mice demonstrated a 61% reduction in circulating VEGF levels compared with septic Ad-Flt1-control (**Fig. 6A**).

To assay for endothelial activation, real-time PCR was performed to measure mRNA expression of E-selectin, intercellular adhesion molecule (ICAM)-1 and vascular cell adhesion molecule (VCAM)-1 in tissues from mice 6 h following injection of PBS (control) or LPS. Compared with wild-type littermate controls, LPS-treated DSCR-1$^{-/-}$ mice demonstrated super-induction of E-selectin in the heart and lung, ICAM-1 in heart, and VCAM-1 in lung. In contrast, LPS-mediated induction of cell adhesion molecules was attenuated by overexpression of DSCR-1s (data not shown).

I have recently shown that hyper-activation of the VEGF-calcineurin-NFAT pathway triggers apoptosis in DSCR-1-deficient tumor endothelial cells (Minami et al., 2009). Given that DSCR-1$^{-/-}$ mice have elevated circulating levels of VEGF level (see **Fig. 6A**), I hypothesized that endotoxemia may result in increased endothelial cell apoptosis in DSCR-1$^{-/-}$ mice. To test this hypothesis, TUNEL assay was carried out in tissue sections from the heart and lung of LPS-treated DSCR-1-null mice and their wild-type littermates. Endotoxemic wild-type mice demonstrated a small number of TUNEL-positive endothelial cells in the heart, and even fewer in the lung. However, in DSCR-1$^{-/-}$ mice, LPS administration resulted in a significant increase in the number of TUNEL-positive cells in both organs (Minami et al., 2009).

Finally in survival studies, LPS-treated DSCR-1$^{-/-}$ mice demonstrated markedly increased mortality compared with endotoxemic wild-type littermates (**Fig.6B**, *left*). In contrast, Ad-mediated overexpression of DSCR-1s conferred a survival advantage compared with Ad-Flt1-control (**Fig. 6B**, *right*). Taken together, these findings suggest that inflammatory induced DSCR-1s obtains a critical role in the host response.

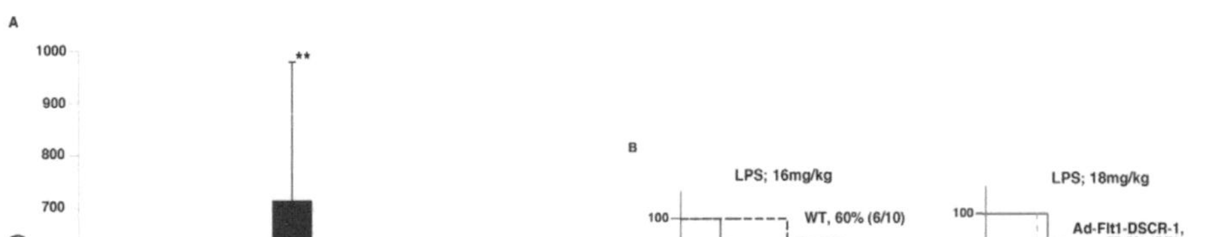

Fig. 6. DSCR-1 modulates inflammatory VEGF expression and sepsis mortality. *A,* Blood was harvested for plasma, and VEGF levels were measured using ELISA. *P<0.001, **P<0.01 compared with wild type or Ad-Flt1-control (cont), n=10. *B,* Survival studies in mice administrated LPS. Percentages of mice (surviving/total) are indicated.

3.4 DSCR-1s attenuates tumor progression

Having established an inhibitory role for DSCR-1 on inflammation *in vivo*, I next study the functional relevance of angiogenesis, tumor growth, and tumor metastasis *in vivo*. Adenovirus mediated locally DSCR-1 expression in vascular demonstrated significant reduction of the blood vessel formation in a matrigel-plug, compared to the Ad-control treated-plug vascularity. In a xenograft model with B16 melanoma and Lewis lung carcinoma revealed that DSCR-1 overexpression statistically significant (more than 70%) reduction of the tumor growth, in the parallel for the reduction of the vessel density from DSCR-1 treated tumor. Subsequently, to test whether DSCR-1 stable expression in the vascular endothelium inhibit the tumor growth, the transgenic mice was generated containing the endothelial cell specific Tie 2 promoter-linked DSCR-1s cDNA constract. Two independent transgenic lines indicate the vascular-specific DSCR-1s expression, both of which delayed the tumor growth at the early step, up to the tumor mass ≈1,500 cm^3. Cryosection of the xenografted tumor and immunostained with anti-PECAM1 antibody revealed the reduction of the vascular density in vascular specific DSCR-1s transgenic mice compared with wild type control mice. Taken together, DSCR-1s expressed in endothelial cells *in vivo* would function as an anti-angiogenic molecule. Stable expression of the DSCR-1s would lead the endogenous anti-tumor activities.

3.5 DSCR-1s attenuates tumor metastasis

During the study for the DSCR-1s promoter activity *in vivo*, by using the tumor metastasis model, we found the DSCR-1s promoter was already active in the lung microvascular endothelium, before the tumor metastasis colony had not yet observed. This DSCR-1s-*lacZ* activity in endothelial lining of lung was clearly abolished by systemic treatment with cyclosporine A. In addition, we have previously shown that stimuli induced DSCR-1 auto-inhibited inflammation in HUVEC (Minami et al., 2004; Minami et al., 2006). Thus, I hypothesized two things; DSCR-1s promoter would be useful for the marker for the pre-metastatic condition, and the DSCR-1s stable expression would overcome the tumor metastasis. At first, to test the latter thing, mice were injected intravenously with $2x10^5$ B16 melanoma cells. Three days later, mice were administrated with adenovirus containing Flt-1 promoter-DSCR-1s, or the control into the lung via the airway with vapor infection. Twenty days after the B16-F10 injection, lungs were harvested and photographed. There was no difference in body weight between the experimental and control groups (data not shown). The Ad-Flt1-Control group exhibited significant endothelial cell surface invaded-melanoma metastasis and the lungs showed significant swelling (**Fig. 7A**). In contrast, the Ad-Flt1-DSCR-1s group exhibited little B16 melanoma metastasis and showed no significant lung swelling. To semi-quantify the metastasis rate, the melanoma-growing area per whole surface was calculated. Compared with control, Ad-Flt1-DSCR-1s treatment resulted in statistically significant reduction (54%) of the B16 melanoma metastasis (**Fig. 7B**). In addition to DSCR-1s's ability to inhibit B16 melanoma metastasis to lung, DSCR-1s treated lung showed a significant reduction in the expression of the inflammatory adhesion molecules, VCAM-1 and E-selectin. It has been reported that endothelial cells expressed VCAM-1 and E-selectin positively influence cancer cell adhesion and migration to lung (Biancone et al., 1996; Fukuda et al., 2000; Futakuchi et al., 2004). Our performed metastasis assays, however, could not distinguish whether reduction in these adhesion molecules attenuated tumor metastasis, or reduced tumor cell migration to lung inhibited inflammation and adhesion molecule induction. We have reported DSCR-1s strongly attenuates adhesion molecule expression in cultured endothelial cells (Minami et al., 2006). Moreover, DSCR-1 stably expressed in cultured endothelial cells significantly blocked B16 melanoma attachment to the endothelial cell surface (data not shown), suggesting that the blunting of adhesion molecule expression by DSCR-1s might be a critical factor in the inhibition of tumor metastasis. Collectively, These data suggest that DSCR-1s stable expression inhibits the inflammatory coordinated pre-metastatic niche formation, resulting the strong interfering of the onset of tumor metastasis to lung.

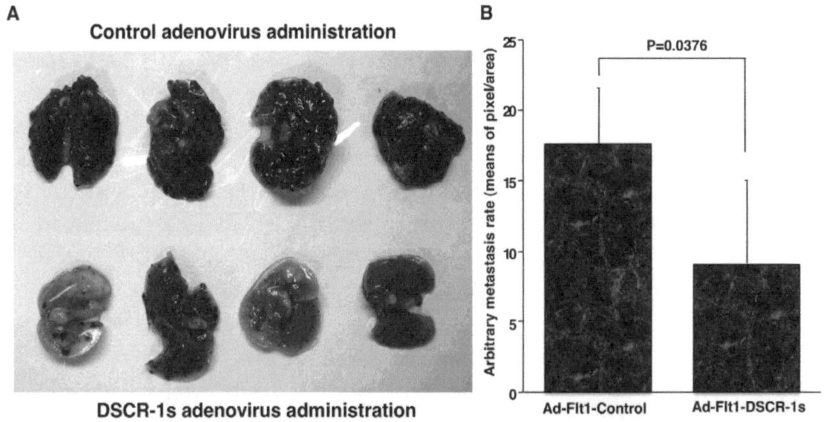

Fig. 7. Endothelial specific DSCR-1s overexpression downregulates the tumor metastasis to lung. *A*, after 20 days for B16-F10 injection administrated either Ad-Flt1-control or Ad-Flt1-DSCR-1s, lungs were harvested, washed and photographed. *B*, to quantify the metastasis rate, metastasis area from the whole surface lung was calculated by using Image J software. Data are expressed as means and standard deviations; n=10.

3.6 Lacking DSCR-1 results with controversy

While our findings reported here lend further evidence toward DSCR-1s as a negative regulator of NFAT-calcineurin signaling *in vivo*, the exact function of DSCR-1 is not without controversy. It has been reported that in CHO cells cultured *in vitro*, a portion of the phosphorylated form of DSCR-1 associated with the 14-3-3 protein, which competitively activated calcineurin activity (Abbasi et al., 2006). However, in a separate report it was shown that phosphorylation of DSCR-1 markedly decreased its stability (Genesca et al., 2003), likely leading to degradation, and thus an increase in calcineurin activity. In endothelial cells, we observed that the non-phosphorylated form of DSCR-1, which we consider to be the pre-active form, was the dominant form during the early phase response to VEGF or thrombin. The phenotype exhibited by the DSCR-1 whole gene knockout mice shows exacerbated constitutively active calcineurin-dependent cardiac hypertrophy, whereas cardiac hypertrophy in response to pressure overload and chronic adrenergic stimulation was blunted in these mice (Vega et al., 2003). In addition, double knockout mice of DSCR-1 and modulator of calcineurin interacting protein (MCIP) 2 also resulted in calcineurin facilitation, although it is difficult to distinguish the relative contribution between DSCR-1 and MCIP2 in these events (Sanna et al., 2006). It light of previous results and the results presented here suggesting differing expression patterns and functions of the DSCR-1s and 1L isoforms, it is plausible that the phenotype of the DSCR-1 null mice results from the complex deletion of both DSCR-1L and DSCR-1s isoforms. Qin et.al., recently reported DSCR-1s inhibited vascular growth and capillary tube formation, consistent with our findings, whereas DSCR-1L induced NFATc transcriptional activity and endothelial cell growth (Qin et al., 2006). Using siRNA or adenoviral miRNA in endothelial cells or in mice *in vivo*, respectively, I recently showed that the DSCR-1s promoter is specifically activated through NFATc1, c2, c3 and GATA-2 (Minami et al., 2009), whereas DSCR-1L, which lacks the NFAT consensus region, is regulated by Notch and glucocorticoid signaling (Mammucari et al., 2005). The lack of such elements in the DSCR-1L promoter, suggest that once DSCR-1L is expressed, the tightly regulated calcineurin-NFATc-DSCR-1s feedback loop may be broken, owing to a lack of NFATc regulation of the DSCR-1L promoter. I also cannot rule out the possibility that the DSCR-1 exon 1 has an as yet 'undetermined' function. Interestingly, in an attempt to understand this regulatory system, an attractive computationally simulated threshold model was shown by Shin, et. al (Shin et al., 2006), in which low-level stimulus causes weak NFAT activation, resulting in only minor DSCR-1s upregulation, and at a level not sufficient to block the target calcineurin (under the threshold). Continuing stimulus facilitates the dissociation of the calcineurin-DSCR-1 complex, so that DSCR-1 appears as an activator of calcineurin.

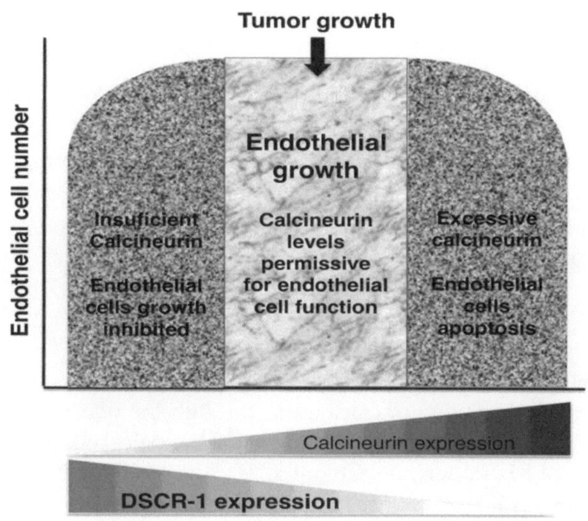

Fig. 8. Schmatic model of the balance of the endothelial cell growth

Interestingly in the endothelial cells, Sandra.et.al., indicated that DSCR-1-/- mice demonstrated reduced blood vessel formation in Matrigel, cornel micropocket, and tumor xenograft assays (Ryeom et al., 2008). DSCR-1-/- endothelial cells displayed hyper-activation of the calcineurin/NFAT pathway and increased sensitivity to VEGF signaling. However, rather than inducing cell proliferation, VEGF-mediated activation of calcineurin/NFAT in DSCR-1-/- endothelial cells 're-routed' downstream signaling, resulting in increased apoptosis, which thus explains the paradoxical reduction in neovascularization. Collectively, considered with the data from DSCR-1 stable expression and null mutation, calcineurin/NFAT activity and DSCR-1s expression level was tightly regulated, resulting the balance would define the endothelial cell growth, viability and tumor angiogenesis (**Fig. 8**). Future animal studies of DSCR-1 function should be performed by endothelial cell-specific knockout mice targeting either DSCR-1s or DSCR-1L separately.

4. Conclusion

DSCR-1 was identified by the study with vascular activation. DSCR-1 was highest induced by VEGF treatment in primary cultured endothelial cells. Previously, DSCR-1 was simply termed by the localization of the human chromosome 21. However, DSCR-1 indeed highly expressed in Down syndrome individuals, and clearly upregulated with NFAT activation in cells. Moreover, combined with same 21st chromosome encoded protein; 'DYRK1A', DSCR-1 strongly feedback attenuated the NFAT activation, resulting the pathogenesis of Down syndrome. I show here that DSCR-1s is highly expressed during embryonic vascular development, and then largely downregulated in adult, yet was highly activated predominantly in endothelium in response to the administration of VEGF or LPS. Stimulated DSCR-1s worked in the auto-inhibition of endothelial cell activation and inflammation. It has still unanswered problems with understanding the phenotypes from DSCR-1 lacking condition, and pathogenesis from DSCR-1L overexpression in neuron. However, based on this knowledge, I believe that DSCR-1s stable expression or the way of DSCR-1s stabilization may lend itself to therapeutic manipulation in vasculopathic disease states, including tumor angiogenesis, metastasis, and inflammation.

5. Acknowledgement

This study was supported by the Leading-edge Research Promotion fund from Japan Society for the Promotion of Science, and in part supported by a Grant-in-Aid for Scientific Research on Innovative Areas from ministry of Education, Culture, Sports, Science, and Technology in Japan and in part by Mochida Memorial and Sankyo Science Foundation in Japan. I am grateful to Dr. Junichi Suehiro (The University of Tokyo, Japan) for providing the ChIP-seq information with NFATc1.

6. References

Abbasi, S., Lee, J.D., Su, B., Chen, X., Alcon, J.L., Yang, J., Kellems, R.E., and Xia, Y. (2006). Protein kinase-mediated regulation of calcineurin through the phosphorylation of modulatory calcineurin-interacting protein 1. The Journal of biological chemistry 281, 7717-7726.

Arron, J.R., Winslow, M.M., Polleri, A., Chang, C.P., Wu, H., Gao, X., Neilson, J.R., Chen, L., Heit, J.J., Kim, S.K., et al. (2006). NFAT dysregulation by increased dosage of DSCR1 and DYRK1A on chromosome 21. Nature 441, 595-600.

Baek, K.H., Zaslavsky, A., Lynch, R.C., Britt, C., Okada, Y., Siarey, R.J., Lensch, M.W., Park, I.H., Yoon, S.S., Minami, T., et al. (2009). Down's syndrome suppression of tumour growth and the role of the calcineurin inhibitor DSCR1. Nature 459, 1126-1130.

Beals, C.R., Sheridan, C.M., Turck, C.W., Gardner, P., and Crabtree, G.R. (1997). Nuclear export of NF-ATc enhanced by glycogen synthase kinase-3. Science 275, 1930-1934.

Biancone, L., Araki, M., Araki, K., Vassalli, P., and Stamenkovic, I. (1996). Redirection of tumor metastasis by expression of E-selectin in vivo. The Journal of experimental medicine 183, 581-587.

Cook, C.N., Hejna, M.J., Magnuson, D.J., and Lee, J.M. (2005). Expression of calcipressin1, an inhibitor of the phosphatase calcineurin, is altered with aging and Alzheimer's disease. J Alzheimers Dis 8, 63-73.

Cvetkovic, B., Yang, B., Williamson, R.A., and Sigmund, C.D. (2000). Appropriate tissue- and cell-specific expression of a single copy human angiotensinogen transgene specifically targeted upstream of the HPRT locus by homologous recombination. The Journal of biological chemistry 275, 1073-1078.

Fuentes, J.J., Pritchard, M.A., and Estivill, X. (1997). Genomic organization, alternative splicing, and expression patterns of the DSCR1 (Down syndrome candidate region 1) gene. Genomics 44, 358-361.

Fukuda, M.N., Ohyama, C., Lowitz, K., Matsuo, O., Pasqualini, R., Ruoslahti, E., and Fukuda, M. (2000). A peptide mimic of E-selectin ligand inhibits sialyl Lewis X-dependent lung colonization of tumor cells. Cancer research 60, 450-456.

Futakuchi, M., Ogawa, K., Tamano, S., Takahashi, S., and Shirai, T. (2004). Suppression of metastasis by nuclear factor kappaB inhibitors in an in vivo lung metastasis model of chemically induced hepatocellular carcinoma. Cancer science 95, 18-24.

Genesca, L., Aubareda, A., Fuentes, J.J., Estivill, X., De La Luna, S., and Perez-Riba, M. (2003). Phosphorylation of calcipressin 1 increases its ability to inhibit calcineurin and decreases calcipressin half-life. The Biochemical journal 374, 567-575.

Graef, I.A., Chen, F., and Crabtree, G.R. (2001). NFAT signaling in vertebrate development. Curr Opin Genet Dev 11, 505-512.

Gwack, Y., Sharma, S., Nardone, J., Tanasa, B., Iuga, A., Srikanth, S., Okamura, H., Bolton, D., Feske, S., Hogan, P.G., et al. (2006). A genome-wide Drosophila RNAi screen identifies DYRK-family kinases as regulators of NFAT. Nature 441, 646-650.

Hesser, B.A., Liang, X.H., Camenisch, G., Yang, S., Lewin, D.A., Scheller, R., Ferrara, N., and Gerber, H.P. (2004). Down syndrome critical region protein 1 (DSCR1), a novel VEGF target gene that regulates expression of inflammatory markers on activated endothelial cells. Blood 104, 149-158.

Isner, J.M., and Losordo, D.W. (1999). Therapeutic angiogenesis for heart failure. Nat Med 5, 491-492.

Liu, X., Zhao, D., Qin, L., Li, J., and Zeng, H. (2008). Transcription enhancer factor 3 (TEF3) mediates the expression of Down syndrome candidate region 1 isoform 1 (DSCR1-1L) in endothelial cells. The Journal of biological chemistry 283, 34159-34167.

Lott, I.T. (1982). Down's syndrome, aging, and Alzheimer's disease: a clinical review. Annals of the New York Academy of Sciences 396, 15-27.

Mammucari, C., Tommasi di Vignano, A., Sharov, A.A., Neilson, J., Havrda, M.C., Roop, D.R., Botchkarev, V.A., Crabtree, G.R., and Dotto, G.P. (2005). Integration of Notch 1 and calcineurin/NFAT signaling pathways in keratinocyte growth and differentiation control. Developmental cell 8, 665-676.

Minami, T., and Aird, W.C. (2005). Endothelial cell gene regulation. Trends in cardiovascular medicine 15, 174-184.

Minami, T., Donovan, D.J., Tsai, J.C., Rosenberg, R.D., and Aird, W.C. (2002). Differential regulation of the von Willebrand factor and Flt-1 promoters in the endothelium of hypoxanthine phosphoribosyltransferase-targeted mice. Blood 100, 4019-4025.

Minami, T., Horiuchi, K., Miura, M., Abid, M.R., Takabe, W., Noguchi, N., Kohro, T., Ge, X., Aburatani, H., Hamakubo, T., et al. (2004). Vascular endothelial growth factor- and thrombin-induced termination factor, Down syndrome critical region-1, attenuates endothelial cell proliferation and angiogenesis. The Journal of biological chemistry 279, 50537-50554.

Minami, T., Kuivenhoven, J.A., Evans, V., Kodama, T., Rosenberg, R.D., and Aird, W.C. (2003). Ets motifs are necessary for endothelial cell-specific expression of a 723-bp Tie-2 promoter/enhancer in Hprt targeted transgenic mice. Arteriosclerosis, thrombosis, and vascular biology 23, 2041-2047.

Minami, T., Miura, M., Aird, W.C., and Kodama, T. (2006). Thrombin-induced autoinhibitory factor, Down syndrome critical region-1, attenuates NFAT-dependent vascular cell adhesion molecule-1 expression and inflammation in the endothelium. The Journal of biological chemistry 281, 20503-20520.

Minami, T., Yano, K., Miura, M., Kobayashi, M., Suehiro, J., Reid, P.C., Hamakubo, T., Ryeom, S., Aird, W.C., and Kodama, T. (2009). The Down syndrome critical region gene 1 short variant promoters direct vascular bed-specific gene expression during inflammation in mice. J Clin Invest 119, 2257-2270.

Okada, Y., Yano, K., Jin, E., Funahashi, N., Kitayama, M., Doi, T., Spokes, K., Beeler, D.L., Shih, S.C., Okada, H., et al. (2007). A three-kilobase fragment of the human Robo4 promoter directs cell type-specific expression in endothelium. Circulation research 100, 1712-1722.

Qin, L., Zhao, D., Liu, X., Nagy, J.A., Hoang, M.V., Brown, L.F., Dvorak, H.F., and Zeng, H. (2006). Down syndrome candidate region 1 isoform 1 mediates angiogenesis through the calcineurin-NFAT pathway. Mol Cancer Res 4, 811-820.

Reynolds, L.E., Watson, A.R., Baker, M., Jones, T.A., D'Amico, G., Robinson, S.D., Joffre, C., Garrido-Urbani, S., Rodriguez-Manzaneque, J.C., Martino-Echarri, E., et al. Tumour angiogenesis is reduced in the Tc1 mouse model of Down's syndrome. Nature 465, 813-817.

Roizen, N.J., and Patterson, D. (2003). Down's syndrome. Lancet 361, 1281-1289.

Ryan, M.J., and Sigmund, C.D. (2003). HPRT targeting: "Ets" a powerful tool for investigating endothelial-cell specific gene expression. Arteriosclerosis, thrombosis, and vascular biology 23, 1960-1962.

Ryeom, S., Baek, K.H., Rioth, M.J., Lynch, R.C., Zaslavsky, A., Birsner, A., Yoon, S.S., and McKeon, F. (2008). Targeted deletion of the calcineurin inhibitor DSCR1 suppresses tumor growth. Cancer Cell 13, 420-431.

Salvolini, E., Orciani, M., Lucarini, G., Vignini, A., Tranquilli, A.L., and Di Primio, R. VEGF and nitric oxide synthase immunoexpression in Down's syndrome amniotic fluid stem cells. Eur J Clin Invest 41, 23-29.

Sanna, B., Brandt, E.B., Kaiser, R.A., Pfluger, P., Witt, S.A., Kimball, T.R., van Rooij, E., De Windt, L.J., Rothenberg, M.E., Tschop, M.H., et al. (2006). Modulatory calcineurin-interacting proteins 1 and 2 function as calcineurin facilitators in vivo. Proceedings of the National Academy of Sciences of the United States of America 103, 7327-7332.

Shin, S.Y., Choo, S.M., Kim, D., Baek, S.J., Wolkenhauer, O., and Cho, K.H. (2006). Switching feedback mechanisms realize the dual role of MCIP in the regulation of calcineurin activity. FEBS letters 580, 5965-5973.

Vega, R.B., Rothermel, B.A., Weinheimer, C.J., Kovacs, A., Naseem, R.H., Bassel-Duby, R., Williams, R.S., and Olson, E.N. (2003). Dual roles of modulatory calcineurin-interacting protein 1 in cardiac hypertrophy. Proceedings of the National Academy of Sciences of the United States of America 100, 669-674.

Yano, K., Liaw, P.C., Mullington, J.M., Shih, S.C., Okada, H., Bodyak, N., Kang, P.M., Toltl, L., Belikoff, B., Buras, J., et al. (2006). Vascular endothelial growth factor is an important determinant of sepsis morbidity and mortality. The Journal of experimental medicine 203, 1447-1458.

Yano, K., Okada, Y., Beldi, G., Shih, S.C., Bodyak, N., Okada, H., Kang, P.M., Luscinskas, W., Robson, S.C., Carmeliet, P., et al. (2008). Elevated levels of placental growth factor represent an adaptive host response in sepsis. The Journal of experimental medicine 205, 2623-2631.

7

Down Syndrome and Vascular Disease: DSCR1 and NFAT Signaling

Monica Y. Lee and Brian R. Wamhoff
University of Virginia, Robert M. Berne Cardiovascular Research Center
U.S.A.

1. Introduction

Down Syndrome (DS) is one of the most common genetic disorders to date, occurring in 1 out of every 800-1000 live births (Egan *et al.* 2004; Roizen & Patterson, 2003; Stoll *et al.* 1990). DS patients often display several developmental and cognitive deficiencies. Common phenotypes of DS patients include congenital heart disease, dysmorphic physical features, and early-onset Alzheimer's disease (AD). Since the discovery in 1959 that DS occurs from an extra copy of human chromosome 21 (hChr21) (Lejeune J, Gautier & Turpin, 1959), questions arose whether a 1.5-fold increase in a gene or set of genes were responsible for the phenotypes associated with DS. Sequence analysis of hChr21 indentified over 225 genes and/or predicted genes (Hattori *et al.* 2000). With the recent advances in sequencing, the gene content of hChr21 is now estimated to exceed 300 genes (Roizen & Patterson, 2003). While typically characterized by complete trisomy of hChr21, several DS cases, however, demonstrate that partial trisomy of hChr21 is enough to elicit the phenotypes associated with DS (Stoll *et al.* 1990), hence arising the concept of a Down Syndrome Critical Region (DSCR). The DSCR theory suggests that enhanced expression of a few genes located in this critical chromosomal region (between markers D21S17 and D21S55 (Delabar *et al.* 1993; Korenberg *et al.* 1994)) are responsible for some, if not all, of the features of DS. Olson LE *et al* show, however, that triplication of this region alone is not enough to fully manifest the phenotypes associated with DS (Olson *et al.* 2004; Olson *et al.* 2007). These findings contradict the longstanding DSCR theory, indicating that the genetic instability seen with hChr21 triplication is not merely from excess gene expression. Rather, the functional interactions occurring within a set of overexpressed genes may explain the various phenotypes observed in DS.

Many of the triplicate genes on hChr21 are implicated in several diseases. Cohorts of genes, interestingly, have been associated with pathologies that appear to be more common for DS individuals. A group of at least 16 genes on hChr21 have been correlated with a role in energy and reactive oxygen species (ROS) metabolism (Roizen & Patterson, 2003). Several studies have linked mitochondrial dysfunction and metabolic disorders with DS (Arbuzova, Hutchin & Cuckle, 2002). *In vitro,* DS neurons were observed to have 3- to 4-fold increases in reactive oxygen species compared to control cells, with elevated rates of consequent cell apoptosis (Busciglio & Yankner, 1995). Degeneration of DS neurons was rescued by administration of free-radical scavengers, suggesting DS neurons are unable to efficiently metabolize ROS. DS patients are also evidenced to have increased mitochondrial superoxide production compared to control groups (Capone *et al.* 2002). In addition, Busciglio J *et al.* show altered processing of the amyloid precursor protein (APP) in DS astrocytes and neurons (Busciglio *et al.* 2002). Elevated levels of APP, a gene also located on hChr21, have been associated with AD progression. Given that DS patients invariably display the characteristic plaques and tangles suggestive of AD (Hardy & Selkoe, 2002), this 1.5-fold increase in particular hChr21-located genes may explain the metabolic-related diseases associated with DS patients.

Another cohort of at least 10 genes located on hChr21 have been demonstrated to influence the central nervous system (CNS), and may hence play a role in the neuropathogenesis of DS (Capone, 2001). Considering the major phenotypes of DS patients include altered brain development, neuronal loss, and Alzheimer's-like neuropathology, the identification of CNS-related genes is not surprising. As demonstrated by these two gene clusters, phenotypic outcome is dependent not only on genotype but also on successive protein interactions. It is therefore possible that additional sets of genes, when in excess as a result of trisomy hChr21, lead to the manifestation of other DS-related pathologies, such as vascular-related pathologies.

2. Clinical observations and chapter overview

While developmental and behavioral disorders have been extensively studied in adults with DS, relatively little is known regarding their propensity to vascular-related diseases. Several intriguing clinical observations relating to the vasculature have been reported amongst DS patients over the last several decades. Unlike the aforementioned developmental deficits of DS individuals, DS patients appear to have a unique advantage in the context of several vascular pathologies.

2.1 Cancer incidence in DS patients

While adults with DS have been shown to have a higher incidence of leukemia compared to the general public, the risk of solid tumors appear to be strikingly low in individuals with DS (Hasle, Clemmensen & Mikkelsen, 2000). A population-based study on causes of mortality in over 17,000 DS patients showed a significant lack of malignant neoplasms as a cause of death (Yang, Rasmussen & Friedman, 2002). These findings suggest that individuals with DS express possible tumor-suppressor genes on hChr21, such that trisomy of a set of genes results in an antineoplastic effect on solid tumors. It is possible that these set of genes modulate a common biological mechanism that is critical for tumorigenesis and/or cancer progression.

2.2 Atherosclerosis in DS patients

A post-mortem, observational study published in 1977 found that 40-66 year old patients with DS displayed an almost complete absence of atherosclerotic plaque formation in arteries, compared to those without DS (Murdoch *et al.* 1977). Additional population studies in DS patients have found consistent results (Draheim, Geijer & Dengel, 2010; Yla-Herttuala *et al.* 1989), leading one to speculate that an unidentified factor(s) specific to DS patients explains the near absence of atherosclerotic plaque formation. Considering the vascular similarities between tumorigenesis and atherosclerosis, it is possible these events are driven by a shared molecular mechanism.

2.3 Other vascular pathologies in DS patients

Studies focusing on vascular tone show that DS patients have extremely low percentages of hypertension (Kerins *et al.* 2008). Significant decreases in both systolic and diastolic pressures were observed in DS patients when compared to reference populations (Morrison *et al.* 1996; Richards & Enver, 1979). Low blood pressures have also been observed in Alzheimer's disease (AD) (Burke *et al.* 1994; Landin *et al.* 1993), suggesting the mechanisms driving AD contribute to the observed hypotensive tendencies of DS patients. The already mentioned propensity for DS patients to develop AD, in addition to blood pressure levels similar to that of AD patients, strongly suggests a shared genetic contribution(s) of hChr21-located genes.

The observed decrease in solid tumor growth, lack of atherosclerotic plaque formation, and hypotensive nature of DS adults indicates onset of these vascular disorders may share an underlying molecular mechanism. This chapter will aim to discuss the observed differences in the vasculature of DS patients based on current literature to date. As of now, there is no concrete evidence distinguishing DS patients from non-DS patients on a genetic level concerning vascular anomalies. Correlative studies, however, suggest DS individuals harness a genetic advantage in regard to vascular health and disease.

3. Tumorigenesis in Down Syndrome

The molecular mechanisms underlying oncogenesis are undoubtedly one of the most intricate processes to date. Accumulation of multiple genomic mutations leads to the dysregulation of cell signaling pathways that are critical for controlling basic cellular functions including cell growth, survival, and cell fate. The extensive cross-talk between various signaling cascades highlights the sophisticated communication that transpires during cancer development and progression.

3.1 Calcium/calcineurin/NFAT signaling

Calcium (Ca^{2+}) fluxes are involved in multiple cell processes such as cell metabolism, membrane transport, cell permeability, and apoptosis. Changes in intracellular Ca^{2+} levels affect downstream gene expression and cell function through various mechanisms. In particular, intracellular Ca^{2+} concentrations often regulate kinase and phosphatase activity through the Ca^{2+}-binding protein, calmodulin (CaM). Increases in intracellular Ca^{2+} have been demonstrated in various cell types to activate the Ca^{2+}/CaM-dependent serine-threonine protein phosphatase, calcineurin (Cn). The Cn pathway is critical for the transduction of many extracellular, adaptive stimuli. Activated Cn subsequently dephosphorylates target proteins, including the nuclear factor of activated T-cells (NFATc1-c4) family of transcription factors (**Figure 1**). The NFAT family was originally identified in lymphocytes for its role in cytokine gene expression. While first identified in immune cells, recent findings show NFAT proteins are ubiquitously expressed. NFAT at the basal state are localized to the cytoplasm in an inactive form, with more than 20 identified phosphorylation sites (Okamura *et al.* 2000). CaM/Cn-mediated dephosphorylation of NFAT promotes nuclear translocation and target gene transcription (**Figure 1**). As downstream effectors of the Cn signaling pathway, NFAT-dependent gene transcription influences a range of cellular functions, including endothelial cell migration (Minami *et al.* 2004), skeletal muscle differentiation (Rothermel *et al.* 2000), cardiac valve development (Lange, Molkentin & Yutzey, 2004), and vascular smooth muscle cell adaptation (Crabtree & Olson, 2002; Horsley& Pavlath, 2002; Lee *et al.* 2010).

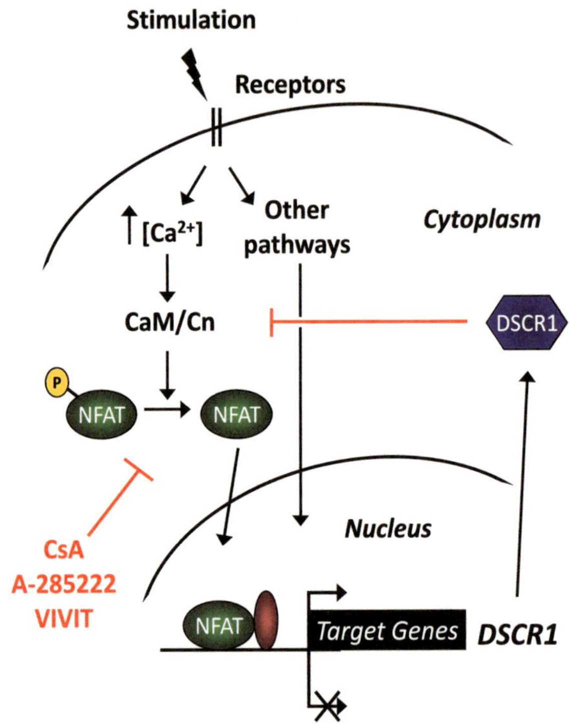

Fig. 1. The Cn/NFAT signaling pathway. calmodulin (CaM), calcineurin (Cn), cyclosporin A (CsA) (adapted from Viola, J.B.P., 2005)

Given the versatility of NFAT activation, it is not surprising that solid tumors and haematological malignances are correlated with overexpression of NFATc isoforms. For example, pancreatic carcinomas display elevated levels of NFATc1 for transcriptional activation of the c-myc oncogene (Buchholz *et al.* 2006). Studies using human breast carcinoma cell lines also show NFATc2 expression promotes carcinoma migration and invasion (Jauliac *et al.* 2002). The increased NFATc activity in malignant cells suggests activation of downstream NFATc targets is critical for tumor progression. Cyclooxygenase-2 (COX2/PTGS2) has been reported by several groups as an NFAT-dependent gene in non-lymphoid tissues, including endothelial cells (Hernandez *et al.* 2001), mesangial cells (Sugimoto *et al.* 2001), and vascular smooth muscle cells (Pritchard, Jr. *et al.* 1994). As an enzyme involved in prostaglandin formation, COX2 expression plays an important role in cell survival and angiogenesis. A gain-of-function approach shows that forced overexpression of COX2 alone is enough to induce mammary gland tumorigenesis (Liu *et al.* 2001). On the converse, inhibition of COX2 significantly reduces colon tumor incidence and multiplicity in a dose-dependent manner (Reddy *et al.* 2000). These findings strongly support the notion that tumor growth/invasion necessitates an abundance of COX2 levels. The increased expression of COX2 in a multitude of cancer lines (*i.e.* gastric, esophageal, breast, bladder, cervical, colorectal, endometrial (Brown & DuBois, 2005; Duque, Fresno & Iniguez, 2005b)) have thus launched the production of several COX2 inhibitors with therapeutic potential. It is, however, important to note the importance of COX2 in other cell types. Unlike the constitutively expressed COX1 isoform, COX2 expression occurs in a limited number of cell types, primarily in response to cytokines, inflammatory mediators, and tissue damage (Lipsky *et al.* 2000). The inducible nature of COX2 activation results in prostaglandin formation, including prostacyclin, a vasodilator and a potent inhibitor of platelet aggregation. Prostacylin formation in vascular endothelial cells thus provides a mechanism by which the thrombotic response in platelet activation can be regulated (Rudic *et al.* 2005). Hence, COX2 expression is necessary to maintain vascular health. While COX2-selective inhibitors may attenuate tumor angiogenesis, COX2 antagonists will undoubtedly shift eicosanoid balance toward a prothrombotic state, promoting the risk for cardiovascular events (Mukherjee, Nissen & Topol, 2001). Targeting other proteins involved in Cn/NFAT signaling aside from COX2 may yield similar anti-neoplastic results.

Tumor survival and growth is highly-dependent on a vascular system for delivery of essential nutrients and oxygen. A tumor's vasculature also provides a mechanism by which aberrant cells can disseminate and metastasize to other organs. Without a constant blood supply, tumor volumes tend to remain 1-2mm^3 in size (Brown & DuBois, 2005). Angiogenesis is a multi-step process that involves migration, proliferation, and differentiation of both endothelial and vascular smooth muscle cells for generation of mature vessels. Tumor cells can facilitate an 'angiogeneic switch' by altering gene transcription and the surrounding microenvironment. Somatic mutations of various proto-oncogenes and/or tumor suppressor genes offset the balance between activators and inhibitors of angiogenesis, ultimately favoring angiogenic activity (Hanahan & Weinberg, 2000). Pro-angiogeneic gene expression is induced by a number of physiological stimuli, such as hypoxia. Cells in hypoxic conditions produce the hypoxia-inducible factor (HIF) transcription factor, where expression of HIF-1 results in Vascular Endothelial Growth Factor (VEGF) transcription (Forsythe *et al.* 1996). VEGF, a major stimulator of angiogenesis, is a potent endothelial mitogen involved in both physiological and pathological blood vessel formation. VEGF is critical for proper embryonic vasculogenesis, as even heterozygous VEGF-deficient mice display abnormal blood vessel formation and consequent embryonic lethality (Carmeliet *et al.* 1996). While necessary for proper blood vessel development, excess VEGF can result in pathological angiogenesis. HIF-1-mediated VEGF expression and activation of other angiogenesis-related genes exemplifies the adaptive responses seen in tumor survival and growth. VEGF has also been demonstrated to induce COX2 expression in a Cn/NFAT-dependent manner (Duque, Fresno & Iniguez, 2005c). As previously mentioned, COX2 expression is critical for tumor cell migration and tube formation. The emerging role of NFAT signaling in oncogenesis is further highlighted, as pharmacological inhibition of NFAT blocks VEGF-stimulated COX2 expression and subsequent cell proliferation and/or angiogenesis both *in vitro* and *in vivo (*Hernandez *et al. 2001).* These results imply activation of Cn/NFAT signaling is required for the formation of new blood vessels, where regulation of angiogenesis is dependent on a local balance between angiogenic factors and inhibitors. The identification of Cn/NFAT activators and downstream NFAT target genes in the last few decades has therefore helped elucidate the biological mechanisms underlying oncogenesis.

3.2 DSCR1 in cancer progression

Cancer incidence for all solid tumors and malignancies have been shown in multiple DS population studies to be significantly lower in DS patients compared to control groups (Hasle *et al.* 2000; Yang *et al.* 2002). Interestingly, a large focus has been placed on the role of the Down Syndrome Candidate Region 1 (DSCR1/RCAN1/MCIP1) gene in cancer progression. Located on hChr21, DSCR1 has been demonstrated as a negative feedback regulator of Cn/NFAT signaling through physical binding to the catalytic subunit of Cn (Fuentes *et al.* 2000) (**Figure 1**). In endothelial cells, VEGF and thrombin stimulation dramatically upregulate DSCR1 expression in a Cn/NFAT dependent manner (Iizuka *et al.* 2004; Minami *et al.* 2004). Several studies in endothelial cells have shown that DSCR1 overexpression inhibits NFAT transcriptional activity, suppresses NFAT nuclear accumulation, and attenuates NFAT-dependent inflammatory marker gene expression, such as COX2 (Hesser *et al.* 2004; Yao & Duh, 2004). Studies also show DSCR1 overexpression in endothelial cells reduces vascular density in matrigel plugs *in vitro* and in tumor growth in mice (Minami *et al.* 2004). Lastly, functional data indicate constitutive expression of DSCR1 impairs endothelial cell proliferation and tube formation (Minami *et al.* 2004). Taken together, VEGF and thrombin-mediated endothelial cell proliferation/vascularization induces expression of DSCR1 as a mechanism to negatively regulate the angiogenic processes.

Researchers have attempted to explain the lack of tumorigenesis in the DS population through use of genetically modified mice. Comparative mapping between mice and humans identify that hChr21 is genetically homologous to mouse chromosome 16 (mChr16) (Reeves & Citron, 1994). Thus, mice exhibiting trisomy of mChr16 (Ts16) were originally developed to study DS. Ts16 mice, however, die *in utero* and therefore pose as a limitation. In addition, several genes located on mChr16 are found on human chromosomes other than hChr21. The observed embryonic lethality as well as gene dosage imbalances resulted in generation of the Ts65Dn mouse (Reeves *et al.* 1995). The Ts65Dn mouse model reflects partial trisomy of hChr21, where mice have been reported to display a variety of phenotypes, including behavioral abnormalities consistent with DS (Reeves *et al.* 1995). Ts65Dn mice are now widely used to study DS at all stages of development.

A recent publication highlights the suppression of tumor growth seen in DS individuals using two different models: 1) the Ts65Dn mouse and 2) a DSCR1-transgenic mouse. Ts65Dn mice possess extra genetic information including the DSCR1 gene – Ts65Dn mice exhibit a 1.7-fold increase in DSCR1 protein expression compared to diploid controls (Baek *et al.* 2009). Baek KH *et al* demonstrate that both lung carcinoma and melanoma cell growth was significantly suppressed in Ts65Dn mice, when compared to control groups (Baek *et al.* 2009). Under the transplantable tumor model, Ts65Dn mice also display significant decreases in tumor growth and microvessel density (Baek *et al.* 2009). Similar results were seen when using DSCR1-transgenic mice, suggesting that one extra copy of DSCR1 is sufficient for tumor growth suppression. Given that hChr21 contains over 200 genes, however, it is likely that other genes act in concert with DSCR1 to facilitate tumor suppressive effects. Another gene of interest includes Dual-specificity tyrosine-(Y)-phosphorylation regulated kinase (DYRK1A), a nuclear serine/threonine kinase located on hChr21. DYRK1A phosphorylates several transcription factors including NFAT. DYRK1A can therefore reduce Cn/NFAT-dependent transcription through its ability to export nuclear NFAT. Baek KH *et al* also show that endothelial cells overexpressing DSCR1 together with DYRK1A demonstrate an even greater suppression of VEGF-mediated cell proliferation (Baek *et al.* 2009). Future work by Baek KH *et al* will focus on additional hChr21-located genes known to suppress tumor angiogenesis through alternate mechanisms (Ryeom, Baek & Zaslavsky, 2009), such as COLLAGEN XVIII (COL18A1), a precursor to the angiogenesis inhibitor endostatin, and ADAMTS1, a metalloproteinase known to regulate the anti-angiogeneic function of thrombospondin-1 (Iruela-Arispe, Carpizo & Luque, 2003;

Zaslavsky *et al.* 2010). In summary, the tumorigenic protective effects seen in DS adults may be due to increased expression of select hChr21-located genes, including DSCR1.

4. Atherosclerosis in Down Syndrome

Atherosclerosis progression is a complex process involving several cell types, multiple biological mechanisms, and environmental factors. The pathogenesis of atherosclerotic plaque formation is highly dependent on hemodynamic flow patterns (DeBakey, Lawrie & Glaeser, 1985; Vanderlaan, Reardon & Getz, 2004), thrombotic processes, and inflammatory signaling cascades (Lusis, 2000). Atherosclerosis is one of the leading causes of mortality in Westernized societies, and thus several cardiovascular risk factors have been identified over the last few decades in an effort to predict cardiovascular events. Given that atherosclerosis is characterized by accumulation of lipids in the large arteries, it is not surprising that elevated plasma triglyceride levels have been demonstrated as a direct propagator of cardiovascular disease (Austin, Hokanson & Edwards, 1998; Hokanson & Austin, 1996). Other plasma measurements indicative of cardiovascular risk include reduced levels of high-density lipoprotein (HDL) (Assmann *et al.* 1996; Gordon *et al.* 1977), and elevated serum levels of C-reactive protein (CRP), an indicator of inflammation (Mendall *et al.* 1996). High values for body mass index have also been demonstrated as a measure of cardiovascular risk (Berenson *et al.* 1998).

Atherosclerotic cardiovascular disease has been associated with metabolic syndrome, which includes several clinical disorders such as obesity, insulin resistance, glucose intolerance, hypertension, and dyslipidemia (Moller & Kaufman, 2005). Consistent with the aforementioned metabolic deficiencies associated with DS patients, individuals with DS also exhibit impaired lipid metabolism (Ishihara *et al.* 2009). In addition, DS patients have lower levels of low-density lipoprotein receptor (LDLR) expression compared to adults without DS (Corsi *et al.* 2005). Interestingly, lack of or dysfunctional LDLR expression results in familial hypercholesterolemia, a genetic disease characterized by elevated cholesterol levels and premature coronary artery disease (Brown & Goldstein, 1976). LDLR-null mice have since been generated and is now a widely used atherosclerotic mouse model (Ishibashi *et al.* 1993; Wouters *et al.* 2005). Lastly, DS patients exhibit significantly elevated levels of plasma triglycerides, low levels of HDL, high levels of CRP, and high levels of total body fat (Corsi *et al.* 2005; Draheim *et al.* 2010; Nishida *et al.* 1977). Taken together, these findings imply DS adults are surely at risk for cardiovascular events. DS patients, however, are significantly less susceptible to cardiovascular disease. A comparison of intimal-to-medial thickness (IMT) of the common carotid artery in DS adults show significantly lower IMT ratios when compared to control groups (Draheim *et al.* 2010). These findings corroborate the observational findings in 1977 where DS patients were proposed to be an "an atheroma-free model" (Murdoch *et al.* 1977). One can speculate that DS patients thus express an altered gene expression profile where an additional copy of hChr21-located genes results in protection against atheroma formation, despite the many validated plasma indicators of cardiovascular risk. Similar to the identified gene clusters responsible for the metabolic and developmental deficiencies in DS patients, it is highly likely that a cohort of genes located on hChr21 is responsible for the protective effects against cardiovascular disease. Identification of these genes will therefore provide a therapeutic direction as we continue to understand the etiology behind atherosclerotic plaque formation.

4.1 Vascular smooth muscle and atherogenesis

At the cellular level, atherosclerosis progression is characterized by lipid accumulation and fibrous lesion formation in large arteries, resulting in chronic arterial wall inflammation. The release of cytokines and growth factors induce vascular smooth muscle cells (SMC) to undergo a process known as phenotypic modulation, whereby an adult, contractile SMC alters its expression profile to facilitate cell proliferation, migration, and/or inflammatory cell recruitment (Shin *et al.* 2008) (**Figure 2**). Phenotypic modulation is a key event underlying atherogenesis and in-stent restenosis that involves several signaling cascades, including the Cn/NFAT pathway. Activation of Cn/NFAT signaling has been shown to induce vascular SMC proliferation and migration in response to receptor tyrosine kinase and G-protein-coupled receptor agonists, respectively (Liu, Dronadula & Rao, 2004; Yellaturu *et al.* 2002). Cn/NFAT activity is also critical for vessel wall assembly (Graef *et al.* 2001). Cyclosporin A (CsA) and the VIVIT peptide are commonly used Cn and NFAT inhibitors, respectively (**Figure 1**). A third pharmacological compound, A-285222, also inhibits Cn/NFAT signaling (Lee *et al.* 2010; Nilsson *et al.* 2007). Inhibition of Cn/NFAT signaling through use of either CsA or A-285222 attenuates Cn/NFAT-mediated SMC migration and proliferation *in vitro* (unpublished, **Figure 1**). Previous literature also shows that blocking Cn/NFAT signaling *in vivo* significantly inhibits vascular-injury-induced neointima formation (Liu *et al.* 2005), supporting the notion that Cn/NFAT signaling is intimately involved in the smooth muscle response to vascular injury. While NFAT-dependent gene regulation has been widely studied in lymphocytes, cardiac and skeletal muscle, the lack of known NFAT target genes in SMCs limits our understanding of Cn/NFAT signaling in vascular remodeling.

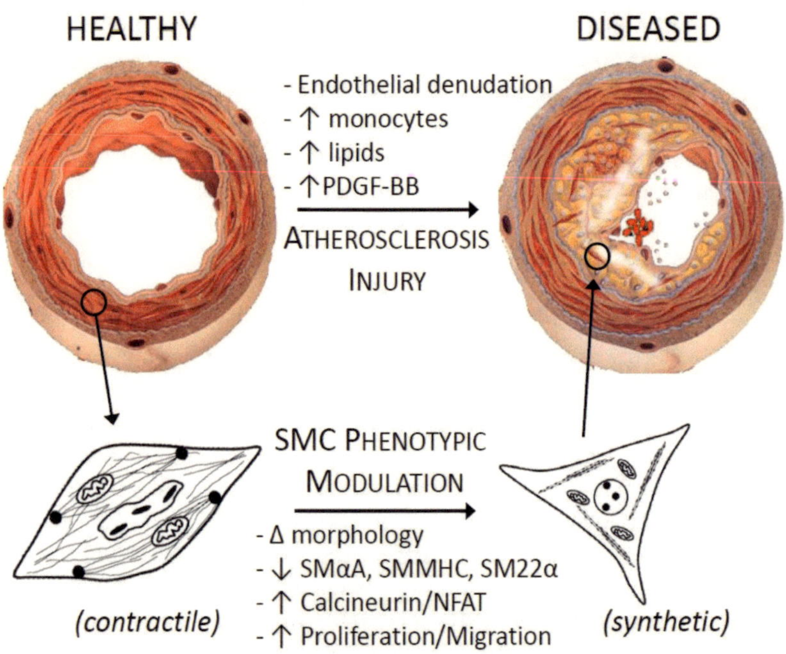

Fig. 2. The interplay between SMC phenotypic modulation and Cn/NFAT signaling in vascular disease.

4.2 Identification of DSCR1 using integrative genomics

We recently developed an unbiased, top-down, integrative genomics approach to determine downstream targets of Cn/NFAT activation in vascular SMCs (Lee *et al.* 2010). In brief, whole-genome expression data sets were analyzed to identify differentially upregulated genes in human, mouse, and rat SMCs. Comparison between control and phenotypic modulatory stimuli identified 63 species-conserved, upregulated genes. Differentially upregulated genes were then compared against an *in silico* NFAT-ome (a list of gene promoters containing at least one species-conserved physical NFAT binding site), yielding 18 potential Cn/NFAT-dependent genes. Use of pharmacological Cn/NFAT inhibitors substantiated the NFAT-dependent role for COX2, a previously identified Cn/NFAT dependent gene, and revealed the Cn/NFAT-dependent property of DSCR1 in vascular SMCs (Lee *et al.* 2010). DSCR1 has been reported in other cell types to function as a negative feedback regulator of Cn/NFAT signaling (**Figure 1**). Both gain- and loss-of-function studies were conducted to determine the role of DSCR1 in vascular SMCs. Overexpression of DSCR1 resulted in decreased NFAT transcriptional activity and reduced expression of other Cn/NFAT-dependent genes, such as COX2. Conversely, knockdown of endogenous DSCR1 enhanced NFAT transcriptional activity suggesting DSCR1 also functions as a negative regulator in vascular SMCs (Lee *et al.* 2010). Lastly, analysis of *in vivo* whole-genome expression arrays found significant DSCR1 upregulation with acute vascular injury in mouse carotid arteries, regardless of strain type (Lee *et al.* 2010). The significant induction of DSCR1 exemplifies its functional importance and may be critical for modulating the vascular injury response. Similarly, an extra copy of the DSCR1 gene in DS patients may function in an atheroprotective manner through its ability to negatively regulate Cn/NFAT signaling. The recent study highlighting significantly less tumor growth in DSCR1-transgenic mice (Baek *et al.* 2009) fosters the regulatory role of DSCR1 in Cn/NFAT-mediated cell growth. It is possible DSCR1 functions in both endothelial cells and vascular SMCs as a modulator of cell proliferation, thereby providing a shared mechanism underlying tumorigenesis and atheroma formation.

4.3 Ongoing research

Several studies are currently underway in an effort to understand the functional role of DSCR1 in SMC phenotypic modulation and atherosclerotic plaque formation. DSCR1-deficient mice have since been obtained and are proving to be instrumental as we continue to elucidate the role of DSCR1 in atherogenesis. DSCR1-related family members, however, have been identified in most eukaryotic organisms. In humans, DSCR1 family members include DSCR1-like 1 (DSCR1L1/ZAKI-4/RCAN2) and DSCR1-like 2 (DSCR1L2/RCAN3) (Strippoli *et al.* 2000). Interestingly, DSCR1L1 mimics the inhibitory effects of DSCR1 on Cn signaling in endothelial cells and inhibits angiogenesis (Gollogly, Ryeom & Yoon, 2007). In lymphocytes, DSCR1L2 blocks nuclear NFAT translocation and inhibits NFAT-dependent cytokine gene expression (Mulero *et al.* 2007). Given the functional overlap between the DSCR1 family members, global DSCR1-/- mouse models may possibly exhibit compensation by DSCR1L1 and/or DSCR1L2. In addition, DSCR1 plays a critical role in each of the major cell types seen with atherogenesis and will therefore be difficult to attribute our findings as a vascular SMC-specific response. Until a SMC-specific conditional knock-out mouse study is carried out, a conservative approach must be taken when interpreting results gathered from DSCR1-null mice given the complexities surrounding

DSCR1 expression and regulation in other cell types. Nonetheless, the data gathered will provide a better understanding of DSCR1 function.

Apolipoprotein E (ApoE) is critical for lipoprotein metabolism. Defects in ApoE expression can consequently increase plasma cholesterol and triglyceride levels. Hence, targeted mutagenesis of the ApoE gene in mice promotes elevated serum cholesterol levels, where combination with a high fat/cholesterol diet results in massive accumulation of cholesterol and causative atherosclerotic lesion formation. DSCR1$^{-/-}$; ApoE$^{-/-}$-double knockout mice have been generated in an effort to study how the absence of DSCR1 affects atherosclerotic plaque formation. These double-null mice have been placed on a 20-week, high fat/cholesterol diet to ensure plaque formation, where atherosclerotic plaque size will be quantified and compared against proper control groups. Given the literature to date, we predict atherosclerotic lesion formation and size to significantly increase in DSCR1$^{-/-}$; ApoE$^{-/-}$ double-null mice. The absence of DSCR1, a negative regulator of Cn/NFAT activity, should in theory promote SMC proliferation and infiltration into the neointima. A recent publication, however, emphasizes the dual role of DSCR1, suggesting DSCR1 is necessary for both Cn/NFAT activation and self-regulation (Liu, Busby & Molkentin, 2009). This effect has been demonstrated in cardiomyocytes and hypertrophy, an adaptive response driven by Cn and NFATc4 signaling (De Windt *et al.* 2001; Molkentin *et al.* 1998). Several groups have shown an attenuation of cardiac hypertrophy with overexpression of DSCR1 (Rothermel *et al.* 2001). DSCR1$^{-/-}$; DSCR1L1$^{-/-}$ double-null mice were thus hypothesized to demonstrate significantly greater cardiac hypertrophy. DSCR1$^{-/-}$; DSCR1L1$^{-/-}$ double-null mice, however, exhibit the reverse response - cardiac hypertrophy is impaired in response to adrenergic stimulation or exercise, similar to responses seen in calcineurin Aβ-/- mice (Sanna *et al.* 2006). These results suggest a basal level of DSCR1 is necessary to properly activate Cn/NFAT signaling. The DSCR1 yeast homolog, RCN1/CBP1, has also been functionally characterized as a facilitator of Cn/NFAT signaling (Kingsbury & Cunningham, 2000). The notion that DSCR1 may also activate Cn/NFAT signaling highlights the elaborate nature of this protein, suggesting that the paradoxical function of DSCR1 depends on initial protein concentrations (Shin *et al.* 2006). It is thus possible we may instead observe a decrease in atherosclerotic lesion formation in the DSCR1$^{-/-}$; ApoE$^{-/-}$ double-null mice. With this in mind, we have also placed DSCR1$^{+/-}$; ApoE$^{-/-}$ mice to observe how DSCR1 haploinsufficiency affects plaque formation. The presence of one DSCR1 allele will allow for minimal DSCR1 expression, yet also test the effects of reduced DSCR1 expression on lesion formation.

We are also performing several *in vitro* assays on primary aortic SMC cultures from DSCR1$^{-/-}$ mice to determine the consequences of DSCR1 absence on cell functionality. With our recent findings demonstrating DSCR1 as a negative regulator of Cn/NFAT signaling in vascular SMCs (Lee *et al.* 2010), one would hypothesize that DSCR1-null vascular SMCs to exhibit increased cell proliferation in response to phenotypic modulatory stimuli. Preliminary data, however, show a reduced proliferative response in DSCR1-null vascular SMCs when stimulated with either platelet-derived growth factor (PDGF-BB) or serum (unpublished). These initial results support the emerging dual role of DSCR1, suggesting basal levels of DSCR1 is necessary for Cn/NFAT activation. While our model cannot fully explain the almost complete absence of atheroma formation in DS patients, our results will not only help elucidate the functional role of DSCR1 in atherogenesis, but also provide insight on the effects of trisomy 21 through a single gene approach.

5. Vascular tone and Down Syndrome

Enzyme activity of endothelial nitric oxide synthase (eNOS) plays a critical role in determining vascular tone through its ability to generate nitric oxide (NO) and consequently affect vascular smooth muscle contraction. Regulation of eNOS enzymatic activity is a highly dynamic system involving several kinases and phosphatases with significant downstream effects on NO-signaling (Duran, Breslin & Sanchez, 2010). While phosphorylation of eNOS is typically associated with enzyme activation, several groups demonstrate that dephosphorylation of eNOS can also trigger eNOS activation and subsequent NO production (Harris *et al.* 2001; Kou, Greif & Michel, 2002; Thomas, Chen & Keaney, Jr., 2002). The Cn phosphatase has been shown to target several proteins aside from NFAT, including eNOS (Kou *et al.* 2002). While the absolute role of DSCR1 is unknown in the vasculature, recent literature suggests DSCR1 plays a vital role in vessel contraction. DSCR1$^{-/-}$ mice have been reported to exhibit an attenuated vasocontriction response with phenylephrine treatment compared to appropriate controls (Riper *et al.* 2008). Riper DV *et al* speculate that the altered vascular constriction in DSCR1$^{-/-}$ mice may be due to Cn dysregulation, thereby facilitating excess endothelial NO production. Based on the proposed mechanism, overexpression of DSCR1 should then limit NO formation and promote vasoconstriction. As stated earlier, however, adults with DS are significantly hypotensive when compared to control groups (Morrison *et al.* 1996; Richards & Enver, 1979). Although the attenuated vasoconstriction response in DSCR1$^{-/-}$ mice may contradict the hypertensive nature of DS patients, the account by Riper DV *et al* is the first publication to date revealing a potential role of DSCR1 in vascular tone.

It is also important to note that these observations of a weakened vasoconstriction response in DSCR1$^{-/-}$ mice reflect those of mesenteric rather than carotid arteries. While the underlying effects of NO on smooth muscle and vascular tone may be synonymous between the differing vascular beds, vasoconstriction could be regulated through different mechanisms. The effect of vascular bed type is further exemplified by the fact that while DS patients may be significantly hypotensive, they are also at an increased risk of developing pulmonary arterial hypertension (PAH) (Cua *et al.* 2007). The observed increase in PAH incidence amongst DS individuals may be due to several factors such as chronic upper airway obstruction (Jacobs, Gray & Todd, 1996) and abnormal pulmonary vasculature growth (Chi, 1975). Vascular tone therefore appears to depend not only on the vascular bed of interest but also on peripheral influences. In addition, basal levels of DSCR1 may be required for proper Cn/NFAT function, as previously described. Future contractility studies in haploinsufficient DSCR1$^{+/-}$ mice may thus provide clarity on the true role of DSCR1 in vascular tone. This study clearly demonstrates the widespread effect of DSCR1 loss, where dysregulation of Cn/NFAT activity in the endothelium alters paracrine signaling molecule production, creating invariable effects on neighboring cell types. The prevalent nature of DSCR1 prompts consideration for cell-cell interaction effects as we continue to decipher DSCR1 function in vascular disease.

6. NFAT regulation and other considerations

The importance of calcium signaling, NFATc transcriptional regulation, and ensuing downstream gene expression is increasingly evident. Adequate and controlled Cn/NFAT signaling is necessary, as dysregulation results in several vascular pathologies. Both the versatility in DNA binding and the presence of multiple NFAT family members suggest NFAT proteins have a more extensive role than originally anticipated. A few notable features of NFAT are brought to attention below.

NFAT transcription factors bind to DNA in a rather versatile manner. The promiscuous nature of NFAT-DNA binding suggests the presence of other binding partners. The most common and well-documented binding partner of NFAT is AP-1, a transcription factor comprised of Fos- and Jun- family proteins (Rao, Luo & Hogan, 1997). Several groups have demonstrated the need for cooperative NFAT-AP1 binding for optimal target gene transcription (Hogan *et al.* 2003). In addition to AP-1, NFAT has been shown to interact with other transcription factors involved in cell growth and differentiation, including GATA4, MEF2, and FOXP3 (Crabtree & Olson, 2002; Wu *et al.* 2006). Several groups have also noted the presence of multiple NFAT binding sites in validated NFAT-target gene promoters, such as interleukin-2 (Randak *et al.* 1990), interleukin-4 (Chuvpilo *et al.* 1993), and DSCR1 (Harris, Ermak & Davies, 2005). These multiple NFAT binding domains most likely confer a synergistic effect between NFAT-containing complexes and thereby promote efficient gene transcription (Rao *et al.* 1997). Thus, NFAT proteins may serve as 'coincidence detectors' (Crabtree & Olson, 2002) that can integrate information from multiple signaling pathways to coordinate gene expression.

The ubiquitous nature of NFAT amongst various cell types and processes demonstrates the broad-range effects of NFAT activity. While functional redundancy has been noted between the different NFAT isoforms, differences in tissue distribution (Rao *et al.* 1997), evidence of multiple splice variants, and distinguishing phenotypes of NFAT-deficient mice suggest NFAT proteins may in fact possess unique isoform-specific functions. For example, while NFATc1 and NFATc2 share 72% sequence agreement and demonstrate functional similarities, genetic deletion for either NFATc isoform results in divergent mouse phenotypes. Whereas NFATc2$^{-/-}$ mice are viable and demonstrate an enhanced immune response (Duque, Fresno & Iniguez, 2005a), NFATc1$^{-/-}$ mice display abnormal cardiac valve development and consequent embryonic lethality (de la Pompa *et al.* 1998). Variations between NFAT proteins is further seen where targeted disruption of NFATc3, but not NFATc4, significantly reduces Cn transgene-induced cardiac hypertrophy (Wilkins *et al.* 2002). The disparate outcomes from NFATc genetic deletions as well as the ability for NFATc isoforms to compensate one another limits the use of NFATc-specific knock-out mice.

Recent data have also challenged the longstanding premise viewing NFAT as a transcriptional activator. Several groups have in fact demonstrated the dual role of NFAT as both a gene activator and silencer (Robbs *et al.* 2008). NFATc1 and NFATc2 have been shown to repress cyclin-dependent kinase 4 (Horsley *et al.* 2008) and cyclinA2 (Carvalho *et al.* 2007) expression, respectively. NFATc2 has also been demonstrated as a negative regulator of cyclin B1 and cyclin E in lymphocytes (Caetano *et al.* 2002). The nonoverlapping functions and apparent gene silencing effects of individual NFATc proteins further complicates our understanding of Cn/NFAT signaling. NFAT is clearly involved in maintaining a balance between cell quiescence and cell proliferation – the two fundamental biological mechanisms underlying tumorigenesis and atherosclerosis.

7. Conclusions

The Cn/NFAT signaling cascade is undoubtedly a major determinant of cell growth and differentiation. Regulation of Cn/NFAT signaling is a critical determinant of neoplastic and cardiovascular risk. With DSCR1 now known as an endogenous regulator of Cn/NFAT signaling, several groups have successfully manipulated downstream gene expression and cell function by altering DSCR1 levels. The observation that DS patients exhibit significantly less tumor growth and arterial plaque formation cannot be mere coincidence, but rather evidence supporting the notion that these large-scale, vascular-related pathologies share an underlying mechanism. This is further reinforced by the fact that DSCR1 and other candidate antiangiogenic genes found on hChr21 are of growing attention. A more comprehensive analysis of hChr21-located genes may therefore provide direction as we continue to elucidate the mechanisms underlying tumorigenesis and atherosclerotic plaque formation.

8. References

Arbuzova, S., Hutchin, T. & Cuckle, H. (2002). Mitochondrial dysfunction and Down's syndrome. *Bioessays* 24(8):681-684.

Assmann, G., Schulte, H., von, E.A. & Huang, Y. (1996). High-density lipoprotein cholesterol as a predictor of coronary heart disease risk. The PROCAM experience and pathophysiological implications for reverse cholesterol transport. *Atherosclerosis* 124 Suppl:S11-S20.

Austin, M.A., Hokanson, J.E. & Edwards, K.L. (1998). Hypertriglyceridemia as a cardiovascular risk factor. *Am J Cardiol.* 81(4A):7B-12B.

Baek, K.H., Zaslavsky, A., Lynch, R.C., Britt, C., Okada, Y., Siarey, R.J., Lensch, M.W., Park, I.H., Yoon, S.S., Minami, T., Korenberg, J.R., Folkman, J., Daley, G.Q., Aird, W.C., Galdzicki, Z. & Ryeom, S. (2009). Down's syndrome suppression of tumour growth and the role of the calcineurin inhibitor DSCR1. *Nature* 459(7250):1126-1130.

Berenson, G.S., Srinivasan, S.R., Bao, W., Newman, W.P., III, Tracy, R.E. & Wattigney, W.A. (1998). Association between multiple cardiovascular risk factors and atherosclerosis in children and young adults. The Bogalusa Heart Study. *N.Engl.J Med.* 338(23):1650-1656.

Brown, J.R. & DuBois, R.N. (2005). COX-2: a molecular target for colorectal cancer prevention. *J Clin.Oncol.* 23(12):2840-2855.

Brown, M.S. & Goldstein, J.L. (1976). Familial hypercholesterolemia: A genetic defect in the low-density lipoprotein receptor. *N.Engl.J Med.* 294(25):1386-1390.

Buchholz, M., Schatz, A., Wagner, M., Michl, P., Linhart, T., Adler, G., Gress, T.M. & Ellenrieder, V. (2006). Overexpression of c-myc in pancreatic cancer caused by ectopic activation of NFATc1 and the Ca2+/calcineurin signaling pathway. *EMBO J* 25(15):3714-3724.

Burke, W.J., Coronado, P.G., Schmitt, C.A., Gillespie, K.M. & Chung, H.D. (1994). Blood pressure regulation in Alzheimer's disease. *J Auton.Nerv.Syst.* 48(1):65-71.

Busciglio, J., Pelsman, A., Wong, C., Pigino, G., Yuan, M., Mori, H. & Yankner, B.A. (2002). Altered metabolism of the amyloid beta precursor protein is associated with mitochondrial dysfunction in Down's syndrome. *Neuron* 33(5):677-688.

Busciglio, J. & Yankner, B.A. (1995). Apoptosis and increased generation of reactive oxygen species in Down's syndrome neurons in vitro. *Nature* 378(6559):776-779.

Caetano, M.S., Vieira-de-Abreu, A., Teixeira, L.K., Werneck, M.B., Barcinski, M.A. & Viola, J.P. (2002). NFATC2 transcription factor regulates cell cycle progression during lymphocyte activation: evidence of its involvement in the control of cyclin gene expression. *FASEB J* 16(14):1940-1942.

Capone, G., Kim, P., Jovanovich, S., Payne, L., Freund, L., Welch, K., Miller, E. & Trush, M. (2002). Evidence for increased mitochondrial superoxide production in Down syndrome. *Life Sci.* 70(24):2885-2895.

Capone, G.T. (2001). Down syndrome: advances in molecular biology and the neurosciences. *J Dev.Behav.Pediatr.* 22(1):40-59.

Carmeliet, P., Ferreira, V., Breier, G., Pollefeyt, S., Kieckens, L., Gertsenstein, M., Fahrig, M., Vandenhoeck, A., Harpal, K., Eberhardt, C., Declercq, C., Pawling, J., Moons, L., Collen, D., Risau, W. & Nagy, A. (1996). Abnormal blood vessel development and lethality in embryos lacking a single VEGF allele. *Nature* 380(6573):435-439.

Carvalho, L.D., Teixeira, L.K., Carrossini, N., Caldeira, A.T., Ansel, K.M., Rao, A. & Viola, J.P. (2007). The NFAT1 transcription factor is a repressor of cyclin A2 gene expression. *Cell Cycle* 6(14):1789-1795.

Chi, T.P.L. (1975). The pulmonary vascular bed in children with Down syndrome. *J Pediatr.* 86(4):533-538.

Chuvpilo, S., Schomberg, C., Gerwig, R., Heinfling, A., Reeves, R., Grummt, F. & Serfling, E. (1993). Multiple closely-linked NFAT/octamer and HMG I(Y) binding sites are part of the interleukin-4 promoter. *Nucleic Acids Res.* 21(24):5694-5704.

Corsi, M.M., Malavazos, A.E., Passoni, D. & Licastro, F. (2005). LDL receptor expression on T lymphocytes in old patients with Down syndrome. *Immun.Ageing* 2(1):3.

Crabtree, G.R. & Olson, E.N. (2002). NFAT signaling: choreographing the social lives of cells. *Cell* 109 Suppl:S67-S79.

Cua, C.L., Blankenship, A., North, A.L., Hayes, J. & Nelin, L.D. (2007). Increased incidence of idiopathic persistent pulmonary hypertension in Down syndrome neonates. *Pediatr.Cardiol.* 28(4):250-254.

de la Pompa, J.L., Timmerman, L.A., Takimoto, H., Yoshida, H., Elia, A.J., Samper, E., Potter, J., Wakeham, A., Marengere, L., Langille, B.L., Crabtree, G.R. & Mak, T.W. (1998). Role of the NF-ATc transcription factor in morphogenesis of cardiac valves and septum. *Nature* 392(6672):182-186.

De Windt, L.J., Lim, H.W., Bueno, O.F., Liang, Q., Delling, U., Braz, J.C., Glascock, B.J., Kimball, T.F., del Monte, F., Hajjar, R.J. & Molkentin, J.D. (2001). Targeted inhibition of calcineurin attenuates cardiac hypertrophy in vivo. *Proc.Natl Acad.Sci U.S.A* 98(6):3322-3327.

DeBakey, M.E., Lawrie, G.M. & Glaeser, D.H. (1985). Patterns of atherosclerosis and their surgical significance. *Ann.Surg.* 201(2):115-131.

Delabar, J.M., Theophile, D., Rahmani, Z., Chettouh, Z., Blouin, J.L., Prieur, M., Noel, B. & Sinet, P.M. (1993). Molecular mapping of twenty-four features of Down syndrome on chromosome 21. *Eur.J Hum Genet* 1(2):114-124.

Draheim, C.C., Geijer, J.R. & Dengel, D.R. (2010). Comparison of intima-media thickness of the carotid artery and cardiovascular disease risk factors in adults with versus without the Down syndrome. *Am J Cardiol.* 106(10):1512-1516.

Duque, J., Fresno, M. & Iniguez, M.A. (2005a). Expression and function of the nuclear factor of activated T cells in colon carcinoma cells: involvement in the regulation of cyclooxygenase-2. *J Biol Chem.* 280(10):8686-8693.

Duque, J., Fresno, M. & Iniguez, M.A. (2005b). Expression and function of the nuclear factor of activated T cells in colon carcinoma cells: involvement in the regulation of cyclooxygenase-2. *J Biol Chem.* 280(10):8686-8693.

Duque, J., Fresno, M. & Iniguez, M.A. (2005c). Expression and function of the nuclear factor of activated T cells in colon carcinoma cells: involvement in the regulation of cyclooxygenase-2. *J Biol Chem.* 280(10):8686-8693.

Duran, W.N., Breslin, J.W. & Sanchez, F.A. (2010). The NO cascade, eNOS location, and microvascular permeability. *Cardiovasc.Res.* 87(2):254-261.

Egan, J.F., Benn, P.A., Zelop, C.M., Bolnick, A., Gianferrari, E. & Borgida, A.F. (2004). Down syndrome births in the United States from 1989 to 2001. *Am J Obstet.Gynecol.* 191(3):1044-1048.

Forsythe, J.A., Jiang, B.H., Iyer, N.V., Agani, F., Leung, S.W., Koos, R.D. & Semenza, G.L. (1996). Activation of vascular endothelial growth factor gene transcription by hypoxia-inducible factor 1. *Mol Cell Biol* 16(9):4604-4613.

Fuentes, J.J., Genesca, L., Kingsbury, T.J., Cunningham, K.W., Perez-Riba, M., Estivill, X. & de la, L.S. (2000). DSCR1, overexpressed in Down syndrome, is an inhibitor of calcineurin-mediated signaling pathways. *Hum Mol Genet* 9(11):1681-1690.

Gollogly, L.K., Ryeom, S.W. & Yoon, S.S. (2007). Down syndrome candidate region 1-like 1 (DSCR1-L1) mimics the inhibitory effects of DSCR1 on calcineurin signaling in endothelial cells and inhibits angiogenesis. *J Surg.Res* 142(1):129-136.

Gordon, T., Castelli, W.P., Hjortland, M.C., Kannel, W.B. & Dawber, T.R. (1977). High density lipoprotein as a protective factor against coronary heart disease. The Framingham Study. *Am J Med.* 62(5):707-714.

Graef, I.A., Chen, F., Chen, L., Kuo, A. & Crabtree, G.R. (2001). Signals transduced by Ca(2+)/calcineurin and NFATc3/c4 pattern the developing vasculature. *Cell* 105(7):863-875.

Hanahan, D. & Weinberg, R.A. (2000). The Hallmarks of Cancer. *Cell* 100(1):57-70.

Hardy, J. & Selkoe, D.J. (2002). The amyloid hypothesis of Alzheimer's disease: progress and problems on the road to therapeutics. *Science* 297(5580):353-356.

Harris, C.D., Ermak, G. & Davies, K.J. (2005). Multiple roles of the DSCR1 (Adapt78 or RCAN1) gene and its protein product calcipressin 1 (or RCAN1) in disease. *Cell Mol Life Sci* 62(21):2477-2486.

Harris, M.B., Ju, H., Venema, V.J., Liang, H., Zou, R., Michell, B.J., Chen, Z.P., Kemp, B.E. & Venema, R.C. (2001). Reciprocal phosphorylation and regulation of endothelial nitric-oxide synthase in response to bradykinin stimulation. *J Biol Chem.* 276(19):16587-16591.

Hasle, H., Clemmensen, I.H. & Mikkelsen, M. (2000). Risks of leukaemia and solid tumours in individuals with Down's syndrome. *Lancet* 355(9199):165-169.

Hattori, M., Fujiyama, A., Taylor, T.D., Watanabe, H., Yada, T., Park, H.S., Toyoda, A., Ishii, K., Totoki, Y., Choi, D.K., Groner, Y., Soeda, E., Ohki, M., Takagi, T., Sakaki, Y., Taudien, S., Blechschmidt, K., Polley, A., Menzel, U., Delabar, J., Kumpf, K., Lehmann, R., Patterson, D., Reichwald, K., Rump, A., Schillhabel, M., Schudy, A., Zimmermann, W., Rosenthal, A., Kudoh, J., Schibuya, K., Kawasaki, K., Asakawa, S., Shintani, A., Sasaki, T., Nagamine, K., Mitsuyama, S., Antonarakis, S.E., Minoshima, S., Shimizu, N., Nordsiek, G., Hornischer, K., Brant, P., Scharfe, M., Schon, O., Desario, A., Reichelt, J., Kauer, G., Blocker, H., Ramser, J., Beck, A.,

Klages, S., Hennig, S., Riesselmann, L., Dagand, E., Haaf, T., Wehrmeyer, S., Borzym, K., Gardiner, K., Nizetic, D., Francis, F., Lehrach, H., Reinhardt, R. & Yaspo, M.L. (2000). The DNA sequence of human chromosome 21. *Nature* 405(6784):311-319.

Hernandez, G.L., Volpert, O.V., Iniguez, M.A., Lorenzo, E., Martinez-Martinez, S., Grau, R., Fresno, M. & Redondo, J.M. (2001). Selective inhibition of vascular endothelial growth factor-mediated angiogenesis by cyclosporin A: roles of the nuclear factor of activated T cells and cyclooxygenase 2. *J Exp Med.* 193(5):607-620.

Hesser, B.A., Liang, X.H., Camenisch, G., Yang, S., Lewin, D.A., Scheller, R., Ferrara, N. & Gerber, H.P. (2004). Down syndrome critical region protein 1 (DSCR1), a novel VEGF target gene that regulates expression of inflammatory markers on activated endothelial cells. *Blood* 104(1):149-158.

Hogan, P.G., Chen, L., Nardone, J. & Rao, A. (2003). Transcriptional regulation by calcium, calcineurin, and NFAT. *Genes and Development* 17(18):2205-2232.

Hokanson, J.E. & Austin, M.A. (1996). Plasma triglyceride level is a risk factor for cardiovascular disease independent of high-density lipoprotein cholesterol level: a meta-analysis of population-based prospective studies. *J Cardiovasc.Risk* 3(2):213-219.

Horsley, V., Aliprantis, A.O., Polak, L., Glimcher, L.H. & Fuchs, E. (2008). NFATc1 balances quiescence and proliferation of skin stem cells. *Cell* 132(2):299-310.

Horsley, V. & Pavlath, G.K. (2002). Nfat: ubiquitous regulator of cell differentiation and adaptation. *The Journal of Cell Biology* 156(5):771-774.

Iizuka, M., Abe, M., Shiiba, K., Sasaki, I. & Sato, Y. (2004). Down syndrome candidate region 1, a downstream target of VEGF, participates in endothelial cell migration and angiogenesis. *J.Vasc Res.* 41(4):334-344.

Iruela-Arispe, M.L., Carpizo, D. & Luque, A. (2003). ADAMTS1: a matrix metalloprotease with angioinhibitory properties. *Ann.N.Y.Acad.Sci.* 995:183-190.

Ishibashi, S., Brown, M.S., Goldstein, J.L., Gerard, R.D., Hammer, R.E. & Herz, J. (1993). Hypercholesterolemia in low density lipoprotein receptor knockout mice and its reversal by adenovirus-mediated gene delivery. *J Clin.Invest* 92(2):883-893.

Ishihara, K., Amano, K., Takaki, E., Ebrahim, A.S., Shimohata, A., Shibazaki, N., Inoue, I., Takaki, M., Ueda, Y., Sago, H., Epstein, C.J. & Yamakawa, K. (2009). Increased lipid peroxidation in Down's syndrome mouse models. *J Neurochem.* 110(6):1965-1976.

Jacobs, I.N., Gray, R.F. & Todd, N.W. (1996). Upper airway obstruction in children with Down syndrome. *Arch.Otolaryngol.Head Neck Surg.* 122(9):945-950.

Jauliac, S., Lopez-Rodriguez, C., Shaw, L.M., Brown, L.F., Rao, A. & Toker, A. (2002). The role of NFAT transcription factors in integrin-mediated carcinoma invasion. *Nat Cell Biol* 4(7):540-544.

Kerins, G., Petrovic, K., Bruder, M.B. & Gruman, C. (2008). Medical conditions and medication use in adults with Down syndrome: a descriptive analysis. *Downs.Syndr.Res.Pract.* 12(2):141-147.

Kingsbury, T.J. & Cunningham, K.W. (2000). A conserved family of calcineurin regulators. *Genes and Development* 14(13):1595-1604.

Korenberg, J.R., Chen, X.N., Schipper, R., Sun, Z., Gonsky, R., Gerwehr, S., Carpenter, N., Daumer, C., Dignan, P., Disteche, C. & . (1994). Down syndrome phenotypes: the consequences of chromosomal imbalance. *Proc.Natl.Acad.Sci.U.S.A* 91(11):4997-5001.

Kou, R., Greif, D. & Michel, T. (2002). Dephosphorylation of endothelial nitric-oxide synthase by vascular endothelial growth factor. Implications for the vascular responses to cyclosporin A. *J Biol Chem.* 277(33):29669-29673.

Landin, K., Blennow, K., Wallin, A. & Gottfries, C.G. (1993). Low blood pressure and blood glucose levels in Alzheimer's disease. Evidence for a hypometabolic disorder? *J Intern.Med.* 233(4):357-363.

Lange, A.W., Molkentin, J.D. & Yutzey, K.E. (2004). DSCR1 gene expression is dependent on NFATc1 during cardiac valve formation and colocalizes with anomalous organ development in trisomy 16 mice. *Developmental Biology* 266(2):346-360.

Lee, M.Y., Garvey, S.M., Baras, A.S., Lemmon, J.A., Gomez, M.F., Schoppee Bortz, P.D., Daum, G., LeBoeuf, R.C. & Wamhoff, B.R. (2010). Integrative genomics identifies DSCR1 (RCAN1) as a novel NFAT-dependent mediator of phenotypic modulation in vascular smooth muscle cells. *Hum Mol Genet* 19(3):468-479.

Lejeune J, Gautier, M. & Turpin, R. (1959). Etude des chromosomes somatiques de neuf enfants mongoliens. *Compte Rendu d'Acad Sci* (248):1721-1722.

Lipsky, P.E., Brooks, P., Crofford, L.J., DuBois, R., Graham, D., Simon, L.S., van de Putte, L.B. & Abramson, S.B. (2000). Unresolved issues in the role of cyclooxygenase-2 in normal physiologic processes and disease. *Arch.Intern.Med.* 160(7):913-920.

Liu, C.H., Chang, S.H., Narko, K., Trifan, O.C., Wu, M.T., Smith, E., Haudenschild, C., Lane, T.F. & Hla, T. (2001). Overexpression of cyclooxygenase-2 is sufficient to induce tumorigenesis in transgenic mice. *J Biol Chem.* 276(21):18563-18569.

Liu, Q., Busby, J.C. & Molkentin, J.D. (2009). Interaction between TAK1-TAB1-TAB2 and RCAN1-calcineurin defines a signalling nodal control point. *Nat Cell Biol* 11(2):154-161.

Liu, Z., Dronadula, N. & Rao, G.N. (2004). A novel role for nuclear factor of activated T cells in receptor tyrosine kinase and G protein-coupled receptor agonist-induced vascular smooth muscle cell motility. *J Biol Chem* 279(39):41218-41226.

Liu, Z., Zhang, C., Dronadula, N., Li, Q. & Rao, G.N. (2005). Blockade of Nuclear Factor of Activated T Cells Activation Signaling Suppresses Balloon Injury-induced Neointima Formation in a Rat Carotid Artery Model. *Journal of Biological Chemistry* 280(15):14700-14708.

Lusis, A.J. (2000). Atherosclerosis. *Nature* 407(6801):233-241.

Mendall, M.A., Patel, P., Ballam, L., Strachan, D. & Northfield, T.C. (1996). C reactive protein and its relation to cardiovascular risk factors: a population based cross sectional study. *BMJ* 312(7038):1061-1065.

Minami, T., Horiuchi, K., Miura, M., Abid, M.R., Takabe, W., Noguchi, N., Kohro, T., Ge, X., Aburatani, H., Hamakubo, T., Kodama, T. & Aird, W.C. (2004). Vascular endothelial growth factor- and thrombin-induced termination factor, Down syndrome critical region-1, attenuates endothelial cell proliferation and angiogenesis. *J Biol Chem* 279(48):50537-50554.

Molkentin, J.D., Lu, J.R., Antos, C.L., Markham, B., Richardson, J., Robbins, J., Grant, S.R. & Olson, E.N. (1998). A calcineurin-dependent transcriptional pathway for cardiac hypertrophy. *Cell* 93(2):215-228.

Moller, D.E. & Kaufman, K.D. (2005). Metabolic syndrome: a clinical and molecular perspective. *Annu.Rev.Med.* 56:45-62.

Morrison, R.A., McGrath, A., Davidson, G., Brown, J.J., Murray, G.D. & Lever, A.F. (1996). Low blood pressure in Down's syndrome, A link with Alzheimer's disease? *Hypertension* 28(4):569-575.

Mukherjee, D., Nissen, S.E. & Topol, E.J. (2001). Risk of cardiovascular events associated with selective COX-2 inhibitors. *JAMA* 286(8):954-959.

Mulero, M.C., Aubareda, A., Schluter, A. & Perez-Riba, M. (2007). RCAN3, a novel calcineurin inhibitor that down-regulates NFAT-dependent cytokine gene expression. *Biochim.Biophys.Acta* 1773(3):330-341.

Murdoch, J.C., Rodger, J.C., Rao, S.S., Fletcher, C.D. & Dunnigan, M.G. (1977). Down's syndrome: an atheroma-free model? *Br.Med.J* 2(6081):226-228.

Nilsson, L.M., Sun, Z.W., Nilsson, J., Nordstrom, I., Chen, Y.W., Molkentin, J.D., Wide-Swensson, D., Hellstrand, P., Lydrup, M.L. & Gomez, M.F. (2007). Novel blocker of NFAT activation inhibits IL-6 production in human myometrial arteries and reduces vascular smooth muscle cell proliferation. *AJP - Cell Physiology* 292(3):C1167-C1178.

Nishida, Y., Akaoka, I., Nishizawa, T., Maruki, M. & Maruki, K. (1977). Hyperlipidaemia in patients with Down's syndrome. *Atherosclerosis* 26(3):369-372.

Okamura, H., Aramburu, J., Garcia-Rodriguez, C., Viola, J.P., Raghavan, A., Tahiliani, M., Zhang, X., Qin, J., Hogan, P.G. & Rao, A. (2000). Concerted dephosphorylation of the transcription factor NFAT1 induces a conformational switch that regulates transcriptional activity. *Mol Cell* 6(3):539-550.

Olson, L.E., Richtsmeier, J.T., Leszl, J. & Reeves, R.H. (2004). A chromosome 21 critical region does not cause specific Down syndrome phenotypes. *Science* 306(5696):687-690.

Olson, L.E., Roper, R.J., Sengstaken, C.L., Peterson, E.A., Aquino, V., Galdzicki, Z., Siarey, R., Pletnikov, M., Moran, T.H. & Reeves, R.H. (2007). Trisomy for the Down syndrome 'critical region' is necessary but not sufficient for brain phenotypes of trisomic mice. *Hum Mol Genet* 16(7):774-782.

Pritchard, K.A., Jr., O'Banion, M.K., Miano, J.M., Vlasic, N., Bhatia, U.G., Young, D.A. & Stemerman, M.B. (1994). Induction of cyclooxygenase-2 in rat vascular smooth muscle cells in vitro and in vivo. *Journal of Biological Chemistry* 269(11):8504-8509.

Randak, C., Brabletz, T., Hergenrother, M., Sobotta, I. & Serfling, E. (1990). Cyclosporin A suppresses the expression of the interleukin 2 gene by inhibiting the binding of lymphocyte-specific factors to the IL-2 enhancer. *EMBO J* 9(8):2529-2536.

Rao, A., Luo, C. & Hogan, P.G. (1997). Transcription factors of the NFAT family: regulation and function. *Annu.Rev Immunol* 15:707-747.

Reddy, B.S., Hirose, Y., Lubet, R., Steele, V., Kelloff, G., Paulson, S., Seibert, K. & Rao, C.V. (2000). Chemoprevention of colon cancer by specific cyclooxygenase-2 inhibitor, celecoxib, administered during different stages of carcinogenesis. *Cancer Res.* 60(2):293-297.

Reeves, R.H. & Citron, M.P. (1994). Mouse chromosome 16. *Mamm.Genome* 5 Spec No:S229-S237.

Reeves, R.H., Irving, N.G., Moran, T.H., Wohn, A., Kitt, C., Sisodia, S.S., Schmidt, C., Bronson, R.T. & Davisson, M.T. (1995). A mouse model for Down syndrome exhibits learning and behaviour deficits. *Nat Genet* 11(2):177-184.

Richards, B.W. & Enver, F. (1979). Blood pressure in Down's syndrome. *J Ment.Defic.Res.* 23(2):123-135.

Riper, D.V., Jayakumar, L., Latchana, N., Bhoiwala, D., Mitchell, A.N., Valenti, J.W. & Crawford, D.R. (2008). Regulation of vascular function by RCAN1 (ADAPT78). *Arch.Biochem.Biophys.* 472(1):43-50.

Robbs, B.K., Cruz, A.L., Werneck, M.B., Mognol, G.P. & Viola, J.P. (2008). Dual roles for NFAT transcription factor genes as oncogenes and tumor suppressors. *Mol Cell Biol* 28(23):7168-7181.

Roizen, N.J. & Patterson, D. (2003). Down's syndrome. *Lancet* 361(9365):1281-1289.

Rothermel, B., Vega, R.B., Yang, J., Wu, H., Bassel-Duby, R. & Williams, R.S. (2000). A Protein Encoded within the Down Syndrome Critical Region Is Enriched in Striated Muscles and Inhibits Calcineurin Signaling. *Journal of Biological Chemistry* 275(12):8719-8725.

Rothermel, B.A., McKinsey, T.A., Vega, R.B., Nicol, R.L., Mammen, P., Yang, J., Antos, C.L., Shelton, J.M., Bassel-Duby, R., Olson, E.N. & Williams, R.S. (2001). Myocyte-enriched calcineurin-interacting protein, MCIP1, inhibits cardiac hypertrophy in vivo. *Proceedings of the National Academy of Sciences* 98(6):3328-3333.

Rudic, R.D., Brinster, D., Cheng, Y., Fries, S., Song, W.L., Austin, S., Coffman, T.M. & FitzGerald, G.A. (2005). COX-2-derived prostacyclin modulates vascular remodeling. *Circulation Research* 96(12):1240-1247.

Ryeom, S., Baek, K.H. & Zaslavsky, A. (2009). Down's syndrome: protection against cancer and the therapeutic potential of DSCR1. *Future.Oncol.* 5(8):1185-1188.

Sanna, B., Brandt, E.B., Kaiser, R.A., Pfluger, P., Witt, S.A., Kimball, T.R., van Rooij, E., De Windt, L.J., Rothenberg, M.E., Tschop, M.H., Benoit, S.C. & Molkentin, J.D. (2006). Modulatory calcineurin-interacting proteins 1 and 2 function as calcineurin facilitators in vivo. *Proc.Natl Acad.Sci U.S.A* 103(19):7327-7332.

Shin, S.Y., Choo, S.M., Kim, D., Baek, S.J., Wolkenhauer, O. & Cho, K.H. (2006). Switching feedback mechanisms realize the dual role of MCIP in the regulation of calcineurin activity. *FEBS Letters* 580(25):5965-5973.

Shin, S.Y., Yang, J.M., Choo, S.M., Kwon, K.S. & Cho, K.H. (2008). System-level investigation into the regulatory mechanism of the calcineurin/NFAT signaling pathway. *Cellular Signalling* 20(6):1117-1124.

Stoll, C., Alembik, Y., Dott, B. & Roth, M.P. (1990). Epidemiology of Down syndrome in 118, 265 consecutive births. *Am J Med.Genet Suppl* 7:79-83.

Strippoli, P., Lenzi, L., Petrini, M., Carinci, P. & Zannotti, M. (2000). A new gene family including DSCR1 (Down Syndrome Candidate Region 1) and ZAKI-4: characterization from yeast to human and identification of DSCR1-like 2, a novel human member (DSCR1L2). *Genomics* 64(3):252-263.

Sugimoto, T., Haneda, M., Sawana, H., Isshiki, K., Maeda, S., Koya, D., Inoki, K., Yasuda, H., Kashiwagi, A. & Kikkawa, R. (2001). Endothelin-1 Induces Cyclooxygenase-2 Expression Via Nuclear Factor of Activated T-Cell Transcription Factor in Glomerular Mesangial Cells. *Journal of the American Society of Nephrology* 12(7):1359-1368.

Thomas, S.R., Chen, K. & Keaney, J.F., Jr. (2002). Hydrogen peroxide activates endothelial nitric-oxide synthase through coordinated phosphorylation and dephosphorylation via a phosphoinositide 3-kinase-dependent signaling pathway. *J Biol Chem.* 277(8):6017-6024.

Vanderlaan, P.A., Reardon, C.A. & Getz, G.S. (2004). Site specificity of atherosclerosis: site-selective responses to atherosclerotic modulators. *Arteriosclerosis, Thrombosis, and Vascular Biology* 24(1):12-22.

Wilkins, B.J., De Windt, L.J., Bueno, O.F., Braz, J.C., Glascock, B.J., Kimball, T.F. & Molkentin, J.D. (2002). Targeted disruption of NFATc3, but not NFATc4, reveals an intrinsic defect in calcineurin-mediated cardiac hypertrophic growth. *Mol Cell Biol* 22(21):7603-7613.

Wouters, K., Shiri-Sverdlov, R., van Gorp, P.J., van Bilsen, M. & Hofker, M.H. (2005). Understanding hyperlipidemia and atherosclerosis: lessons from genetically modified apoe and ldlr mice. *Clin Chem Lab Med.* 43(5):470-479.

Wu, Y., Borde, M., Heissmeyer, V., Feuerer, M., Lapan, A.D., Stroud, J.C., Bates, D.L., Guo, L., Han, A., Ziegler, S.F., Mathis, D., Benoist, C., Chen, L. & Rao, A. (2006). FOXP3 controls regulatory T cell function through cooperation with NFAT. *Cell* 126(2):375-387.

Yang, Q., Rasmussen, S.A. & Friedman, J.M. (2002). Mortality associated with Down's syndrome in the USA from 1983 to 1997: a population-based study. *Lancet* 359(9311):1019-1025.

Yao, Y.G. & Duh, E.J. (2004). VEGF selectively induces Down syndrome critical region 1 gene expression in endothelial cells: a mechanism for feedback regulation of angiogenesis? *Biochem.Biophys.Res Commun.* 321(3):648-656.

Yellaturu, C.R., Ghosh, S.K., Rao, R.K., Jennings, L.K., Hassid, A. & Rao, G.N. (2002). A potential role for nuclear factor of activated T-cells in receptor tyrosine kinase and G-protein-coupled receptor agonist-induced cell proliferation. *Biochem.J* 368(Pt 1):183-190.

Yla-Herttuala, S., Luoma, J., Nikkari, T. & Kivimaki, T. (1989). Down's syndrome and atherosclerosis. *Atherosclerosis* 76(2-3):269-272.

Zaslavsky, A., Baek, K.H., Lynch, R.C., Short, S., Grillo, J., Folkman, J., Italiano, J.E., Jr. & Ryeom, S. (2010). Platelet-derived thrombospondin-1 is a critical negative regulator and potential biomarker of angiogenesis. *Blood* 115(22):4605-4613.

Part 2

Down Syndrome Models

8

Down Syndrome Model of Alzheimer's Disease: Beyond Trisomy 21Nondisjunction

Antoneta Granic and Huntington Potter
University of South Florida
USA

1. Introduction

Alzheimer's disease (AD), the most common type of dementia in old age, is a complex, multifactorial neurodegenerative disorder currently affecting 35,6 million people in either familial (genetic) or sporadic form, whose prevalence is expected to quadruple worldwide by the year 2050 (Alzheimer's Disease International, 2010; Ferri et al., 2005). While genetic or early-onset AD accounts for only 5% of all cases (Cummings, 2004), 95% of sporadic or late-onset AD is attributed to the interaction between advancing age, environmental factors (Grant, et al., 2002; Tanzi & Bertram, 2001), and to the few risk-enhancing genetic polymorphisms discovered so far (Bertram & Tanzi, 2004). Autosomal dominant mutations in the amyloid precursor protein (APP), presenilin 1 (PS1), and presenilin 2 (PS2) are linked to early-onset (familial) AD (FAD, Hardy, 2009). A combination of bio-psycho-social factors, especially if experienced at midlife, such as abnormal glucose and cholesterol metabolism, cerebral hypoperfusion, hypertension, physical and mental inactivity, diet, head injury, depression and small social networks are thought to contribute to sporadic AD initiation and development (reviewed in Flicker, 2010; Bendlin et al., 2010; Hughes & Ganguli, 2009). There is a temporal gap between clinical and pathological manifestation of Alzheimer's dementia; AD has a long prodromal phase and many clinically silent older adults are experiencing substantial pathological burden (Elias et al., 2000; Small et al., 2000). Common clinical manifestation of AD include memory impairment and dysfunctions in several cognitive domains such as language, problem solving, executive function, visuospatial skills, and others along with changes in personality and behavior (Maurer & Hoyer, 2006).

1.1 Neuropathology of Alzheimer's disease

The brain pathology of AD is characterized by extracellular deposits of the amyloid-beta peptide (Aβ), a main constituent of senile plaques, and intracellular accumulation of the hyperphosphorylated protein tau (p-tau) (Selkoe, 1999; 2001). The central hypothesis of AD, the amyloid cascade hypothesis, posits that an imbalance between Aβ production, aggregation and clearance from the brain is the initiating event in the disease process leading to synaptic loss, neuronal degeneration, inflammation, senile plaque formation and dementia (Blennow, de Leon, & Zetterberg, 2006; Hardy, 2006; Hardy & Selkoe, 2002; Lee et al., 2004; Potter et al., 2001).

The main constituent of the extracellular senile plaques is a highly neurotoxic Aβ42 isoform of Aβ protein, produced by consecutive action of two cleaving proteases, β- (BACE-1) and γ-secretase, from a larger transmembrane protein, the Amyloid Precursor Protein (APP) (Hardy, 2009; Haass & Selkoe, 1993; Wolfe, 2003) within cholesterol rich membrane domains (Wahrle et al., 2002). A number of biochemical and genetic studies have indicated that oligomerization or polymerization of Aβ peptide driven by inflammation-induced proteins is a crucial step in AD pathogenesis (Potter et al., 2001; Hardy, 2006). Aβ42 self-aggregates and forms insoluble plaque deposits that include dystrophic neurites, activated microglia and reactive astrocytes (Itagati et al., 1989) which express a number of proinflammatory proteins (Akiyama et al., 2000; Potter et al., 2001). Furthermore, Aβ induces increased phosphorylation of the intracellular protein tau, resulting in destabilization of microtubules (MT) (Small & Duff, 2008). The evidence from transgenic mice and human studies indicates that not only extracellular, but also intracellular Aβ accumulates in diseased neurons and contributes to dementia progression by affecting the function of mitochondria, calcium ion channels and synapses (La Ferla, Green, and Oddo, 2007; Li et al., 2007). It is still unclear which toxic species of the Aβ peptide are most damaging to the neurons or whether the process of aggregation itself is detrimental to neuronal membranes.

Neurofibrillary tangles (NFTs) are the second major pathological hallmark in AD, which result from abnormally aggregated tau protein filling the intracellular space of the neurons. In AD brain, tau gets hyperphosphorylated, detaches from microtubules and forms paired helical filaments, which cause disruption in neuronal signaling, synaptic failure, impaired nutrient trafficking and neuronal death (Alonso et al., 2006; Grundke-Iqbal et al., 1986). Furthermore, oxidative damage as a consequence of free radical and reactive oxygen species (ROS) attacks has been observed in post-mortem AD brains in the form of oxidized lipids and proteins, mutated DNA, and mitochondrial damage (Floyd & Hensley, 2002). Formation of amyloid plaques and neurofibrillary tangles is not only associated with neuronal and synaptic loss, and depletion of neurotransmitters (Scheff, et al., 2006; Selkoe, 1999; 2004), but with abnormal axonal transport of key molecules and organelles important for neural cells survival and communication early in the disease process (Stokin et al., 2005; Stokin & Goldstein, 2006). Neurons, with their long axons, branched dendrites and large cell surface are especially vulnerable to energy and/or oxygen deprivation, impaired movement of molecules, and neurotoxins observed in AD pathology (Mattson & Magnus, 2006). The development of early diagnosis and successful treatments of AD will be greatly aided by a complete understanding of the pathological pathway that leads to formation of misfolded proteins, inflammation and neurodegeneration.

1.2 The Down syndrome model of Alzheimer's disease

The discovery that Down syndrome (DS) patients who live beyond the age of 30 or 40 develop neuropathology indistinguishable from the one observed in classic AD (Glenner & Wang, 1984; Olson & Shaw, 1969; Wisniewski et al., 1988) provided an important insight into AD pathogenesis, shifting the focus on nondisjunction of human chromosome 21 (HSA21) where the APP gene resides (Goldgaber et al. 1987; Neve et al., 1988; Petterson et al., 1988; Tanzi et al., 1987), and on the consequence of the gene overexpression in DS (Epstein, 1990). The fact that an extra copy of APP and subsequent 50% increase in gene dosage due to trisomy 21 in every cell of the body in DS individuals is sufficient to cause AD later in life instigated research on common biological links between AD and DS (Potter, 1991, 2008; Geller & Potter, 1999). Trisomy 21 results in altered APP processing and in an increased ratio of more amyloidogenic Aβ42 over Aβ40 (Teller et al., 1996), similar to the process observed in animal models of AD and in patients harboring mutations in FAD genes, PS1, PS2 and APP (Haas & De Stooper, 1999; Hardy & Selkoe, 2002; Suzuki et al., 1994; Wolfe, 2003).

Several biochemical and genetic studies have shown that both sporadic and familial AD patients, including those carrying FAD mutations, are abnormal in one or more aspects of the cell cycle (Arendt et al., 1996; Geller & Potter, 1999; Potter, 1991; Varvel et al., 2008; Yang et al., 2001; 2006; Yang & Herrup, 2007; reviewed in Nagy, 2005; Obrenovic et al., 2003; Potter, 2004, 2008). The universal presence of AD pathology in DS individuals and the occurrence of an aberrant cell cycle in the brains of FAD mouse models and AD patients, led us to hypothesize that a slow accumulation of aneuploid, including trisomy 21 cells through defective mitosis and chromosome mis-segregation in central and peripheral tissues over the course of life of an individual could cause or at least help promote late-onset Alzheimer's (Potter, 1991; 2008). The extra copy of chromsome 21 that in full human trisomy of DS leads to neurodegeneration and dementia, could account for both genetic and sporadic AD, depending upon whether the chromosomal instability and mosaic aneuploidy was induced by a genetic (familial) mutation or by environmental insults. We further postulated that the microtubule disfunction likely responsible for the mitotic defects and genomic instability in AD could be linked to altered APP production and increased Aβ levels, probably affecting other aspects of neuronal physiology and function (Borysov et al., 2011; Granic et al., 2010; Potter, 2008).

The Down syndrome model and chromosome mis-segregation/microtubule disfunction hypothesis of AD made several predictions (Geller & Potter, 1999; Potter, 2008):

1. Alzheimer's patients should harbor a small number of aneuploid, including trisomy 21 cells in their somatic tissues. Altered genomic stability and development of trisomy 21 mosaicism would contribute to dementia onset and neurodegeneration but at slower pace than in DS due to the modulating effect of mostly disomic cells in the body.
2. Mutations that cause familial AD should occur in genes that encode proteins directly or indirectly involved in the cell cycle and chromosome segregation.
3. There should be alternations in microtubules, mitotic spindle apparatus and mitosis-related proteins in AD cells that could lead to aneuploidy, including trisomy 21 mosaicism.

In the past twenty years, compelling epidemiological and molecular evidence from our and other laboratories has been accumulated to test all three predictions. Together, the evidence suggests a link between pathological changes observed in the brains of DS and AD individuals and chromosomal instability and mosaic aneuploidy, including nondisjunction of HSA21 which likely contributes to dementia initiation and/or progression, with important implications for AD diagnosis and therapy.

2. The epidemiology of trisomy 21 mosaicism in Alzheimer's disease

Early epidemiological evidence indicating that chromosome mis-segregation and trisomy 21 mosaicism might be implicated in AD pathogenesis came for the studies showing a significantly higher number of Down syndrome offspring born in some families with FAD mutations (Heston et al., 1981; Heyman et al., 1983). The studies that failed to confirm this association reported to have too small sample sizes to observe statistically significant results (Amaducci et al., 1986; Chandra et al., 1987) suggesting that larger scale studies are needed to establish a connection between a higher frequency of DS children in families with genetic forms of AD. An important result that provided support for the trisomy 21 model of AD came from a retrospective study of young mothers (aged <35) showing a five-fold greater risk of developing AD later in life compared to either older DS mothers or the general population (Schupf et al., 1994; 2001). Schupf and her colleagues interpreted this phenomenon as a novel form of 'accelerated aging'. In the light of our trisomy 21 model of AD, we postulated that the young DS mothers were most likely mosaic for chromosome 21 and had a predisposition for genomic instability, which resulted in DS progeny and their own increased risk of AD later in life. Indeed, a recent study by Migliore et al. (2006; 2009) confirmed the susceptibility to aneuploidy and trisomy 21 nondisjunction in young mothers of DS children. Case studies of patients with trisomy 21 mosaicism and no intellectual impairments of the DS type who developed AD by the age of 40 demonstrated that a small percentage of chromosomal instability is sufficient to result in early-onset AD (Hardy, et al., 1989; Ringman et al. 2008; Schapiro et al., 1989). Similarly, a slow accumulation of a low number of trisomy 21 cells over the life span may lead and/or contribute to the pathogenesis of both genetic and sporadic form of AD.

In order to directly test if Alzheimer's patients harboured mis-segregated including trisomy 21 cells, we and others have used fluorescence *in situ* hybridization (FISH), a cytogenetic technique that allows one to detect the number of copies of a particular chromosome in both metaphase and interphase cells (Ried, 1998) with great sensitivity and specificity. This method is especially suitable for poorly and non-dividing cells, or for the cells with a very low level of aneuploidy (e.g., lymphocytes). In our early study of chromosome mis-segregation in AD, we found more than twice the frequency of trisomy 21 in skin fibroblasts of AD patients (p=0.007) compared to age-matched controls, which was not related to the age of affected individuals (Figure 1, Geller & Potter, 1999). A small parallel study of chromosome 18 nondisjunction showed a similar increase in aneuploidy, indicating that the mitotic defect likely affected all chromosomes. The AD fibroblasts in our study included those with sporadic (late-onset) AD and those carrying a familial AD mutation in PS1, PS2, or APP which are now known to cause early AD onset and altered APP processing (e.g., Li et al., 1995; Schellenberg et al., 1993; Rogaev et al. 1995).

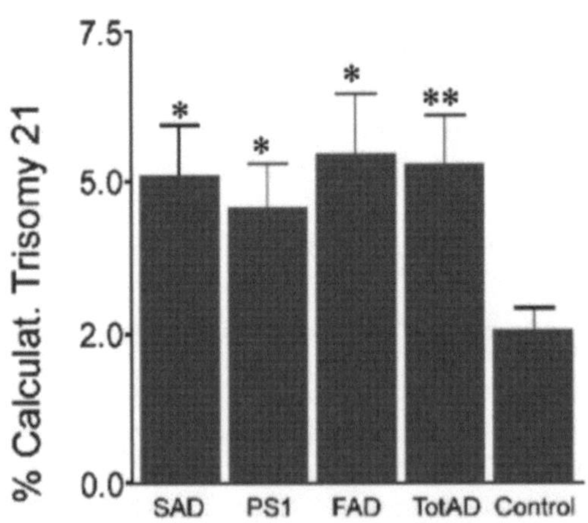

Fig. 1. AD fibroblasts, including those with PS1 or PS2 mutation (FAD) and those of sporadic origin (SAD) showed increased trisomy 21, *p < 0.01; **p < 0.001. (Used with permission from Geller & Potter, 1999, *Neurobiology of Disease*).

Trisomy 21 mosaicism and chromosome mis-segregation have also been observed among peripheral blood lymphocytes (Migliore 1997; 1999; Trippi et al., 2001), buccal cells (Thomas & Fenech, 2008), and neurons from sporadic AD patients (Arendt et al., 2010; Iourov et al., 2009; Mosch et al., 2007; Yang et al., 2001). Specifically, AD brains harbor up to 35% of hyperploid, including trisomy 21 and other tetrasomic neurons which are detectable at mild stages of the disease before any evident neuronal loss (Arendt et al., 2010; Iourov et al. 2009). The presence of tetrasomic neurons as explained by some reseachers, may indicate re-entry into an incomplete cell cycle and selective vulnerability to cell death of post-mitotic, mosaic neurons as an important pathogenic event in AD (Arendt et al., 2010; Obrenovich et al., 2003; Varvel et al., 2008; Vincent et al., 1996; Yang & Herrup, 2007). In our studies of AD mosaicism (Boeras et al., 2008; Geller & Potter, 1999; Granic et al., 2010), we failed to observe statistically significant induction of tetrasomic cells in sporadic and familial models of AD, but rather pronounced accumulation of trisomy cells in both peripheral and brain tissues. A larger scale cytogenetic autopsy and biopsy study, preferably at the single cell level is needed to further elucitate the type and extent of pathologic genetic instability in AD and other neurodegenerative diseases.

In summary, several laboratories confirmed that trisomy 21 mosaicism is commonly associated with AD. Moreover, there is an indication of a dose response effect in which full trisomy 21 in DS individuals elicits AD-like pathology by age 20 and by middle age in familial AD and even later in sporadic Alzheimer's patients, who also belonged to the trisomy 21 mosaic group found to have an increased frequency of DS children before the age of 35. The recent discovery of families that develop early-onset inherited AD only because the APP gene on one chromosome 21 is duplicated (McNaughton et al., 2010; Rovelet-Lecrux et al., 2006; Sleegers et al., 2006) indicates that the extra copy of the APP gene and consequent overproduction of Aβ peptide is the likely cause of AD in both Down syndrome and trisomy 21 mosaic individuals.

2.1 Mitotic defects in Alzheimer's disease

Along with the studies described above, separate lines of investigations provided independent evidence that other mitotic defects and mitosis-specific proteins may be present in the cells of AD patients (reviewed in Potter, 2004). For instance, the mitotic spindles in dividing AD cells exhibit abnormalities and susceptibility to premature centromere division (PCD) and micronucleation upon chemically induced (e.g., colchicines) microtubule damage (e.g., Fitzgerald et al., 1986; Potter et al., 1995; Trippi et al., 2001). The event of PCD, in which individual sister chromatids are separated by a clear gap and not connected at the centromeres, has been observed in patients prone to genomic instability and chromosome mis-segregation, and recently confirmed in neurons of individuals with sporadic AD (Spremo-Potparević et al., 2008).

Further evidence linking cell cycle defects with AD pathogenesis came for the finding that both APP and the microtubule-stabilizing tau protein get increasingly phosphorylated during mitosis (Suzuki et al., 1994; Pope et al., 1994; Padmanabhan et al., 2011). Also, phospho-tau and other mitosis-specific phospho-proteins are overexpressed in AD but not in normal brains (e.g., Arendt et al., 1996; Vincent et al., 1996; Nagy et al., 1997), indicating a cycling stage of AD neurons. The idea of unscheduled cycle in fully differentiated neurons challenged the dogma of their post-mitotic nature and the inability to replicate (Rakic, 1985). To date, the evidence drawn from animal models of AD and autopsy studies of human brains indicates that reactivation of the cell cycle and DNA duplication (e.g., Yang et al.,

2001) in the vulnerable population of AD neurons may present a fundamental initiator of AD pathogenesis (Nagy, 2005; Vincent et al., 1996; Varvel et al., 2008; Yang & Herrup, 2007; Yang et al., 2006) present before deposition of fibrilar Aβ and neuronal death, and could also lead to chromosome mis-segregation and aneuploidy.

3. Presenilin and APP mutations induced aneuploidy

The finding that fibroblast cultures from patients carrying autosomal dominant mutations in the PS1, PS2 or APP gene harbour chromosomal instability and trisomy 21 mosaicism provided the first indication that FAD genes are likely to be involved in mitosis and chromosome mis-segregation, or to be associated with structures and proteins of the cell cycle (Geller & Potter, 1999).

Indeed, we and others have confirmed a major location of PS1 and PS2 proteins in dividing cells in the centromeres, the nuclear envelope, and the kinetochores during interphase (Li et al., 1997; Honda et al., 2000). Further support for a mitotic function of presenilins comes from studies showing inhibition of the cell cycle (Janicki & Montero, 1999) and increased sensitivity to apoptosis (Vito et al., 1996; Wolozin et al., 1996) in the cells carrying a mutated PS gene. Furthermore, polymorphisms in the PS1 gene have been associated with an increased risk of AD (Wragg et al., 1996; Higuchi et al., 1996; Scott et al., 1996) and with an increase of DS offspring via a meiosis II defect (Petersen et al., 2000; Lucarelli et al., 2004) as a more direct confirmation of PS1 involvement in the cell cycle.

Further research should be directed at discovering the mechanism by which the mutant presenilins influence chromosome segregation. One possibility supported by the data collected so far points to inability of altered presenilin proteins to properly link the chromosomes to the nuclear envelope and to release them at the appropriate time during mitosis, which may lead to chromosome mis-segregation and other cell cycle abnormalities. Another possibility discussed further below links PS mutations to altered processing of APP and increased production of neurotoxic Aβ42 as a likely effector molecule responsible for cell cycle defects, including mitotic spindle abnormalities and chromosome mis-segregation (Boeras et al., 2008; Borysov et al., 2011, Granic et al., 2010). Similarly, APP is also found to localize to the centrosomes and nuclear membrane in dividing cells (Nizzari et al., 2007; Zitnik et al., 2006), and to get increasingly phosphorylated during the cell cycle (Padmanabhan et al., 2011).

In a series of *in vivo* and *in vitro* experiments we investigated the role of mutated PS1 and APP genes and their proteolytic product, the Aβ peptide in chromosome mis-segregation and trisomy 21 mosaicism. All assays, tissues and cells from transgenic mice carrying AD mutations and the cells transfected with FAD genes or treated with Aβ peptide yielded comparable results: overexpression of FAD genes *in vivo* and *in vitro* and exposure to Aβ peptide induced chromosome instability and trisomy 21 mosaicism through several defects in mitotic spindle apparatii and dysfunction of microtubule assembly (Boeras et al., 2008; Borysov et al., 2011; Granic et al., 2010; Potter et al., 2008).

3.1 Presenilin and APP mutations induced aneuploidy in transgenic mice

We asked whether chromosome mis-segregation and trisomy 21 mosaicism observed in human fibroblasts with PS1 or APP mutations could be mimicked in peripheral and brain tissues of FAD-transgenic mice. For example, whole brains from PS1 (M146l and M146V) and APP (V717) mutant mice and non-transgenic littermates were processed to yield primary cultures. The isolated neurons were hybridized with a mouse chromosome 16 BAC probe (Kulnane et al., 2002), followed by immunocytochemistry to stain for neurons. Most cells were disomic with two copies of chromosome 16; while the neurons from PS1 mutant and PS1 knock in mice exhibited up to 4% of trisomy 16 (data not shown, Boeras et al, 2008), the APP-transgenic mice had about 6.5% of trisomies (Figure 2, Granic et al., 2010).

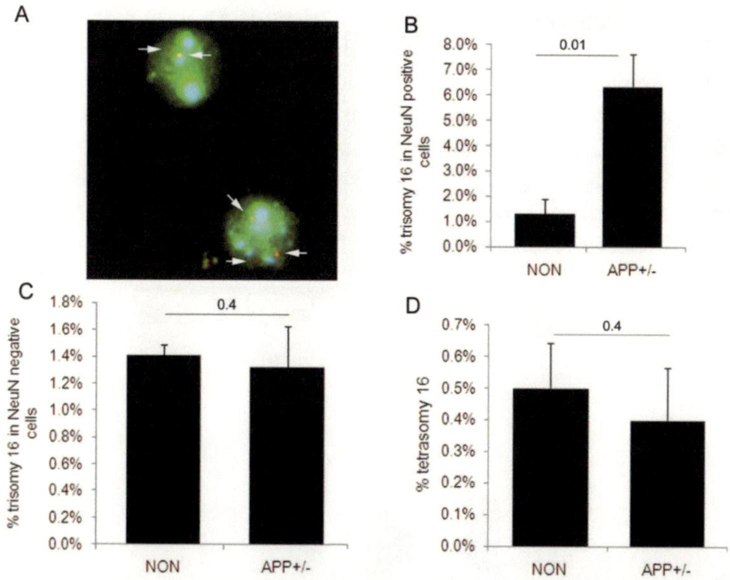

Fig. 2. Quantitative FISH analysis revealed significantly higher levels of trisomy 16 in APP mice (A & B) compared to controls but no tetrasomy (D) and no induction of aneuploidy in non-neuronal cells (C). (Used with permission from Granic et al., 2010, *Molecular Biology of the Cell*).

3.2 Presenilin and APP mutations induced aneuploidy in transfected cells

To determine whether the aneuploidy observed in FAD-transgenic and knock-in mice was caused directly by mutated genes and not by some other factors, parallel cultures of the hTERT-HME1, an immortalized primary mammary epithelial cell line with a stable karyotype (Clontech) were transiently transfected with WT-PS1, mutant PS1 (M146L), mutant APP (K595N/M596L and V642I or V717) and control empty vector (pcDNA3 and paG3). FISH was used to assess the levels of aneuploidy for chromosome 21 and 12. Overexpression of FAD-genes induced between 2-3% of trisomy 21 and/or trisomy 12 (Boeras et al., 2008; Granic et al., 2010), and about 30% of total aneuploidy in metaphase cells within 48 hours (Boeras et al., 2008). These results indicated that an aneugenic effect of FAD-mutations likely affected all chromosomes with random gains and losses of whole chromosomes, and that chromosome mis-segregation was not restricted only to the cells expressing mutated genes, but extended to nearby, non-transfected cells. We hypothesized that Aβ peptide itself found at increased levels in both familial and sporadic AD might be the probable effector molecule interfering with mitosis and chromosome segregation (Boeras et al., 2008; Potter, 2008). Lastly, immunocytochemistry of PS1-transfected cells revealed several abnormalities in the mitotic spindles, with disarrayed microtubules, multiple centosomes and lagging chromosomes as the most prominent spindle malformations (Boeras et al., 2008).

3.3 Aβ induced aneuploidy and the role of tau

Sequential cleavage of the APP protein with β- and presenilin/γ-secretase enzymes yields more amyloidogenic Aβ42 peptide as a central event in AD pathogenesis. We proposed to test the role of Aβ in genomic instability and trisomy 21 induction. Led by our initial observation that more cells became aneuploid than are transfected and express FAD genes, we examined the aneugenic effect of Aβ peptide in culture. hTERT-HME cells treated with 1μM Aβ40 and Aβ42 develop more than 20% aneuploid metaphases and about 2% trisomy 21 and 12 cells within the 48 hours of exposure compared to 6% and less than 1% of the cells treated with various control peptides (Figure 3, Granic et al., 2010). These results indicated that AD might be a self-propagating disorder in which the product of FAD mutations and trisomy 21, the Aβ peptide, further induces chromosome segregation and generation of trisomy 21 cells.

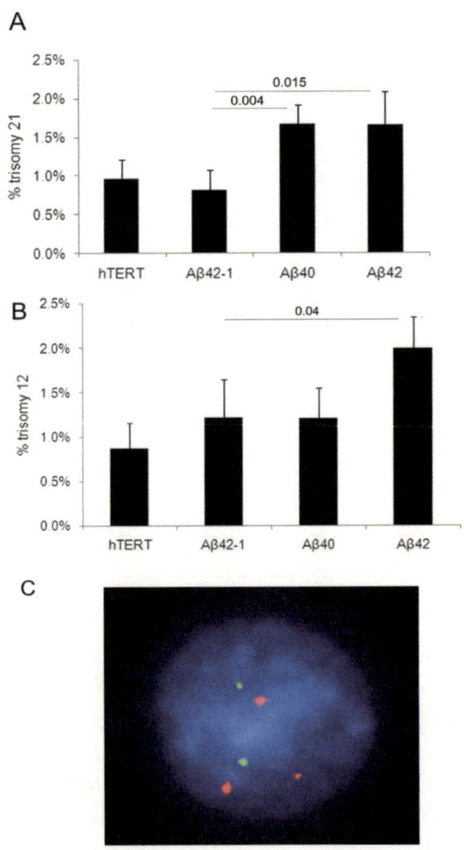

Fig. 3. Quantitative FISH analysis with a dual color probe revealed an increased induction of trisomy 21 (SpectrumOrange, Vysis) and trisomy 12 (SpectrumGreen) in Aβ treated hTERT-HME cells (A-C). (Used with permission from Granic et al., 2010, *Molecular Biology of the Cell*).

To investigate the mechanism by which Aβ exerts its aneugenic effect on dividing cells, we analyzed the peptide's other toxic activities especially those related to microtubule function. Several lines of investigation have indicated that Aβ induces and requires downstream changes/defects in microtubules (MT) to exert its neurodegenerative activity. Numerous *in vitro* and *in vivo* studies have shown that Aβ induces phosphorylation of tau (e.g., Small & Duff, 2008), and that Aβ toxicity depends on the presence of tau (Rappaport et al., 2002). Therefore, we investigated the role of tau in Aβ induced aneuploidy. Splenocytes prepared from normal, Tau+/-, Tau -/- mice were treated with Aβ peptide and analyzed for aneuploidy 48 hours later. Knocking out one or even more effectively both copies of Tau induced up to 5% aneuploidy (trisomy 16). However, the Aβ aneugenic effect was greatly attenuated in the cells lacking Tau but not in normal cells, indicating that Aβ induced chromosome mis-segregation requires tau protein and disrupts normal tau-stabilizing microtubule function. In a series of studies, Borysov et al. (2011) have shown that Aβ42 peptide added to *Xenopus* egg extracts impairs the structure and stability of mitotic spindles, and inhibits three motor kinesins, Eg5, KIF4A, and MCAK, required for normal mitotic spindle function and proper chromosome segregation.

Recently, we have shown that overexperssion of APP prevents the localization of low density lipoprotein receptor (LDLR) from the Golgi to the cell membrane (Abisambra et al., 2010). This latest finding led us to hypothetize that neurons exposed to Aβ in AD brains may also fail to localize other key receptors to the cell membrane, including those for neurotrophins and neurotransmitters, causing neuronal disfunction and dementia. Future studies are under way to confirm if the interference with microtubule function by Aβ will cause defects in neuroplasticity through mis-localization of the receptors away from the plasma membrane, as well as contributing to defective neurogenesis leading to dysfunctional, aneuploid, including trisomy 21 neurons prone to Aβ overproduction and neurodegeneration.

4. How trisomy 21 mosaicism may lead to Alzheimer's disease

Several potential mechanisms could explain how trisomy 21 mosaicism could lead to AD (Potter, 1991; 2004; 2008). For instance, aneuploidy cells might be prone to cell death and neurodegeneration (Arendt et al., 2010), similar to cortical neurons in DS brains that undergo spontaneous apoptosis (Busciglio & Yankner, 1997). Apoptosis could also indirectly affect APP processing and Aβ levels in mosaic AD brain. The support for the latter hypothesis comes from the finding that embryonic DS brains and adult sera contain a higher ratio of neurotoxic Aβ42 over Aβ40 peptide (Teller et al., 1996). Also, trisomy 21 microglia overexpress inflammatory proteins and begin an inflammatory cascade that promotes Aβ fibrilization (Potter et al., 2001). Finally, aneuploidy in AD may arise from a defect in microtubule function which may lead to poor protein, neurotransmitters and nutrient trafficking (Cash et al., 2003). Trisomy 21 may be both a cause and an effect of microtubule dysfunction generating a feed-forward loop further promoting AD progression.

5. Implications of the trisomy 21 model of Alzheimer's disease for diagnosis and therapy

The mechanistic implication of the results discussed in this review is that an early step in Alzheimer's disease pathogenesis may be the development of genomic instability and trisomy 21, contributing to progression of dementia. The search for more effective diagnoses should take into account the events of mitotic defects in peripheral and central tissues of individuals at risk. Chromosome analysis and detection of low levels of trisomy 21 in skin fibroblasts or buccal cells in patients during the pre-clinical phase of dementia could be a potential diagnostic test. Another implication of the data presented above that trisomy 21 in AD may be the initiating event in disease pathogenesis also suggests new approaches to treatments (Potter, 2004). For example, drugs that would repair the mitotic defects and strengthen the fidelity of the chromosome segregation could be searched for and used prophylactically. Further, aneugenic environmental agents that cause chromosome instability could be identified and counteracted with drugs that restore genomic homeostasis. Another more difficult but equally effective approach to therapy would be to detect and remove mis-segregated cells from the body by exploiting their unique cell biology and/or gene expression.

To summarize, the results from several laboratories over the past twenty years have shown that Alzheimer's patients are prone to genomic instability accumulating about 2-3 fold more trisomy 21 cells throughout the body compared to age matched healthy controls. The precise mechanism by which these abnormal cells arise during the life span of an individual and how or whether they contribute to disease initiation and progression are subjects of active investigation. The better understanding of these novel findings has the potential to contribute to the development of future diagnoses and therapies for Alzheimer's disease.

6. Summary

Convincing epidemiological and molecular evidence has been accumulating that link pathological changes observed in the brains of both Down syndrome individuals and neurodegeneration in Alzheimer's disease to chromosomal instability and trisomy 21 mosaicism. The results from several laboratories indicate that errors in mitosis, specifically mis-segregation of somatic chromosomes in peripheral and brain tissues of AD patients may play an important role in both early (familial) and late (sporadic) onset of disease. Here, we proposed a unifying hypothesis for Alzheimer's and Down syndrome neurodegeneration—development of a mosaic population of aneuploid, including trisomy 21 cells and alternation in genomic stability may lead to classic AD neuropathology observed in both diseases. The evidence for this hypothesis include: a) cells from familial and sporadic AD patients exhibit mis-segregated, including trisomy 21 cells in brain, blood, mucosa and skin, and harbour abnormalities in several aspects of the cell cycle that may contribute to aneuploidy and neurodegeneration; b) overexpression of mutated Alzheimer's genes, presenilin 1 and APP, in cellular and transgenic mouse models induce aneuploidy, including trisomy 21; and c) Aβ peptide is the likely effector molecule responsible for disruption of proper functioning of microtubules and mitotic spindle integrity leading to mitotic defects and apoptosis. The possibility that many cases of Alzheimer's disease are mosaic for trisomy 21 opens new approaches for diagnosis and therapy.

7. Acknowledgment

Our work was supported by the Byrd Alzheimer's Institute, the Eric Pfeiffer Chair for Research on Alzheimer's Disease, the Alzheimer's Association, and the National Institute on Aging grant No. AG25711. We thank Dr. Bruce Lamb for the chromosome 16 BAC probe and Dr. Karen Duff for PS1 transgenic mice. Figure 1 was reprinted from the publication 'Chromosome missegregation and trisomy 21 mosaicism in Alzheimer's disease', *Neurobiology of Disease,* Vol. 6, No. 3, (December, 1998), pp. 167-179, Geller, L. N., & Potter, H. (1999), copyright (1998), with permission from Elsevier. Figure 2 and Figure 3 were reprinted from the publication 'Alzheimer Aβ peptide induces chromosome mis-segregation and aneuploidy, including trisomy 21: requirement for tau and APP. *Molecular Biology of the Cell,* Vol. 21, No. 4, (December, 2009), pp. 511-520, copyright (2009), with the permission from the Molecular Biology of the Cell.

8. References

Abisambra, J. F., Fiorelli, T., Padmanabhan, J., et al. (2010). LDLR expression and localization are altered in mouse and human cell culture models of Alzheimer's disease. *PLoS ONE,* Vol. 5, No. 1, (January, 2010), pp. e8556

Akiyama, H., Barger, S., Barnum, S., et al. (2000). Inflammation and Alzheimer's disease. *Neurobiology of Aging,* Vol. 21, No. 3, (May, 2000), pp.383-421

Alonso, A del C., Li, B., Grudke-Iqbal, & Igbal. K (2006). Polymerization of hyperphosphorylated tau into filaments eliminates its inhibitory activity. *Proceedings of the National Academy of Science of the USA,* Vol. 103, .23, (June, 2006), pp. 8864-8869

Amaducci, L. A., Fratiglioni, L., Rocca, W. A., et al. (1986). Risk factors for clinically diagnosed Alzheimer's disease : a case-control study of an Italian population. *Neurology,* Vol. 36, No. 7, (July, 1986), pp. 922-931

Alzheimer's Disease International (2010). World Alzheimer Report 2010, In: *Alzheimer's Disease International,* 12.12.2010, Available from: http://www.alz.co.uk/research/files/WorldAlzheimerReport2010ExecutiveSummary

Arendt, T., Brückner, M. K., Mosch, B., et al. (2010). Selective cell death of hyperploid neurons in Alzheimer's disease. *The American Journal of Pathology,* Vol. 177, No. 1, (July, 10), pp. 15-20

Arendt, T., Rodel., L., Gartner, U., et al. (1996). Expression of the cyclin-dependent kinase inhibitor p16 in Alzheimer's disease. *Neuroreports,* Vo. 7, No. 18, (November, 1996), pp. 3047-3049

Bendlin, B. B., Caresson, C. M., Gleason, C. E., et al. (2010). Midlife predictors of Alzheimer's disease. *Maturitas,* Vol. 65, No. 2, (February, 2010), pp. 131-137

Bertram, L., & Tanzi, R. E. (2005). Alzheimer's disease: one disorder, too many genes? *Human Molecular Genetics,* Vol.13 Spec, No. 1,(April, 2004), pp. R135-141

Blennow, K., de Leon, M., & Zetterberg, H. (2006). Alzheimer's disease. *The Lancet,* Vol. 368, No. 9533, (July, 2006), pp. 387-403

Boeras, D. I., Granic, A., Padmanabhan, J., et al. (2008). Alzheimer's presenilin 1 causes chromosome missegregation and aneuploidy. *Neurobiology of Aging,* Vol. 29, No 3, (December, 2006), pp. 319-328

Borysov, S.I., Granic, A., Padmanabhan, J., Walczak, C. E., & Potter, H. (2011). Alzheimer Aβ disrupts the mitotic spindle and directly inhibits mitotic microtubule motors. *Cell Cycle,* Vol. 10, No. 9, (May, 2011), pp.1-14.

Busciglio, J., & Yankner, B. A. (1996). Apoptosis and increased generation of reactive oxygen species in Down syndrome neurons in vitro. *Nature*, Vol. 378, No. 6559, (December, 1995), pp. 776-779

Cash, A. D., Aliev, G., Siedlak, S. L., et al. (2003). Microtubule reduction in Alzheimer's disease and aging is independent of tau filament formation. *American Journal of Pathology*, Vol. 162, No. 5, (May, 2003), pp. 1623-1627

Chandra, V., Philipose, V., Bell, P. A., et al. (1987). Case-control study of probable Alzheimer's disease. *Neurology*, Vol. 37, No. 8, (August, 1987), pp. 1295-1300

Cummings, J. L. (2004). Alzheimer's disease. *New England Journal of Medicine*, Vol. 351, No. 1, (July 2004), pp. 56-67

Elias, M. F., Beiser, A., Wolf, P. A., et al. (2000). The preclinical phase of Alzheimer disease: A 22-year prospective study of Framingham cohort. *Archives of Neurology*, Vo. 57, No. 6, (June, 2000), pp. 808-813

Epstein, C. J. (1990). The consequences of chromosome imbalance. *American Journal of Medical Genetics: Supplement*, Vol. 7, No. 31-7, (n.d), pp. 31-37

Ferri, C. P., Prince, M., Brayne, C., Brodaty H., et al. (2005). Alzheimer's Disease International. Global prevalence of dementia: a Delphi consensus study. *Lancet*, Vol. 366, No. 9503, (December, 2005), pp. 2112-2117

Fitzgerald, P. H., Archer, S. A., & Morris, C. M. (1986). Evidence for the repeated primary non-disjunction of chromosome 21 as a result of premature centromere division (PCD). *Human Genetics*, Vol. 72, No. 1, (January, 1986), pp. 58-62

Flicker, J. (2010). Modifiable lifestyle risk factors for Alzheimer's disease. *Journal of Alzheimer's Disease*, Vol. 20, No. 3, (n.d.), pp. 803-811

Floyd, R. F., & Hensley, K. (2002). Oxidative stress in brain aging: Implications for therapeutics of neurodegenerative diseases. *Neurobiology of Aging*, Vol. 23, No. 5, (September, 2002), 795-807

Geller, L. N., & Potter, H. (1999). Chromosome missegregation and trisomy 21 mosaicism in Alzheimer's disease. *Neurobiology of Disease*, Vol. 6, No. 3, (December, 1998), pp. 167-179

Glenner, G. G., & Wang, C. W. (1984). Alzheimer's disease and Down's syndrome: sharing of a unique cerebrovascular amyloid fibril protein. *Biochemical and Biophysiological Research Communications*, Vol. 122, No. 3, (August, 1984), 1131-1135

Goldgaber, D., Lerman, M. J., McBride, O. W., et al. (1987). Characterization and chromosomal localization of cDNA encoding brain amyloid of Alzheimer's disease. *Science*, Vol. 235, No. 4791, (February, 1987), pp 877-880

Granic, A., Padmanabhan, J., Norden, M., & Potter, H. (2010). Alzheimer Aβ peptide induces chromosome mis-segregation and aneuploidy, including trisomy 21: requirement for tau and APP. *Molecular Biology of the Cell*, Vol. 21, No. 4, (December, 2009), pp. 511-520

Grant, W. B., Campbell, A., Itzhaki, R. F., et al. (2002). The significance of environmental factors in the etiology of Alzheimer's disease. *Journal of Alzheimer's Disease*, Vol. 4, No. 3, (June, 2002), pp. 179-189

Grundke-Iqbal, I., Iqbal, K., Quinlan, M., et al. (1986). Microtubule associated protein tau. A component of Alzheimer paired helical filaments. *The Journal of Biological Biochemistry,* Vol. 261, No. 13, (May, 1986), pp. 6084-6089

Hardy, J. (2006). Alzheimer's disease: the amyloid cascade hypothesis: an update and reappraisal. Alzheimers Disease, Vol. 9, No. 3 (Suppl), pp. 151-153

Hardy, J. (2009). The amyloid hypothesis for Alzheimer's disease: a critical reappraisal. *Journal of Neurochemistry,* Vol. 110, No. 4, (August, 2009), pp. 1129-1134

Hardy, J., Goate, A., Owen, M., et al. (1989). Presenile dementia associated with mosaic trisomy 21 in a patient with Down syndrome child. *Lancet,* Vol. 2, No. 8665, (September, 1989), pp. 743

Haass, C., & Selkoe, D. J. (1993). Cellular processing of beta-amyloid precursor protein and the genesis of amyloid beta-peptide. *Cell,* Vol. 75, No. 6, (December, 1993), pp. 1039-1042

Heston, L. L., Mastri, A. R., Anderson, V. E., et al. (1981). Dementia of Alzheimer type. *Archives of Genetic Psychiatry,* Vol. 38, No. 10, (October, 1981), pp. 1081-1090

Heyman, A., Wilkinson, W., Hurwitz, B., et al. (1983). Alzheimer's disease; genetic aspects and associated clinical disorders. *Annals of Neurology,* Vol. 14, No. 5, (November, 1983), pp. 507-515

Higuchi, S., Muramatsu, T., Matsushita, S. et al. (1996). Presenilin-1 polymorphism and Alzheimer's disease. *Lancet,* Vol. 347, No. 9009, (April, 1996), pp. 1186

Honda, T., Nihonmatsu, N., Yasutake, K., et al. (2000). Familial Alzheimer's disease-associated mutations block translocation of full-length presenilin 1 to the nuclear envelope. *Neuroscience Research,* Vol. 37, No. 2, (June, 2000), pp. 101-11

Hughes, T. F., & Ganguli, M. (2009). Modifiable risk factors for late-life cognitive impairment and dementia. *Current Psychiatry Reviews,* Vol. 5, No. 2, (May, 2009), pp. 73-92

Itagaki, S., McGreer, P. L., Akiyama, H., et al. (1989). Relationship of microglia and astrocytes to amyloid deposits of Alzheimer disease. *Journal of Immunology,* Vol. 24, No. 3, (October, 1989), pp. 173-182

Iourov, I. Y., Vorsanova, S. G., Liehr, T., et al. (2009). Aneuploidy in the normal, Alzheimer's disease and ataxia-telangiectasia brain: differential expression and pathological meaning. *Neurobiology of Disease,* Vol. 34, No. 2, (May, 2009), pp. 212-220

Janicki, S. M. & Monteiro, M. J. (1999). Presenilin overexpression arrests cells in the G1 phase of the cell cycle: arrest potentiated by the Alzheimer's disease PS2 (N141I) Mutant. *American Journal of Pathology,* Vol. 155, No. 1, (July, 1999), pp. 135-144

Kulnane, L. S., Lehman, E. J., Hock, B. J., et al. (2002). Rapid and efficient detection of transgene homozygosity by FISH of mouse fibroblasts. *Mammalian Genome,* Vol. 13, No. 4, (April, 2002), pp. 223-226

LaFerla, F. M., Green, K. N., & Oddo, S. (2007). Intracellular amyloid-β in Alzheimer's disease. *Nature Reviews Neuroscience,* Vol. 8, No. 7, (July, 2007), pp. 499-509

Lee, H. G., Casadesus, G., Zhu X, et al. (2004). Challenging the amyloid cascade hypothesis: senile plaques and amyloid-beta as protective adaptations to Alzheimer disease. *Annals of the New York Academy of Science,* Vol. 1019, No. 1-4, (June, 2004), pp. 1-4

Li, J., Ma, J., & Pottre, H. (1995). Identification and expression analysis of a potential familial Alzheimer's disease gene on chromsome 1 related to AD3. *Proceedings of the National Academy of Science of the USA,* Vo. 92, No. 26, (December, 1995), pp. 12180-12184

Li, J., Xu, M., Zhou, H., Ma, et al. (1997). Alzheimer presenilins in the nuclear membrane, interphase kinetochores, and centrosomes suggest a role in chromosome segregation. *Cell,* Vol. 90, No. 5, (September, 1997), pp. 917-927

Li, M., Chen, L., Lee, D. H., et al. (2007). The role of intracellular amyloid beta in Alzheimer's disease. *Progress in Neurobiology,* Vol. 83, No. 3, (October, 2007), pp. 131-139

Lucarelli, P., Piciullo, A., Palmarino, M., et al. (2004). Association between presenilin 1-48C/T polymorphism and Down syndrome. *Neuroscience Letters,* Vol. 367, No. 1, (August, 2004), pp. 88-91

Mattson, M. P. & Magnus, T. (2006). Ageing and neuronal vulnerability. *Nature Reviews of Neuroscience,* Vol. 7, No. 4, (April, 2006), pp. 278-294

Maurer, K. & Hoyer, S. (2006). Alzheimer revisited: differences in origin of the disease carrying his name. *Journal of Neuronal Transmission,* Vol. 113, No. 11, (November, 2006), pp. 1645-1658

McNaughton, D., Knight, W., Guerreiro, R., et al. (2010). Duplication of amyloid precursor protein (APP), but not prion protein (PRNP) gene is a significant cause of early onset dementia in a large UK series. *Neurobiology of Aging,* Epub ahead of print, (December 2010), Article in Press

Migliore, L., Botto, N., Scarpato, R., et al. (1999). Preferential occurrence of chromosome 21 malsegregation in peripheral blood lymphocytes of Alzheimer disease patients. *Cytogenetics and Cell Genetics,* Vol. 87, No. 1-2, (n.d.), pp. 41-46

Migliore, L., Testa, A., Scarpato, R., et al. (1997). Spontaneous and induced aneuploidy in peripheral blood lymphocytes of patients with Alzheimer's disease. *Human Genetics,* Vol. 101, No. 3, (December, 1997), pp. 299-305

Migliore, L., Boni, G., Bernardini, F., et al. (2006). Susceptibility to chromosome malsegregation in lymphocytes of women who had a Down syndrome child in young age. *Neurobiology of Aging,* Vol. 27, No. 5, (May, 2006), pp. 710-716

Migliore, L., Migheli, F., & Coppedé, F. (2009). Susceptibility to aneuploidy in young mothers of Down syndrome children. *ScientificWorldJournal,* Vol. 9, (October, 2009), pp. 1052-1060

Mosch, B., Morawski, M., Mittag, A., et al. (2007). Aneuploidy and DNA replication in the normal human brain and Alzheimer's disease. *Journal of Neuroscience,* Vol. 27, No. 26, (June, 2007), pp. 6859-6867

Nagy, Z. (2005). The last neuronal division: a unifying hypothesis for the pathogenesis of Alzheimer's disease. *Journal of Cellular and Molecular Medicine,* Vol. 9, No. 3, pp. (July-September, 2005), 531-541

Nagy, Z., Esiri, M. M., Cato, A. M., et al. (1997). Cell cycle markers in the hippocampus in Alzheimer's disease. *Acta Neuropathologica,* Vol. 94, No. 1, (July, 1997), pp. 6-15

Neve, R. L., Finch, E. A., & Dawes, L. R. (1988). Expression of the Alzheimer amyloid precursor gene transcripts in the human brain. *Neuron,* Vol. 1, No. 8, (October, 1988), pp. 669-677

Nizzari, M., Venezia, V., Bianchini, P., et al. (2007). Amyloid precursor protein and presenilin 1 interaction studied by FRET in human H4 cells. *Annals of the New York Academy of Science*, Vol. 1096, (January, 2007), pp. 249-257

Obrenovic, M. E., Raina, A. K., Ogawa, O., et al. (2003). Alzheimer's disease - a new begining, or final exit? In: *Cell Cycle Mechanisms and Neuronal Cell death,* Copani, A. & Nicoletti, F. (eds.), pp. 79-93, Landes Bioscience, Austin, TX

Olson, M. I. & Shaw, C. M. (1969). Presenile dementia and Alzheimer's disease in mongolism. *Brain,* Vol. 92, No. 1, (March, 1969), pp.147-156

Padmanabhan, J., Levy, M., & Pottre, H. (2011). Cell cycle-dependent phosphorylation, distribution, and processing of amyloid precursor protein (In submission).

Petterson, D., Gardiner, K., Kao, F-T., et al. (1988). Mapping of the gene encoding the β-amyloid precursor protein and its relationship to the Down syndrome region of chromosome 21. *Proceedings of the National Academy of Science of the USA,* Vol. 85, No. 21, (November, 1988), 8266-8270

Pope, W. B., Lambert, M. P., Leypold, B., et al. (1994). Microtubule-associated protein tau is hyperphosphorylated during mitosis in the human neuroblastoma cell line SH-SY5Y. *Experimental Neurology,* Vol. 126, No. 2, (April, 1994), pp. 185-194

Potter, H. (1991). Review and hypothesis: Alzheimer disease and Down syndrome chromosome 21 nondisjunction may underlie both disorders. *American Journal of Human Genetics,* Vol. 48, No. 6, (June, 1991), pp. 1192-1200

Potter, H. (2004). Cell cycle and chromosome segregation defects in Alzheimer's disease. In: *Cell Cycle Mechanisms and Neuronal Cell Death,* Copani, A. & Nicoletti, F. (eds.), pp. 55-78, Landes Bioscience, Austin, TX

Potter, H. (2008). Down syndrome and Alzheimer's disease: two sides of the same coin. *Future Neurology,* Vol. 3, No. 1, (n.d.), pp. 29-37, 1479-6708

Potter H, Ma J, Das S, et al. (1995). Beyond β-protein: New steps in the pathogenic pathway to Alzheimer's disease. In: *Research Advances in Alzheimer's Disease and Related Disorders,* Iqbal, K., Mortimer, J. A., Winblad, B. & Wisniewski, H. M. (eds), pp. 643-654, John Wiley and Sons Ltd, New York

Potter H., Wefes, I. M., & Nilsson L. N. G. (2001). The inflammation-induced pathological chaperones ACT and apoE are necessary catalysts of Alzheimer amyloid formation. *Neurobiology of Aging,* Vol. 22, No. 6, (November, 2001), pp. 923-930

Rakic, P. (1985). Limits of neurogenesis in primates. *Science,* Vol. 227, No. 4690, (March, 1985), pp. 1054-1056

Rapoport, M., Dawson, H. N., Binder, L. I., et al. (2002). Tau is essential to beta-amyloid-induced neurotoxicity. *Proceedings of the National Academy of Science of the USA,* Vol. 99, No. 9, (April, 2002), pp. 6364-6369

Ried, T. (1998). Interphase cytogenetics and its role in molecular diagnostics of solid tumors. *American Journal of Pathology,* Vol. 152, No. 2, 325-327

Ringman, J. M., Rao, P. N., Lu, P. H. et al. (2008). Mosaicism for trisomy 21 in a patient with young-onset dementia: a case report and brief literature review. *Archives of Neurology,* Vol. 65, No. 3, (March, 2008), pp. 412-415

Rogaev, E. I., Sherrington, R., Rogaeva, E. A., et al. (1995). Familial Alzheimer's disease in kindreds with missense mutations in a gene on chromsome 1 related to the

Alzheimer's disease type 3 gene. *Nature*, Vol. 376, No. 6543, (August, 1995), pp. 775-778

Rowe, I. F., Ridler, M. A. C., Gibberd, F. B., et al. (1989). Presenile dementia associated with mosaic trisomy 21 in a patient with a Down syndrome child. *Lancet*, Vol. 2, No. 8656, (July, 1989), pp. 229

Rovelet-Lecrux, A., Hannequin D, Raux G., et al. (2006). APP locus duplication causes autosomal dominant early-onset Alzheimer disease with cerebral amyloid angiopathy. *Nature Genetics*, Vol. 38, No. 1, (January, 2006), pp. 11-12

Scheff, S. W., Price, D. A., Schmitt, F. A., & Mufson, E. J. (2006). Hippocampal synaptic loss in early Alzheimer's disease and mild cognitive impairment. *Neurobiology of Aging*, Vol. 27, No. 10, (October, 2006), pp. 1372-1384

Schupf, N., Kapell, D., Lee, J. H., Ottman, R. & Mayeux, R. (1994). Increased risk of Alzheimer's disease in mothers of adults with Down's syndrome. *Lancet*, Vol. 344, No. 8919, (August, 1994), pp. 353-356

Schumpf, B., Kapell, D., Nightingale, J. H., Lee, J., Mohlenhoff, Bewley, S., et al. (2001). Specificity of the fivefold increase in AD in mothers of adults with Down syndrome. *Neurology*, Vol. 57, No. 6, (September, 2001), 979-984

Scott, W. K., Growdon, J. H., Roses, A. D. et al. (1996). Presenilin-1 polymorphism and Alzheimer's disease. *Lancet*, Vol. 347, No. 9009, (April, 1996), pp. 1186-1187

Selkoe, D. J. (1999). Translating cell biology into therapeutic advances in Alzheimer's disease. *Nature*,Vol. 399, No. 6738, (June, 1999), pp. A23-A31

Selkoe, D. J. (2001). Alzheimer's disease: genes, proteins, and therapy. *Physiological Reviews*,Vol. 81, No. 2, (April, 2001), pp. 742-760

Selkoe, D. J. (2004). Cell biology of protein misfolding: the examples of Alzheimer's and Parkinson's disease. *Nature Cell Biology*, Vol. 6, pp. No. 11, (November, 2004), pp. 1054-1061

Small, S. A.,. & Duff, K. (2008). Linking Abeta and tau in late-onset Alzheimer's disease: a dual pathway hypothesis. *Neuron*, Vol. 60, No. 4, (November, 2008), pp. 534-542

Small, B. J., Fratiglioni L., Viitanen, M., et al. (2000). The course of cognitive impairment in preclinical Alzheimer's disease. Three- and 6-year follow-up of a population based sample. *Archives of Neurology*, Vol. 57, No. 6, (June, 2000), pp. 839-844.

Sleegers, K., Brouwers, N., Gijselinck, I., et al. (2006). APP duplication is sufficient to cause early onset Alzheimer's dementia with cerebral amyloid angiopathy. *Brain*, Vol. 129, No. 11, (November, 2006), pp. 2977-2983

Spremo-Potparević, B., Živković, L., Djelić, N., et al. (2008). Premature centomere division of the X chromosome in neurons in Alzheimer's disease. *Journal of Neurochemistry*, Vol. 106, No. 5, (September, 2008), pp. 2218-2223

Stokin, G. B., & Goldstein, S. B. (2006). Axonal transport and Alzheimer's disease. *Annual Reviews of Biochemistry*, Vol. 75, No. 607-27, (n.d), pp. 607-627

Stokin, G. B., Lillo, C., Falzone, T. L., Brusch, R. G., Rockenstein, E., et al. (2005). Axonopathy and transport deficits early in the pathogenesis of Alzheimer's disease. *Science*, Vol. 307, No. 5713, (February, 2005), pp. 1282-1288

Suzuki, N., Cheung, T. T., Cai, X.-D., et al. (1994). An increased percentage of long amyloid β-protein by familial amyloid β-protein precursor (βAPP_{717}) mutants. *Science*, Vol. 264, No. 5163, (May, 1994), pp. 1336-1340

Suzuki, T., Oishi, M., Marshak, D. R., et al. (1994). Cell cycle-dependent regulation of the phosphorylation and metabolism of the Alzheimer amyloid precursor protein. *The EMBO Journal* Vol. 13, No. 5, (March, 1994), pp. 1114-1122

Tanzi, R. E., & Bertram, L. (2001). New frontiers in Alzheimer's disease genetics. *Neuron*, Vol. 32, No. 2, (October, 2001), pp. 181-184

Tanzi, R. E., Gusella, J. F., Watkins, P. C., et al. (1987). Amyloid β-protein gene cDNA, mRNA distributions, and genetic linkage near the Alzheimer locus. *Science*, Vol. 235, No. 4791, (February, 1987), pp. 880-884

Teller, J. K., Russo, C., deBusk, L. M., et al. (1996). Presence of soluble amyloid β-peptide precedes amyloid plaque fromation in Down syndrome. *Nature Medicine*, Vol. 2, No. 1, (January, 1996), pp. 93-95

Thomas, P., & Fenech, M. (2008). Chromosome 17 and 21 aneuploidy in buccal cells is increased with ageing and in Alzheimer's disease. *Mutagenesis*, Vol. 23, No. 1, (January, 2008), pp. 57-65.

Trippi, F., Botto, N., Scarpato, R., et al. (2001). Spontaneous and induced chromosomal damage in somatic cells of sporadic and familial Alzheimer's disease patients. *Mutagenesis*, Vol. 16, No.4, (July, 2001), 321-327

Varvel, N. H., Bhaskar, K., Patil, A. R., Pimplikar, S. W., Herrup, K., & Lamb, B. T. (2008). Abeta oligomers induce neuronal cell cycle events in Alzheimer's disease. *Journal of Neuroscience*, Vol. 28, No. 43, (October, 2008), pp. 10786-10793

Vincent, I., Rosado, M. & Davies, P. (1996). Mitotic mechanisms in Alzheimer's Disease? *Journal of Cell Biology*, Vol. *132*, No. 3, (February, 1996), pp. 423-425

Vito, P., Wolozin, B., Ganjei, J. K. et al. (1996). Requirement of the familial Alzheimer's disease gene *PS2* for apoptosis. Opposing effect of ALG-3. *Journal of Biological Chemistry*, Vol. 271, No. 49, (December, 1996), pp. 31025-31028

Wahrle, S., Das, P., Nyborg, A. C., et al. (2002). Cholesterol dependent gamma-secretase activity is buoyant in cholesterol rich membrane microdomains. *Neurobiology of Disease*, Vol. 9, No. 1, (February, 2002), pp. 11-23

Wisniewski, H. M., Rabe, A., Wisniewski K. E. (1988). Neuropathology and dementia in people with Down's syndrome. In: *Molecular Neuropathology of Aging*, Davies, P. & Finch, C. (eds.), pp. 399-413, Cold Spring Harbor Laboratory, New York, USA

Wolfe, M. S. (2003). The secretases of Alzheimer's disease. *Current Topics in Developmental Biology*, Vol. 54, No. 233-61, (n.d.), pp. 233-261

Wolozin, B., Iwasaki, K., Vito, P. et al. (1996). Participation of presenilin 2 in apoptosis: enhanced basal activity conferred by an Alzheimer mutation. *Science*; Vol. 274, No. 5293, (December, 1996), pp. 1710-1713

Wragg, M., Hutton, M., & Talbot, C. (1996). Genetic association between intronic polymorphism in presenilin-1 gene and late-onset Alzheimer's disease. Alzheimer's Disease Collaborative Group. *Lancet*, Vol. 347, No. 9000, (February, 1996), pp. 509-512

Yang, Y., Geldmacher, D.S. & Herrup, K. (2001). DNA replication precedes neuronal cell death in Alzheimer's disease. *Journal of Neuroscience,* Vol. 21, No. 8, (April, 2001), pp. 2661-2668

Yang, Y., & Herrup, K. (2007). Cell division in the CNS: Protective response or lethal event in post-mitotic neurons? *Biochimica et Biophysica Acta,* Vol. 1772, No. 4, (April, 2007), 457-466

Yang, Y., Varvel, N. H., Lamb, B. T. & Herrup, K. (2006). Ectopic cell cycle events link human Alzheimer's disease and amyloid precursor protein transgenic mouse models. *Journal of Neuroscience,* Vol. 26, No. 3, (January, 2006), pp. 775-784

Zitnik, G., Wang, L., Martin, G. M., et al. (2006). Localization of eddogenous APP/APP-proteolytic products are consistent with microtubular transport. *Journal of Molecular Neuroscience,* Vol. 31, No. 1, (n.d.), pp. 59-68

9

Deficiency of Adult Neurogenesis in the Ts65Dn Mouse Model of Down Syndrome

Pavel V. Belichenko and Alexander M. Kleschevnikov
University of California, San Diego, School of Medicine, La Jolla, California
USA

1. Introduction

Neurogenesis in the mammalian adult brain is a well established phenomenon (for the recent reviews see Carpentier & Palmer, 2009; Kaneko & Sawamoto, 2009; Rodriguez & Verkhratsky, 2011) that is important in both young and aging brain (Galvan & Jin, 2007; Rao et al., 2006). The subventricular zone, subgranular layer of the dentate gyrus (DG), and cortex are the main sites of adult neurogenesis (Gould et al., 1999; Luskin & Boone, 1994; Palmer et al., 2000; Seki et al., 2007; Yoneyama et al., 2011). Newly-born neurons during adult neurogenesis have the ability to integrate into previously established neuronal networks (Kee et al., 2007; Markakis & Gage, 1999; Sandoval et al., 2011). Alteration of neurogenesis under different experimental and pathological conditions has been described to a great extent (Rodriguez & Verkhratsky, 2011; Sandoval et al., 2011; Winner et al., 2011; Yoneyama et al., 2011; Yu et al., 2009). Significant decreases of neurogenesis have been found in neurodevelopmental (Contestabile et al., 2007; Guidi et al., 2008, 2010) and in neurodegenerative diseases (Rodriguez & Verkhratsky, 2011). Numerous studies provide evidence that a lack of neurogenesis significantly diminishes plasticity in the adult brain and interferes with learning and memory (reviewed in Koehl & Abrous, 2011; Mongiat & Schinder, 2011). Different mechanisms have been proposed to regulate neurogenesis in the adult brain, including brain injury (Kernie & Parent, 2010; Moriyama et al., 2011), ischemia (Kernie & Parent, 2010; Kreuzberg et al., 2010), and inflammation (Voloboueva et al., 2010).

One of the least studied factors that affects neurogenesis are chromosomal aberrations. Down syndrome (DS) results from the extra copy of chromosome 21 occurring with a prevalence of 1 in 733 live births (Canfield et al., 2006). Subjects with DS show developmental regression, diminished cognitive ability, and autonomic dysfunction (Antonarakis & Epstein, 2006; Chapman & Hesketh, 2000). The DS brain is severely affected showing a reduction in both overall size and of particular areas (frontal cortex, hippocampus, cerebellum, and brainstem) due to a reduced number of neurons (Aylward et al., 1997, 1999; Kesslak et al., 1994; Pinter et al., 2001; Raz et al., 1995; Wisniewski et al., 1984).

1.1 Neurogenesis in subjects with DS

Very little data is available describing neurognesis in subjects with DS. In hippocampal DG and neocortex of fetuses with DS the number of proliferating cells was found to be significantly reduced (Contestabile et al., 2007). These reductions were mainly due to a reduced number of cycling cells in S phase (Contestabile et al., 2007). Both a reduction in neurogenesis and significantly higher incidence of apoptotic cell death in the hippocampal region of fetuses with DS has been noted (Guidi et al., 2008). Also, trisomy 21 significantly modify cell phenotypes producing higher numbers of cycling cells going to a glial phenotype and less cells expressing neuronal markers (Guidi et al., 2008). Detailed analysis of the consequences of both reduced neurogenesis and increased apoptosis in fetuses with DS, revealed a severe reduction in the volume and cell number of investigated brain areas (Guidi et al., 2008). More recently, significant neurogenesis impairments were also revealed in the cerebellum of fetuses with DS (Guidi et al., 2010). However, apoptotic cell death was similar in the cerebellum in fetuses with DS vs. controls (Guidi et al., 2010). The differences between the levels of apoptosis in hippocampus vs. cerebellum in fetuses with DS points to different mechanisms for the reduced cell number in hippocampus and cerebellum in DS. For the hippocampus, a reduction of neurogenesis, increased apoptosis and changing cell phenotypes in favor of glia may underlie reduced cell number in fetuses with DS. As for the cerebellum, only a reduction in neurogenesis may be the main factor in decreased cerebellar volume in fetuses with DS.

1.2 Neurogenesis in mouse models of DS

Taking to account that this subject is very important for the neurobiology of DS, only a few papers addressed neurogenesis in mouse models of DS (Bianchi et al., 2010; Chakrabarti et al., 2007; Clark et al., 2006; Contestabile et al., 2007; Lorenzi & Reeves, 2006; Rueda et al., 2005). It was noted that in prenatal and newborn Ts65Dn mice neurogenesis was significantly reduced (Chakrabarti et al., 2007; Contestabile et al., 2007; Lorenzi & Reeves, 2006). At postnatal day 2 cell proliferation in Ts65Dn mice, assessed 2 hours after single injection of bromodeoxyuridine (BrdU) was significantly reduced (Contestabile et al., 2007); similar results were revealed at postnatal day 15 (Bianchi et al., 2010). However in young adult Ts65Dn mice the results are conflicting (Clark et al., 2006; Rueda et al., 2005). Similar procedures in young (3-5 months) Ts65Dn mice shows no difference in hippocampal cell proliferation and survival (Rueda et al., 2005). However, in aged (13-15 months) Ts65Dn mice, cell proliferation in the hippocampus (Rueda et al., 2005) and in the subventricular zone (Bianchi et al., 2010) were significantly reduced. Finally, Clark et al. (2006) found a difference in DG neurogenesis in young (2-5 months) Ts65Dn mice.

It seems that genetic dissections of mouse partial trisomy 16 (Ts65Dn model) did not restore reduced neurogenesis. Indeed, Ts1Cje and Ts2Cje mouse models of DS showed a similar degree of impairment in adult neurogenesis (Hewitt et al., 2010; Ishihara et al., 2010).

To solve these conflicting results in DS mouse models a recent study was initiated to examine young adult neurogenesis, and we also expanded this study to include DG, cortex and corpus callosum (CC) at three different levels. We chose to investigate whether or not trisomy has any affect on neurogenesis in Ts65Dn mice. To carry out this work we injected BrdU in 2N and Ts65Dn mice. Combining BrdU immunoreactivity and high resolution confocal microscopy, we examined the number of BrdU-positive (BrdU+) neurons in DG, cortex and CC at three different levels: rostral, middle and caudal. Comparing 2N and Ts65Dn mice, we discovered significant decreases in the density of BrdU+ cells in trisomic mice in the cortex and DG. We found that the number of cells per cluster was significantly reduced in both the rostral and the caudal parts of DG in the Ts65Dn vs. 2N. This change resulted in reduced cell density in the caudal DG, while the density of clusters was not altered. Our findings are evidence for decreased neurogenesis in young adult cortex and DG of Ts65Dn mice and indicate neurogenesis as a potential target for pharmacological intervention to avert neuronal plasticity in individuals with DS.

2. Materials and methods

All experiments were conducted in accordance with the National Institutes of Health guidelines for the care and use of animals and with an approved animal protocol from the Stanford University Institutional Animal Care and Use Committee. All efforts were made to minimize animal stress and discomfort.

2.1 Mice husbandry

Details of maintenance and using Ts65Dn mouse colony were described previously (Belichenko et al., 2004). The Ts65Dn mouse colony was maintained for more than 10 generations by crossing B6EiC3Sn-Ts(17^{16})65Dn females (Jackson Laboratory, Bar Harbor, ME) with B6EiC3Sn F1/J A/a males (Jackson Laboratory). This breeding scheme was used because trisomic mice breed very poorly or not at all when inbred; the B6C3 background has been the most successful. To distinguish 2N from Ts65Dn mice, genomic DNA was extracted from tail samples. A quantitative PCR protocol (provided by The Jackson laboratory) was used to measure Mx1 gene expression, which is present in three copies in Ts65Dn. Each mouse was genotyped twice. Male littermates mice were used in all studies at ages 2-3 months.

2.2 BrdU injections and immunofluorescent staining

In the beginning of experiment we weighed mice. Each animal was injected once a day for 6 consecutive days with 5-bromo-2'-deoxyuridine (BrdU, 10 mg/ml in saline, i.p.) (Cat. # B9285, Sigma-Aldrich Corp., St. Louis, MO, USA) to a final dose of 50 mg/kg body weight. Twenty four hours after the last injection, animals were deeply anesthetized with sodium pentobarbital (200 mg/kg i.p.) (Abbott Laboratories, North Chicago, IL, USA), again weighed, and transcardially perfused for 1 minute with 0.9% sodium chloride (10 ml) and then for 20 minutes with 4% paraformaldehyde in 0.1 M phosphate-buffered saline (PBS), pH 7.4 (200 ml). After perfusion, the brain was immediately removed and postfixed for another 24 hours. The weight of the entire brain (including the olfactory bulbs, cerebellum, and brainstem along with the cervical spinal cord through C1–C2) was recorded. The brain was then sectioned coronally at 100-μm with a Vibratome (series 1000, TPI Inc., St. Louis, MO, USA), and sections were placed in 0.9% NaCl solution. Immunofluorescence method with anti-BrdU antibody was used to reveal BrdU+ cells as follows. Free-floating sections were rinsed twice in saline (0.9 % NaCl) for 10 min at RT, and then pretreated with 1M HCl for 30 minutes at 37°C. Sections were neutralized by rinsing 3 times in PBS and then pre-incubated in a solution of 0.1 M PBS containing 5% non-fat milk and 0.3% Triton-X 100 (PBS+), for 1 hour at room temperature. Then sections were incubated overnight at 4°C with primary rat anti-BrdU antibody (Cat. #MCA2060, Serotec, Raleigh, NC, USA) at a dilution 1:100 in PBS+. Sections were rinsed in PBS (20 minutes, three changes) and incubated for 1 hour at room temperature with biotinylated donkey anti-rat IgG (1:200; Jackson ImmunoResearch Labs, West Grove, PA). After being rinsed with PBS (20 minutes, three changes), sections were incubated with FITC-conjugated streptavidin (1:500; Jackson

ImmunoResearch Labs, West Grove, PA) for 1 hour at room temperature. Following further careful rinsing, the sections were mounted on microscope glass slides and coverslipped with 90% glycerol in PB.

2.3 Confocal microscopy imaging, cell quantification, cluster and statistical analyses

To study cell proliferation and clustering in 2N and Ts65Dn mice we used confocal microscopy imaging of BrdU+ cells in the cortex, hippocampus and CC. Confocal imaging of brain slices labeled with one fluorophores was performed as previously described (Belichenko et al., 2004). In brief, slices with BrdU+ cells were examined and scanned in a Radiance 2000 confocal microscope (BioRad, Hertfordshire, United Kingdom) attached to a Nikon Eclipse E800 fluorescence microscope. LaserSharp software (Bio Rad) was used to establish optimal conditions for collecting images. The laser was an argon/krypton mixed gas laser with exciting wavelengths for FITC (488 λ). The emission was registered with HQ515/30 "green" filter. Sections with FITC staining of BrdU immunoreactivity were studied under the following optimal conditions: the lens was a x10 objective (Nikon; Plan Fluor x10/0.30); laser power was 10%; the zoom factor was 1; scan speed was 500 lines per second; each optical section was the result of 3 scans followed by Kalman filtering; the size of the image was 512 x 512 pixels (i.e., 1208 x 1208 μm).

LazerPix software (Bio Rad) analysis of confocal images was used to measure the area or length of investigated brain structures, and for quantitative analysis of BrdU+ cells. Three slices per mouse (500 μm apart) were used. The location of each coronal section was designated based on its relative position to bregma in mm (Hof et al., 2000). Rostral section was corresponded to bregma -1.60 mm level, middle section – to bregma -2.10 mm level, and caudal section to bregma -2.60 mm level. Entire DG at these three different locations was imaged. CC was imaged from midline and then for 1200 μm to the left or right extension at the same three different locations. Based on mouse brain atlas (Hof et al., 2000), cortex were correspondent to motor cortex at rostral and middle sections and to visual cortex at caudal section). Images from the both the left and right side for each mouse brain were analyzed. To count number of BrdU+ cells, we first outlined the area of interest and measure area or length (in a case of DG). Next, for each image, the intensity thresholds were estimated by analyzing the distribution of pixel intensities in the image areas that did not contain immunoreactivity. This value, the background threshold, was then subtracted and number of BrdU+ cells was counted. In addition each BrdU+ cells were traced manually and their XY coordinates were exported to Excel. The number of BrdU+ cell in each hemisphere was expressed for DG as per 100-μm length of neurogenic subgranule zone, and for cortex and CC as per 1 mm^2. We also counted the occurrence of BrdU+ cell clusters. To quantify the number of clusters we used previously established criteria (Palmer et al., 2000), where cluster was defined as a contiguous group of cells separated by less than 25 μm. Special macro was design in Excel program for cluster counting. For every section, X and Y coordinates of individual BrdU+ cell were recorded using LaserPix software (BioRad). Distance between all pairs of the BrdU+ cells within one section were calculated using an Excel Microsoft macro, and the cells with distances < 25 μm were regarded as belonging to a cluster. All analyses were performed by the same investigator blinded to mice genotype.

Digital images were imported, enhanced for brightness and contrast, assembled and labeled in Adobe Photoshop CS2 9.0.2, and archived. Figures were printed with a Phaser 7300 color printer (Tektronix by Xerox, Norwalk, CT).

The data for body and brain weights, total number of BrdU+ cells, their coordinates and cluster evaluations were exported to Excel (Microsoft, Redmond, WA) and statistical comparisons were performed using two-way analysis of variance (ANOVA) and for two samples using two-tailed Student's *t*-tests. All results are expressed as mean ± SEM, and P values < 0.05 were considered to be significant.

3. Results

3.1 Body and brain weights

The body weight of 2N and Ts65Dn mice at 2-3 months was similar (2N: 31.1 ± 1.6 g, n = 6; Ts65Dn = 26.7 ± 2.3 g, n = 5; $P = 0.14$). The brain weight was also unchanged (2N: 0.43 ± 0.01 g, n = 6; Ts65Dn = 0.43 ± 0.01 g, n = 5; $P = 0.60$). Of note, there was no effect of the BrdU injection on changes in body weight during 6 day injections since no significant differences were found between 2N and Ts65Dn mice (2N: -0.60 ± 0.29 g, n = 6; Ts65Dn = -0.20 ± 0.51 g, n = 5; $P = 0.49$). These mice also showed no aversive or any other neurological symptoms during injection.

3.2 Changes in BrdU+ cells number and in cell cluster density in Ts65Dn mice

We examined the density of BrdU+ cells in DG of hippocampus, cortex and CC in 2N and Ts65Dn male mice (Table 1, Figs. 1, 2). The BrdU+ cells were bright fluorescent, allowing for a detailed quantitative analysis by confocal microscopy (Figs. 1a, 2a). For this analysis, the number of BrdU+ cells per 100 μm length of subgranule zone for DG or per 1 mm^2 area of cortex or CC was counted to define cell density (Table 1). In addition we measured the number of cell cluster, the number of BrdU+ cells per cluster and the frequency distribution of BrdU+ cells per cluster (Table 1; Figs. 1 d,e; 2 d,e).

Comparing BrdU+ cell densities in 2N and Ts65Dn mice, there was a statistically significant decrease in the caudal part of DG (by 27%) and in the rostral part of motor cortex (by 36%; $P < 0.01$; Table 1). Interestingly, BrdU+ neurons in the inferior blade were on average 30% fewer than in the superior blade for 2N, and 23% fewer for Ts65Dn mice ($P < 0.01$; Table 1). BrdU+ cell density were similar for CC in 2N and Ts65Dn mice, and 33% more in caudal then rostral CC for 2N mice ($P < 0.01$; Table 1).

Comparing BrdU+ cell cluster densities in 2N and Ts65Dn mice, there was a statistically significant decrease in the rostral part of motor cortex (by 29%; $P < 0.01$; Table 1). In the inferior blade there were on average 9% fewer than in superior blade for 2N, and 25% fewer for Ts65Dn mice ($P < 0.05$; Table 1). Interestingly, in the DG the BrdU+ cell cluster density was not different in 2N and Ts65Dn mice (Table 1).

We next quantified the number of cells per cluster (Table 1). As compared to 2N mice, significantly lower numbers of BrdU+ cells per cluster were present in rostral (mainly due to superior blade, $P < 0.003$; Table 1) and in the caudal part of DG in Ts65Dn mice ($P = 0.03$; Table 1), and in the rostral part of motor cortex in Ts65Dn mice ($P < 0.01$; Table 1). Comparing the superior and inferior blades in 2N mice, numbers of cells per cluster were ~1.5 times higher in the rostral and middle parts of the superior blade of the DG in 2N mice ($P < 0.02$; Table 1).

In conclusion, significant differences in the number of BrdU+ cells, cell cluster densities, and in number of BrdU+ cells per cluster were evident for Ts65Dn mice as compared to their 2N cohorts. These findings are evidence for reduced neurogenesis in both DG and cortex due to mouse chromosome 16 trisomy.

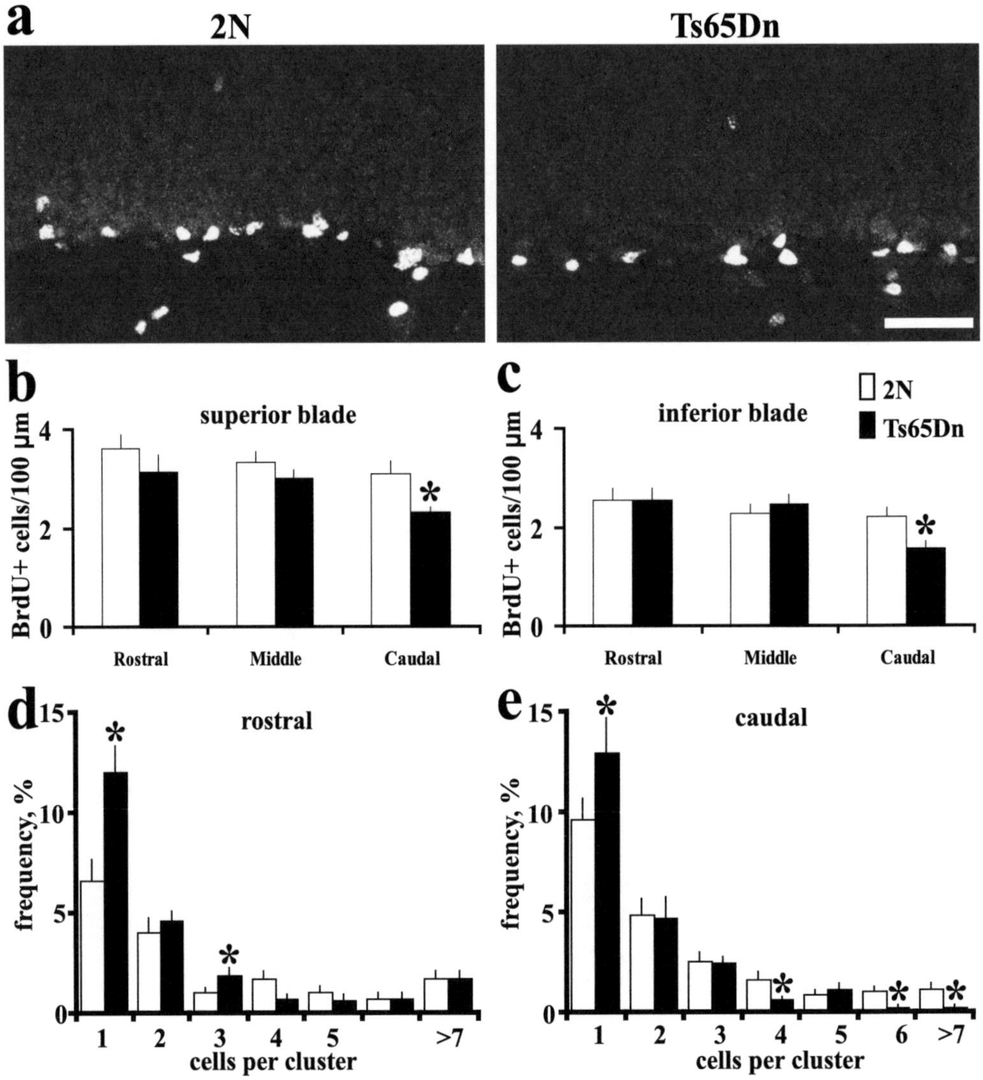

Fig. 1. Morphometry of BrdU+ cells in dentate gyrus in 2N and Ts65Dn mice. (a) Confocal image of BrdU+ cells in caudal part of dentate gyrus of 2N and Ts65Dn mice. BrdU+ cell density in superior (**b**) and inferior blades (**c**) of dentate gyrus. Note a significant reduction of BrdU+ cell in caudal DG in Ts65Dn mice. The number of cells per cluster in rostral (**d**) and caudal (**e**) part of DG. Scale bar = 50 µm.

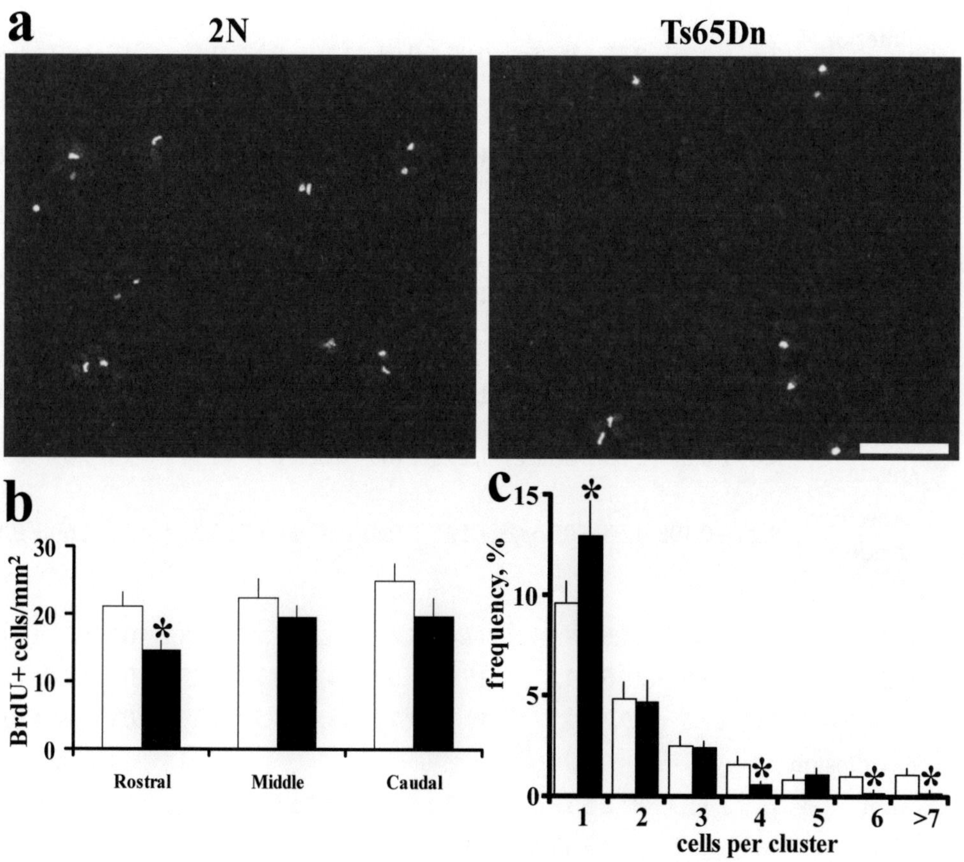

Fig. 2. Neurogenesis in cortex in 2N and Ts65Dn mice. (a) Confocal image of BrdU+ cells in the rostral part of cortex of 2N and Ts65Dn mice. (**b**) BrdU+ cell density in cortex. Note significant reduction of BrdU+ cell in rostral cortex in Ts65Dn mice. (**c**) The number of cells per cluster in rostral part of cortex. Scale bar = 100 μm.

	cell density		cluster density		# cells per cluster	
	2N	Ts65Dn	2N	Ts65Dn	2N	Ts65Dn
Dentate gyrus						
Rostral						
Total	3.06 ± 0.27	2.87 ± 0.25	1.01 ± 0.08	1.22 ± 0.09	3.05 ± 0.22	2.39 ± 0.16a
Superior blade	3.61 ± 0.29	3.13 ± 0.36	1.02 ± 0.11	1.25 ± 0.09	3.69 ± 0.29	2.47 ± 0.21a
Inferior blade	2.55 ± 0.25b	2.55 ± 0.25	0.99 ± 0.08	1.19 ± 0.13	2.65 ± 0.29b	2.42 ± 0.37
Middle						
Total	2.88 ± 0.17	2.77 ± 0.15	1.21 ± 0.05	1.17 ± 0.08	2.56 ± 0.20	2.52 ± 0.12
Superior blade	3.33 ± 0.21	3.01 ± 0.17	1.23 ± 0.05	1.24 ± 0.09	3.01 ± 0.26	2.66 ± 0.12
Inferior blade	2.28 ± 0.18b	2.46 ± 0.20c	1.19 ± 0.08	1.08 ± 0.14	1.96 ± 0.17b	2.51 ± 0.34
Caudal						
Total	2.73 ± 0.19	2.00 ± 0.08a	1.13 ± 0.04	1.10 ± 0.08	2.59 ± 0.31	2.01 ± 0.12a
Superior blade	3.09 ± 0.27	2.31 ± 0.12a	1.21 ± 0.07	1.22 ± 0.10	2.84 ± 0.27	1.69 ± 0.16a
Inferior blade	2.20 ± 0.19b	1.55 ± 0.15a,c	1.10 ± 0.06b	0.92 ± 0.07c	2.21 ± 0.22	1.69 ± 0.16a
Cortex						
Rostral	21.1 ± 2.2	14.6 ± 1.4a	14.4 ± 1.4	10.2 ± 1.2a	1.46 ± 0.04	1.24 ± 0.05a
Middle	22.3 ± 2.9	19.5 ± 1.8	15.9 ± 1.5	14.9 ± 1.7	1.25 ± 0.03	1.22 ± 0.02
Caudal	25.0 ± 2.5	19.7 ± 2.7	14.9 ± 1.7	13.9 ± 1.7	1.30 ± 0.03	1.26 ± 0.04
Corpus callosum						
Rostral	74.7 ± 11.3	87.2 ± 12.6	56.7 ± 3.1	53.0 ± 5.6	1.15 ± 0.05	1.16 ± 0.03
Middle	96.1 ± 15.8	77.3 ± 13.4	64.1 ± 7.2	62.6 ± 7.6	1.28 ± 0.07	1.22 ± 0.03
Caudal	111.2 ± 11.8b	105.1 ± 16.1	73.8 ± 7.3	73.2 ± 9.4	1.36 ± 0.06	1.32 ± 0.04

The number of mice used was as follows: 2N/Ts65Dn = 6/5.

Each value represents the mean ± SEM.

BrdU+ cells and clusters densities are expressed as: for FD per 100 μm length of subgranule zone, for cortex and CC per 1 mm^2.

a, $P < 0.05$, significantly different from 2N mice.

b, $P < 0.05$, significantly different between 2N mice.

c, $P < 0.05$, significantly different between Ts65Dn mice.

Table 1. Morphometry of BrdU+ cells in 2N and Ts65Dn mice

4. Discussion

Numerous studies have shown that adult neurogenesis is affected by various neurodegenerative diseases such as Alzheimer's, Parkinson's, and Huntington's diseases (reviewed in Curtis et al., 2011; Kaneko & Sawamoto, 2009; Rodriguez & Verkhratsky, 2011; Winner et al., 2011). Alteration of neurogenesis in neurodevelopmental disorders were studied to a lesser extent in DS (Contestabile et al., 2007; Guidi et al., 2008, 2010), autism spectrum disorders (Greco et al., 2011; Wegiel et al., 2010), including Rett syndrome (Ronnett et al., 2003). Studies to understand the neurobiology of DS have benefited from the ability to examine mouse models of the disorder (Belichenko et al., 2004; 2007; 2009; Kleschevnikov et al., 2004; Popov et al., 2011). Previous studies demonstrated that trisomy in Ts65Dn mouse model of DS resulted in alteration of hippocampal long-term potentiation (LTP) (Kleschevnikov et al., 2004; Siarey et al., 1997). Significant alteration of neurogenesis could be one of the contributing factors to diminished plasticity in DS. Interestingly, studies involving mice to different enrichments or pharmacotherapies enhanced both neurogenesis and learning (Deng et al., 2010; Mongiat & Schinder, 2011; Saxe et al., 2006; Shors et al., 2002; Singer at al., 2011), including Ts65Dn mice (Bianchi et al., 2010). Moreover, manipulations that stimulate adult neurogenesis in mice also increase LTP (van Praag et al., 1999).

Our study in the Ts65Dn mouse model of DS presents novel evidence of altered neurogenesis in adult young mice (2-3 months of age). Significant increases in the number of clusters containing single BrdU+ cells in Ts65Dn mice point to severely affected cell proliferation. Our present data are in agreement with previous data (Clark et al., 2006) and conflicting with Rueda et al. (2005) data on young adult Ts65Dn mice. The discrepancy with the Rueda et al. (2005) results likely result from several factors including the different gender of mice (we used only male mice and no gender of studied mice were mentioned in Rueda et al., 2005), the different brain areas investigated (we studied rostral, middle, and caudal parts of hippocampus, cortex and CC separately, while in Rueda et al. (2005) the entire hippocampus was studied). The BrdU injection protocol was also different. We used standard a procedure with BrdU injection during 6 days, while Rueda et al., (2005) used a 12 days injection approach.

The majority of BrdU+ cells in adult brain during the proliferation phase formed clusters (Palmer et al., 2000; Seki et al., 2007). Data on neurogenesis in adult rat hippocampus suggests that newly-born cells appeared to stay in clusters for a few days and then migrate from clusters (Seki et al., 2007). Currently, little is known about the molecular mechanisms of cluster formation. Previous reports suggested that cell clustering supports intercellular contacts and/or signals that encourage neurogenesis (Seki et al., 2007). It is possible that the initial formation of a cluster is triggered by a certain factor, which is not affected in Ts65Dn mice. Thus, we have similar cluster density in Ts65Dn vs. 2N mice. The 'just-divided' cells could be divided further, thus resulting in a cluster (Seki et al., 2007). However, this could be only accomplished when the cell is going through all cycles. Indeed, as was shown previously (Contestabile et al., 2008) that the dividing in Ts65Dn cells are 'stuck' in S phase, thus decreasing the probability of cell cycle re-entry. This delay could suspend the second and the following divisions, thus resulting in a reduced number of the newly-born cells per cluster. Interestingly, we observed that the number of cells per cluster was reduced only in the rostral and caudal, but not in the middle part of the Ts65Dn hippocampus. The exact nature of this phenomenon is not clear yet, but may result from differences in the structure and function of hippocampus along the rostro-caudal axis. Indeed, neuronal network architecture is different in hippocampus (Witter et al., 2000).

Reduction in the number of cells per cluster leads to a reduction of total number of newly-born neurons in the Ts65Dn hippocampus. It was shown previously that LTP in the DG depends strongly on neurogenesis, and that a blockade of neurogenesis results in reduced synaptic plasticity (Snyder et al., 2001). Because we observed that LTP in the DG of Ts65Dn mice is significantly diminished (Kleschevnikov et al., 2004), it is tempting to assume that reduced neurogenesis is one of the factors contributing to this abnormality. It is clear that alteration in prenatal growth of the cortex and hippocampus in trisomic mice is due to a longer cell cycle and reduced neurogenesis (Chakrabarti et al., 2007; Contestabile et al., 2007).

We further propose that alteration of neurogenesis may also affect the balance between excitation and inhibition. Indeed, the putative young neurons are completely unaffected by GABA(A) inhibition (Wang et al., 2000). Reduced number of such disinhibited neurons in DG of Ts65Dn mice could thus result in elevation of the overall efficiency of the inhibitory system (Belichenko et al., 2009; Kleschevnikov et al., 2004). The excitatory/inhibitory neuron ratio could be affected also in other bran regions. The new granule cells of the DG, olfactory bulb, and cerebellum and the new cells in cortex are constantly produced during adult neurogenesis. However, there are many differences between these cells. For example, in the olfactory bulb and neocortex the newly-born cells are mainly inhibitory (GABAergic) (reviewed in Cameron & Dayer, 2008). Reduced neurogenesis in these regions could result in relative disinhibition and, thus, could be regarded as a factor contributing to epilepsy in DS (Goldberg-Stern et al., 2001; Menendez, 2005; Pueschel et al., 1991). In contrast, DG and cerebellar granule cells are excitatory (glutamatergic). However, this question needs to be studied in greater detail. The influence of chromosomal aberration on the transition from proliferating stage to differentiated stage into either glutamatergic or GABA-ergic neurons should be also studied.

Numerous factors can be implicated in the control of adult neurogenesis, including chromosomal aberrations. Although the exact mechanism(s) of influence of partial or complete trisomy on neurogenesis is not known, we can extract some data from the scattered information. Impaired neurogenesis has been described not only in Ts65Dn (Rueda et al., 2005; Clark et al., 2006; Lorenzi and Reeves, 2006; Constestabile et al., 2007; Chakrabarti et al., 2007; Bianchi et al., 2010) and Ts2Cje (Ishihara et al., 2010) mouse models of DS, but also in TsCje1 mice (Hewitt et al., 2010; Ishihara et al., 2010) with smaller triplicated chromosomal region. Genetic dissection approaches (Ts65Dn vs. Ts1Cje) point out to the same genes in smaller triplicated region, i.e. I*tsn1, Dyrk1A, Olig2* may involve in neurogenesis (Hewitt et al., 2010; Ishihara et al., 2010). It has been proposed that overexpressions of Dyrk1A in trisomic segment may be responsible for impaired neurogenesis in Ts65Dn, Ts2Cje, and Ts1Cje mouse models of DS (Canzonetta et al., 2008; Ishihara et al., 2010). These authors also suggest that altered neurogenesis in the Ts1Cje mouse is due to a reduction in neuronal progenitors and neuroblasts rather than neural stem cells (Hewitt et al., 2010). The further identification and characterization of triplicated genes in altered neurogenesis may significantly contribute to understanding the neurobiology of DS and may lead to the development of pharmacotherapy for DS.

5. Conclusion

Down syndrome (DS) is a neurodevelopmental disorder caused by the triplication of chromosome 21. Few studies have explored neurogenesis in mouse models of DS and these have produced conflicting results on the alteration of neurogenesis. Using confocal microscopy analysis we have examined adult neurogenesis in the hippocampus (dentate gyrus, DG), motor cortex and corpus callosum (CC) of male wild-type (2N) and Ts65Dn mice at age 2-3 months. In Ts65D we found significant decreases in the BrdU+ cells density in DG and motor cortex. BrdU+ cell cluster density were higher in rostral motor cortex in Ts65Dn. Number of BrdU+ cells per cluster were significantly lower in DG and motor cortex of Ts65Dn mice, mainly due to the presence of single cell clusters. Density of BrdU+ cells was significantly lower in the inferior than in the superior blade of DG. Thus, we show for the first time a lower density of BrdU+ cells in Ts65Dn mice. Our findings are evidence on a deficiency of adult neurogenesis in Ts65Dn mouse model of DS. Moreover, we propose a correlation of the present data with our previously published data on alteration of LTP due to excessive inhibition in Ts65Dn mouse model of DS. The new findings can shed light on possible mechanisms underlying the changes in the Ts65Dn neurogenesis, synaptic structure and function that were described previously. Based on our data and recent studies we reasonable suggested that new complex therapies should improve neurogenesis, and as consequence also learning and memory.

6. Acknowledgments

We thank Dr. Theo D. Palmer and Dr. William C. Mobley for their critical inputs in the beginning of this work. We also thank Michael Maloney for critically reading the article. This work was supported by the Larry L Hillblom Foundation and by the Down Syndrome Research and Treatment Foundation.

7. References

Antonarakis, S.E. & Epstein, C.J. (2006). The challenge of Down syndrome. *Trends Mol Med,* Vol. 12, No. 10, pp. 473-479.

Aylward, E.H., Li, Q., Habbak, Q.R., Warren, A., Pulsifer, M.B., Barta, P.E., Jerram, M. & Pearlson, G. (1997). Basal ganglia volume in adults with Down syndrome. *Psychiatry Res,* Vol. 74, No. 2, pp. 73-82.

Aylward, E.H., Li, Q., Honeycutt, N.A., Warren, A.C., Pulsifer, M.B., Barta, P.E., Chan, M.D., Smith, P.D., Jerram, M. & Pearlson, G.D. (1999). MRI volumes of the hippocampus and amygdala in adults with Down's syndrome with and without dementia. *Am J Psychiatry,* Vol. 156, No. 4, pp. 564-568.

Belichenko, P.V., Kleschevnikov, A.M., Masliah, E., Wu, C., Takimoto-Kimura, R., Salehi, A. & Mobley, W.C. (2009). Excitatory-inhibitory relationship in the fascia dentata in the Ts65Dn mouse model of Down syndrome. *J Comp Neurol,* Vol. 512, No. 4, pp. 453-466.

Belichenko, P.V., Kleschevnikov, A.M., Salehi, A., Epstein, C.J. & Mobley, W.C. (2007). Synaptic and cognitive abnormalities in mouse models of Down syndrome: exploring genotype-phenotype relationships. *J Comp Neurol,* Vol. 504, No. 4, pp. 329-345.

Belichenko, P.V., Masliah, E., Kleschevnikov, A.M., Villar, A.J., Epstein, C.J., Salehi, A. & Mobley, W.C. (2004). Synaptic structural abnormalities in the Ts65Dn mouse model of Down Syndrome. *J Comp Neurol,* Vol. 480, No. 3, pp. 281-298.

Bianchi, P., Ciani, E., Guidi, S., Trazzi, S., Felice, D., Grossi, G., Fernandez, M., Giuliani, A., Calza, L. & Bartesaghi, R. (2010). Early pharmacotherapy restores neurogenesis and cognitive performance in the Ts65Dn mouse model for Down syndrome. *J Neurosci,* Vol. 30, No. 26, pp. 8769-8779.

Cameron, H.A. & Dayer, A.G. (2008). New interneurons in the adult neocortex: small, sparse, but significant? *Biol Psychiatry,* Vol. 63, No. 7, pp. 650-655.

Canfield, M.A., Honein, M.A., Yuskiv, N., Xing, J., Mai, C.T., Collins, J.S., Devine, O., Petrini, J., Ramadhani, T.A., Hobbs, C.A. & Kirby, R.S. (2006). National estimates and race/ethnic-specific variation of selected birth defects in the United States, 1999-2001. *Birth Defects Res A Clin Mol Teratol,* Vol. 76, No. 11, pp. 747-756.

Canzonetta, C., Mulligan, C., Deutsch, S., Ruf, S., O'Doherty, A., Lyle, R., Borel, C., Lin-Marq, N., Delom, F., Groet, J., Schnappauf, F., De Vita, S., Averill, S., Priestley, J.V., Martin, J.E., Shipley, J., Denyer, G., Epstein, C.J., Fillat, C., Estivill, X., Tybulewicz, V.L., Fisher, E.M., Antonarakis, S.E. & Nizetic, D. (2008). DYRK1A-dosage imbalance perturbs NRSF/REST levels, deregulating pluripotency and embryonic stem cell fate in Down syndrome. *Am J Hum Genet,* Vol. 83, No. 3, pp. 388-400.

Carpentier, P.A. & Palmer, T.D. (2009). Immune influence on adult neural stem cell regulation and function. *Neuron,* Vol. 64, No. 1, pp. 79-92.

Chakrabarti, L., Galdzicki, Z. & Haydar, T.F. (2007). Defects in embryonic neurogenesis and initial synapse formation in the forebrain of the Ts65Dn mouse model of Down syndrome. *J Neurosci,* Vol. 27, No. 43, pp. 11483-11495.

Chapman, R.S. & Hesketh, L.J. (2000). Behavioral phenotype of individuals with Down syndrome. *Ment Retard Dev Disabil Res Rev,* Vol. 6, No. 2, pp. 84-95.

Clark, S., Schwalbe, J., Stasko, M.R., Yarowsky, P.J. & Costa, A.C. (2006). Fluoxetine rescues deficient neurogenesis in hippocampus of the Ts65Dn mouse model for Down syndrome. *Exp Neurol,* Vol. 200, No. 1, pp. 256-261.

Contestabile, A., Fila, T., Ceccarelli, C., Bonasoni, P., Bonapace, L., Santini, D., Bartesaghi, R. & Ciani, E. (2007). Cell cycle alteration and decreased cell proliferation in the hippocampal dentate gyrus and in the neocortical germinal matrix of fetuses with Down syndrome and in Ts65Dn mice. *Hippocampus,* Vol. 17, No. 8, pp. 665-678.

Curtis, M.A., Kam, M. & Faull, R.L. (2011). Neurogenesis in humans. *Eur J Neurosci,* Vol. 33, No. 6, pp. 1170-1174.

Deng, W., Aimone, J.B. & Gage, F.H. (2010). New neurons and new memories: how does adult hippocampal neurogenesis affect learning and memory? *Nat Rev Neurosci,* Vol. 11, No. 5, pp. 339-350.

Galvan, V. & Jin, K. (2007). Neurogenesis in the aging brain. *Clin Interv Aging,* Vol. 2, No. 4, pp. 605-610.

Goldberg-Stern, H., Strawsburg, R.H., Patterson, B., Hickey, F., Bare, M., Gadoth, N. & Degrauw, T.J. (2001). Seizure frequency and characteristics in children with Down syndrome. *Brain Dev,* Vol. 23, No. 6, pp. 375-378.

Gould, E., Reeves, A.J., Graziano, M.S. & Gross, C.G. (1999). Neurogenesis in the neocortex of adult primates. *Science,* Vol. 286, No. 5439, pp. 548-552.

Greco, C.M., Navarro, C.S., Hunsaker, M.R., Maezawa, I., Shuler, J.F., Tassone, F., Delany, M., Au, J.W., Berman, R.F., Jin, L.W., Schumann, C., Hagerman, P.J. & Hagerman, R.J. (2011). Neuropathologic features in the hippocampus and cerebellum of three older men with fragile X syndrome. *Mol Autism,* Vol. 2, No. 1, pp. 2.

Guidi, S., Bonasoni, P., Ceccarelli, C., Santini, D., Gualtieri, F., Ciani, E. & Bartesaghi, R. (2008). Neurogenesis impairment and increased cell death reduce total neuron number in the hippocampal region of fetuses with Down syndrome. *Brain Pathol,* Vol. 18, No. 2, pp. 180-197.

Guidi, S., Ciani, E., Bonasoni, P., Santini, D. & Bartesaghi, R. (2010). Widespread Proliferation Impairment and Hypocellularity in the Cerebellum of Fetuses with Down Syndrome. *Brain Pathol,* Vol. No., pp. 1-13.

Hewitt, C.A., Ling, K.H., Merson, T.D., Simpson, K.M., Ritchie, M.E., King, S.L., Pritchard, M.A., Smyth, G.K., Thomas, T., Scott, H.S. & Voss, A.K. (2010). Gene network disruptions and neurogenesis defects in the adult Ts1Cje mouse model of Down syndrome. *PLoS One,* Vol. 5, No. 7, pp. e11561.

Hof, P.R., Young, W.G., Bloom, F.E., Belichenko, P.V. & Celio M.R. (2000) *Comparative Cytoarchitectonic Atlas of the C57Bl/6 and 129/Sv Mouse Brains.* Elsevier, Amsterdam.

Ishihara, K., Amano, K., Takaki, E., Shimohata, A., Sago, H., Epstein, C.J. & Yamakawa, K. (2010). Enlarged brain ventricles and impaired neurogenesis in the Ts1Cje and Ts2Cje mouse models of Down syndrome. *Cereb Cortex,* Vol. 20, No. 5, pp. 1131-1143.

Kaneko, N. & Sawamoto, K. (2009). Adult neurogenesis and its alteration under pathological conditions. *Neurosci Res,* Vol. 63, No. 3, pp. 155-164.

Kee, N., Teixeira, C.M., Wang, A.H. & Frankland, P.W. (2007). Preferential incorporation of adult-generated granule cells into spatial memory networks in the dentate gyrus. *Nat Neurosci,* Vol. 10, No. 3, pp. 355-362.

Kernie, S.G. & Parent, J.M. (2010). Forebrain neurogenesis after focal Ischemic and traumatic brain injury. *Neurobiol Dis,* Vol. 37, No. 2, pp. 267-274.

Kesslak, J.P., Nagata, S.F., Lott, I. & Nalcioglu, O. (1994). Magnetic resonance imaging analysis of age-related changes in the brains of individuals with Down's syndrome. *Neurology,* Vol. 44, No. 6, pp. 1039-1045.

Kleschevnikov, A.M., Belichenko, P.V., Villar, A.J., Epstein, C.J., Malenka, R.C. & Mobley, W.C. (2004). Hippocampal long-term potentiation suppressed by increased inhibition in the Ts65Dn mouse, a genetic model of Down syndrome. *J Neurosci,* Vol. 24, No. 37, pp. 8153-8160.

Koehl, M. & Abrous, D.N. (2011). A new chapter in the field of memory: adult hippocampal neurogenesis. *Eur J Neurosci,* Vol. 33, No. 6, pp. 1101-1114.

Kreuzberg, M., Kanov, E., Timofeev, O., Schwaninger, M., Monyer, H. & Khodosevich, K. (2010). Increased subventricular zone-derived cortical neurogenesis after ischemic lesion. *Exp Neurol,* Vol. 226, No. 1, pp. 90-99.

Lorenzi, H.A. & Reeves, R.H. (2006). Hippocampal hypocellularity in the Ts65Dn mouse originates early in development. *Brain Res,* Vol. 1104, No. 1, pp. 153-159.

Luskin, M.B. & Boone, M.S. (1994). Rate and pattern of migration of lineally-related olfactory bulb interneurons generated postnatally in the subventricular zone of the rat. *Chem Senses,* Vol. 19, No. 6, pp. 695-714.

Markakis, E.A. & Gage, F.H. (1999). Adult-generated neurons in the dentate gyrus send axonal projections to field CA3 and are surrounded by synaptic vesicles. *J Comp Neurol,* Vol. 406, No. 4, pp. 449-460.

Menendez, M. (2005). Down syndrome, Alzheimer's disease and seizures. *Brain Dev,* Vol. 27, No. 4, pp. 246-252.

Mongiat, L.A. & Schinder, A.F. (2011). Adult neurogenesis and the plasticity of the dentate gyrus network. *Eur J Neurosci,* Vol. 33, No. 6, pp. 1055-1061.

Moriyama, M., Fukuhara, T., Britschgi, M., He, Y., Narasimhan, R., Villeda, S., Molina, H., Huber, B.T., Holers, M. & Wyss-Coray, T. (2011). Complement Receptor 2 Is Expressed in Neural Progenitor Cells and Regulates Adult Hippocampal Neurogenesis. *J Neurosci,* Vol. 31, No. 11, pp. 3981-3989.

Palmer, T.D., Willhoite, A.R. & Gage, F.H. (2000). Vascular niche for adult hippocampal neurogenesis. *J Comp Neurol,* Vol. 425, No. 4, pp. 479-494.

Pinter, J.D., Eliez, S., Schmitt, J.E., Capone, G.T. & Reiss, A.L. (2001). Neuroanatomy of Down's syndrome: a high-resolution MRI study. *Am J Psychiatry,* Vol. 158, No. 10, pp. 1659-1665.

Popov, V.I., Kleschevnikov, A.M., Klimenko, O.A., Stewart, M.G. & Belichenko, P.V. (2011). Three-dimensional synaptic ultrastructure in the dentate gyrus and hippocampal area CA3 in the Ts65Dn mouse model of down syndrome. *J Comp Neurol,* Vol. 519, No. 7, pp. 1338-1354.

Pueschel, S.M., Louis, S. & McKnight, P. (1991). Seizure disorders in Down syndrome. *Arch Neurol,* Vol. 48, No. 3, pp. 318-320.

Rao, M.S., Hattiangady, B. & Shetty, A.K. (2006). The window and mechanisms of major age-related decline in the production of new neurons within the dentate gyrus of the hippocampus. *Aging Cell,* Vol. 5, No. 6, pp. 545-558.

Raz, N., Torres, I.J., Briggs, S.D., Spencer, W.D., Thornton, A.E., Loken, W.J., Gunning, F.M., McQuain, J.D., Driesen, N.R. & Acker, J.D. (1995). Selective neuroanatomic abnormalities in Down's syndrome and their cognitive correlates: evidence from MRI morphometry. *Neurology,* Vol. 45, No. 2, pp. 356-366.

Rodriguez, J.J. & Verkhratsky, A. (2011). Neurogenesis in Alzheimer's disease. *J Anat,* Vol. No., pp. 1-12.

Ronnett, G.V., Leopold, D., Cai, X., Hoffbuhr, K.C., Moses, L., Hoffman, E.P. & Naidu, S. (2003). Olfactory biopsies demonstrate a defect in neuronal development in Rett's syndrome. *Ann Neurol,* Vol. 54, No. 2, pp. 206-218.

Rueda, N., Mostany, R., Pazos, A., Florez, J. & Martinez-Cue, C. (2005). Cell proliferation is reduced in the dentate gyrus of aged but not young Ts65Dn mice, a model of Down syndrome. *Neurosci Lett,* Vol. 380, No. 1-2, pp. 197-201.

Sandoval, C.J., Martinez-Claros, M., Bello-Medina, P.C., Perez, O. & Ramirez-Amaya, V. (2011). When are new hippocampal neurons, born in the adult brain, integrated into the network that processes spatial information? *PLoS One,* Vol. 6, No. 3, pp. e17689.

Saxe, M.D., Battaglia, F., Wang, J.W., Malleret, G., David, D.J., Monckton, J.E., Garcia, A.D., Sofroniew, M.V., Kandel, E.R., Santarelli, L., Hen, R. & Drew, M.R. (2006). Ablation of hippocampal neurogenesis impairs contextual fear conditioning and synaptic plasticity in the dentate gyrus. *Proc Natl Acad Sci U S A,* Vol. 103, No. 46, pp. 17501-17506.

Seki, T., Namba, T., Mochizuki, H. & Onodera, M. (2007). Clustering, migration, and neurite formation of neural precursor cells in the adult rat hippocampus. *J Comp Neurol,* Vol. 502, No. 2, pp. 275-290.

Shors, T.J., Townsend, D.A., Zhao, M., Kozorovitskiy, Y. & Gould, E. (2002). Neurogenesis may relate to some but not all types of hippocampal-dependent learning. *Hippocampus,* Vol. 12, No. 5, pp. 578-584.

Siarey, R.J., Stoll, J., Rapoport, S.I. & Galdzicki, Z. (1997). Altered long-term potentiation in the young and old Ts65Dn mouse, a model for Down Syndrome. *Neuropharmacology,* Vol. 36, No. 11-12, pp. 1549-1554.

Singer, B.H., Gamelli, A.E., Fuller, C.L., Temme, S.J., Parent, J.M. & Murphy, G.G. (2011). Compensatory network changes in the dentate gyrus restore long-term potentiation following ablation of neurogenesis in young-adult mice. *Proc Natl Acad Sci U S A,* Vol. 108, No. 13, pp. 5437-5442.

Snyder, J.S., Kee, N. & Wojtowicz, J.M. (2001). Effects of adult neurogenesis on synaptic plasticity in the rat dentate gyrus. *J Neurophysiol,* Vol. 85, No. 6, pp. 2423-2431.

van Praag, H., Christie, B.R., Sejnowski, T.J. & Gage, F.H. (1999). Running enhances neurogenesis, learning, and long-term potentiation in mice. *Proc Natl Acad Sci U S A,* Vol. 96, No. 23, pp. 13427-13431.

Voloboueva, L.A., Lee, S.W., Emery, J.F., Palmer, T.D. & Giffard, R.G. (2010). Mitochondrial protection attenuates inflammation-induced impairment of neurogenesis in vitro and in vivo. *J Neurosci,* Vol. 30, No. 37, pp. 12242-12251.

Wang, S., Scott, B.W. & Wojtowicz, J.M. (2000). Heterogenous properties of dentate granule neurons in the adult rat. *J Neurobiol,* Vol. 42, No. 2, pp. 248-257.

Wegiel, J., Kuchna, I., Nowicki, K., Imaki, H., Marchi, E., Ma, S.Y., Chauhan, A., Chauhan, V., Bobrowicz, T.W., de Leon, M., Louis, L.A., Cohen, I.L., London, E., Brown, W.T. & Wisniewski, T. (2010). The neuropathology of autism: defects of neurogenesis and neuronal migration, and dysplastic changes. *Acta Neuropathol,* Vol. 119, No. 6, pp. 755-770.

Winner, B., Kohl, Z. & Gage, F.H. (2011). Neurodegenerative disease and adult neurogenesis. *Eur J Neurosci,* Vol. 33, No. 6, pp. 1139-1151.

Wisniewski, K.E., Laure-Kamionowska, M. & Wisniewski, H.M. (1984). Evidence of arrest of neurogenesis and synaptogenesis in brains of patients with Down's syndrome. *N Engl J Med,* Vol. 311, No. 18, pp. 1187-1188.

Witter, M.P., Wouterlood, F.G., Naber, P.A. & Van Haeften, T. (2000). Anatomical organization of the parahippocampal-hippocampal network. *Ann N Y Acad Sci,* Vol. 911, No., pp. 1-24.

Yoneyama, M., Shiba, T., Hasebe, S. & Ogita, K. (2011). Adult Neurogenesis Is Regulated by Endogenous Factors Produced During Neurodegeneration. *J Pharmacol Sci,* Vol. No., pp. 1-8.

Yu, Y., He, J., Zhang, Y., Luo, H., Zhu, S., Yang, Y., Zhao, T., Wu, J., Huang, Y., Kong, J., Tan, Q. & Li, X.M. (2009). Increased hippocampal neurogenesis in the progressive stage of Alzheimer's disease phenotype in an APP/PS1 double transgenic mouse model. *Hippocampus,* Vol. 19, No. 12, pp. 1247-1253.

Part 3

Neurologic, Urologic, Dental and Allergic Disorders

10

Dermatological Manifestations of Down Syndrome

Dominguez-Cruz JJ and Bueno Delgado MA
Virgen del Rocío Universitary Hospital, Sevilla
Spain

1. Introduction

Down syndrome (DS) is increased frequency of some common dermatoses and associated with rare dermatological disorders. With the increasing life span and number of DS patients in the population, dermatologists are more likely to encounter skin manifestations associated with DS. Subjects with DS have high rates of infections and autoimmune phenomena. The immunological disturbances in DS (High IgG and low IgM levels, reduced total T-lymphocyte numbers, high CD8+ and low CD4+ count, decreased chemotaxis,...) could be implicated in some higher cutaneous manifestations.

In this chapter, it has been exposed the dermatological disorders associated with DS. Very few studies in the literature have studied dermatological manifestations of DS. Newer reports are mostly in the form of case reports highlighting the rare dermatological findings. Dermatologic manifestation in DS has been studied in 6 major surveys but the results are not concordant. These studies differ in some aspects (age range, living conditions of the study group,...). Daneshpazhooh *et al* studied 100 children with DS with a mean age of 11.2 years; Carter and Jegasothy examined 213 institutionalized patients with ages between 12 and 48 years old; Ercis *et al* studied 71 children who live with their families; Polenghi *et* al observed adults with ages between 14 and 53 years old; Schepis *et al* examined 203 patients from infancy till adulthood with a mean age of 11.7 years; and Sureshbabu *et al* studied 95 patients with a mean age of 11.9 years, ranging from 6 months to 40 years.

These dermatologic disorders can be separated in manifestations that could be, or not, associated to immunological alterations (Table 1).

Associated to immunological alterations	Probably not associated to immunological alterations
Atopic dermatitis *Seborrhoeic dermatitis* *Alopecia areata* *Vitiligo* *Infections* - *Onychomycosis* - *Scabies*	*Anetoderma* *Milia-like calcinosis cutis* *Acanthosis nigricans* *Syringomas elastosis perforans serpiginosa* *Leukaemia cutis* *Acrocyanosis* *Cutis marmorata* *Keratodermatoses*

Table 1. Dermatological manifestations of Down's syndrome associates or probably not associated to immunological alterations

2. Dermatological manifestations that could be associated to immunological alterations

2.1 Atopic dermatitis

Atopic dermatitis (AD) is a chronic inflammatory skin condition that appears to involve a genetic defect in the proteins supporting the epidermal barrier. AD affects approximately 5-20% of children worldwide. The incidence of AD appears to be increasing. Onset tends to occur during childhood and gradually diminishes with age, although it can persist or even appear in adults. The term AD was coined by Wise and Sulzberger in 1933 to define an entity characterized by dry skin, pruritus, erythematous lesions, and a chronic recurrent course. Currently, the terms AD and atopic eczema are used and both are acceptable.

Its prevalence has increased 3-fold or 4- fold in recent decades in some countries. According to the International Study of Asthma and Allergies in Childhood, during a minimum period of 1 year, the prevalence of symptoms of AD in 6- or 7-year-old children presented great variability between different geographic areas. Thus, prevalence was almost 20% in England or Australia but less than 2% in China or Iran. There is a higher prevalence in urban areas than in rural ones in developed countries, and higher social classes are more affected. Regarding the disease by sex, a study of 12- to 16-year-olds found a higher prevalence among girls (25.7%) than among boys (17%). The onset of AD occurred during the first 6 months of life in 45% of children, in the first year in 60%, and in the first 5 years in more than 85%.

One study diagnosed AD in 56.5% of DS, and another a prevalence of more than 50%. The high reported prevalence of AD, in some studies, could be an overestimate and isolated signs such as facial dermatitis and generalized xerosis could easily be misinterpreted as AD.

Pathogenesis of AD is complex; several factors are involved, many of which are still not well understood. Likewise, it has yet to be determined how these factors might interact with one another origin of atopic eczema seems to involve a feedback cycle: pruritus and mechanical damage caused by scratching leads to the production of proinflammatory cytokines (interleukin [IL]-1, IL-18, tumor necrosis factor, granulocyte-macrophage colony stimulating factor) that recruit leukocytes to the skin.

Different leukocyte populations are activated through different processes; on induction by dendritic cells, the lymphocytes differentiate via the Th2 pathway; these dendritic cells also show increased antigen-presenting capacity and bind to the IgE-antigen complex. The IgE antigen complex in turn induces mast cell accumulation and activation. The activated Th2 cells release IL-4 and IL-13, which suppress the production of antimicrobial peptides. Viruses, bacteria, and fungi take advantage of these reduced peptide levels, colonizing the skin and releasing proinflammatory products (superantigens, proteoglycans, and lipoteichoic acid) that amplify leukocyte activation. This activation increases the release of inflammatory mediators, such as proteases and IL-31, which perpetuate pruritus.

Increased prevalence of childhood AD in developed countries has led to the appearance of many theories on the possible involvement of environmental factors. Increases in the prevalence of allergic disease probably depend more on environmental factors than on other individual characteristics.

The diagnosis of AD is based on a constellation of signs and symptoms. There is no laboratory "gold standard" for the diagnosis of AD. In a majority of the cases, the diagnosis is quite easy. Establishing firm diagnostic criteria for all forms of AD is difficult due to the clinical and pathophysiological heterogeneity. Atopic individuals can also suffer from other dermatitis or dermatoses, and because every dermatitis in an atopic individual need not be AD. Hanifin and Rajka for the first time proposed a systematic approach toward the standardization of the diagnosis of AD by incorporating three major/basic and 23 minor features. They suggested that a diagnosis of AD can be established if 3 of the major and 3 of the minor criteria are present. (Table 2).

Major	Minor
1. *Pruritus* 2. *Typcial morphology and distribution:* - *Flexural lichenification or linearity in adults* - *Facial and extensor involvement in infants and children* 3. *Chronic or chronically relapsing dermatitis* 4. *Personal or family history of atopy (asthma, AR, atopic dermatitis)*	1. *Xerosis* 2. *Ichthyosis/palmar hyperlinearity/keratosis pilaris* 3. *Immediate (type 1) skin test reactivity* 4. *Elevated serum IgE* 5. *Early age at onset* 6. *Tendency toward cutaneous infections (esp. Staph. aureus and Herpes simplex)/impaired cell-mediated immunity* 7. *Tendency toward nonspecific hand or foot dermatitis* 8. *Nipple eczema* 9. *Cheilitis* 10. *Recurrent conjuntivitis* 11. *Dennie-Morgan infraorbital folds* 12. *Keratoconus* 13. *Anterior subcapsular cataracts* 14. *Orbital darkening* 15. *Facial pallor/facial erythema* 16. *Pityriasis alba* 17. *Anterior neck folds* 18. *Itch when sweating* 19. *Intolerance to wool or lipid solvents* 20. *Perifollicular accentuation* 21. *Food intolerance* 22. *Course influenced by environmental/emotional factors* 23. *White dermographism/delayed blanch*

Table 2. Diagnostic criteria of Hanifin and Rajka Diagnosis of AD can be established if 3 of the major and 3 of the minor criteria are present

In DS, the skin in infancy is usually soft, but soon becomes dry, thick, and rough, with patchy lichenification. The reported frequency of xerosis differs from 9.8 percent to 85 percent in various studies. Sureshbabu *et al* observed disorders lichenification as the most common disorder, seen in 52.6% of DS patients, with a peak incidence in the 5-10 year age group. High incidence of AD reported by Carter *et al* (56.5%) and cited in some major review articles contrast with Sureshbabu *et al* study which none of subjects fulfilled the criteria of Hanifin and Rajka for AD. Two studies observed 3% and 4.9% for the prevalence of AD in

DS using the criteria of Rajka and Hanifin, These results are in favour of the opinion that AD is not as common as previously thought when using the acknowledged diagnostic criteria of Rajka and Hanifin.

In the treatment of AD, topical corticosteroids are considered the gold standard for assessment of other treatments. The potency and formulation employed depends on the area to be treated and the chronicity of the lesions. Areas with have undergone lichenification requiring stronger formulations. One application per day is sufficient, as treatment twice a day confers no advantage while increasing the likelihood of adverse reactions. Adverse reactions are well known and frequently overestimated by patients and their family members, even though the new formulations have a demonstrated lower risk of causing cutaneous atrophy than the older ones and that several studies have found a far lower incidence of local and systemic complications.

Application of topical antibiotics in combination with corticosteroid therapy has advantages compared to topical corticosteroids. Fusidic acid appears to be the topical antibacterial treatment of choice, due to its low minimum inhibitory concentration and its good penetration.

Topical calcineurin inhibitors have proven to be effective in the treatment of AD. Topical tacrolimus seems to have an efficacy similar to high-potency corticosteroids, whereas pimecrolimus is substantially weaker. Controlled pediatric studies have confirmed the superior efficacy of topical tacrolimus compared to pimecrolimus and hydrocortisone. There appear to be no significant differences between the response of children to concentrations of 0.03% and 0.1%. Neither tacrolimus nor pimecrolimus cause cutaneous atrophy, but they can cause other adverse reactions such as local itching-burning sensation when being applied, which is an added discomfort for the skin of children with AD.

Use of emollients is widely recognized as a basic measure in the treatment and prevention of flares of AD. It has been shown that their use in combination with topical corticosteroids accelerates healing and decreases the total dose of corticosteroids required to resolve the flare.

Dietary restrictions have proven effective in the case of children with egg-specific IgE, but not for other foods which have the same effect. It seems reasonable to establish diets that avoid food proven to cause an allergic response using the radioallergosorbent test, although the most relevant test would be the challenge test, which in many cases cannot be performed. Psychological care is recommended to help deal with the emotional needs of patients with atopic dermatitis, and should be based on providing education and information on the clinical and preventable aspects of the disease. One study found that this type of intervention reduced anxiety scores.

Short-course systemic corticosteroids are recommended to control acute flares of AD, taking into account that new flares are frequent after stopping treatment. Their long term use in children is not recommended. Little evidence exists to support using oral antihistamines in AD. Other systemic treatments to AD are: Cyclosporine A, azathioprine, interferon, light therapy or intravenous immunoglobulins. Biologic treatment has recently appeared in the field of dermatology and has shown some potential.

2.2 Seborrhoeic dermatitis

Seborrhoeic dermatitis (SD) is a common, chronic dermatoses of unknown aetiology, characterized by scaling and redness occurring primarily in the areas with the highest concentration of sebaceous glands such as the scalp, face (mid-facial region), and certain areas of the trunk, such as the mid-thoracic and interscapular areas and the area around the buttocks. On the scalp, it generally appears first as small patches of scales, progressing to involve the entire scalp with exfoliation of excessive amounts of dry scales.

It affects around 1% to 3% of the immunocompetent adult population, with a higher prevalence in men than women. Although it can appear at any age, the highest prevalence is observed in individuals aged 30 to 60 years and in the first 3 months of life in the infantile form of the disease.

Clinically, the disease is characterized by erythema and flaking of the skin in the affected area. Lesions are well delimited, reddish, and covered with oily yellowish-white scales. On the scalp, in the milder form of the disease, the scales are small, dry, and whitish, and they detach easily and spontaneously in steady amounts. In the more severe form of the disease, plaques are observed that range in size from a few centimeters to areas covering a large part of the scalp; they are made up of thick dry scales. On the face they are found in the eyebrows, around the nose, at the edge of the scalp, and on the inner surface of the auricle. In the thorax, the lesions are rounded, well delimited, and reddish brown; they are located on the medial part of the chest and on the back, between the shoulder blades. All of these forms are associated with varying degrees of itching. In adults, the course of SD involves periods of remission and exacerbation, irrespective of the treatments administered. Outbreaks are common under conditions of emotional stress, fatigue, and depression.

While the disease rarely causes serious complications, it always leads to a marked esthetic deterioration that leads to emotional and social difficulties for the affected individual.

The etiology of seborrheic dermatitis is not fully understood but is known to involve various factors. Increased secretion by the sebaceous glands favours the development of microorganisms of the genus *Malassezia*, which are responsible for the symptoms.

It appears more frequently in patients with neurological disorders such as Parkinson disease, in those suffering from depression, and in patients with AIDS. One study, by Carter and Jegasothy, found a 36% prevalence of SD in DS patients and another was found a similar prevalence (Ercis *et* 31%; mostly during the first year of life). SD was seen in 4.2% of DS by Sureshbabu *et al. al.* SD is commonly seen in patients with immunodeficiency. High prevalence of *pityrosporum folliculitis* in DS patients could have a pathogenic role.

A diet rich in animal fats and lacking in vegetables, as well as alcohol consumption can also potentiate the appearance of lesions. Topical corticosteroids are the first choice treatment for SD. Others drugs can currently be used to minimize the effects of this dermatologic disease: antifungals, keratolytics, tar or pyrithione derivatives, and selenium sulfate. Many of these treatments have been tested as both monotherapy and in combination.

2.3 Alopecia areata

Alopecia areata (AA) is a recurrent nonscarring type of hair loss that can affect any hair-bearing area. Clinically, AA can manifest many different patterns. Although medically benign, AA can cause tremendous emotional and psychosocial distress in affected patients and their families.

AA is a genetically determined, immune-mediated disorder of the hair follicle with an estimated lifetime risk of approximately 2%, making it one of the most common autoimmune diseases

AA is characterized by patchy hair loss on the scalp, which can eventually involve the entire scalp (*alopecia totalis*) or the entire body (*alopecia universalis*). The onset of the disease can be sudden, its progression is unpredictable, and it can be recurrent throughout life. It is thought that AA represents a breakdown in immune privelege with the subsequent unable to function of the hair follicle by T lymphocytes. AA has a deeply disturbing psychologic impact on affected individuals. It shows a spectrum of severity that ranges from patchy localized hair loss on the scalp to the complete absence of hair everywhere on the body.

Treatment of AA may induce hair growth, but usually does not change the course of the disease. When treatment is stopped, hair loss recurs. Many patients with one or two small patches can be managed without treatment and with reassurance of the benign nature of the condition. Treatment with topical and oral steroids, topical minoxidil, topical cyclosporine, and photo-dynamic therapy has been found no long-term benefit of these interventions. In patients with persistent hair loss and less than 50% scalp involvement, intralesional corticosteroid therapy is the first-line treatment. Patients with more than 50% hair loss can be treated with topical immunotherapy using diphenyl-cyclopropenone or squaric acid. *Alopecia totalis* and *alopecia universalis* have the worst prognosis, with fewer than 10% of patients recovering.

AA occurs in approximately 0.1% of the general but a recognized association of AA with DS exists and it was reported between 20% to 1.4% prevalence. Sureshbabu *et al* saw in 9.4% of DS with AA. Female predilection was observed by Carter and Jegasothy but not in other studies. AA was observed in 3% of DS patients in the study of Schepis *et al*, with the usual age of onset in middle childhood (5-10 years). AA, in DS patients, is usually severe and refractory to the standard treatments.

2.4 Vitiligo

Vitiligo is a hypopigmentation disorder where the loss of functioning melanocytes causes the appearance of white patches on the skin. It occurs when melanocytes, the cells responsible for skin pigmentation, die or are unable to function. The cause of vitiligo is unknown, but research suggests that it may arise from autoimmune, genetic, oxidative stress, neural, or viral causes. Vitiligo is an autoimmune disease characterized by melanocyte loss, which results in patchy depigmentation of skin and hair, and is associated with an elevated risk of other autoimmune diseases. It is a genetically complex disorder involving multiple susceptibility genes and unknown environmental triggers. Recent data provide strong evidence supporting an autoimmune pathogenesis of vitiligo. Genetic factors also appear to play a role in the etiopathogenesis of vitiligo as 20% to 30% of patients have a family history of the disorder. Vitiligo is associated with other autoimmune diseases (Addison´s disease, hyperthyroidism and pernicious anemia).

Vitiligo affects 1% of the world population, but the prevalence has been reported as high as 4% in some South Asian, Mexican and American populations. Vitiligo can develop at any age, but several studies report that 50% of cases appear before the age of 20 years old. Only one study investigated the association between vitiligo and DS found a prevalence of 1.9%. 75% of this also had AA. However, Sureshbabu *et al* did not observed an incidence significantly higher in DS people.

Flat areas of normal-feeling skin without any pigment appear suddenly or gradually. These areas have a darker border. The edges are well defined but irregular. Vitiligo most often affects the face, elbows and knees, hands and feet, and genits. It affects both sides of the body equally. Vitiligo is more noticeable in darker-skinned people because of the contrast of white patches against dark skin. No other skin changes occur. Sometimes, the use of Wood's light can improve to see lesions. In some cases, a skin biopsy may be needed to rule out other causes of pigment loss.

Vitiligo is difficult to treat. As vitiligo can have a major effect on quality of life, treatment can be considered and should preferably begin early when the disease is active. Current treatment modalities are directed towards stopping progression of the disease and achieving repigmentation. Therapies include corticosteroids, topical immunomodulators, phototherapy, surgery, combination therapies and depigmentation of normall pigmented skin. Topical corticosteroids can be used for localized vitiligo. The use of topical immunomodulators seems to be equally effective as topical steroids, especially when used in the face and neck region. Narrowband ultraviolet-B therapy seems to be superior to psoralen ultraviolet-A. Depigmentation therapy can be considered if vitiligo affects more than 60% to 80% of the body.

2.5 Onychomycosis

Onychomycosis is one of the most prevalent fungal infections in the population with a higher rate of treatment failures. Onychomycosis is a frequent nail disease caused by dermatophytes, yeasts, and nondermatophyte molds. *Trichophyton rubrum, T mentagrophytes,* and *Epidermophyton floccosum* are the most common etiologic agents worldwide.

Onychomycosis may be classified into several types: distal subungual, white superficial, proximal subungual, endonyx, and total dystrophic. Distal subungual onychomycosis, the most common type, involves the nail bed and, subsequently, the nail plate. White superficial onychomycosis usually manifests as superficial white patches with distinct edges on the surface of the nail plate. Proximal subungual onychomycosis results when the fungal organism enters via the cuticle and the ventral aspect of the proximal nail fold. In endonyx onychomycosis, fungal organisms invade the nail plate without resulting nail bed hyperkeratosis, onycholysis, or nail bed inflammatory changes. In total dystrophic onychomycosis, complete dystrophy of the nail plate occurs; these changes may be primary or secondary.

Diagnosis is corroborated by direct microscopic examination, culture, and histomycology. Treatment is based on oral antifungals. Systemic treatment for onychomycosis includes terbinafine, an allylamine that is primarily fungicidal, and itraconazole, a triazole that is primarily fungistatic. Both represent a major therapeutic advancement over griseofulvin in the treatment of this condition.

For toenail infection, terbinafine is usually taken continuously for 12 weeks, whereas itraconazole is taken either continuously or intermittently that is 1 week in 4 weeks for the same period. Because therapeutic concentration of itraconazole is believed to persist in the nail for a considerable time after systemic treatment is stopped, intermittent therapy with higher daily doses to achieve and maintain therapeutic concentration might be an effective alternative to continuous treatment.

Such intermittent treatment is widely used currently to treat onychomycosis and is claimed to be as effective for this condition as both continuous itraconazole and continuous terbinafine

Although both itraconazole and terbinafine are well tolerated and highly effective drugs, continuous terbinafine is more effective than intermittent itraconazole at achieving mycological cure of toenail onychomycosis.

There is a higher frequency of onychomycosis in DS patients. It has been reported prevalence of 67,8% to 4,4%. A low incidence of infection was seen in Sureshbabu *et al* study in contrast to Carter *et al* who reported a high prevalence of fungal infections. Schepis *et al* also reported a relatively low figure for onychomycosis and tinea corporis. Fungal infections may have been over diagnosed in the past or may be caused by poor hygienic conditions.

2.6 Scabies

Scabies (caused by *Sarcoptes scabiei*) is probably one of the most common parasitic infections, usually spread by bodily contact, though other contaminated objects can also infect. There is severe itching, usually worse at night, with lesions (mostly excoriated burrows) on the fingerwebs, volar wrists, buttocks, Scabies is an infestation caused by human itch mite, Sarcoptes scabiei, which infests some 300 million persons each year and is one of the most common causes of itching dermatoses throughout the world. Gravid female mite measuring 0.3 to 0.4 mm in length burrows superficially beneath the stratum corneum for a month, depositing two or three eggs a day. Nymphs that hatch from these eggs mature in about 2 weeks through a series of molts and then emerge as adults to the surface of the skin, where they mate and subsequently reinvade the skin of the same or another host. Transfer of newly fertilized female mites from person to person occurs by intimate personal contact and is facilitated by crowding, uncleanliness and sexual promiscuity.

The most commonly used to treatment scabies is permethrin 5% cream which applied all over the body. The whole family or sexual partners of infected people should be treated, even if they do not have symptoms. Creams are applied as a one-time treatment or they may be repeated in 1 week. Wash underwear, towels, and sleepwear in hot water. Vacuum the carpets and upholstered furniture. For difficult cases, oral Ivermectin 200-400 µgr/Kg may be used.

Other creams include benzyl benzoate, sulfur in petrolatum, and crotamiton. Lindane is rarely used because of its side effects.

Itching may continue for 2 weeks or more after treatment begins, but it will disappear if the infection is over.

Patients with DS seem predisposed to crusted scabies. Immunological dysfunction has been proposed as one factor for this propensity. However, Norwegian scabies can appear as isolated or epidemic conditions but no cases were recorded in some studies

3. Other dermatological manifestations that would not be associated to immunological alterations

3.1 Anetoderma

Anetoderma is a rare benign dermatosis caused by a loss of mid-dermal elastic tissue resulting in well-circumscribed areas of pouchlike herniations of flaccid skin. It has been hypothesized that a congenital malformation of elastic fibres in this population may be responsible for anetoderma.

Sureshbabu *et al* observed anetoderma in 3.2% of DS. Schepis *et al* reported 3.9% of patients having anetoderma in their study. It has been hypothesized that a congenital malformation of elastic fibers in this population may be responsible for anetoderma secondary to chronic folliculitis. Anetoderma is due to elastolysis probably induced by leukocytes or bacteria during the recurrent inflammatory events

3.2 Milia-like calcinosis cutis

Milia-like idiopathic calcinosis cutis (MICC) is a rare entity. Only few cases have been reported so far. Two-thirds of these have been associated with Down syndrome.

MICC is a micronodular, whitish, acral, calcified lesion. Laboratory tests are usually within normal range (including serum calcium and phosphate, urinary calcium and parathyroid hormone). The term MICC was introduced in the literature by Smith *et al* who described a 6-year-old child affected by DS. Some additional cases of MICC have been reported in children or adolescents affected by DS.

Milia-like idiopathic calcinosis cutis has long been regarded as a peculiar subtype of idiopathic calcinosis cutis. The pathogenesis of the disorder remains unclear. The pathogenesis of MICC in association with DS is unclear. Higher concentrations of calcium in sweat have been found in DS, which may lead to sweat-duct calcification

3.3 Acanthosis nigricans

Acanthosis nigricans (AN) is a skin disorder in which there is darker, thick, velvety skin in body folds and creases. Obesity can lead to AN, as can some endocrine disorders. It is often found in people with obesity-related diabetes Some drugs, particularly hormones such as human growth hormone or oral contraceptives, can also cause AN. Because AN usually only changes the skin's appearance, no treatment is needed. It is important, however, to treat any underlying medical problem that may be causing these skin changes. When AN is related to obesity, losing weight often improves the condition.

AN was seen by Sureshbabu *et al* in 8,4% of DS. The increased incidence of AN in adults is more than in children, but this fact may be attributed to the fact that all these patients were obese with a high BMI (> 30).

3.4 *Elastosis perforans serpiginosa*

Elastosis perforans serpiginosa (EPS) is characterized clinically by papules and keratotic plaques and histologically by focal elastosis of the dermis and transepidermal elimination of abnormal elastic fibers. It is a rare skin disease classified as a primary perforating dermatosis similar to reactive perforating collagenosis. It was given the current denomination of EPS by Dammert and Putkonen.

The incidence of EPS has yet to be established, although looks like higher in DS people. Around 90% of patients develop symptoms of the disease prior to 30 years of age, the majority between 6 and 20 years of age; however, age at onset may range from 5 to 89 years, as reported in the literature. Approximately 75% of those affected are male.

Etiopathogenesis is as yet unclear. It is believed that the focal inflammation in the dermis, which has a biochemical or mechanical origin, may induce the formation of epidermal and follicular channels to expulse abnormal elastic fibers considered irritants.

The disorder can present with papules and erythematous or normochromic, keratotic, asymptomatic or pruriginous plaques grouped in an annular, arciform or serpiginous pattern, surrounded by satellite lesions. They have umbilicated centers from which dermal material is eliminated. The lesions are characteristically symmetrical except in cases associated with DS.

Various forms of treatment have been indicated; however, management of the disease is difficult and there is no standard treatment. There have been reports of therapeutic success using cryotherapy with liquid nitrogen and oral isotretinoin.

3.5 Others

It also has been reported higher prevalence of other skin alterations I DS patients: syringomas, leukaemia cutis, acrocyanosis and cutis marmorata, keratodermatoses… However, none all studies have observed them; for example Sureshbabu *et al* did not see syringoma, milia-like calcinosis cutis, leukemia cutis, elastosis perforans serpiginosa, carotenemia, or vascular instability; they referred that may relate to the fact that their study was not hospital based, unlike other previous studies. Other miscellaneous cutaneous lesions were probably coincidentally seen in the studies, concordant with that seen in the general population.

4. Conclusions

DS is increased frequency of some common dermatoses. Some dermatologic manifestation in DS can been in relation with their immunological alterations. Skin alterations of DS have been observed by few studies. Their management is equal to rest patient, but they can occasionally be more resistant to conventional treatment, for example AA.

AD is one of the most frequent skin diseases associated a DS. However, perhaps this high association observed in first studies could be overestimated. Newer studies, which have used criteria of Hanifin and Rajka to diagnostic AD, does not show so higher incidence of AD in DS. SD can be more extensive than in other patients.

Some immunologic skin diseases, as vitiligo and AA, have been reported with high incidence in DS. Also, fungal infection and scabies has been observed with higher prevalence in DS than rest population. However, scabies in DS could be overestimated in some studies with patients under epidemic conditions.

MICC y EPS are rare skin alterations observed more frequently in DS. AN, frequently associated to overweight, can usually been observed in patients with IMC>30. Other miscellaneous cutaneous lesions were probably coincidentally seen in every study.

5. References

[1] Madan V, Williams J, Lear JT. Dermatological manifestations of Down's syndrome. Clin Exp Dermatol. 2006 ;31:623-9.

[2] Barankin B, Guenther L. Dermatological manifestations of Down's syndrome. J Cutan Med Surg. 2001;5:289-93.

[3] Ercis M, Balci S, Atakan N. Dermatologic manifestations of 71 Down syndrome children admitted to a clinical genetics unit. Clin Genet. 1996;50:317-20

[4] Carter DM, Jegasothy BV. Alopecia areata and Down syndrome. Arch Dermatol. 1976;112:1397-9.

[5] Polenghi MM, Plattoni F, Orsini GB, et al. Dermatologic disorders in Down syndrome. Am J Med Genet 1990; 7:324.

[6] Schepis C, Barone C, Siragusa M et al. An updated survey on skin conditions in Down syndrome. Dermatology 2002;205: 234-8.

[7] Daneshpazhooh M, Nazemi TM, Bigdeloo L, Yoosefi M. Mucocutaneous findings in 100 children with Down syndrome. Pediatr Dermatol. 2007;24:317-20.

[8] Liyanage S, Barnes J. The eye and Down's syndrome. British Br J Hosp Med. 2008;11:632-4.

[9] Aase JM: The physical examination: Hands and feet - Minor variants; in Aase JM (ed): Diagnostic Dysmorphology. New York, Plenum Medical Book Co, 1990, p. 236-237.

[10] Valia RG, Valia AR., IADVL Textbook of dermatology, 2rd ed. Mumbai: Bhalani Publishing House, 2001. p. 121-122

[11] Sureshbabu R, Kumari R, Ranugha S, Sathyamoorthy S, Udayashankar C, Oudeacoumar P.Phenotypic and dermatological manifestations in Down Syndrome. Dermatology Online Journal 2011;17:3

[12] Zeligman I, Scalia SP. Dermatologic manifestations of mongolism. A M A Arch Dermatol Syphil 1954: 69: 342-344.

[13] Pueschel SM. Clinical aspects of Down syndrome from infancy to adulthood. Am J Med Genet 1990; 7 (suppl):52-56.

[14] Howells G. Down's syndrome and the general practitioner. JR Coll Gen Pract 1989; 39: 470-475.

[15] Van Schrojensterin Lantman-de Valk HMJ, Haveman MJ, Crebolder HFJM. Comorbidity in people with Down's syndrome: a criteria-based analysis. J Intellect Disabil Res 1996; 40:385-399.

[16] Hanifin JM, Rajka G. Diagnostic features of atopic dermatitis. Acta Dermatol Venerol 1980;92(Suppl.):44-47.

[17] Scherbenske JM, Benson PM, Rotchford JP. Cutaneous and ocular manifestations of Down syndrome. J Am Acad Dermatol 1990; 22: 933-8.

[18] Schepis C, Barone C, Siragusa M. Prevalence of atopic dermatitis in patients with Down syndrome: a clinical survey. J Am Acad Dermatol 1997; 36: 1019-21.

[19] Hart RW, Setlow RB. Correlation between deoxyribonucleic acid excision-repair and life-span in a number of mammalian species. Proc Natl Acad Sci USA 1974; 71:2169-73.

[20] Butterworth T, Leoni EP, Beerman H, et al. Cheilitis of mongolism. J Invest Dermatol 1960; 35:347-352.

[21] Hatamochi A, Ueki H. Successful treatment of alopecia areata with dinitrochlorobenzene in a patient with Down's syndrome. J Dermatol 1984; 11: 191-3.

[22] Freedberg IM, Eisen AZ, Wolff K, Austen KF, Goldsmith LA, Katz SI, editors. Fitzpatrick's dermatology in general medicine. 6th ed. New York: McGraw-Hill; 2003. p. 1199

[23] Bieber T. 1. Atopic dermatitis. N Engl J Med 2008; 358:1483–1494.

[24] Levy RM, Gelfand JM, Yan AC. The epidemiology of atopic dermatitis. Clin Dermatol 2003; 21: 109–115.

[25] Cookson W. The immunogenetics of asthma and eczema: a new focus on the epithelium. Nat Rev Immunol 2004;4: 978–988.

[26] Taïeb A. Hypothesis: from epidermal barrier dysfunction to atopic disorders. Contact Dermatitis 1999; 41: 177–180.

[27] Halkjaer LB, Loland L, Buchvald FF, Agner T, Skov L,Strand M, et al. Development of atopic dermatitis during the first 3 years of life: the Copenhagen Prospective Study

on asthma in childhood cohort study in high-risk children. Arch Dermatol 2006; 142: 561–566.

[28] Wang CY, Lai CS, Chen GY, Cheng YW, Chen WC. Comparative analysis of the prevalence of atopic dermatitis in elementary schoolchildren in Kaohsiung and Penghu County. Dermatol Sinica 2006; 24: 94–101.

[29] Lee YL, Li CW, Sung FC, Guo YL. Increasing prevalence of atopic eczema in Taiwanese adolescents from 1995 to 2001. Clin Exp Allergy 2007; 37: 543–551.

[30] Lee YL, Li CW, Sung FC, Yu HS, Sheu HM, Guo YL. Environmental factors, parental atopy and atopic eczema in primary-school children: a cross-sectional study in Taiwan. Br J Dermatol 2007; 157: 1217–1224.

[31] Kao CC, Huang JL, Ou LS, See LC. The prevalence, severity and seasonal variations of asthma, rhinitis and eczema in Taiwanese schoolchildren. Pediatr Allergy Immunol 2005; 16: 408–415.

[32] Vichyanond P, Sunthornchart S, Singhirannusorn V, Ruangrat S, Kaewsomboon S, Visitsunthorn N. Prevalence of asthma, allergic rhinitis and eczema among university students in Bangkok. Respir Med 2002; 96: 34–38.

[33] Illi S, von Mutius E, Lau S, Nickel R, Gruber C, Niggemann B, et al. The natural course of atopic dermatitis from birth to age 7 years and the association with asthma. J Allergy Clin Immunol 2004; 113: 925–931.

[34] Bousquet J, Van Cauwenberge P, Khaltaev N. Allergic rhinitis and its impact on asthma. J Allergy Clin Immunol 2001; 108: S147–334.

[35] Arruda LK, Sole D, Baena-Cagnani CE, Naspitz CK. Risk factors for asthma and atopy. Curr Opin Allergy Clin Immunol 2005; 5: 153–159.

[36] Gupta AK, Bluhm R, Cooper EA, Summerbell RC, Batra R. Seborrheic dermatitis. Dermatol Clin. 2003;21:401-12.

[37] Schwartz RA, Janusz CA, Janniger CK. Seborrheic dermatitis: an overview. Am Fam Physician. 2006;74:125-30.

[38] Picardi A, Abeni D. Stressful life events and skin diseases: disentangling evidence from myth. Psychother Psychosom.2001;70:118-36.

[39] Gupta AK, Nicol KA. Seborrheic dermatitis of the scalp: etiology and treatment. J Drugs Dermatol. 2004;3:155-8.

[40] Mastrolonardo M, Diaferio A, Logroscino G. Seborrheic dermatitis, increased sebum excretion, and Parkinson's disease: a survey of (im)possible links. Med Hypotheses. 2003;60: 907-11.

[41] Jones-Caballero M, Penas PF, García-Díez A, Badía X, Chren MM. The Spanish version of Skindex-29. Int J Dermatol. 2000;39:907-12.

[42] Gupta AK, Bluhm R. Seborrheic dermatitis. JEADV. 2004;18:13-26.

[43] Alkhalifah A, Alsantali A, Wang E, McElwee KJ, Shapiro J.Alopecia areata update: part II. Treatment. J Am Acad Dermatol. 2010:62:191-202.

[44] Harries MJ, Sun J, Paus R, King LE Jr. Management of alopecia areata. BMJ. 2010; 23-41.

[45] Friedli A, Harms M. Alopecia areata. Ther Umsch. 2002;59:233-7.

[46] Alkhateeb A, Fain PR, Thody A, Bennett DC, et al. Epidemiology of vitiligo and associated autoimmune diseases in Caucasian probands and their families. Pigment cell res. 2003;16(3):208–214.

[47] Delamere FM, Sladden MM, Dobbins HM, Leonardi-Bee J. Interventions for alopecia areata. Cochrane Database Syst Rev. 2008 Apr 16;(2):CD004413.
[48] Garg S, Messenger AG. Alopecia areata: evidence-based treatments. Semin Cutan Med Surg. 2009;28:15-8.
[49] Gauthier Y, Cario Andre M, Taïeb A. A critical appraisal of vitiligo etiologic theories. Is melanocyte loss a melanocytorrhagy? Pigment Cell Res. 2003;16(4):322–332.
[50] Esfandiarpour I, Ekhlasi A, Farajzadeh S, Shamsadini S. The efficacy of pimecrolimus 1% cream plus narrow-band ultraviolet B in the treatment of vitiligo: A double-blind, placebo-controlled clinical trial. J Dermatolog Treat. In press 2008.
[51] 35. El Mofty M, Mostafa W, Esmat S. Narrow band Ultraviolet B 311 nm in the treatment of vitiligo: two right-left comparison studies. Photodermatol Photoimmunol Photomed. 2006;22(1):6–11.
[52] Yones SS, Palmer RA, Garibaldinos TM, Hawk JL. Randomized double-blind trial of treatment of vitiligo: effi cacy of psoralen-UV-A therapy vs Narrowband-UV-B therapy. Arch Dermatol. 2007;143(5): 578–584.
[53] Arca E, Tastan HB, Erbil AH, Sezer E, Koc E, Kurumlu Z. Narrow-band ultraviolet B as monotherapy and in combination with topical calcipotriol in the treatment of vitiligo. J Dermatol. 2006;33(5):338–343.
[54] Passeron T, Ortonne JP. Use of the 308-nm excimer laser for psoriasis and vitiligo. Clin Dermatol. 2006;24(1):33–42
[55] Hadi S, Tinio P, Al-Ghaithi K, et al. Treatment of vitiligo using the 308-nm excimer laser. Photomed Laser Surg. 2006;24(3):354–357.
[56] Passeron T, Ostovari N, Zakaria W. Topical tacrolimus and the 308-nm excimer laser: a synergistic combination for the treatment of vitiligo. Arch Dermatol. 2004;140(9):1065–1069.
[57] Goldinger SM, Dummer R, Schmid P, et al. Combination of 308-nm xenon chloride excimer laser and topical calcipotriol in vitiligo. J Eur Acad Dermatol Venereol. 2007;21(4):504–508.
[58] Schepis C, Siragusa M. Secondary anetoderma in people with Down's syndrome. Acta Derm Venereol 1999;79:245.
[59] Gupta AK. Types of onychomycosis. Cutis. 2001 Aug;68:4-7.
[60] Derby R, Rohal P, Jackson C, Beutler A, Olsen C. Novel treatment of onychomycosis using over-the-counter mentholated ointment: a clinical case series. J Am Board Fam Med. 2011;24:69-74.
[61] Krob AH, Fleischer AB Jr, D'Agostino R Jr, Feldman SR.Terbinafine is more effective than itraconazole in treating toenail onychomycosis: results from a meta-analysis of randomized controlled trials. J Cutan Med Surg. 2003;7:306-11.
[62] Trivedi NA, Shah PC. A meta-analysis comparing efficacy of continous terbinafine with intermittent itraconazole for yoenal onychomycosis. Indian J Dermatol. 2010; 55: 198–199.
[63] Gilmore SJ. Control strategies for endemic childhood scabies. PLoS One. 2011;6:e15990.
[64] Schepis C, Siragusa M, Alberti A. Guess what! Milia-like idiopathic calcinosis cutis. Eur J Dermatol. 2000;10:637-8.

[65] Pereira AC, Baeta IG, Costa Júnior SR, Gontijo Júnior OM, Vale EC. Elastosis perforans serpiginosa in a patient with Down's syndrome. An Bras Dermatol. 2010;85:691-4.

11

Down Syndrome and Periodontal Disease

Ahmed Khocht
Temple University, School of Dentistry
United States

1. Introduction

Periodontal diseases are inflammatory diseases of the supporting structures of the teeth (Cochran, 2008; Kornman, 2008). They are initiated by periodontopathic bacteria and result in progressive destruction and loss of the periodontium (Cochran, 2008; Kornman, 2008). Progression of periodontal disease eventually leads to tooth loss (Chambrone, et al., 2010). Periodontal diseases are multifactorial with complex pathogenesis (Cochran, 2008; Kornman, 2008).

Plaque bacteria trigger a host inflammatory response in the gingival tissues (Kornman, 2008). Neutrophils migrate from within the gingival tissues towards the gingival crevice and build a barrier wall against the bacteria (Kornman, 2008). Within the gingival connective tissue, the gingival macrophages and fibroblasts produce inflammatory cytokines (e.g. interleukin-1 and tumor necrosis factor- alpha) that activate collagenases and other degrading enzymes (Kornman, 2008). These enzymes when released and activated destroy the gingival collagen. Lymphocytes are recruited to the gingival lesion to initiate an adaptive immune response and help with containing the infection (Kornman, 2008). With persistence of the microbial infection, the inflammatory changes in the gingival tissues expand apically and reach the alveolar bone (Cochran, 2008). Inflammatory mediators such as interleukin-1, interleukin-6, tumor necrosis factor alpha and prostaglandins induce osteoclasogenesis (Cochran, 2008). Increased inflammatory activity disrupts the normal balance of bone formation/resorption and results in alveolar bone loss (Cochran, 2008).

Periodontal disease is a serious and morbid oral condition among Down-syndrome (DS) affected individuals (Morgan, 2007). Gingivitis and periodontitis start early in life and their severity increases with age (Reuland-Bosma, et al., 1988). Periodontal disease advances rapidly in DS individuals and is characterized by severe gingival inflammation, loss of periodontal attachment and radiographic alveolar bone loss (Agholme, et al., 1999; Saxen, et al., 1977). Heavy amounts of plaque and calculus are often present (Morgan, 2007). Periodontal disease is an important cause of tooth loss among DS individuals (Reuland-Bosma, et al., 2001).

The exact reason (or reasons) for this increased susceptibility to periodontitis is (are) not known. Understanding the pathogenesis of periodontitis in DS individuals would greatly help with the management and control of the destructive process associated with the disease and help DS affected individuals retain their teeth hopefully throughout their lifetime.

Previously researchers have investigated factors usually associated with periodontitis such as subgingival plaque microbial composition, immune and inflammatory responses *individually* in DS affected individuals. The individual factors investigated were never collectively evaluated together to provide an overall understanding of the pathogenesis of periodontitis in individuals with DS. The objective of this chapter is to review in a systematic fashion all the involved factors previously reported *together* to generate a hypothetical collective model of the pathogenesis of periodontal disease in individuals with DS. Such a model would enhance our understanding of periodontal disease development/progression in this vulnerable group, would help with disease management, would identify gaps in knowledge, and would provide enlightenment for future research endeavors.

In this review I have searched the available dental/medical literature for studies investigating the main factors suspected in the increased susceptibility to periodontitis in DS individuals. I have summarized the main findings from these studies and used this information to generate a hypothetical model of the pathogenesis of periodontitis in DS individuals.

2. Methods

The methodology applied in this review covers the literature search strategy, inclusion and exclusion criteria for choosing articles, screening of articles and quality assessment of the selected articles.

2.1 Search strategy

Electronic searching was performed using the following databases: MEDLINE (1948-2011) and PubMed. The search terms that were used related to the subject groups of interest: Down syndrome and mental retardation; the oral condition: gingivitis, periodontitis, periodontal disease, gingiva, periodontium, tooth loss; etiological factors: microbiological (dental plaque, subgingival plaque, periodontopathic bacteria), immune factors (neutrophils, lymphocytes, antibody production) and inflammatory factors (cytokines, prostaglandins, metalloproteinases) and the type of study: comparative study, randomized controlled trial, or review. The search was limited to English language literature. The electronic search was supplemented by checking bibliographies of review papers. One hundred forty five articles were initially identified.

2.2 Inclusion criteria

Studies were included if they met the following minimum criteria:

1. Human subjects with Down syndrome.
2. Clinical measures of periodontal status.
3. Microbiological, immune or inflammatory measures.
4. Comparison of DS subjects to a control/comparison group(s).
5. Written in English.

2.3 Exclusion criteria

Editorial letters, historical reviews and descriptive studies such as case reports were excluded. In addition, studies that did not specifically address the main focus of the search or duplicated other studies were also excluded.

2.4 Screening and selection of papers

At first the articles were screened by title and abstract. A review of abstracts based on the criteria above led to initial consideration of 32 articles. Then full text was retrieved either electronically or in printed format. Further review of full texts resulted in inclusion of 20 articles.

2.5 Quality assessment

Systematic reviews need to assess the methodological *quality* of the included studies (Pai, et al., 2004). Quality within the context of this chapter refers to the minimization of bias. An objective of this assessment was to judge the strength of the scientific evidence with higher score given to studies free of bias. To minimize bias, the comparison group needs to be matched as close as possible to the DS group. In addition, the evaluated parameters should be assessed in the same manner between the groups. Studies with an adequately matched control group were scored higher than studies that used population data or previously collected data for comparison.

The instrument used for judging articles for this chapter was based freely on the use of STROBE methodology (von Elm, et al., 2007) evaluating the following parameters:

- Down syndrome diagnosis: clearly stated and explained.
- Inclusion of a comparison group: well matched (age, gender, race) or not.
- Periodontal parameters: how periodontitis was defined and measured. Adequate if clinical attachment level was reported. Inadequate when only periodontal probing depth or radiographic measurements are reported.
- Laboratory methodology to assess microbial, immune or inflammatory factors: was the methodology clearly explained. Was the methodology appropriate or not.
- Examiner calibration: adequate if reported, inadequate if not reported.
- Descriptive information: characteristics of study participants (number of subjects, gender, mean and range of age) were clearly presented.
- Confounders identified: confounders that may affect periodontal status such as age, gender, and plaque levels were clearly defined.
- Data analysis: adequate when multivariate analysis adjusting for confounders was presented. Inadequate if only bivariate analysis was presented.

The studies included in the review were scored as follows:

- Score 1: when all the parameters presented above were reported in the study.
- Score 2: when only DS diagnosis, inclusion of a comparison group, clinical periodontal measures and laboratory measures were reported.
- Score 3: other than score 1 and 2.

3. Results

A total of 20 articles were selected, 5 articles related to microbiological evaluations, 3 articles related to neutrophil function, 3 articles related to gingival cellular immunity, 4 articles related to antibody production and 5 articles related to degrading enzymes and inflammatory mediators. All selected articles met the minimum inclusion criteria previously described. Two articles were scored as 1, fifteen articles were scored as 2 and three articles were scored as 3.

Nineteen out of the twenty selected studies were designed as cross-sectional case-controlled studies. Thus in addition to the DS group, they included a matched comparison group of either medically healthy and periodontally healthy individuals or a comparison group with mental disability other than DS. One study was longitudinal (Zaldivar-Chiapa, et al., 2005).

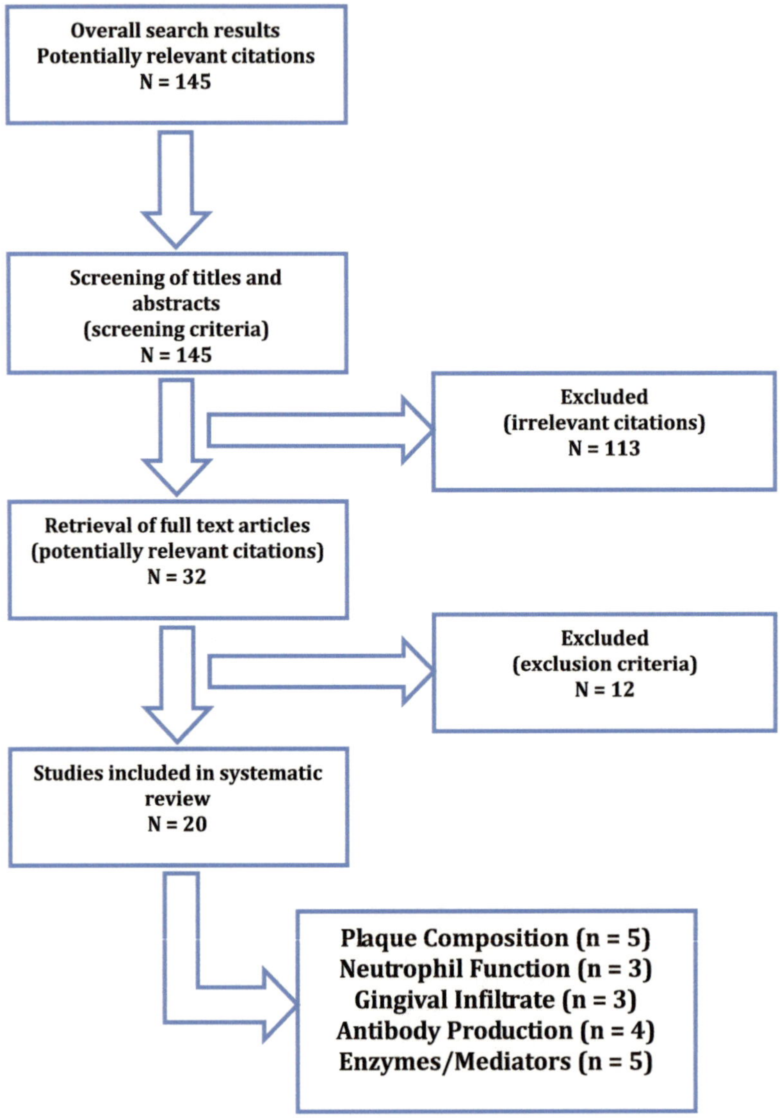

Fig. 1. Summary of search strategy.

Down subjects in most of the studies were either children or young adults. Few of the selected studies included DS adults (Amano, et al., 2001; Chaushu, et al., 2007; Komatsu, et al., 2001; Sakellari, et al., 2005; Sohoel, et al., 1995).

3.1 Summary of study methodologies

Microbiology studies employed a variety of techniques including culturing, polymerase chain reaction and checkerboard DND-DNA hybridization techniques to investigate the composition of subgingival plaque. All the studies attempted to compare the subgingival plaque composition of DS individuals to a matched comparison group. In addition some studies attempted to determine at what age important periodontopathic bacteria become detectable in DS individuals. A few studies attempted to investigate the association between presence of periodontopathic bacteria and clinical periodontal parameters in DS individuals. Neutrophil function studies mainly focused on neutrophil chemotaxis. Neutrophil chemotaxis was measured by the Boyden chamber method. All selected studies compared neutrophil chemotaxis of DS individuals to a matched comparison group. One of the studies investigated the relation between neutrophil chemotaxis measures with clinical and radiographic periodontal measures.

Gingival cellular immunity studies examined the immune cellular composition, expression of HLA Class II antigens on the surfaces of immune cells and gamma/delta T-cell receptor-bearing lymphocytes in discarded gingival tissues from DS individuals. Indirect immunofluorescent techniques were used to examine the gingival tissues. All the selected studies compared the gingival tissue cellular findings in DS individuals to medically and periodontally healthy individuals.

The selected antibody production studies focused on specific antibodies against some important periodontopathic bacteria. The studies examined either serum antibody titers or salivary antibody levels. All selected studies used an enzyme-linked immunosorbent assay (ELISA). Four of the selected studies compared the antibody serum titer or saliva levels in DS individuals to matched controls. One study made the comparison to a normal adult reference serum pool.

The selected studies investigating degrading enzymes and inflammatory mediators mainly focused on matrix metalloproteinases (MMP) activity in gingival fluid. One study examined cultured fibroblast MMP activity. Two studies examined prostaglandin E2 (PGE2) and one study examined interleukin-1 (IL-1) in gingival fluid. All selected studies compared their findings in DS individuals with non-DS controls. MMP activity was assessed with a variety of techniques including gel electrophoresis, Western blot analysis and ELISA. PGE2 was assessed with a radio-immuno-assay and IL-1 with ELISA.

3.2 Summary of study findings

A summary of all selected articles and their main findings is presented in the following tables:

3.2.1 Subgingival plaque composition studies

Author	Scr.	DS	CG	Measures	Findings
Barr-Agholme 1992	2	37	37	Levels of *Aggregatibacter (Actinobacillus) actinomycetemcomitans*, *Capnocytophaga* and *Porphyromonas gingivalis* were determined in subgingival plaque samples.	*A. actinomycetemcomitans* was detected in the subgingival plaque in 35% of the DS adolescents and in 5% of the controls. On site level, *A. actinomycetemcomitans* and *Capnocytophaga* were more frequent in the subgingival plaque samples of DS children than in those of controls.

Author	Scr.	DS	CG	Measures	Findings
Amano 2000	2	60 Yng.	60	Ten periodontal pathogens were surveyed in subgingival plaque samples using a polymerase chain reaction.	All of the pathogens were detected with greater frequency in the DS children. *Tannerella forsythia* (*Bacteroides forsythus*), *Treponema denticola, Prevotella nigrescens,* and *Campylobacter rectus* were significantly prevalent throughout all age brackets of the DS children. The occurrence of *Porphyromonas gingivalis* was also significant in the DS subjects over 5 years old.
Amano 2001	2	67 Adt.	41	Ten periodontal pathogens were surveyed in subgingival plaque samples using a polymerase chain reaction.	No significant differences were observed in the bacterial profiles between the two groups.
Sakellari 2005	1	70	121 NC 76 MR	Clinical parameters and microbiological analysis by "checkerboard" DNA-DNA hybridization.	Important periodontal pathogens including *Porphyromonas gingivalis, Tannerella forsythia* (*Bacteroides forsythus*) and *A. actinomycetemcomitans* colonize these subjects earlier and at higher levels.
Reuland-Bosma 2001	2	17	17	Prevalence and proportions of the putative periodontal pathogens *A. actinomycetemcomitans, Porphyromonas gingivalis, Prevotella intermedia, Tannerella forsythia (Bacteroides forsythus), Peptostreptococcus micros, Fusobacterium nucleatum* and *Campylobacter rectus* in the subgingival plaque were determined using anaerobic culture techniques.	No differences in the prevalence of distinct suspected periodontopathic bacteria and bacterial subgingival composition between the DS group and the comparison group could be established.

Scr = score, DS = number of DS group, CG = number of comparison group, Yng = young, Adt = adult, NC = normal controls, MR = mental retardation not Down.

Table 1. Summarizes the findings of the subgingival plaque composition studies.

3.2.2 Neutrophil function studies

Author	Scr.	DS	CG	Measures	Findings
Izumi 1989	2	14	14	Periodontal clinical measures, radiographic measures and neutrophil chemotaxis.	DS patients showed significantly lower chemotaxis than healthy volunteers. Bone loss in DS subjects was inversely proportional to the chemotactic index.
Yavuzyilm-az 1993	2	15	15	Clinical periodontal parameters, chemotaxis and random migration of neutrophils.	The random migration and chemotaxis of neutrophils from DS subjects were significantly decreased in comparison with the control group.
Zaldivar-Chiapa 2005 Longitudinal	2	14	9	Clinical parameters and neutrophil function.	Neutrophil chemotaxis, phagocytic activity, and production of super-oxide anion were significantly decreased in the DS patients.

Scr = score, DS = number of DS group, CG = number of comparison group.

Table 2. Summarizes the neutrophil function studies.

3.2.3 Gingival immune response studies

Author	Scr.	DS	CG	Measures	Findings
Sohoel 1992	3	16	12	Indirect immune-fluorescence used to study immune cellular composition of gingival tissues from DS individuals.	Denser inflammatory infiltrate in DS individuals. Counting showed different cell distribution and cell profiles between DS subjects and non-DS subjects.
Sohoel 1995	3	16	14	Expression of HLA Class II antigens on the surfaces of immune cells.	Increased frequency of HLA Class II (HLA-expression on inflammatory cells and on keratinocytes of the oral gingival epithelium) in chronic periodontitis of DS patients compared to sections from non-DS subjects.
Sohoel 1995	3	NR	NR	Assessment of Gamma/delta T-cell receptor-bearing lymphocytes in gingival tissues.	Gamma/delta T-cell receptor-bearing lymphocytes are decreased in inflamed gingival tissues of DS individuals.

Scr = score, DS = number of DS group, CG = number of comparison group, NR = not reported.

Table 3. Summarizes the gingival immune cellular response studies.

3.2.4 Antibody production studies

Author	Scr.	DS	CG	Measures	Findings
Santos 1996	2	16	10	Circulating antibody titers to *A. actinomycetemcomitans*.	Significant differences were noted between the control group and the DS subjects (p = 0.05), with the DS periodontitis group having the highest response, followed by the DS gingivitis group and normal controls, respectively. The DS groups were not significantly different.
Morinushi 1997	3	75	RSP	Antibody titers to *Porphyromonas gingivalis (Pg), Prevotella intermedia (Pi), Treponema denticola (Td), Fusobacterium nucleatum (Fn), Selenomonas sputigena (Sel), A. actinomycetemcomitans (Aa)*, and *Streptococcus mitis (Mi)*.	IgG antibody titers to *Pg, Aa, Sel*, and *Mi* increased significantly with increasing gingival inflammtion score. Furthermore, the IgG antibody titers to *Pg* were higher ($P < 0.05$) in the most extensive disease group compared to the DS no-disease group. The IgG antibody titers to *Pg* at early puberty were significantly higher when compared to preschool children.
Barr-Agholme 1998	2	20	19	Salivary levels of immunoglobulins sIgA, IgM, and IgG subclass distribution and albumin, quantified by enzyme-linked immunosorbent assay.	The immunoglobulin levels of sIgA, IgM, the sum of IgG subclasses, and the concentration of albumin did not differ significantly between the 2 groups. However, the proportion of IgG1 expressed as percentage of the sum of total IgG was significantly higher ($P < 0.01$) in the Down syndrome group compared to controls. On the contrary, the proportion of IgG2, IgG3, and IgG4 subclasses in saliva did not differ between the 2 groups.
Chaushu 2007	2	40	39	The levels of total IgA, and specific antibodies to three common oral pathogens (*Porphyromonas gingivalis, Actinobacillus (Aggregatibacter) actinomycetemcomitans* and *Streptococcus mutans*) were analyzed.	The median secretion rates of the specific antibodies in whole and parotid saliva were 70-77% and 34-60% (respectively) lower in young DS individuals as compared to young controls and farther 77-100% and 75-88% (respectively) lower in old DS compared to young DS.

Scr = score, DS = number of DS group, CG = number of comparison group, RSP = reference serum pool.

Table 4. Summarizes the antibody production studies.

3.2.5 Inflammatory mediator studies

Author	Scr.	DS	CG	Measures	Findings
Halinen 1996	2	9	9	Clinical periodontal measures and matrix metalloproteinase (MMP-8 and -9) activities in saliva and in gingival crevicular fluid.	The endogenously active collagenase and total collagenase activities were slightly higher in GCF of DS children compared to healthy controls. GCF collagenase of DS patients was human neutrophil collagenase (MMP-8 or collagenase-2), in DS patients, but not in controls. Salivary collagenase in DS was high when compared to controls but of the same MMP-8 type as in control saliva.
Barr-Agholme 1997	2	15	15	Levels of prostaglandin E2 (PGE2) and interleukin-1 beta (IL-1 beta) were determined in gingival crevicular fluid.	The mean level of PGE2 in GCF was significantly higher ($P < 0.05$) in the Down syndrome group than in the control group. In GCF samples collected from sites characterized as non-inflamed, the mean level of PGE2 was significantly higher ($P < 0.001$) in the Down syndrome group than in the controls. The mean level of PGE2 in samples from inflamed sites, on the other hand, did not differ between the two groups. The mean level of IL-1 beta was not significantly higher in the Down syndrome group than in the controls.
Komatsu 2001	2	9	9	Enzyme activity and the mRNA expression pattern of matrix metalloproteinases (MMPs) of cultured gingival fibroblasts (GF) and fresh gingival tissues.	The production of the active type of MMP-2 in GF from Down's syndrome patients (D-GF) was found to be significantly higher ($P < 0.05$) than that of the control GF (C-GF) at the protein level.
Tsilingaridis 2003	2	18	14	Levels of prostaglandin E2 (PGE2), leukotriene B4 (LTB4), and matrix metalloproteinase-9 (MMP-9) in gingival crevicular fluid.	The mean levels of PGE2, LTB4, and MMP-9 were significantly ($P<0.05$) higher in GCF from Down syndrome patients compared to controls.
Yamazaki-Kubota 2010	1	14	14	Matrix metalloproteinase (MMP-8 and MMP-2) activity in gingival crevicular fluid.	Levels of MMP-2 and MMP-8 in Down's syndrome patients were higher than those in healthy control subjects.

Scr = score, DS = number of DS group, CG = number of comparison group.

Table 5. Summarizes the inflammatory mediator studies.

4. Discussion

Periodontal disease is a common problem among DS individuals with an estimated prevalence between 58% and 96% for those under 35 years of age (Morgan, 2007). The disease starts early in life and progresses with age eventually leading to tooth loss (Reuland-Bosma, et al., 2001; Saxen, et al., 1977; Saxen & Aula, 1982). Periodontal disease in DS individuals adversely impacts on the quality of their life (Amaral Loureiro, et al., 2007). The increased prevalence and severity of periodontal disease in DS individuals inspired many researchers to investigate the various factors that might be involved.

Periodontal diseases are initiated by bacterial plaque build-up in the dentogingival region (Kornman, 2008). It is well documented that DS individuals have difficulty with maintaining adequate oral hygiene levels and thus tend to harbor high levels of bacterial plaque on their teeth (Cohen, et al., 1961; Khocht, et al., 2010; Sakellari, et al., 2005). In addition, DS individuals following oral hygiene instructions have reduced ability to master adequate plaque control (Sakellari, et al., 2001). It was often surmised that mental disability associated with DS is an important factor in their reduced ability to maintain adequate oral hygiene and consequently increases their susceptibility to periodontitis (Desai, 1997; Morgan, 2007). Our group (Khocht, et al., 2010) recently showed in a multivariate model including traditional risk factors for periodontitis combined with mental disability that loss of periodontal attachment in DS individuals was not associated with mental disability. Thus other factors associated with DS might be involved.

It is well documented that DS is associated with immune deficiencies and host response impairment (Kusters, et al., 2009; Reuland-Bosma, et al., 1988). Infections, in particular respiratory infections are an important cause of death in DS individuals (Thase, 1982). The most likely reason for this increased susceptibility to infection and reduced immunity in DS individuals is an increased dosage of a protein product or products encoded by chromosome 21. Several proteins important in immune function are encoded on chromosome 21. Examples include superoxide dismutase (SOD), carbonyl reductase (NADPH) (Lemieux, et al., 1993) and integrin beta-2 (CD18). Increased SOD and NADPH production is associated with increased oxidative stress and tissue injury in DS individuals (Akinci, et al., 2010; Strydom, et al., 2009). Aberrant expression of CD18 integrin on immune cell surfaces in DS individuals may be associated with altered lymphocyte function (Kusters, et al., 2009; Taylor, 1987). The IL10RB component of the IL-10 receptor (involved with resolution of inflammation) is encoded by chromosome 21 and its function may be altered in DS individuals (Glocker, et al., 2009). In addition, it seems that interleukin-1 (IL-1) is upregulated indirectly by some chromosome 21 based genes (Mrak & Griffin, 2004). IL-1 is an important immune/inflammatory mediator. Its increased production in DS individuals was associated with brain tissue damage (Mrak & Griffin, 2004).

Since periodontitis is initiated by bacterial infections, indeed it is conceivable that altered immunity in DS individuals may be the primary reason for their increased susceptibility to periodontal infections. Perhaps reduced immunity in DS individuals would make it easier for virulent periodontopathic microbial species to colonize their subgingival plaque. If true, such elevated microbial presence, unchallenged and unchecked, would induce an intense inflammatory reaction within the gingival tissues. Increased gingival inflammation within the gingival tissues would lead to elevated production of degrading enzymes and alter bone remodeling. The end result of these inflammatory induced changes would be the loss and destruction of the periodontium and eventually tooth loss. Several studies (microbiological, immune and inflammatory) attempted to investigate these hypotheses.

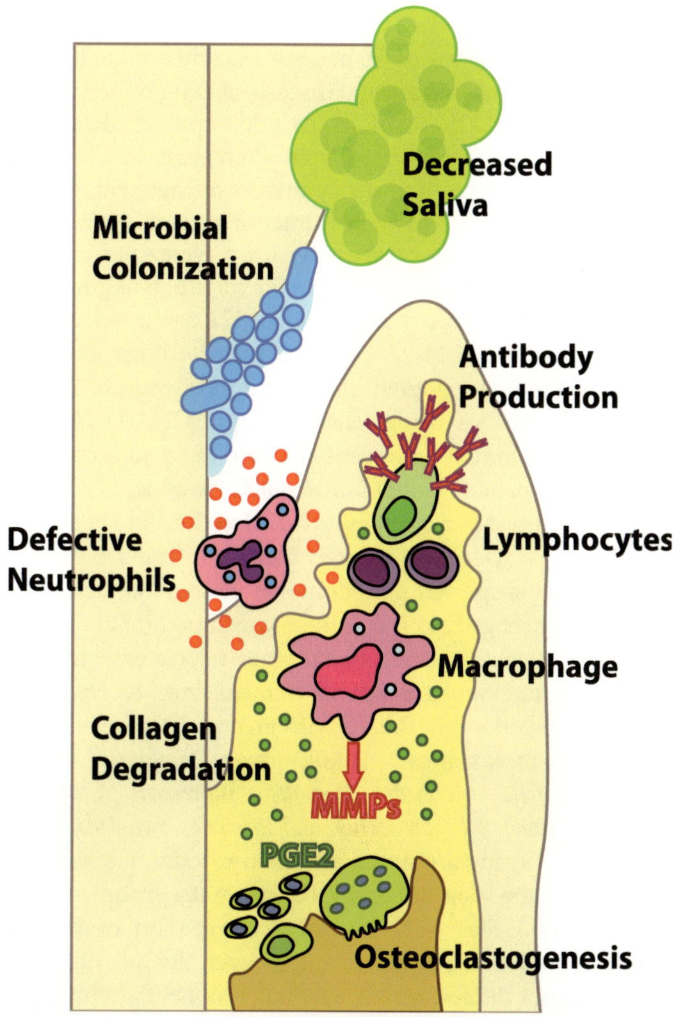

Fig. 2. The above schematic illustrates the main findings of the selected articles. Decreased salivary flow and associated decreased salivary antibody production. Neutrophils with defective chemotaxis incapable of reaching the target pathogens. Early colonization of the dentogingival region with periodntopathic bacteria. Gingival marginal tissues heavily infiltrated with immune cells such as macrophages and lymphocytes. Antigen presenting cells active in processing and presenting microbial antigens. Robust humoral antibody production. Macrophages and other gingival cells engaged in producing degrading enzymes (MMPs). Collagen degradation. Tissue injury and release of prostaglandins (PGE2). Increased osteoclastic activity and alveolar bone loss.

4.1 Microbiological studies

Barr-Agholme et al. (1992) reported increased presence of *Aggregatibacter* (*Actinobacillus*) *actinomycetemcomitans, Capnocytophaga and Porphyromonas gingivalis* in subgingival plaque of *adolescents* with DS. *A. Actinomycetemcomitans* was detected in 35% of patients with DS compared to 5% in the healthy, age and sex matched controls. The authors suggested that this increased frequency of *A. actinomycetemcomitans* indicated an altered microbial composition in the subgingival plaque of DS patients as compared to healthy controls.

Amano et al. (2000) found various periodontal disease-causing bacteria present in *very young* DS patients. The authors reported that various periodontopathic bacteria could colonize the teeth in the very early childhood of DS patients. Pathogens in DS patient's subgingival plaque were detected with far greater frequency than in the age-matched controls. This may be the reason why these DS patients have such intense gingival inflammation. The authors concluded that periodontopathic pathogens establish a presence at a very early age, and that certain bacteria, like *P. gingivalis*, play a key role in the initiation of gingival inflammation.

Sakellari et al. (2005) evaluated seventy DS patients, 121 age-matched healthy individuals and 76 patients with cerebral palsy. Full-mouth recordings of clinical periodontal parameters were assessed and subgingival plaque samples were taken from the Ramfjord teeth and analysed for 14 species using "checkerboard" DNA-DNA hybridization. They reported that important periodontal pathogens colonize these subjects earlier and at higher levels compared with age-matched healthy individuals and patients with cerebral palsy.

Reuland-Bosma et al. (2001) compared subgingival microflora in DS adult patients to other mentally retarded individuals. Despite advanced periodontitis in DS patients, no differences in the prevalence of distinct suspected periodontopathic bacteria were established between the DS patients and the control group. The authors concluded that host factors are the most likely explanation for the advanced periodontal disease associated with DS patients.

Amano et al. (2001) took subgingival plaque specimens from 67 DS young adults and 41 age-matched systemically healthy individuals with mental disabilities (MD). The prevalence of *Actinobacillus actinomycetemcomitans, Porphyromonas gingivalis, Bacteroides forsythus, Treponema denticola, Prevotella intermedia, Prevotella nigrescens, Capnocytophaga ochracea, Capnocytophaga sputigena, Campylobacter rectus, and Eikenella corrodens,* were investigated in subgingival plaque samples using a polymerase chain reaction method. The authors found no significant differences in the bacterial profiles between the groups.

The cited microbiological studies indicate early colonization of important periodontal pathogens in children and adolescents with DS. However, the microbial subgingival profile of *adult* DS individuals is not different from matched non-DS individuals. Perhaps reduced immunity in young DS individuals facilitates early colonization in comparison to young non-DS individuals with normal immunity. With age, and a combination of long-term exposure to pathogens and changes in immune response, non-DS individuals may also be susceptible to colonization by periodontal pathogens. However, despite lack of differences in microbial profiles between adult DS and non-DS individuals, adult DS individuals still show greater loss of periodontal attachment (Amano, et al., 2001; Reuland-Bosma, et al., 2001). This suggests that the host response to the same bacteria is different between DS and non-DS individuals. It seems that the immune-inflammatory response in DS is more intense resulting in greater tissue damage. The following studies will investigate this claim.

4.2 Immune dysfunction studies

As we said earlier, DS is associated with immune dysfunction (Kusters, et al., 2009). Various studies investigated different components of the immune system in relation to periodontitis in DS patients. These studies mainly focused on neutrophil function, the gingival immune cellular response and antibody production against periodontopathic bacteria.

4.2.1 Neutrophil function studies

Izumi et al. (1989) found a faulty neutrophil chemotaxis in DS patients. The authors reported that DS patients had significantly lower chemotaxis compared to healthy controls. Since the neutrophils are the main cells involved in the first line of host defense in a bacterial invasion, having a defective neutrophil chemotaxis can lead to the progression of periodontitis. Significant correlations were identified between the amount of bone loss and the age and chemotactic index of the DS patients. The authors found that the rate of periodontal destruction was dependent on the degree of defective chemotaxis.

Yavuzyilmaz et al. (1993) evaluated clinical parameters, chemotaxis and random migration of neutrophils in 15 patients with DS and 15 healthy subjects. Signs of more severe gingival inflammation were present in the DS group. The random migration and chemotaxis of neutrophils were significantly decreased in comparison with the control group.

Zaldivar-Chiapa (2005) examined patients with DS to evaluate the effectiveness of surgical and non-surgical periodontal therapies and to assess their neutrophil immunological status. The population consisted of 14 DS patients, 14 to 30 years old. Surgical and non-surgical periodontal therapies were compared in a split-mouth design. Clinical periodontal parameters were recorded at baseline, post-treatment, 6 months, and 1 year. Neutrophil chemotaxis, phagocytic activity, and production of super-oxide anion were compared between DS patients and healthy controls. Both surgical and non-surgical therapies showed a significant improvement in all the clinical parameters compared to baseline. Neutrophil chemotaxis, phagocytic activity, and production of super-oxide anion were significantly decreased in the DS patients. The authors concluded that the neutrophil impairment does not seem to affect the clinical response to therapy.

All the presented studies showed deficient neutrophil chemotaxis in DS subjects. The reason for impaired neutrophil chemotaxis in DS individuals may be secondary to increased oxidative stress associated with trisomy of chromosome 21 (Akinci, et al., 2010). Oxidative stress may impair internal cell function and disrupt chemotaxis. One study positively correlated such reduced chemotaxis with measures of periodontitis (Izumi, et al., 1989). Another study gave hope that despite reduced neutrophil chemotaxis, periodontal therapy aiming at reducing plaque and correcting periodontal architecture is still helpful (Zaldivar-Chiapa, et al., 2005).

4.2.2 Gingival Immune cellular response

Sohoel et al. (1992) examined the composition of mononuclear cells in the gingival inflammatory infiltrate in DS patients with marginal periodontitis. The authors reported that DS patients had a higher number of cells in the cellular infiltrate of chronic marginal periodontitis (CMP) compared to normal patients. There were also an increased number of CD22+ cells (B lymphocytes), CD3+ cells, CD4+ cells, CD8+ cells, and CD11+ cells (macrophages). There was also a significantly higher CD4+/CD8+ ratio in DS patients when compared to the normal controls, which could indicate active tissue destruction. This study concluded that DS patients have a more pronounced and altered gingival cellular immune response when compare to controls.

Sohoel et al. (1995) investigated the expression of HLA class II antigens in chronic marginal periodontitis (CMP) in patients with DS. Variations in the expression of HLA class II antigens on antigen-presenting cells play an important role in immune regulation. The results of this study indicated an increased frequency of HLA class II antigens in the gingival tissues of CMP DS patients when compared to controls. There were significantly higher numbers of CD1a+ cells and ratios of HLA-DR+/CD1a+ cells and HLA-DP+/CD1a+ cells in the DS group compared to the control group. The authors concluded that there is a highly activated immune response in DS patients.

The same investigators (Sohoel, et al., 1995) also investigated gamma/delta T lymphocytes in gingival tissues of DS individuals. The T-cell receptor (TCR) of gamma/delta T lymphocytes is different from the alpha/beta TCR. The gamma/delta TCR binds to antigens that are intact proteins and antigens that are not presented within class I or class II histocompatibility molecules. The gamma/delta T lymphocytes usually reside within epithelial tissues and encounter antigens on the surface of epithelial cells. The researchers reported that the percentage of gamma/delta T lymphocytes in the gingival tissues of DS subjects was less than 1%.

The presented studies showed an intense presence of a variety of immune cells within the gingival tissues of DS patients with periodontitis. Increased production of HLA class II antigens on the surfaces of antigen producing cells suggests that the cells are locally engaged in specific immune responses. The low presence of gamma/delta T lymphocytes may increase the vulnerability to microbial noxious agents.

4.2.3 Antibody/immunoglobulin production

These studies investigated specific antibodies against periodontopathic bacteria in serum and saliva.

Santos et al. (1996) determined the circulating antibody titers to *Aggregatibacter (Actinobacillus) actinomycetemcomitans (Aa)* in sera of DS and normal patients. Eleven DS patients with periodontitis (pocket depth > 4 mm), five DS patients with gingivitis (inflammation and pocket depth < or = 3 mm), and 10 non-DS healthy subjects had blood drawn and analyzed for antibody response to *Aa*. The authors noted significant differences between the control group and the DS groups ($p = 0.05$), with the DS periodontal group having the highest response, followed by the DS gingivitis and normal controls, respectively.

Morinushi et al. (1997) obtained sera from 75 DS subjects (aged 2 to 18 years) and their gingival health assessed using a modified gingival inflammation index (PMA Index). Antibody titers to *Porphyromonas gingivalis, Prevotella intermedia, Treponema denticola, Fusobacterium nucleatum, Selenomonas sputigena, Actinobacillus actinomycetemcomitans, and Streptococcus mitis* were determined using a micro-ELISA. The average antibody titers to *A. actinomycetemcomitans, S. mitis,* and *F. nucleatum* exceeded those of the normal adult reference serum pool. In addition, IgG antibody titers to *P. gingivalis* , *A actinomycetemcomitans, F. nucleatum, S. sputigena*, and *S. mitis* correlated significantly with the modified PMA scores.

Barr-Agholme et al. (1998) investigated the clinical periodontal conditions and salivary immunoglobulins in patients with DS. The results showed an altered distribution of IgG subclasses in saliva, with an increased amount of IgG1 in DS patients compared to controls. This is in agreement with other studies that show increased IgG1 in DS patients (Kusters, et al., 2009). On the contrary, the proportion of IgG2, IgG3, and IgG4 subclasses in saliva did not differ between the 2 groups. Also, in DS patients with bone loss, it was noted that they have an increased level of sIgA, compared to those DS patients without bone loss.

Chaushu et al. (2007) assessed age-related changes in the salivary-specific humoral immunity of DS subjects. Parotid and whole saliva were collected from a young group of DS, an older group of DS individuals and compared to two age-matched groups of healthy volunteers. The levels of total IgA, and specific antibodies to three common oral pathogens (*Porphyromonas gingivalis, Aggregatibacter (Actinobacillus) actinomycetemcomitans and Streptococcus mutans*) were analyzed. The median secretion rates of the specific antibodies in whole and parotid saliva were 70-77% and 34-60% (respectively) lower in young DS individuals as compared to young controls and farther 77-100% and 75-88% (respectively) lower in old DS compared to young DS.

The presented studies were somewhat controversial and indicated different antibody responses between saliva and serum in DS individuals. While in saliva the antibody response was low in DS individuals, in serum the antibody responses to several periodontopathic bacteria were elevated. The low antibody responses in saliva were associated with decreased salivary flow in DS individuals. The low salivary antibody activity may facilitate the colonization of periodontal pathogens in DS individuals. The elevated antibody titers in DS serum corroborate the gingival immune cellular activity described previously. It demonstrates that DS individuals despite known immune deficiencies are capable of mounting a humoral specific immune response. Such antibodies would find their way into the gingival tissues and fluid and help with containing the microbial damage. Increased antibody levels in gingival tissues may also accentuate the gingival inflammatory response through complement activation.

4.3 Inflammatory response studies

Inflammatory response studies focused on inflammatory mediators and degrading enzymes in gingival crevicular fluid.

4.3.1 Studies investigating inflammatory mediators

Barr-Agholme et al. (1997) investigated the levels of prostaglandin E2 (PGE2) and interleukin-1β (IL-1β) in gingival crevicular fluid (GCF). GCF was collected from both DS patients and healthy controls. They found the mean level of PGE2 in GCF was significantly higher in the DS patients as compared to the controls. This finding suggests an alteration in arachidonic acid metabolism in DS patients. The mean level of IL-1β in the GCF was not significantly higher in the DS patients as compared to the healthy controls. Perhaps the reason the IL-1β levels did not differ between the groups, despite the fact that the gingival inflammation was more severe in the DS group, may be because PGE2 has been reported to down-regulate the production of IL-1β (Kunkel, et al., 1987). This issue has not been revisited since and indeed is worthy of further investigation.

Tsilingaridis et al. (2003) determined the levels of PGE2, LTB4, and MMP-9 in GCF from 18 Down syndrome patients and from 14 controls matched with respect to age and degree of gingival inflammation. Clinical periodontal parameters were recorded including probing depth (PD) and bleeding on probing (BOP). The mean levels of PGE2, LTB4, and MMP-9 were significantly ($P<0.05$) higher in GCF from Down syndrome patients compared to controls. When comparing the two groups, the correlation coefficients for LTB4 to BOP and PD, respectively, as well as for MMP-9 to BOP significantly differed between Down syndrome and controls ($P<0.05$).

4.3.2 Studies investigating degrading enzymes

Halinen et al. (1996) characterized the periodontal status of 9 non-institutionalized DS children 9 to 17 years old relative to their age-matched systemically and periodontally healthy controls. Clinical periodontal parameters were recorded. They also assessed the collagenase and gelatinase activities in the gingival crevicular fluid (GCF) and saliva samples collected from DS patients and from the controls. The endogenously active collagenase and total collagenase activities were slightly higher in GCF of DS children compared to healthy controls. Western blot demonstrated that GCF collagenase of DS patients was human neutrophil collagenase (MMP-8 or collagenase-2). Salivary collagenase in DS was high when compared to controls but of the same MMP-8 type as in control saliva.

Komatsu et al. (2001) examined both the amount present and the enzyme activity of matrix metalloproteinases (MMP-2) in the gingival tissues of Down syndrome patients and controls. The authors reported that there was a significantly higher production of MMP-2 in the cultured gingival fibroblasts of the Down syndrome patients when compared with the controls. In addition, the mRNA expressions of membrane-type I metalloproteinases (MTI-MMP) and MMP-2 were markedly different when the cultured fibroblasts of the DS patients were compared to the controls. This would indicate that the increased amount of active MMP-2 produced in DS could be linked to the simultaneous expression of MTI-MMP, which could also be connected to the cause of periodontal disease that is seen in a majority of DS patients.

Yamazaki-Kubota et al. (2010) investigated levels of matrix metalloproteinase-2 (MMP-2) and matrix metalloproteinase-8 (MMP-8) in gingival crevicular fluid (GCF) and detection of periodontopathic bacteria from subgingival plaque. Samples of GCF and plaque were isolated from central incisors. Levels of MMPs were evaluated by enzyme-linked immunosorbent assay, and periodontopathic bacteria were detected by polymerase chain reaction. Levels of MMP-2 and MMP-8 in DS patients were higher than those in healthy control subjects. In the DS group, increases in these MMPs were observed in GCF from patients with good oral hygiene and absence of bleeding on probing. The detection rate of periodontopathic bacteria in DS patients was higher than that in the control subjects. Surprisingly, MMP-2 levels in sites harbouring *Porphyromonas gingivalis* or *Aggregatibacter (Actinobacillus) actinomycetemcomitans* were lower than in those without these microorganisms.

The cited studies indicate increased matrix metalloproteinase activity in the gingival tissues of DS individuals. The presence of MMP-8 suggests that neutrophils in their frustration to reach their target pathogens release their enzymes extracellularly. Matrix metalloproteinases are involved in the breakdown of the extracellular matrix. Their increased activity in the gingival tissues of DS individuals explains the gingival tissue loss and associated clinical signs (increased probing depth and loss of attachment) described. In addition the increased levels of prostaglandin E2 in combination with increased activity of MMP-9 suggests increased osteoclastic activity and explains the increased alveolar bone loss described in DS individuals.

5. A hypothesized model of the pathogenesis of periodontitis in Down syndrome

The presented articles viewed collectively suggest the following sequence of events in the pathogenesis of periodontitis in DS. Decreased salivary flow accompanied by reduced salivary antibody production and defective neutrophil chemotaxis facilitates early microbial colonization in the dentogingival region and makes it easier for periodontal pathogens to gain a foothold. The heavy microbial presence initiates a strong gingival immune/inflammatory response characterized by the presence of high numbers of macrophages and lymphocytes in the gingival tissues. Antigen presenting cells are active in initiating adaptive immunity (as evidenced by the increased expression of HLA Class II antigens on inflammatory cells) and eventually the production of a strong humoral antibody response. The specific antibodies may help with containing the microbial infection. In addition, macrophages and other gingival resident cells (fibroblasts) seem to be engaged in high production of degrading enzymes. Frustrated neutrophils may release their degrading enzymes extracellularly into the gingival tissues. Tissue injury releases arachidonic acid metabolites (prostaglandins). The degrading enzymes and prostaglandins are involved with periodontal tissue destruction (figure 3).

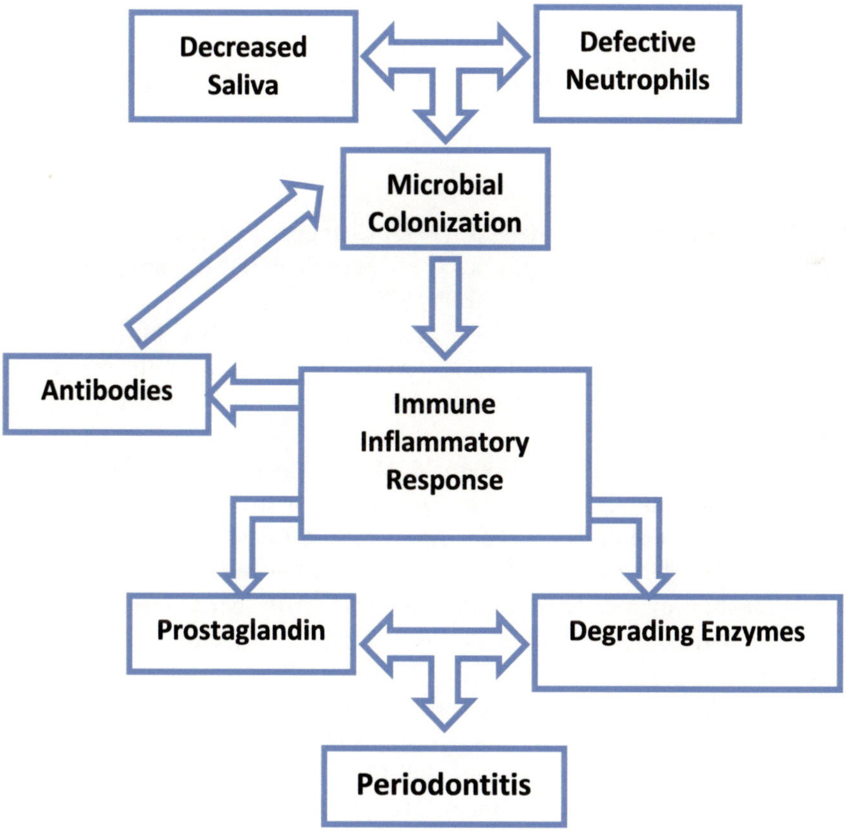

Fig. 3. Hypothesized model of periodontitis pathogenesis in Down syndrome.

6. Conclusions

In summary I have attempted to use the available periodontal literature on periodontitis in DS to construct a hypothesized model of the pathogenesis of the disease. Periodontitis in DS individuals is characterized by an intense and persistent immune/inflammatory response. Viewing this body of literature as a temporal sequence of events suggests that therapies aiming at reduction of microbial colonization could greatly benefit DS individuals by reducing the immune/inflammatory response and associated inflammatory mediators and degrading enzymes. The model also may suggest future therapies such as host response modulation. Strikingly absent from the model is information related to core immune/inflammatory abnormalities associated with DS such as increased oxidative stress, altered integrin expression (and associated altered lymphocyte function), altered IL-10 receptor expression (and possible impact on resolution of inflammation), and increased IL-1 production and their relation to periodontal disease. Further studies are needed to resolve these gaps in knowledge, and to access the implications for everyday periodontal care of this periodontally vulnerable population.

7. Acknowledgement

I would like to express my sincere appreciation to Dr. Ruth Nowjack-Raymer, Dr. Kevin Heaney, Dr. Bobby Turner and Dr. Malvin Janal who led my way into Down syndrome research.

8. References

Agholme, M. B., Dahllof, G. & Modeer, T. (1999) Changes of periodontal status in patients with Down syndrome during a 7-year period. *European Journal of Oral Sciences,* Vol.107, No. 2, (Apr), pp. 82-88, 0909-8836

Akinci, O., Mihci, E., Tacoy, S., Kardelen, F., Keser, I. & Aslan, M. (2010) Neutrophil oxidative metabolism in Down syndrome patients with congenital heart defects. *Environmental & Molecular Mutagenesis,* Vol.51, No. 1, (Jan), pp. 57-63, 1098-2280

Amano, A., Kishima, T., Kimura, S., Takiguchi, M., Ooshima, T., Hamada, S. & Morisaki, I. (2000) Periodontopathic bacteria in children with Down syndrome. *Journal of Periodontology,* Vol.71, No. 2, (Feb), pp. 249-255, 0022-3492

Amano, A., Kishima, T., Akiyama, S., Nakagawa, I., Hamada, S. & Morisaki, I. (2001) Relationship of periodontopathic bacteria with early-onset periodontitis in Down's syndrome. *Journal of Periodontology,* Vol.72, No. 3, (Mar), pp. 368-373, 0022-3492

Amaral Loureiro, A. C., Oliveira Costa, F. & Eustaquio da Costa, J. (2007) The impact of periodontal disease on the quality of life of individuals with Down syndrome. *Down Syndrome: Research & Practice,* Vol.12, No. 1, (Jul), pp. 50-54, 0968-7912

Barr-Agholme, M., Dahllof, G., Linder, L. & Modeer, T. (1992) Actinobacillus actinomycetemcomitans, Capnocytophaga and Porphyromonas gingivalis in subgingival plaque of adolescents with Down's syndrome. *Oral Microbiology & Immunology,* Vol.7, No. 4, (Aug), pp. 244-248, 0902-0055

Barr-Agholme, M., Krekmanova, L., Yucel-Lindberg, T., Shinoda, K. & Modeer, T. (1997) Prostaglandin E2 level in gingival crevicular fluid from patients with Down syndrome. *Acta Odontologica Scandinavica,* Vol.55, No. 2, (Apr), pp. 101-105, 0001-6357

Barr-Agholme, M., Dahllof, G., Modeer, T., Engstrom, P. E. & Engstrom, G. N. (1998) Periodontal conditions and salivary immunoglobulins in individuals with Down syndrome. *Journal of Periodontology,* Vol.69, No. 10, (Oct), pp. 1119-1123, 0022-3492

Chambrone, L., Chambrone, D., Lima, L. A. & Chambrone, L. A. (2010) Predictors of tooth loss during long-term periodontal maintenance: a systematic review of observational studies. *Journal of Clinical Periodontology,* Vol.37, No. 7, (Jul), pp. 675-684, 1600-051X

Chaushu, S., Chaushu, G., Zigmond, M., Yefenof, E., Stabholz, A., Shapira, J., Merrick, J. & Bachrach, G. (2007) Age-dependent deficiency in saliva and salivary antibodies secretion in Down's syndrome. *Archives of Oral Biology,* Vol.52, No. 11, pp. 1088-1096, 0003-9969

Cochran, D. L. (2008) Inflammation and bone loss in periodontal disease. *Journal of Periodontology,* Vol.79, No. 8 Suppl, (Aug), pp. 1569-1576, 0022-3492

Cohen, M. M., Winer, R. A., Schwartz, S. & Shklar, G. (1961) Oral aspects of mongolism. I. Periodontal disease in mongolism. *Oral Surgery, Oral Medicine, Oral Pathology,* Vol.14, No. (Jan), pp. 92-107, 0030-4220

Desai, S. S. (1997) Down syndrome: a review of the literature. *Oral Surgery Oral Medicine Oral Pathology Oral Radiology & Endodontics,* Vol.84, No. 3, (Sep), pp. 279-285, 1079-2104

Glocker, E.-O., Kotlarz, D., Boztug, K., Gertz, E. M., Schaffer, A. A., Noyan, F., Perro, M., Diestelhorst, J., Allroth, A., Murugan, D., Hatscher, N., Pfeifer, D., Sykora, K.-W., Sauer, M., Kreipe, H., Lacher, M., Nustede, R., Woellner, C., Baumann, U., Salzer, U., Koletzko, S., Shah, N., Segal, A. W., Sauerbrey, A., Buderus, S., Snapper, S. B., Grimbacher, B. & Klein, C. (2009) Inflammatory bowel disease and mutations affecting the interleukin-10 receptor. *New England Journal of Medicine,* Vol.361, No. 21, (Nov 19), pp. 2033-2045, 1533-4406

Halinen, S., Sorsa, T., Ding, Y., Ingman, T., Salo, T., Konttinen, Y. T. & Saari, H. (1996) Characterization of matrix metalloproteinase (MMP-8 and -9) activities in the saliva and in gingival crevicular fluid of children with Down's syndrome. *Journal of Periodontology,* Vol.67, No. 8, (Aug), pp. 748-754, 0022-3492

Izumi, Y., Sugiyama, S., Shinozuka, O., Yamazaki, T., Ohyama, T. & Ishikawa, I. (1989) Defective neutrophil chemotaxis in Down's syndrome patients and its relationship to periodontal destruction. *Journal of Periodontology,* Vol.60, No. 5, (May), pp. 238-242, 0022-3492

Khocht, A., Janal, M. & Turner, B. (2010) Periodontal health in Down syndrome: contributions of mental disability, personal, and professional dental care. *Special Care in Dentistry,* Vol.30, No. 3, (May-Jun), pp. 118-123, 1754-4505

Komatsu, T., Kubota, E. & Sakai, N. (2001) Enhancement of matrix metalloproteinase (MMP)-2 activity in gingival tissue and cultured fibroblasts from Down's syndrome patients. *Oral Diseases,* Vol.7, No. 1, (Jan), pp. 47-55, 1354-523X

Kornman, K. S. (2008) Mapping the pathogenesis of periodontitis: a new look. *Journal of Periodontology,* Vol.79, No. 8 Suppl, (Aug), pp. 1560-1568, 0022-3492

Kunkel, S. L., Remick, D. G., Spengler, M. & Chensue, S. W. (1987) Modulation of macrophage-derived interleukin-1 and tumor necrosis factor by prostaglandin E2. *Advances in Prostaglandin, Thromboxane, & Leukotriene Research,* Vol.17A, No. pp. 155-158, 0732-8141

Kusters, M. A. A., Verstegen, R. H. J., Gemen, E. F. A. & de Vries, E. (2009) Intrinsic defect of the immune system in children with Down syndrome: a review. *Clinical & Experimental Immunology,* Vol.156, No. 2, (May), pp. 189-193, 1365-2249

Lemieux, N., Malfoy, B. & Forrest, G. L. (1993) Human carbonyl reductase (CBR) localized to band 21q22.1 by high-resolution fluorescence in situ hybridization displays gene dosage effects in trisomy 21 cells. *Genomics,* Vol.15, No. 1, (Jan), pp. 169-172, 0888-7543

Morgan, J. (2007) Why is periodontal disease more prevalent and more severe in people with Down syndrome? *Special Care in Dentistry,* Vol.27, No. 5, (Sep-Oct), pp. 196-201, 0275-1879

Morinushi, T., Lopatin, D. E. & Van Poperin, N. (1997) The relationship between gingivitis and the serum antibodies to the microbiota associated with periodontal disease in children with Down's syndrome. *Journal of Periodontology,* Vol.68, No. 7, (Jul), pp. 626-631, 0022-3492

Mrak, R. E. & Griffin, W. S. T. (2004) Trisomy 21 and the brain. *Journal of Neuropathology & Experimental Neurology,* Vol.63, No. 7, (Jul), pp. 679-685, 0022-3069

Pai, M., McCulloch, M., Gorman, J. D., Pai, N., Enanoria, W., Kennedy, G., Tharyan, P. & Colford, J. M., Jr. (2004) Systematic reviews and meta-analyses: an illustrated, step-by-step guide. *National Medical Journal of India,* Vol.17, No. 2, (Mar-Apr), pp. 86-95, 0970-258X

Reuland-Bosma, W., Liem, R. S., Jansen, H. W., van Dijk, L. J. & van der Weele, L. T. (1988) Morphological aspects of the gingiva in children with Down's syndrome during experimental gingivitis. *Journal of Clinical Periodontology,* Vol.15, No. 5, (May), pp. 293-302, 0303-6979

Reuland-Bosma, W., van den Barselaar, M. T., van de Gevel, J. S., Leijh, P. C., de Vries-Huiges, H. & The, H. T. (1988) Nonspecific and specific immune responses in a child with Down's syndrome and her sibling. A case report. *Journal of Periodontology,* Vol.59, No. 4, (Apr), pp. 249-253, 0022-3492

Reuland-Bosma, W., van der Reijden, W. A. & van Winkelhoff, A. J. (2001) Absence of a specific subgingival microflora in adults with Down's syndrome. *Journal of Clinical Periodontology,* Vol.28, No. 11, (Nov), pp. 1004-1009, 0303-6979

Sakellari, D., Belibasakis, G., Chadjipadelis, T., Arapostathis, K. & Konstantinidis, A. (2001) Supragingival and subgingival microbiota of adult patients with Down's syndrome. Changes after periodontal treatment. *Oral Microbiology & Immunology,* Vol.16, No. 6, (Dec), pp. 376-382, 0902-0055

Sakellari, D., Arapostathis, K. N. & Konstantinidis, A. (2005) Periodontal conditions and subgingival microflora in Down syndrome patients. A case-control study. *Journal of Clinical Periodontology,* Vol.32, No. 6, (Jun), pp. 684-690, 0303-6979

Santos, R., Shanfeld, J. & Casamassimo, P. (1996) Serum antibody response to Actinobacillus actinomycetemcomitans in Down's syndrome. *Special Care in Dentistry,* Vol.16, No. 2, (Mar-Apr), pp. 80-83, 0275-1879

Saxen, L., Aula, S. & Westermarck, T. (1977) Periodontal disease associated with Down's syndrome: an orthopantomographic evaluation. *Journal of Periodontology,* Vol.48, No. 6, (Jun), pp. 337-340, 0022-3492

Saxen, L. & Aula, S. (1982) Periodontal bone loss in patients with Down's syndrome: a follow-up study. *Journal of Periodontology,* Vol.53, No. 3, (Mar), pp. 158-162, 0022-3492

Sohoel, D. C., Johannessen, A. C., Kristoffersen, T. & Nilsen, R. (1995) Expression of HLA class II antigens in marginal periodontitis of patients with Down's syndrome. *European Journal of Oral Sciences,* Vol.103, No. 4, (Aug), pp. 207-213, 0909-8836

Sohoel, D. C., Jonsson, R., Johannessen, A. C. & Nilsen, R. (1995) Gamma/delta T lymphocytes in marginal periodontitis in patients with Down's syndrome. *Advances in Experimental Medicine & Biology,* Vol.371B, No. pp. 1135-1136, 0065-2598

Sohoel, P. D., Johannessen, A. C., Kristoffersen, T., Haugstvedt, Y. & Nilsen, R. (1992) In situ characterization of mononuclear cells in marginal periodontitis of patients with Down's syndrome. *Acta Odontologica Scandinavica,* Vol.50, No. 3, (Jun), pp. 141-149, 0001-6357

Strydom, A., Dickinson, M. J., Shende, S., Pratico, D. & Walker, Z. (2009) Oxidative stress and cognitive ability in adults with Down syndrome. *Progress in Neuro-Psychopharmacology & Biological Psychiatry,* Vol.33, No. 1, (Feb 1), pp. 76-80, 0278-5846

Taylor, G. M. (1987) Altered expression of lymphocyte functional antigen in Down syndrome. *Immunology Today,* Vol.8, No. 12, pp. 366-369,

Thase, M. E. (1982) Longevity and mortality in Down's syndrome. *Journal of Mental Deficiency Research,* Vol.26, No. Pt 3, (Sep), pp. 177-192, 0022-264X

Tsilingaridis, G., Yucel-Lindberg, T. & Modeer, T. (2003) Enhanced levels of prostaglandin E2, leukotriene B4, and matrix metalloproteinase-9 in gingival crevicular fluid from patients with Down syndrome. *Acta Odontologica Scandinavica,* Vol.61, No. 3, (Jun), pp. 154-158, 0001-6357

von Elm, E., Altman, D. G., Egger, M., Pocock, S. J., Gotzsche, P. C., Vandenbroucke, J. P. & Initiative, S. (2007) The Strengthening the Reporting of Observational Studies in Epidemiology (STROBE) statement: guidelines for reporting observational studies. *Lancet,* Vol.370, No. 9596, (Oct 20), pp. 1453-1457, 1474-547X

Yamazaki-Kubota, T., Miyamoto, M., Sano, Y., Kusumoto, M., Yonezu, T., Sugita, K., Okuda, K., Yakushiji, M. & Ishihara, K. (2010) Analysis of matrix metalloproteinase (MMP-8 and MMP-2) activity in gingival crevicular fluid from children with Down's syndrome. *Journal of Periodontal Research,* Vol.45, No. 2, (Apr), pp. 170-176, 1600-0765

Yavuzyilmaz, E., Ersoy, F., Sanal, O., Tezcan, I. & Ercal, D. (1993) Neutrophil chemotaxis and periodontal status in Down's syndrome patients. *Journal of Nihon University School of Dentistry,* Vol.35, No. 2, (Jun), pp. 91-95, 0029-0432

Zaldivar-Chiapa, R. M., Arce-Mendoza, A. Y., De La Rosa-Ramirez, M., Caffesse, R. G. & Solis-Soto, J. M. (2005) Evaluation of surgical and non-surgical periodontal therapies, and immunological status, of young Down's syndrome patients. *Journal of Periodontology,* Vol.76, No. 7, (Jul), pp. 1061-1065, 0022-3492

12

Dysfunctional Voiding of Non-Neurogenic Neurogenic Bladder: A Urological Disorder Associated with Down Syndrome

Narihito Seki and Nouval Shahab
Department of Urology, Graduate School of Medical Sciences, Kyushu University
Japan

1. Introduction

Down syndrome (DS), the most common chromosomal abnormality with a prevalence of 1 case per 600 live births (Dennis & Marder,2001), has many manifestations that can affect multiple organ systems (American Academy of Pediatrics Comittee on Genetics, 2001; Kallen et al., 1996) including urological abnormalities which have been recognized throughout urinary tract (Ariel et al., 1991; Berg et al.,1960; Ahmed, 1990; Kravtzova et al., 1975; Handel et al., 2003; Kupferman et al., 1996; Bielek et al., 1996; Narashiman & Gupta, 2004; Koksal et al., 2003; Lang et al., 1987; Paulozzi et al., 1997). The extra copy of chromosome 21 has been suggested as an actor underlying the accompanied phenotypic abnormalities in the syndrome (Lejeune, 1959).

Berg et al. described the first cases of urological anomalies associated with DS in their study of 141 DS autopsy cases and found 1 patient (0.7%) with renal agenesis and 5 patients (3.6%) with horseshoe kidney (Berg et al., 1960). Glomerular microcysts, renal hypoplasia and obstructive uropathy have also been recognized as the most common upper urinary tract anomalies in DS and their incidences were reported by Ariel et al. who examined 124 autopsy cases of DS for abnormalities in urinary tract system to be as high as 23.7% (23 of 97 patients), 21.4% (18 of 84 patients), and 6.45% (8 of the 124 cases), respectively (Ariel et al., 1991). In addition, simple renal cysts were also found in 7 of 124 cases (5.6%).

Anomalies in ureteral structure has also been identified in DS (Ariel et al., 1991; Kravtzova et al., 1975; Handel et al., 2003). The incidence of obstructed megaureter or hydroureteronephrosis was reported in 2 of 124 cases (1.6%), while ureteral atresia was seen in 1 of 124 cases (0.8%) (Ariel et al., 1991). In addition, vesicoureteral reflux (Kravtzova et al., 1975), ureterovesical junction and ureteropelvic junction obstructions have also been described in patients with trisomy 21 (Handel et al., 2003).

Trisomy 21 is one of genetic disorders that can also be accompanied by some urological abnormalities in lower urinary tract. Non-neurogenic neurogenic bladder (NNB) has been reported as a functional lower urinary tract abnormality seen in DS. Handel et al. retrospectively reviewed 26 patients with trisomy 21 and found 4 patients (15.4%) with NNB (Handel et al., 2003). Posterior urethral valve has also been identified in patients with trisomy 21 (Bielek et al., 1996; Narashiman & Gupta, 2004; Koksal et al., 2003; Lang DJ et al., 1987). Bielek et al who reviewed 48 cases of posterior urethral valves found 4 patients with

DS (Bielek et al., 1996). Hypospadia has also a higher incidence in patients with the syndrome (Paulozzi et al., 1997).

There is a lack of awareness regarding DS related urological manifestations in daily clinical practice. The associated urological anomalies have received little attention from physicians especially for NNB which often cause the delay in referring the patients for further management. In this chapter we will focus on the NNB which represents voiding dysfunction due to functional bladder outlet obstruction recognized in DS. The discussion will include the evaluation and management of this particular disorder. Urodynamic assessment as the most important part in the diagnosis of NNB will also be described.

2. Dysfunctional voiding of non-neurogenic neurogenic bladder in Down Syndrome

2.1 Historical note

Non-neurogenic neurogenic bladder, the most severe form of dysfunctional voiding, is a pure functional bladder outlet obstruction without any neurological abnormalities which was described by Hinman (Hinman, 1986). However, it was first described by Beer who reported four patients with chronic urinary retention and upper urinary tract changes without any evidence of neurological pathology (Beer, 1915). He observed the disharmony between the detrusor and sphincter muscles in the patients.

Incoordination syndrome of voiding contraction reflex was also found by Laidley (Ladley, 1942). The syndrome was then called "achalasia of the urinary tract". Paquin et al. reported symptoms of dysfunctional voiding with large bladder in 27 children and the term "megacystis syndrome" was used to represent the syndrome (Paquin et al., 1960). Ambrose and Swanson reported the 13 children with hypertonic detrusor contraction without any neurologic lesion and labeled the syndrome as "hypertonic-type neurogenic bladder" (Ambrose & Swanson, 1960).

Hinman & Baumann reported voiding difficulties in children associated with upper urinary tract deterioration without any anatomical obstruction or neurologic lesion with the identified psychological disorder (Hinman & Baumann, 1972). The term "non-neurogenic neurogenic bladder" was introduced in order to emphasize the absence of neurologic lesions. The cases were followed for 15 years and then reported with new term "Hinman syndrome" according to the important of psychological factors which contribute to the syndrome and change the previous term which was not appropriate and cause confusion. However, the underlying psychological disturbances were not recognized in the syndrome as reported by Allan (Allan ,1977).

Non neurogenic-neurogenic syndrome in association with trisomy 21 was first identified by Handel et al. who reviewed 26 children with DS (all boys) and found higher incidence of NNB compare to other urological abnormalities in DS (Handel et al., 2003). Hicks et al reported the first women with NNB associated with DS and also found higher incidence of NNB cases in trisomy 21 (Hicks et al., 2007).

2.2 Epidemiology

The true prevalence of NNB has not been reported. The available prevalence is only based on data obtained from some centers. Groutz et al. reported that NNB was found in 2% of patients who underwent video-urodynamic studies but the real prevalence would be even higher (Groutz et al., 2001). Jorgensen et al. reported lower prevalence of NNB (0.5%) among patients referred for urodynamic evaluation (Jorgensen et al., 1982).

Handel et al. reported a higher incidence of NNB in patients with trisomy 21. Among 26 patients with DS who were reviewed, 4 (15.4%) was reported to have NNB (Handel et al., 2003). Hicks et al also found higher incidence of NNB cases in DS (Hicks et al., 2007).[23] Non-neurogenic neurogenic bladder has been reported not only in infant and children but also in adult patients (Handel et al., 2003; Hicks et al., 2007; Jayanthi et al., 1997; Kai et al., 2007).

2.3 Etiology

The etiology of the disease is not clearly defined. Some evidences suggest overtraining of the pelvic floor to avoid urine loss due to not only various emotional conditions such as depression, phobias, stress, trauma associated with toilet training but also psychiatric diseases, the presence of detrusor overactivity and other associated voiding dysfunctions as an underlying factors which may contribute to cause NNB (Hoebeke et al., 1996; Koff et al., 1979; Goldston & Perlmutter, 1973; Schimtt, 1982; Ellsworth, 1995). The well known mental retardation and psychological problems in patients with DS may also explain the higher incidence of NNB in this trisomy 21.

In normal voiding function, bladder filling is accommodated at low bladder pressures with a bladder outlet that remains closed while bladder emptying requires a coordinated and sustained contraction of the bladder muscle with concomitant relaxation of the external urethral sphincter. The reflex of micturition is controlled by parasympathetic and somatic components of the sacral spinal cord and sympathetic innervation.

In NNB, functional bladder outlet obstruction is caused by active contractions of the voluntary external sphincters during voiding. The inability to inhibit the detrusor contraction reflex as well as overactivity of the external sphincter as compensation has become fundamental characteristics of patients with NNB (Hinman, 1986). The dyssynergistic voiding pattern created by the incoordination between the bladder and sphincter contraction reflex may result in impairment of renal function caused by functional obstruction (obstructive uropathy) due to unacceptable high voiding pressure with potential upper and lower urinary tract deterioration .

2.4 Diagnosis

General history-taking should include relevant questions for the screening of NNB. A thorough patient history will indicate incontinence associated with chronic urinary retention. History-taking in patients with DS is difficult especially in children due to the impairment of cognitive function and should be supplemented by information obtained from the parents. Because of the intelligence level, some of the existence as well as other underlying factors in patients with DS may be masked or neglected resulting in the delay of the diagnosis which often seen in clinical practice (Handel et al., 2003; Kai et al., 2007; Fernandez & Moore., 1986).

Although unerderlying factors could not be found in some cases, It is important to make sure that history taking have already included all the underlying factors of NNB which may guide to the diagnosis (Goldston & Perlmutter, 1973; Schmitt, 1982; Ellsworth et al., 1995). Neurological symptoms and abnormalities will not be present in NNB but should be confirmed by carefully clinical examination. Laboratory results may show elevated serum creatinine and reduce clearance or decreased renal function with or without signs of urinary tract infection in most of the cases.

Ultrasound is useful to evaluate bladder after voiding which can show residual urine volume as well as determine the bladder thickness. In addition, ultrasound is also important to detect the upper urinary tract dilatation with or without dilatation of the ureters as a complication of functional obstruction in NNB. In trisomy 21, this tool is also useful to identify other associated organ anomalies including abnormalities in the kidney.
To diagnose NNB in trisomy 21 patients, other associated anomalies such as Hirschsprung's disease, spinal cord defects, and posterior urethral valves must be excluded first before concluding that they have a functional rather than anatomical obstruction especially those who present with constipation, recurrent urinary tract infections, incontinence and voiding dysfunction (Handel et al., 2003). In order to rule out the neurological lesions, imaging studies of computed tomography (CT) scans and magnetic resonance imaging (MRI) should be performed (Johnson et al., 1992).
Non-neurogenic neurogenic bladder should be suspected if negative results have been confirmed by standard rectal biopsies and urological evaluation demonstrates the absence of anatomical obstruction and neurological evaluation including imaging studies confirms the absence of any neurologic lesions (Handel et al., 2003).

2.4.1 Voiding-cystourethrography

Voiding-cystourethrography is an important radiologic tool to show varying grade of vesico-ureter reflux in some cases of NNB. In addition, it also shows bladder appearance as a result of functional obstruction such as a trabeculated and enlarged bladder with a lot of residual urine still remains in the bladder after voiding without any evidence of mechanical obstruction (Fig. 1).

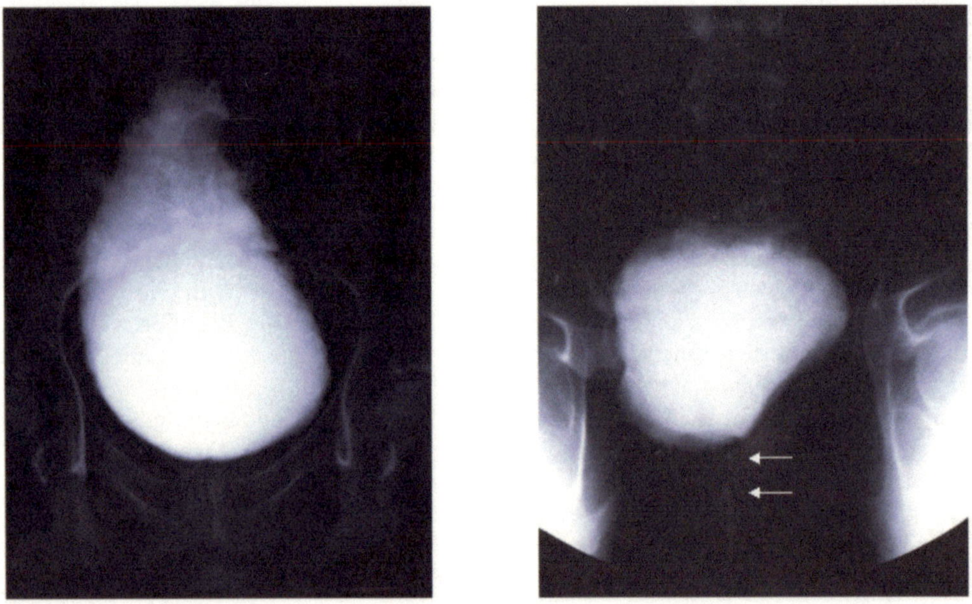

Fig. 1. Voiding cystourethrography shows a deformity of the bladder wall with trabeculation (left) and narrowing of the posterior urethra as pointed by white arrows with significant residual urine (right) without vesico-urethral reflux

In contrast, anatomical obstruction by posterior urethral valve can be identified by posterior urethral dilatation with poor visualization of the anterior urethra. However, it is important to note that the appearance of posterior urethra may entirely normal during early voiding but distended after contraction of the external sphincter as voiding progress which was found in 4 patients who previously diagnosed with NNB as reported by Johnson et al who reviewed the genitourinary images of six boys in whom NNB was diagnosed in the past 5 years (Johnson et al., 1992).

2.4.2 Uroflowmetry

Uroflowmetry is useful for the screening of NNB since it is able to measure the urinary stream during the voiding phase, providing information of bladder and outlet function (Allan & Bright, 1978; Stanton et al., 1983). In uroflowmetry measurement, it is important to pay attention on the the flow pattern beside other important parameters (Vijverberg et al., 1997). Normal urine flow is continuous bell-shaped curve. Continuous plateau shape curve (lower urinary flow rate with prolonged voiding time) is typical for anatomical obstruction. In contrast, functional obstruction is typically reflected by a staccato pattern as interrupted flow of urine occurs due to uninhibited external sphincter contraction and usually demonstrates intermittency with reduced flow rates and prolonged voiding time (Fig. 2). The results also depend on the stage of the disease since the above pattern is hardly ever seen in advance cases with atonia of the bladder and poor detrusor contractility due to decompensated bladder. Uroflowmetry can also be used as a tool for follow-up of bladder training, and biofeedback training (Vijverberg et al., 1997; Hellstrom et al., 1987; Hjalmas, 1988; Griffiths & Scholtmeijer, 1984; Wear et al., 1979).

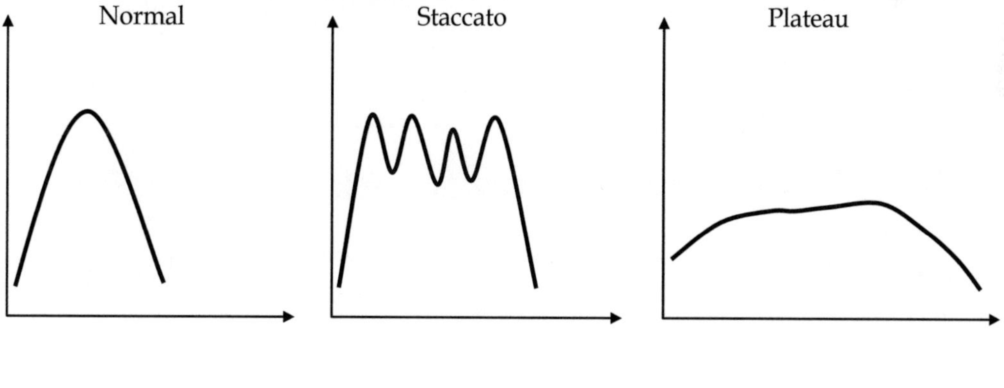

Fig. 2. The illustration of normal and abnormal uroflowmetry patterns.

2.4.3 Urodynamics

Urodynamics study is the gold standard for the diagnosis of patients with voiding dysfunction. (Nitti, 2005) Hypertonicity, instability with impaired external sphincter relaxation during micturation are typical characteristics in patients with NNB (Allan & Bright, 1978). Electromyography (EMG) shows a spastic activity with a high amplitude during voiding phase (Fig. 3).

True detrusor-external sphincter dyssynergia and NNB can be differentiated urodynamically (Rudy & Woodside, 1991). Detrusor-external sphincter dyssynergia is characterized urodynamically by increasing EMG activity during upslope and decreasing activity during down slope of the intravesical pressure tracing during a detrusor contraction. However, NNB is characterized urodynamically by quieting of the EMG during upslope and augmented activity during the down slope of the detrusor contraction.

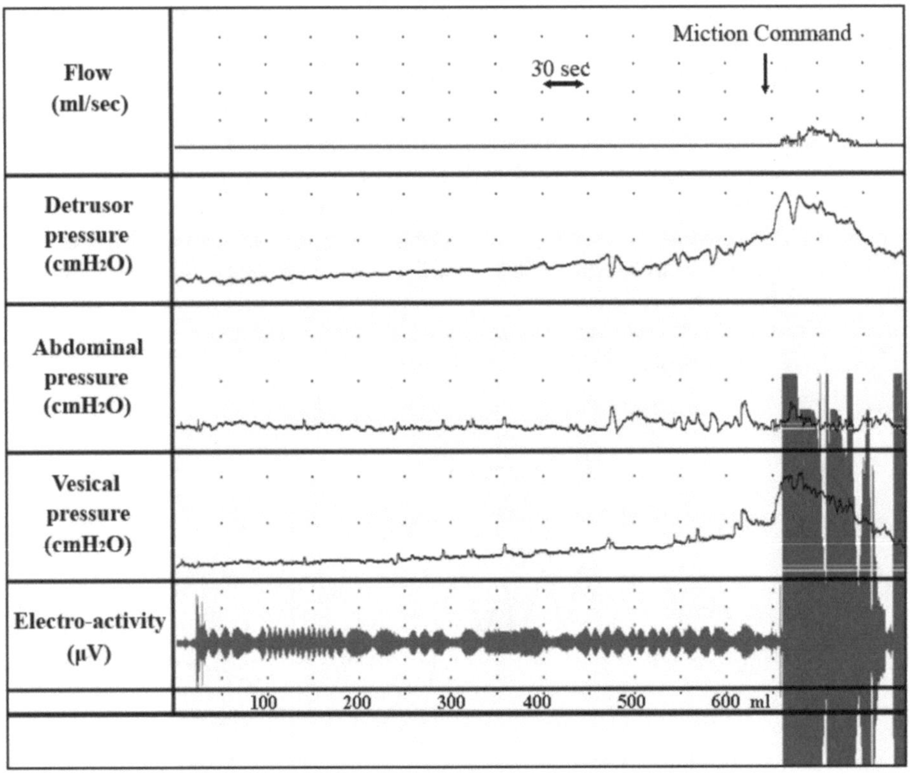

Fig. 3. Urodynamic results indcate a decrease in the bladder sensation without detrusor overactivity. A low urinary flow rate with a high detrusor pressure is shown in the voiding phase. Electromyography shows a spastic activity with a high amplitude during voiding. (Filling rate = 50 ml/min).

2.5 Management

Management of patients with NNB must be focused on the relaxation of external urethral sphincter muscle in order to obtain a more physiological micturation with relaxed sphincter muscle during voiding and to restore the balance of voiding and voluntary sphincter contraction reflex to prevent upper and lower urinary tract deterioration. The additional goals of treatment include prevention of urinary tract infections with proper antibiotics. The management should be addressed to all patients regardless of their intellectual capacity including those with trisomy 21. The intellectual Impairment of patients with DS may cause some difficulties in conducting the treatment.

Anti-cholinergics and alpha blocker therapy either alone or in combination may be useful in the treatment of NNB (Krane & Olsson, 1973; Paul et al., 1999; Bogaert et al., 2004) since significant improvement in emptying was shown in neurogenic cases treated with non selective alpha blocker (Krane & Olsson, 1973). If there is no response to conservative treatment, intermittent catheterization may be required. Trisomy 21 associated NNB patients with abnormal voiding mechanism against a closed sphincter may deal with the difficulty in conducting urethral clean intermittent catheterization due to their intellectual limitation (Handel et al, 2003).

Surgical treatment for renal preservation is also required for social continence. Self-catheterization protocols via the catheterizable stoma may allow trisomy 21 patients with a sufficient intellectual level master such techniques. Patients with NNB who are refractory to conservative treatment or present with an advanced pathological condition may require surgical intervention. Augmentation of the bladder in order to increase the bladder capacity may still be required in those in whom the upper tracts are threatened (Handel et al, 2003).

The use of Botulinum-A toxin injection into detrusor or the external sphincter may help cause striated muscle paralysis and may also restore voiding function especially in those who failed with drug therapy (Schurch et al., 1996). Patients with NNB in DS could also be performed such procedure. This particular treatment is dose dependent and also reversible. Injection may be necessary in every two months.

3. Summary

Children with trisomy 21 have many associated multi organ anomalies including urological abnormalities. Non-neurogenic neurogenic bladder is the most frequent DS associated lower urinary tract disorder. Early diagnosis and prompt management should be conducted in order to prevent upper urinary tract deterioration. According to the high incidence of NND in DS, early and regular sonographic and urodynamic evaluation of the bladder function is mandatory in patients with Down syndrome.

4. References

Ahmed S. 1990. Vesico-ureteric reflux in Down's syndrome: poor prognosis. *Aust N Z J Surg*, Vol. 60, pp. 113-116.

Allen TD. 1977. The non-neurogenic neurogenic bladder. *J Urol*, Vol. 117, pp. 232-238.

Allan TD & Bright T. 1978. Urodynamic patterns in children with dysfunctional voiding problems. *J Urol*, Vol. 119, pp. 247-249.

Ambrose SS, Swanson. 1960. The hypertonic neurogenic bladder in children: its sequelae and management. *J Urol*, Vol. 83, pp. 672-675.

American Academy of Pediatric Committee on Genetics, American Academy of Pediatrics. 2001. Health supervision for children with Down syndrome. *Pediatrics*, Vol. 107, pp. 442-449.

Ariel I, Wells TR, Landing B, Singer DB. 1991. The urinary system in Down's syndrome: a study of 124 autopsy cases. *Pediatr Pathol*, Vol. 11, pp. 879-888.

Beer E. 1915. Chronic retention of urine in children. *JAMA*, Vol 65, pp. 1709-1712.

Berg JM, Crome L, France NE. 1960. Congenital cardiac malformations in mongolism. *Br Heart J*, Vol. 22, pp. 331-346.

Bielek J, Carvajal-Busslinger MI, Bianchetti MG. 1996. Posterior urethral valves in trisomy 21. *Pediatr Nephrol*, Vol. 10, pp. 678.

Bogaert G, Beckers G, Lombaerts R. 2004. The use and rationale of selective alpha blockade in children with non-neurogenic neurogenic bladder dysfunction. International *Braz J Urol*, Vol. 30, pp. 128-134..

Dennis, J. & Marder, E. 2001. Medical management of children with Down's syndrome. *Curr Paediatr*, Vol.11, pp. 57-63.

Ellsworth PI, Merguerian PA, Copening ME. 1995. Sexual abuse: another causative factor in dysfunctional voiding. *J Urol*, Vol. 153, pp. 773-776.

Fernandez J, Moore S. 1986. Continence. Dry at night. *Nurs Times*, Vol. 82, pp. 73-76.

Goldston R, Perlmutter AD. 1973. The urinary manifestations of anxiety in children. *Pediatrics*, Vol. 52, pp. 812-822.

Griffiths DJ, Scholtmeijer RJ. 1984. Place of the free flow curve in the urodynamic investigation of children. *Br J Urol*, Vol. 56, pp. 474-477.

Groutz A, Blaivas JG, Pies C, Sassone AM. 2001. Learned voiding dysfunction (non-neurogenic, neurogenic bladder) among adults. *Neurourol Urodyn*, Vol. 20, pp. 259-268.

Handel LN, Barqawi A, Checa G, Furness PD, Koyle MA. 2003. Males with Down's syndrome and nonneurogenic neurogenic bladder. *J Urol*, Vol. 169, pp. 646-649.

Hellstrom AL, Hjalmas K, Jodal U. 1987. Rehabilitation of the dysfunctional bladder in children: method and 3-year follow-up. *J Urol*, Vol. 138, pp. 847- 849.

Hicks JA, Carson C, Malone PSJ. 2007. Is there an association between functional bladder outlet obstruction and Down's syndrome? *J Pediatr Urol*, Vol. 3, pp. 369-374.

Hinman F Jr, Baumann FW. 1972. Vesical and ureteral damage from voiding dysfunction in boys without neurologic or obstructive disease. *Trans Am Assoc Genitour Surg*, Vol. 64, 116-121.

Hinman F Jr.: Nonneurogenic neurogenic bladder (the Hinman syndrome)-15 years later. 1986. *J Urol*, Vol. 136, pp. 769-777.

Hjalmas K. 1988. Urodynamics in normal infants and children. *Scand J urol Nephrol*; 114(Suppl): 20-27.

Hoebeke P, Van Walle J, Theunis M, De Paepe H, Oosterlinck W, Renson C. 1996. Out-patient pelvic floor therapy in girls with daytime incontinence of dysfunctional voiding. *Urology*, Vol. 48, pp. 923-927.

Jayanthi VR, Khoury AE, McLoire GA, Agarwal SK. 1997. The nonneurogenic neurogenic bladder of early infancy. *J Urol*, Vol. 158, pp. 1281-1285.

Johnson. JF, Hedden RJ, Piccolello ML, Wacksman J. 1992. Distention of the posterior urethra: association with nonneurogenic neurogenic bladder (Hinman syndrome). *Radiology*, Vol. 185, pp. 113-117.

Jorgensen TM, Djurhuus JC, and Schroder HD. 1982. Idiopathic detrusor sphincter dyssynergia in neurologically normal patients with voiding abnormalities. *Eur Urol*, Vol. 8, pp. 107-110.

Kai N, Seki N, Hirata A, Nakamuta S, Naito S. 2007. A female case with Down syndrome and non-neurogenic neurogenic bladder. *Int J Urol*, Vol. 14, pp. 867-868.

Kallen B, Mastroiacovo P, Robert E. 1996. Major congenital malformations in Down syndrome. *Am J Med Genet*, Vol. 65, pp. 160-166.

Koff SA, Lapides J, Piazza DH. 1979. Association of urinary tract infection, reflux with uninhibited bladder contraction and voluntary sphincteric obstruction. *J Urol*, Vol. 122, pp. 373-376.

Koksal IT, Usta M, Erdogru T, et al. 2003. Incidental adult posterior urethral valve without clinical features. *Int Urol Nephrol*, Vol. 35, pp. 227–229.

Krane RJ, Olsson CA. 1973. Phenoxybenzamine in neurogenic bladder dysfunction. II. Clinical consideration. *J Urol*, Vol. 110, pp. 653-656.

Kravtzova GI, Lazjuk GI, Lurie IW. 1975. The malformations of the urinary system in autosomal disorders. *Virchows Arch A Pathol Anat Histol*, Vol. 368, pp. 167-178.

Kupferman JC, Stewart CL, Kaskel FJ, Fine RN. 1996. Posterior urethral valves in patients with Down syndrome. *Pediatr Nephrol*, Vol. 10, pp. 143-146.

Laidley. 1942. Achalasia of the urinary tract in children. *Med J Aust*, Vol. 2, pp. 475-479.

Lang DJ, Van Dyke DC, Heide F, and Lowe PL. 1987. Hypospadias and urethral abnormalities in Down's syndrome. *Clin Pediatr*, Vol. 26, pp. 40-42.

Lejeune J. 1959. Le Mongolism. Premier exemple d'aberration autosomique humaine. *Ann Genet*, Vol. 1, pp. 41-49.

Narashiman KL & Gupta A. 2004 Posterior urethral valves with Down's Syndrome presenting as scrotal urinary sinuses. *Indian Pediatrics*, Vol. 41, pp.1068-1069

Nitti VW. 2005. Pressure flow urodynamic studies: the gold standard for diagnosing bladder outlet obstruction. *Rev Urol, Vol.* 7, (suppl 6), pp. S14-S21.

Paquin AJ Jr, Marshall VF, McGovern JH. 1960. The megacystis syndrome. *J Urol*, pp. 634-639.

Paul FA, Yves LH, Jonathan LM, Mark PC, Anthony JC, Richard CR. 1999. α-Adrenergic blockade in children with neuropathic and non-neuropathic voiding dysfunction. *J Urol*, Vol. 162, pp. 1064-1067.

Paulozzi LJ, Erickson JD, and Jackson RJ. 1997. Hypospadias trends in two US surveillance systems. *Pediatrics*, Vol. 100, pp. 831-834.

Rudy DC, Woodside JR. 1991. Non-neurogenic neurogenic bladder: the relationship between intravesical pressure and the external sphincter electromyogram. *Neurourol urodyn*, Vol. 10, pp. 169-176.

Schmitt BD. 1982. Day time wetting (diurnal enuresis). *Pediatr Clin North Am*, Vol. 29, pp. 9-20.

Schurch B, Hauri D, Rodic B et al. 1996. Botulinum-A toxin as a treatment of detrusor-sfingter dyssynergia: a prospective study in 24 spinal cord injury patients. *J Urol*, Vol. 155, pp. 1023-1029.

Stanton SL, Ozsoy C, Hinton P. 1983. Voiding difficulties in the female: prevalence, clinical and urodynamic review. *Obstet Gynecol*, Vol. 61, pp. 144-147.

Vijverberg MAW, Elzinga-Plomp A, Messer AP, van Gool JD, de Jong TPVM. 1997. Bladder rehabilitation, the effect of a cognitive training program on urge incontinence. *Eur Urol*, Vol. 31, pp. 68-72.

Wear JB, Wear RB, Cleeland C. 1979. Biofeedback in urology using urodynamics: preliminary observation. *J Urol*,Vol. 121, pp. 464-468.

13

Down Syndrome and Epilepsy

A. Nascimento and C. Ortez-González
Servei de Neurologia, Hospital Sant Joan de Déu-Universitat de Barcelona
Fundació Catalana Síndrome de Down Barcelona
Spain

1. Introduction

Down syndrome (DS) is associated with many neurological complications including cognitive deficits, early-onset dementia -which resembles Alzheimer's disease- and seizures. Although seizures and epilepsy were not mentioned in the original description of DS (Down, 1866) the prevalence of seizures in individuals with DS is now known to be higher than in the general population, but lower than in patients with some other types of mental retardation (Corvett et al., 1975). Reported rates of epilepsy in DS range from 1 to 13% (see table 1) (Tatsumo et al., 1984). Individual series are difficult to compare because of differences in inclusion criteria and study populations. The increased seizure susceptibility in DS has been attributed to inherent structural and molecular anomalies of the brain or to associated medical complications, such as cardiovascular abnormalities and recurrent infections.

Medical interventions in DS have resulted in increased longevity, with estimated life expectancy of people with DS in developed countries increasing from an average of 12 years in the 1940s to an average of 57,8 years for women and 61,1 years for men (Bittles et al., 2007). Epilepsy onset in people with DS is age-specific; therefore, because certain complications will arise in childhood and others in adulthood, their occurrence is relevant to paediatric and adult neurologists. This chapter will provide a critical overview of epilepsy in DS.

Authors	No. of patients	Percentage (%)
Romano et al.	113	13.00
Pueschel et al.	405	8.10
Stafstrom et al.	737	6.40

Table 1. Reported incidence of seizures in patients with Down syndrome in the 1990s

2. Epidemiology

Patients with DS show a higher incidence of febrile and non febrile seizures than non-DS individuals. Seizures occur in a bimodal distribution in DS, with 40% of individuals first developing seizures before 1 year of age and another 40% having an onset in their thirties or later (Pueschel et al., 1991). Boys tend to have an earlier age onset, regardless of seizure type, although this may reflect the general male predominance in the infantile spasm group aged less than 1 year at onset. The prevalence of epilepsy increases with age and reaches 46% in those over 50. In general, about 8% of patients with DS have seizure disorders: 47% of them develop partial seizures, 32% infantile spasms and 21% generalized tonic-clonic seizures.

3. Pathophysiology

The mechanisms underlying the increased seizure susceptibility in DS have not yet been completely elucidated. Seizures in infancy have been linked to inherent structural brain abnormalities, such as fewer inhibitory neurons, abnormal cortical lamination, persistent fetal dendritic morphology, and underdeveloped synaptic profiles (Kemper et al., 1988). Concentrations of carbonic anhydrase II, which potentially increases seizure susceptibility, are upregulated in the brains of young children with DS and in a mouse model of the disorder. (Palminello et al., 2008) (Tatsuno et al., 1984).

Altered membrane potassium permeability, which may lead to a decreased voltage threshold for spike generation, smaller hyperpolarization following spikes, or increased action potential duration, has also been documented in patients with DS. Indeed, in the mouse model of trisomy 16, the experimental model of DS, a rapid spike rise and fall was recorded from the dorsal root ganglia neurons (Scott et al., 1981)

In DS there is an overexpression of the 21st chromosome. Many enzymes that are encoded on the extra 21st chromosome are known to be actively transcribed, which results in overexpression of the enzymes, overconsumption of enzymatic substrates and overproduction of metabolic end-products. For example, the superoxide dismutase-1 gene on the 21st chromosome is approximately 50% overexpressed, which decreases levels of superoxide (the enzyme's substrate) and increases levels of hydrogen peroxide (the enzyme's metabolite, end product or output). These primary consequences of genetic overexpression may then produce secondary metabolic adaptations as homeostatic systems attempt to compensate. Thus, decreased levels of superoxide might alter levels of nitric oxide, peroxynitrate, and nitric oxide synthetase, or they may impair aromatic hydroxylation enzymes and thereby impair neurotransmitter synthesis. For another example, increased levels of hydrogen peroxide might induce glutathione peroxidase production and thereby increase selenium requirements. Such genetically driven enzymatic and metabolic disturbances may help explain why individuals with DS appear to be more likely to develop various forms of epilepsy and intractable epilepsy (Smigielska-Kuzia et al. 2009).

Seizures can also be regarded as complications of congenital cardiovascular anomalies in children with DS (Marsh et al., 2009). Moyamoya's disease is a rare vascular complication which seems to occur with a higher frequency in children with DS than in those without it. Moyamoya's disease is characterised by a chronic occlusive cerebrovascular alteration of unknown pathogenesis in which there is progressive stenosis of the supraclinoid portions of the internal carotid arteries. Associated with this stenosis is the formation of convoluted arterial collaterals at the base of the brain. Although the presentation of Moyamoya's disease in adults is haemorrhagic, the presenting symptoms in children are typically ischaemic, with a fixed unilateral neurological deficit or alternating hemiplegia. Some children with Down's syndrome who have Moyamoya's disease also develop seizures or involuntary movements. (Nascimento et al. 2006).

Adult-onset seizures in the absence of dementia are rare in people with DS but might become more frequent in the future because of the extension of the lifespan of people with the disorder. Late-onset seizures in people with DS seem to be associated with a propensity to dementia resembling Alzheimer's disease. The cause of seizures in adults with DS who do not have dementia is not yet clear (Puri, 2001)

Once seizures occur in the course of dementia in patients with DS, functional decline is often rapid, to the point where floor effects preclude further cognitive testing. Seizures are common in people with early-onset Alzheimer's disease associated with genetic defects, including mutations that result in overexpression of amyloid-β, such as those involving presenilin 1 genes. Animals with overexpression of the APP gene have a lower threshold to induced seizures. High concentrations of amyloid-β caused by APP overexpression result in epileptiform activity in vivo, even in the absence of neurodegeneration, suggesting that these high concentrations are a direct cause of epilepsy. (T Llot 2010).

4. Clinical and electrophysiological features

Epilepsy in DS showed a bimodal distribution; in the younger age group, infantile spasms and tonic-clonic seizures with myoclonus are the main finding, whereas older patients often have partial simplex or partial complex seizures as well as tonic-clonic seizures (Pueschel et al., 1991).

4.1 Seizures in infancy and childhood

It is currently known that there is a higher incidence of seizures, particularly infantile spasms, in DS compared to the general population. Few children with DS have their first epileptic attacks after the age of 3. These patients often have partial simplex or partial complex seizures as well as tonic-clonic seizures.

Infantile spasms are an age-dependent epilepsy that most frequently appears in the first year of life, with ictal episodes consisting of spasms that usually occur in clusters (Dulac et al., 1994). There is a characteristic chaotic and high-voltage interictal electroencephalography (EEG) pattern, which, when typical, is called hypsarrhythmia. *West's syndrome* is the term employed when such spasms are concomitant with delayed psychomotor development and EEG hypsarrhythmia. It has been reported that 6.4% of 737 patients with DS had epilepsy, and 12.8% of epileptic patients with DS had West syndrome. In addition, it has been reported that 8.1% of 405 patients with DS had epilepsy in childhood, and 18% of the epileptic patients were diagnosed as having infantile spasms.

Infantile spasms, which often indicate poor prognosis in the general population, do not seem to be associated with difficulties in long-term seizure control in children with DS. However, in children with DS who have infantile spasms, there seems to be a substantial association between treatment and developmental quotient as well as progression to autistic features. There are no long-term studies of the intellectual outcome of children with DS in whom infantile spasms were successfully controlled. In our experience, patients with Down syndrome with infantile spasms and abnormal but non-hypsarrhythmic EEG may have poor disease progression (figure 1 a and b & Figure 2 a and b), with persistence of seizures and severely impaired psychomotor development (Nascimento & Ortez 2009).

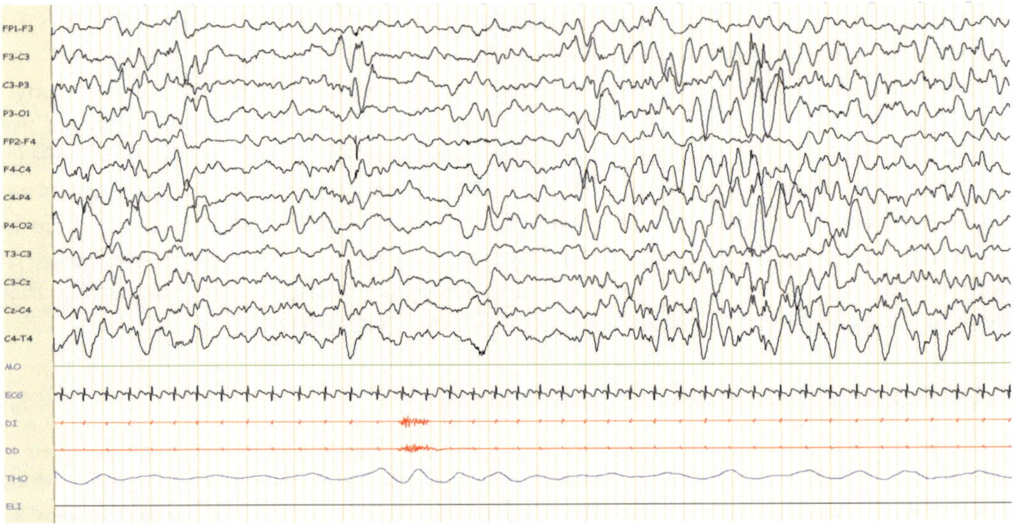

a)

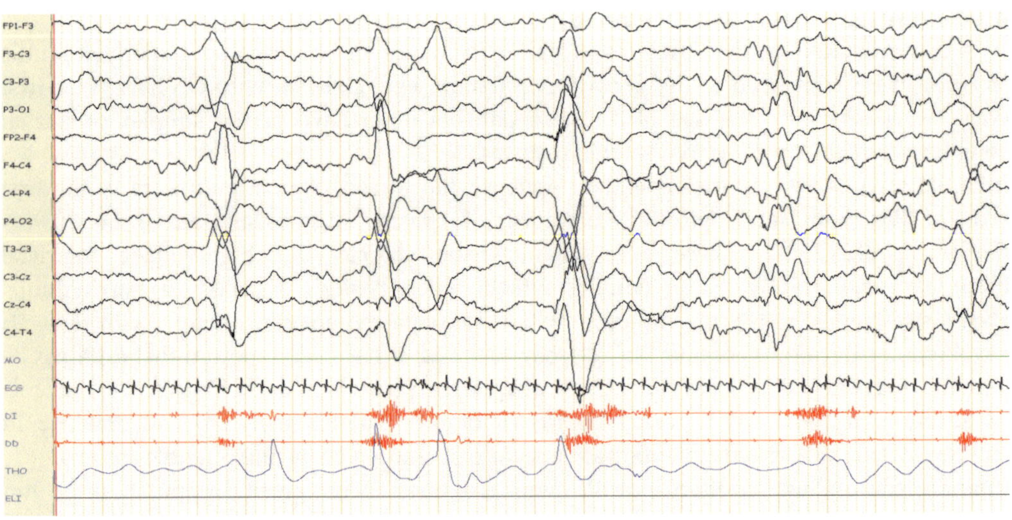

b)

Fig. 1. EEG of an 8m21d boy with DS. a) In a sleep stage, no physiological graphoelements were observed and there were very frequent multifocal paroxysms in the form of high-voltage spike-wave complexes; paroxistic alterations persisted during the waking stage. b) There was an electroclinical episode consisting of the emergence of a high-voltage spike-wave complex clinically accompanied by extension and abduction of the upper limbs and a slight extension of the lower limbs. Note the contraction recorded over both deltoid muscles.

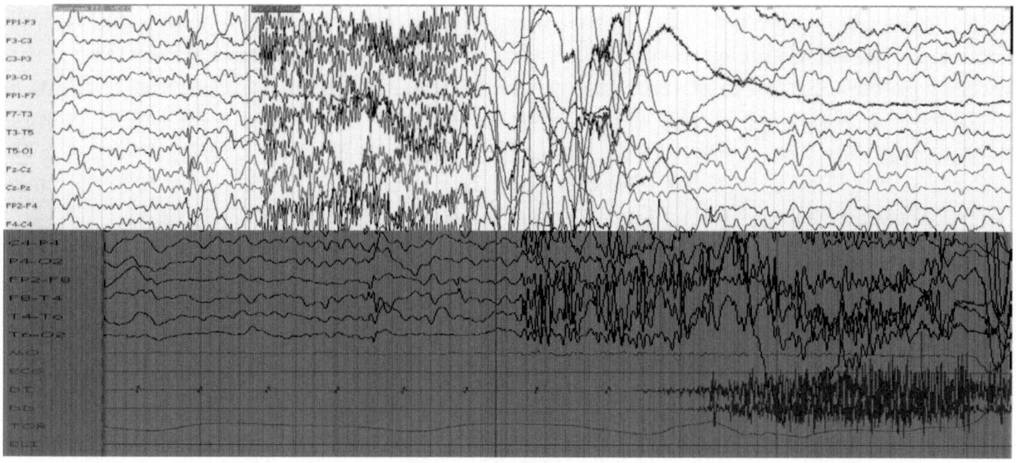

a)

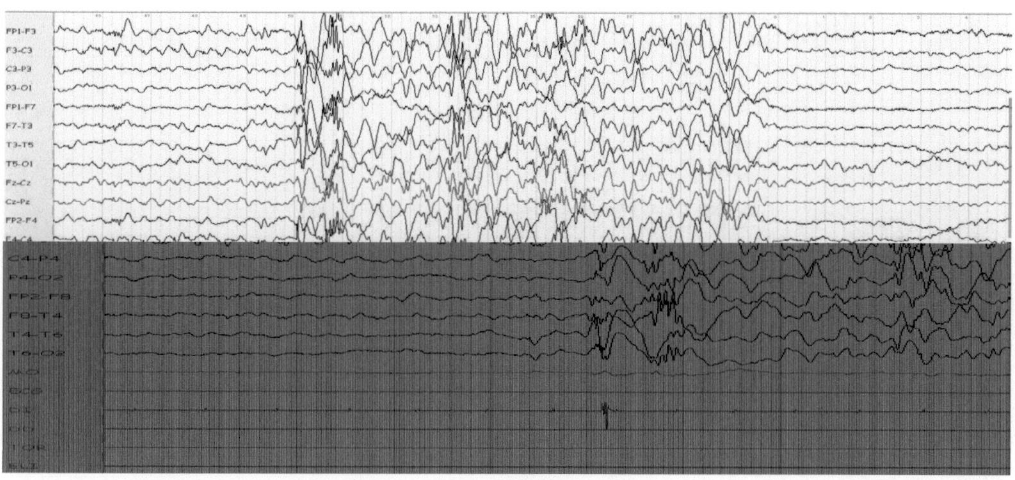

b)

Fig. 2. EEG of a 3-year-old girl with DS initially affected by West's syndrome who then evolved to Lennox-Gastaut syndrome. a) Tonic seizure: Ictal electroencephalography (EEG) shows a diphasic, mid-voltage slow wave, followed by recruiting low-voltage fast activity, replaced by spike and polyspike and wave discharges; tonic contraction was recorded over both deltoid muscles. b) Waking stage: brain activity constituted by an association of delta and theta waves and low-voltage beta rhythms, with a diffuse distribution. Frequent focal paroxysms were observed in the form of spikes and complex spike-waves of irregular medium and high amplitude, located independently in the frontal and parieto-occipital regions of both hemispheres.

There is a chance that DS in association with West's syndrome may evolve to Lennox-Gastaut syndrome (LGS). LGS has classically been defined by the triad of drug-resistant epilepsy with multiple seizure types, typically diurnal atonic as well as atypical absences, and mainly nocturnal tonic seizures; electroencephalography abnormalities, principally diffuse slow spike-wave or polyspike-wave discharges during wakefulness and bursts of diffuse fast rhythms at 10–20 Hz during sleep; mental deterioration of variable severity as well as behavioural disturbances may also occur (Gastaut et al., 1966; Dulac & N'Guyen, 1993). A series of DS patients with late onset LGS has been described, having a higher frequency of reflex seizures and more cognitive impairment (Figure 3). (Ferlazzo et al., 2009)

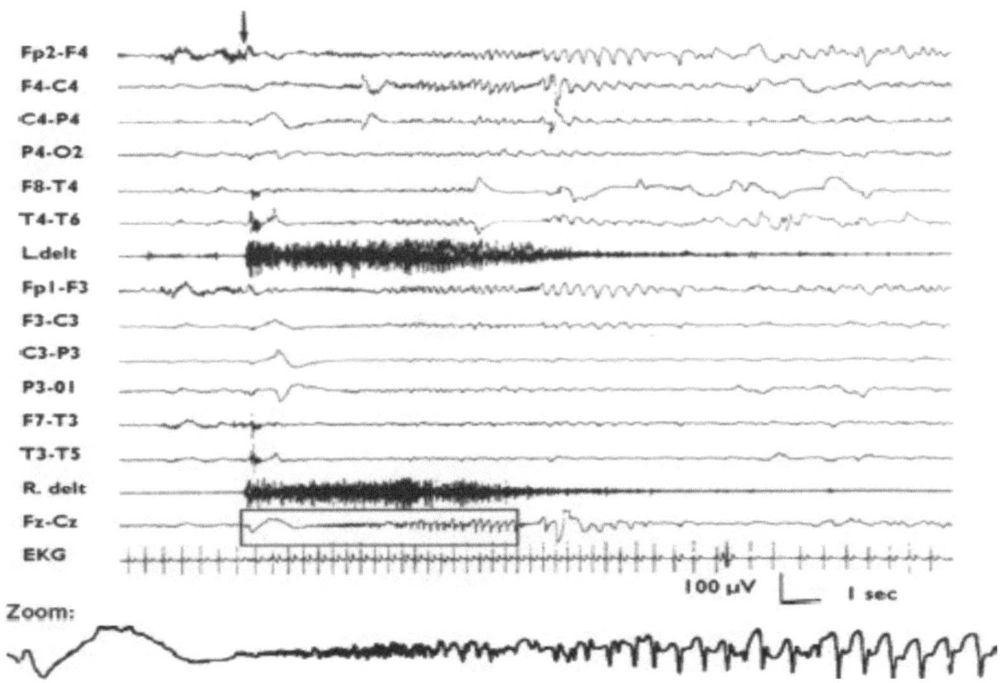

Fig. 3. 7-year-old boy. Tonic seizure triggered by a sudden noise (black arrow). Note the marked tonic contraction recorded over both deltoid muscles. Ictal electroencephalography (EEG) shows a diphasic, mid-voltage slow wave, followed by recruiting low-voltage fast activity, replaced by spike and polyspike and wave discharges, predominant over anterior leads, lasting for about 10 s. Electrocardiography shows an increased heart rate during seizure. Zoom: detail of the ictal discharge recorded over the vertex derivation, where muscular artifacts are less evident. (Ferlazzo et al. 2009)

Why do some infants with DS develop infantile spasms, whereas others with the same disorder do not? The cause has never been fully understood. Naming DS as the "cause" of the infantile spasms may, therefore, be at best inaccurate and at worst totally misleading, suggesting that we understand why the disorder has arisen in that particular child when DS has merely predisposed the child to infantile spasms. Only a few infants with Down syndrome develop infantile spasms, yet Down syndrome is accepted (Eisermann et al., 2003) as a "cause," and frequently such infants are not given a brain scan. As a result, other authors have proposed adopting a terminology that distinguishes the underlying etiology from the cause. According to this scheme, we use the term *proven etiology* to refer to any identified underlying neurological disorder, and employ *cause* as a more specific term that may be a complex and less well-understood sequence or combination of events. Perhaps because of the many different diagnoses that can be made in these infants and the developmental outcomes associated with them, classification into diagnostic groups has been commonly attempted. (Osborne et al., 2010)

The most frequent nomenclature has classified cases as either symptomatic, cryptogenic, or idiopathic, but unfortunately there is no clear definition of these terms (Lux & Osborne, 2005). "Symptomatic" is often used to indicate that a prior disorder exists. "Cryptogenic" is often used to mean that there must be an etiology, but that one has not been found. A recent report of the International League Against Epilepsy (ILAE) Commission on Classification and Terminology also suggests that the terms idiopathic, symptomatic, and cryptogenic should be replaced (Berg et al., 2010). It has suggested broad etiologic categories: genetic, structural–metabolic, and unknown.

4.2 Seizure in adulthood

The prevalence of epilepsy in DS has increased with longevity, reaching 46% in those older than 50. Descriptions of late-onset epilepsy in the absence of dementia in DS patients (LOMEDS) are rare, but since life expectancy of DS patients has markedly increased, LOMEDS may be more frequent than currently acknowledged and should be considered in the differential diagnosis of adult-onset myoclonic epilepsies. The electroclinical features are myoclonic jerks on awakening and generalised tonic-clonic seizures, with generalised spike and wave on EEG, and progressive dementia (Moller et al., 2002).

Familial Alzheimer's dementia (FAD) and progressive myoclonic epilepsy (Unverricht-Lundborg type) are both linked to chromosome 21. In an interesting study of 68 DS adults, it was found that among those with a history of seizures, individuals aged over 45 years were significantly more likely to develop AD than those under 45, and up to 84% of demented individuals with DS developed seizures. It suggests that late-onset epilepsy in DS is associated with AD, while early-onset epilepsy is associated with an absence of dementia (Menéndez, 2005).

Seizures in adults with DS differ from those in adults with Alzheimer's disease who do not have DS: myoclonic seizures usually occur late in the course of Alzheimer's disease whereas partial or tonic–clonic seizures occur in adults with Down's syndrome and are often precursors to cognitive decline. Adults with DS aged over 45 years who have seizures are substantially more likely to develop signs of Alzheimer's disease (Puri et al; 2001). Once seizures occur in the course of dementia in patients with DS, functional decline is often rapid, to the point where floor effects preclude further cognitive testing. Seizures are common in people with early-onset Alzheimer's disease associated with genetic defects, including mutations that result in overexpression of amyloid-β, such as those involving presenilin 1 genes.

Animals with overexpression of the *APP* gene have a lower threshold to induced seizures. High concentrations of amyloid-β caused by *APP* overexpression result in epileptiform activity in vivo, even in the absence of neurodegeneration, suggesting these high concentrations directly as a cause of aberrant neuronal network synchronisation. Slowing of the dominant occipital rhythm seems to be associated with dementia in individuals with DS, and the frequency of dominant occipital activity decreases as cognition deteriorates.

4.3 Seizure in Alzheimer´s and DS

Despite the apparent clinical heterogeneity in aged individuals with DS, age-associated AD-like neuropathology is a consistent feature. This is due to the fact that trisomy 21 leads to a dose-dependent increase in the production of the APP and subsequently the production of the amyloidogenic fragments leading to early and predominant senile plaque formation.

Ten percent of patients with AD have seizures, and another 10% have myoclonus. The incidence of seizures is about 10 times higher than expected in a reference population. Both seizures and myoclonus, individually or together, are manifestations of AD and may be seen at any time in the course of the illness, but myoclonus is often a late manifestation. (Volicer et al., 1995)

4.4 Electroencephalography (EEG) features

Individuals with DS have increased absolute power in all the EEG bands, independent of cognition functions. In the power spectrum of the resting EEG, there is a cognition-related increase in power at theta- and alpha-slowing. Furthermore, in the stimulated EEG, there are several cognition-related abnormalities, such as decreased responses to 12-Hz stimulation and decreased integral of beta- and gamma-band responses, indicative of decreased responsiveness to photic stimulation. Other reports note an increase in power at theta and delta in children with DS during sleep. (S'migielska-Kuzia et al., 2009). There is a significant increase in theta, delta, and beta power and a decrease in alpha compared with non-DS with epilepsy. (Figure 3)

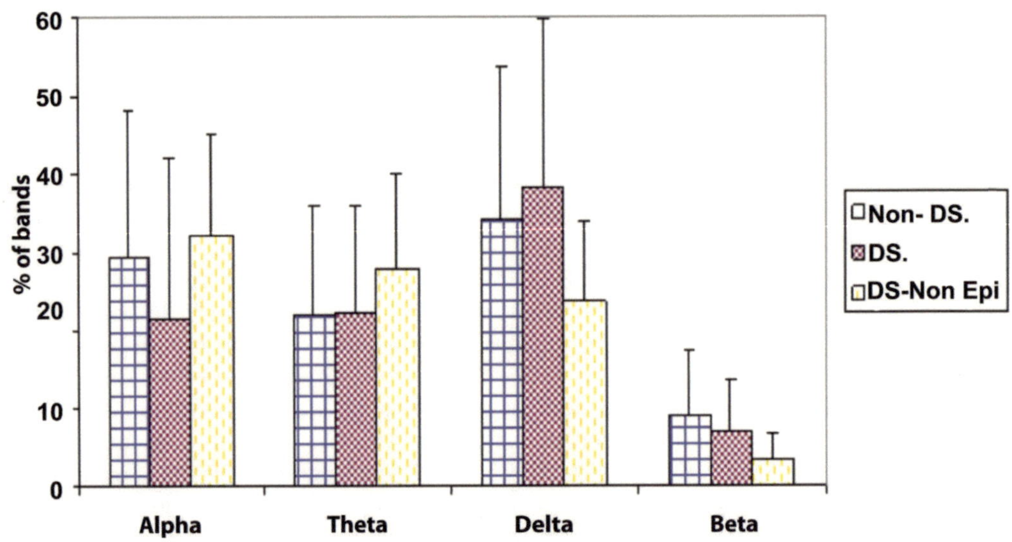

Fig. 3. Spectral power of alpha, theta, delta, and beta bands of DS, n = 12, DS Non-Epilepsy (Non-Epi) n=10 versus Non-DS (epileptic children) n = 28. Alpha Non-DS versus alpha DS P < .001; alpha Non-DS versus alpha DS Non-Epi P = .001; alpha DS versus alpha DS Non-Epi P < .001; theta Non-DS versus theta DS P = .767; theta Non-DS versus theta DS Non-Epi P < .001; theta DS versus theta DS Non-Epi P < .001; delta Non-DS versus delta DS P < .001; delta Non-DS versus delta DS Non-Epi P < .001; delta DS versus delta DS Non-Epi P < .001;beta Non-DS versus beta DS P < .001; beta Non-DS versus beta DS Non-Epi P < .001; beta DS versus beta DS Non-Epi P < .001. (S'migielska-Kuzia et al., 2009)

5. Treatment of epilepsy in DS

The pharmacological treatment of epilepsy in DS is no different from that of other patients diagnosed with epilepsy; the key is proper clinical and electrical classification to guide epilepsy treatment and thereby obtain good therapeutic results.

Although the cognitive profiles of newer antiepileptic drugs (AEDs) are in general better than those of older antiepileptic drugs, neurological adverse events do occur, including somnolence, distractibility, dizziness, and an altered pattern of sleep architecture. Individuals with DS have an unusually high number of side-effects from phenytoin (Tsiouris et al., 2002).

Over time, with the advent of advances in molecular biology, many AEDs have been uncovered, so they have come to be classified as first-, second- and third-generation drugs. (see table 2)

1ª. Generation	2ª. Generation	3ª.Generation
Valproat	Felbamate	Rufinamide
Phenobarbital	Gabapentine	Safinamide
Carbamazepine	Oxcarbamazepine	Eslicarbamazepine
Ethosuximide	Topiramate	Licarbamazepine
Benzodiacepine	Lamotrigine	Estirepentol
Phenytoin	Zonisamide	Bribaracetam, etc.
	Levetiracetam	
	Pregabalin	
	Vigabatrin	

Table 2. Antipileptica drugs by generation

Figures 4 a & b and table 3 describe the different mechanisms of action demonstrated for antiepileptic drugs (AEDs).

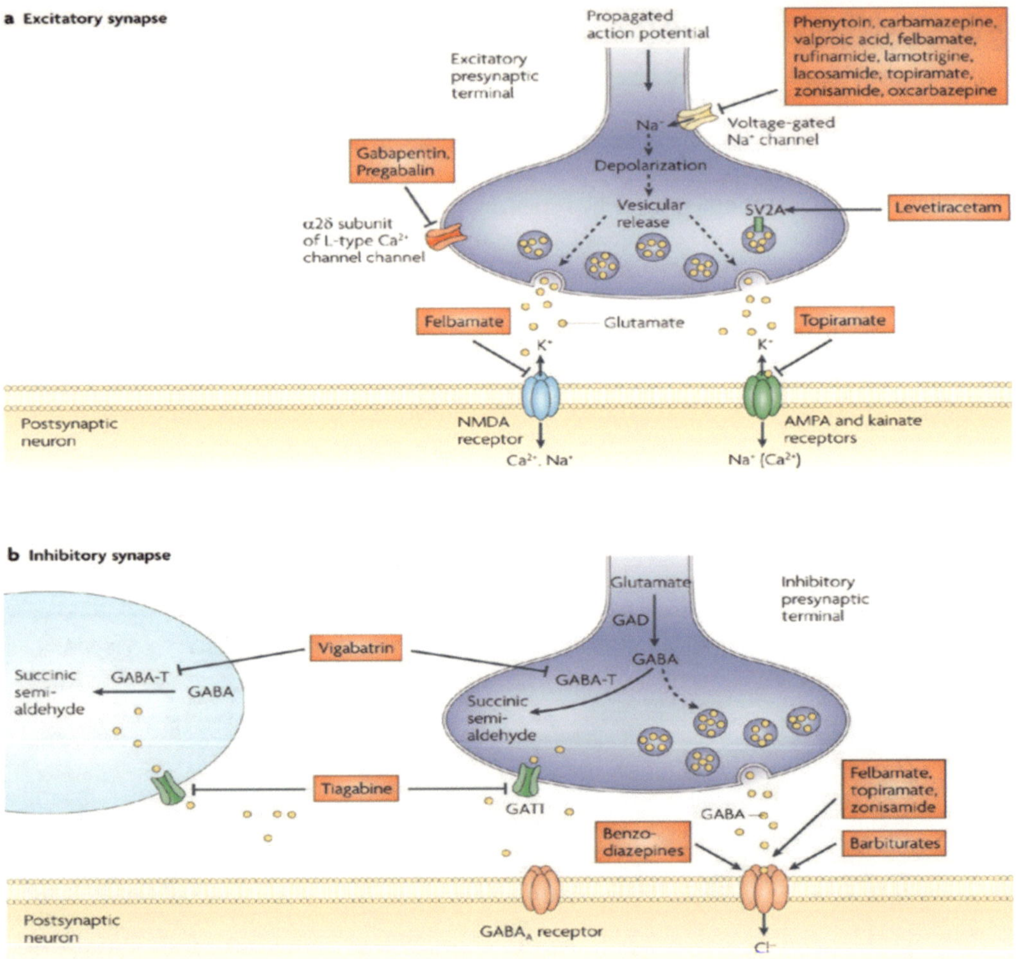

Fig. 4. a& b Proposed mechanisms of action of currently available AEDs at excitatory and inhibitory synapses.

a | Currently available antiepileptic drugs (AEDs) are thought to target several molecules at the excitatory synapse. These include voltage-gated Na^+ channels, synaptic vesicle glycoprotein 2A (SV2A), the α2δ subunit of the voltage-gated Ca^{2+} channel, AMPA (α-amino-3-hydroxy-5-methyl-4-isoxazole propionic acid) receptors, and NMDA (*N*-methyl-D-aspartate) receptors. Many of the AEDs can modulate voltage-gated Na^+ channels. This would be expected to decrease depolarization-induced Ca^+ influx and vesicular release of neurotransmitters. In addition, lacosamide is thought to enhance slow inactivation of voltage-gated Na^+ channels. This effect is different from that of other listed AEDs, which are thought to enhance fast inactivation. Levetiracetam is the only available drug that binds to SV2A, which might have a role in neurotransmitter release. Gabapentin and pregabalin bind to the a2δ subunit of voltage-gated Ca^{2+} channels, which is thought to be associated with a decrease in neurotransmitter release. Excitatory neurotransmission at the postsynaptic membrane can be limited by topiramate (acting on AMPA and kainate receptors) and felbamate (acting on NMDA receptors).

b | AED targets at inhibitory synapses have also been proposed. These include the g-aminobutyric acid (GABA) transporter GAT1 (also known as SLC6A1), which is inhibited by tiagabine, leading to a decrease in GABA uptake into presynaptic terminals and surrounding glia; and GABA transaminase (GABA-T), which is irreversibly inhibited by vigabatrin. This decreases the metabolism of GABA in presynaptic terminals and glial cells. The benzodiazepines, barbiturates, topiramate and felbamate have been found to enhance inhibitory neurotransmission by allosterically modulating $GABA_A$ receptor-mediated Cl^- currents. However, the action of each of these drugs is different and is dependent on the subunit conformation of the $GABA_A$ receptor complex. GAD, glutamic acid decarboxylase. (Bailer & White 2010).

	Blockade of voltage-dependent sodium channels	Increase in brain or synaptic GABA levels	Selective potentiation of $GABA_A$-mediated responses	Direct facilitation or chloride-ion influx	Blockade of calcium channels	Other actions
First generation AEDs.						
Benzodiazepines	-	-	++	-	-	-
Carbamazepine	++	?	-	-	+	+
Ethosuximide	-	-	-	-	++	-
Phenobarbital	-	+	+	++	?	+
Phenytoin	++	-	-	-	?	+
Valproic acid	?	+	?	-	+	++
Second generation AEDs.						
Felbamate	++	+	+	-	+	+
Gabapentin	?	?	-	-	++	?
Lamotrigine	++	+	-	-	++	+
Levetiracetam	-	?	+	-	+	++
Oxcarbamacepine	++	?	-	-	+	+
Pregabalin	-	-	-	-	++	-
Tiagabaline	-	++	-	-	-	-
Topiramate	++	+	+	-	+	+
Vigabatrin	-	++	-	-	-	-
Zonisamide	++	?	-	-	++	+

++ primary action; + secundari action; -, no action described; ?, controversial evidence.

Table 3. Main Mechanism of action of AEDs.

Table 4 describes the different AEDs and the main indication for the type of epilepsy diagnosed. Table 5 describes the AEDs, dose in children and adults and side effects.

FIRST GENERATION AEDs	MAIN INDICATION
Benzodiazepines	Status epilpeticus. Partial an generalizated seizures
Carbamazepine	Partial seizures (with and whithout secondary generalization) and primarily generalized tonic-clonic seizures.
Ethosuximide	Absence seizures, continuous spike – waves during slow sleep.
Phenytoin	Partial seizures (with and whithout secondary generalization) and primarily generalized tonic-clonic seizures. Status epilepticus.
Valproic acid	Generalized and partial seizures. Status epilepticus.
SECOND GENERATION AEDs	MAIN INDICATION
Felbamate	Severe epilepsies, particulary Lennox-Gastaut syndrome, refractory to all other AEDs.
Gabapentin	Partial seizures (with and whithout secondary generalization)
Lamotrigine	Partial and generalized seizures (may aggravate severe myoclonic epilepsy of infancy)
Levetiracetam	Partial and probably generalized seizures.
Oxcarbamacepine	Partial seizures (with and whithout secondary generalization) and primarily generalized tonic-clonic seizures.
Pregabalin	Partial seizures (with and whithout secondary generalization).
Tiagabaline	Partial seizures (with and whithout secondary generalization).
Topiramate	Partial and generalized seizures (efficacy against absence seizures not proven)
Vigabatrin	Infantile spasms and West Sindrome. Partial seizure (with and whithout secondary generalization) refractory to all other AEDs.
Zonisamide	Partial and, probably, generalized seizures.

Table 4. AEDs and the main indication for the type of epilepsy diagnosed

AEDs	Childrens Dose mg/kg/d	Adults Dose mg/day.	Side Effects.
Carbamacepine	15-30	600 – 2000 mg divided into up to 4 doses a day.	Skin rash, if allergic to carbamazepine. Diplopia (double vision), ataxia (unsteadiness) and nausea may occur initially or if the dose is too high.
Clobazam	0,1-0,2	20 - 50 mg divided into 1 or 2 doses a day.	Drowsiness may occur but this drug is less sedating than clonazepam or diazepam. Tolerance may develop.
Clonazepam	0,5-0,8	1 – 4 mg divided into 2 doses a day.	Drowsiness and sedation are quite common but these may wear off.
Ethosuximide	20-35	750 – 1500 mg divided into 2 or 3 doses a day.	Nausea and drowsiness may occur initially or if the dose is too high. Anorexia (weight loss).
Gabapentine	30	1800 – 3600 mg divided into 3 doses a day.	Drowsiness, dizziness, and headache
Levetiracetam	20-60	1000 – 3000 mg divided into 2 doses a day.	Dizziness, drowsiness, irritability, behavioural problems, insomnia, ataxia (unsteadiness), tremor, headache, nausea may occur in high dosages or when doses are increased, but will usually disappear after a few days.
Lamotrigine	5-15 1-5 + VPA	100 - 200mg if taken alone or if also taking sodium valproate. 200 – 400 mg if also taking phenytoin ,	Skin rash if allergic to lamotrigine. Drowsiness, diplopia (double vision), dizziness, headache,

AEDs	Childrens Dose mg/kg/d	Adults Dose mg/day.	Side Effects.
		phenobarbitone or carbamazepine.	insomnia, tremor and flu-like symptoms.
Oxcarbamazepine	15-30	1200 - 2400mg divided into 2 or 3 doses a day.	Skin rash, if allergic to oxcarbazepine. Diplopia (double vision), ataxia (unsteadiness), headache, nausea, confusion and vomiting.
Phenobarbital	3-5	30 – 180 mg divided into 2 doses a day.	Drowsiness may occur initially. Lethargy, sedation and slowing of mental performance may be long-lasting.
Phenytoin	5-10	150 – 600 mg divided into 1 or 2 doses a day.	Skin rash if allergic to phenytoin. Drowsiness, ataxia (unsteadiness) and slurred speech may occur if the dose is too high. Coarsening of facial features, overgrowth of gums, excess hair growth and acne may occur with prolonged therapy (over many years), as can some anaemias.
Topiramate	5-9	Up to 400 mg daily if taken alone. Usually 200 – 400 mg daily if taken with other anti-epileptic drugs, up to 800 mg.	Headache, drowsiness, dizziness, paraesthesia (pins and needles in hands and feet), loss of weight, and kidney stones. Speech disorder, impaired memory and concentration may occur when dose is increased

AEDs	Childrens Dose mg/kg/d	Adults Dose mg/day.	Side Effects.
			but will usually disappear after a few days.
Sodium valproate	20-50	400 - 2000 mg divided into 1 or 2 doses a day.	Drowsiness and tremor are infrequent side effects. Hair loss occurs in some people but is not usually severe and is usually reversible if the dose is reduced. Weight gain may occur. Liver. damage is rare. Sodium valproate has been associated with increased incidence of Polycystic Ovary Syndrome and menstrual irregularitiesthan other AEDs, if taken in pregnancy.
Vigabatrine	50-200	1000 – 4000 mg divided into 1 or 2 doses a day.	Drowsiness, behaviour and mood changes. Psychotic reactions have been reported. Visual field defects have been reported in one in three people taking vigabatrin in the long term.
Zonizamide	4-8	300 - 500mg divided into 1 or 2 doses a day.	Skin rash if allergic to zonisamide. Drowsiness, dizziness, weight loss, kidney stones, confusion, cognitive slowing, agitation, irritability, depression,

Table 5. AEDs, dose in children and adults. Side effects.

6. Conclusions

The findings of the last decade regarding the significant percentage of children with DS and epilepsy (approximately 1 in 10) highlight the importance of the awareness that physicians should start developing about this association so that they can intervene as early as possible when seizures are suspected, to maximize the patient's development and improve quality of life as much as possible.

The diagnosis, classification and treatment of epilepsy in DS must follow the guidelines applied to the general population.

Children with DS have a greater predisposition to epilepsy (specifically to West Syndrome and infantile spasms) attributed to structural and molecular abnormalities. In contrast, in adults with DS, epilepsy is associated with the accumulation of amyloid-β, due to the expression of APP that is observed in DS patients with early-onset Alzheimer-like dementia.

The prognosis of patients with DS and epilepsy will depend on several factors: type of epilepsy, age of initiation, etiology, early diagnosis and treatment's response. Epilepsy in patients with DS, as well as in the general population, in most cases represents an alteration of brain function that can be detrimental to neurological development; this produces a great amount of anxiety and concern in their parents and relatives. For this reason, all of the prognostic factors must be carefully taken into account when considering each individual case. The disease, its control and its management should be discussed in a clear and simple way with the family.

7. Acknowledgments

We would like to express our gratitude to all the patients with DS and their families; to the Library's department of the Fundació Catalana Sindrome de Down whom have made a good work in the translation of this chapter; to the members of the Epilepsy Unit from the Neurolgy Service of Sant Joan de Dèu's Hospital and to our families for their support and time.

8. Reference

Bittles AH, Bower C, Hussain R & Glasson EJ. (2007). The four ages of Down syndrome. *European Journal of Public Health* Vol. 17, No 1, pp 221–25.

Corbett JA, Harris R & Robinson R (1975). Mental retardation and developmental disabilities. In: Wortis J, editor. Epilepsy, New York: Bruner/ Mazel, 1975. pp. 70–111.

Down JLH. (1886). Observations on an ethnic classification of idiots. *London Hosp Clin Lectures Rep* Vol.3, pp. 259–262.

Ferlazzo E Adjien CK, Guerrini R, Calarese T, Crespel A, Elia M, Striano P, Gelisse P, Bramanti P, di Bella P & Genton P. (2009). Lennox-Gastaut syndrome with late-onset and prominent reflex seizures in trisomy 21 patients. Epilepsia. Vol. 50, No.6 , pp 1587-95.

Lott IT & Dierssen M. (2010) Cognitive deficits and associated neurological complications in individuals with Down's syndrome. *Lancet Neurology*; Vol.9, No 6l, pp: 623–33.

Marsh ED & Golden JA (2009). Developing an animal model for infantile spasms: pathogenesis, problems and progress. *Disease Model & Mechanism*. Vol. 2, No. 7, pp 329–35

Menéndez M. (2005) Down syndrome, Alzheimer's disease and seizures. *Brain & Development*. Vol. 6, No. 5, pp 246–252

Moller JC, Hamer HM, Oertel WH & Rosenow F (2002). Late-onset myoclonic epilepsy in Down's syndrome (LOMEDS). *Seizure* . Vol.11, Sup. A, pp 303–5.

Nascimento A, Navarro R, Colomer J & Sola T. (2006) Moyamoya síndrome associated with Down Sindrome: clinical and radiological features. *International Medical Review on Down Sindrome* Vol.10, No. 3 pp 7-11.

Nascimento, A & Ortez, O (2009) Infantile spasms in Downs's syndrome. *International Medical Review on Down Sindrome* Vol.13, No. 2 pp 22-24.

Osborne J, Lux AL, Edwards SW, Hancock E, Johnson AL, Kennedy CR, Newton RW, Verity CM & O'Callaghan FJ. (2010). The underlying etiology of infantile spasms (West syndrome):Information from the United Kingdom Infantile Spasms Study (UKISS) on contemporary causes and their classification. *Epilepsia*. Vol.51 , No.10 , pp 2168-74.

Palminiello S, Kida E, Kaur K, Walus M, Wisniewski KE, Wierzba-Bobrowicz T, Rabe A, Albertini G & Golabek AA. (2008). Increased levels of carbonic anhydrase II in the developing Down syndrome brain. *Brain Research* Vol.1190, No.23, pp 193–205.

Pueschel SM , Louis S & McKnight P (1991) Seizure disorders in Down syndrome. *Archive of Neurology* Vol. 48, No 1, pp 318–20.

Puri BK, Ho KW & Singh I. (2001). Age of seizure onset in adults with Down's syndrome. *International Journal of Clinical Practice* 2001; Vol. 55, No 7, pp 442–44.

Romano C, Tiné A, Fazio G, Rizzo R, Colognola RM, Sorge G, Bergonzi P & Pavone L. (1990). Seizures in patients with trisomy 21. *American Journal of Medical Genetics Supplement*. Vol. 7, No. ,pp 298–300.

Scott BS, Petit TL, Becker LE & Edwards BA.. (1981) Abnormal electric membrane properties of Down's syndrome DRG neurons in cell culture. *Brain Research*.Vol.254, No.2, pp 257-270.

S ´ migielska-Kuzia J, .Sobaniec W, Kułak W & Boćkowski L. (2009). Clinical and EEG Features of Epilepsy in Children and Adolescents in Down Syndrome. *Journal of Child Neurology* Vol. 24, No. 4 pp 416-420.

S ´ migielska-Kuzia J, Sobaniec W, Kułak W, Boćkowski L & Sołowiej E. (2005) Quantitative EEG analysis of REM sleep in children with Down syndrome. *Advances in Medical Science*. Vol.50, No. 1 pp 20-22.

Stafstrom CE, Patxot OF, Gilmore HE & Wisniewski KE (1991). Seizures in children with Down syndrome: etiology, characteristics and outcome. *Developmental Medicine and Child Neurology*. Vol.33, No. 3, pp191–200.

Tatsuno M, Hayashi M, Iwamoto H, Suzuki H & Kuroki Y. (1984). Epilepsy in childhood Down syndrome. *Brain & Development*, Vol.6; No.1, pp 37–44

Tsiouris JA, Patti PJ, Tipu O & Raguthu S. (2002). Adverse eff ects of phenytoin given for late-onset seizures in adults with Down syndrome. *Neurology*. Vol. 59, No.5, 779-80.

Volicer L, Smith S & Volicer BJ. (1995). Effect of seizures on progression of dementia of the Alzheimer type. *Dementia.* Vol. 6, No. 5, pp 258-63.

14

Endocrine and Autonomic Nervous Adaptations during Physical Exercise in Down Syndrome

Véronique ~ Aurélie Bricout
CHU Sud de Grenoble, UF Recherches Cliniques,Université Joseph Fourier UFRAPS, Laboratoire HP2, Grenoble France

1. Introduction

One of the goals of Healthy People 2011 is to increase the quality of life and the years of healthy life of all citizens. As the life expectancy of people with Down Syndrome [DS] increases, changes in body function and structure due to ageing may lead to lead to activity limitations and participation restrictions for this population. The physical conditions seen in people with DS include endocrine dysfunction, cardiovascular disorders, obesity, and musculoskeletal disorders (Finesilver, 2002; Thompson, 1999). These physical problems can have a negative impact on the quality of life, regarding both professional and leisure activities.

Compared with their peers who are not mentally retarded, individuals with DS, regardless of their age, have lower cardiovascular fitness levels (Horvat & Croce, 1995; Tsimaras et al., 2003). This lower level of cardiovascular fitness may be the result of poor eating habits, a sedentary lifestyle, a lack of opportunity for recreational activities, a poor coordination, and a poor motivation for physical activity. In addition, the lack of cardiovascular fitness may be due to or caused by the high obesity rates observed among adults with mental retardation (Draheim et al., 2002). Poor cardiovascular fitness levels also may contribute to an increased risk of heart disease and stroke in adults with mental retardation (Sutherland et al., 2002).

Therefore, involvement in cardiovascular conditioning programs would seem to be essential, however, can the cardiovascular fitness levels of these individuals, be improved with exercise, without major health risks?

If exercise programs seem to be likely to improve the health of adults with DS, thereby increasing their quality of life and life expectancy, yet further research is needed to investigate the effects of exercise on adults, because some autonomic nervous regulations and endocrine adaptations are known to be inadequate in individuals with DS (Baynard et al., 2004; Figueroa et al., 2005; Iellamo et al., 2005; Gouloupoulou et al., 2006; Bricout et al. 2008).

2. Situation of the subject in international literature

One hypothesis explaining the improvements in life expectancy of DS individuals is based on the physical stimulation and psychological standing of these subjects (Eberhard et al., 1989; Draheim et al., 2002). Now, adults with trisomy 21 are living longer than previously and individuals surviving into their sixth or seventh decade of life are encountered (Prasher & Krishnan, 1993). So, there is a need for an overall assessment of the health of adults with trisomy 21, and specifically as the sport activities helps improve the quality of life, and reduce risk factors, it seems important to know the possible effects of physical exercise on the health of these young people with Down syndrome.

In this order, few studies have investigated cardiac and hormonal responses in patients with Down syndrome subjected to acute physical exercise (Murdoch, 1977; Murdoch et al. 1978; Fernhall & Otterstetter, 2003; Baynard et al., 2004; Iellamo et al., 2005; Figueroa et al., 2005; Gouloupoulou et al., 2006). The conclusions of these few studies show that there are inappropriate responses that lead to the appearance of early fatigue, a premature stop of the effort, and/or a limitation to the activity. It was previously suggested that fatigue during exercise, or at least premature stop or the incapacity to do prolonged physical exercise in DS subjects, may partly be explained by a dysfunction of the autonomic nervous system [ANS] (Baynard et al., 2004; Iellamo et al., 2005; Figueroa et al., 2005; Gouloupoulou et al., 2006).

Secondly, others studies have investigated the hormonal adaptation's in specific physical tests and the results of all these works agree to show that heart rate [HR] is lower (-7 to 15 beats per minute) in DS individuals. Specifically, numerous studies hypothesized that the lower catecholamine responses (epinephrine and norepinephrine) in DS population to maximal exercise could explain the weaker heart rate (Fernhall et al., 2009).

These observations are reinforced by the results of a work achieved by Eberhard et al., (1989, 1991) and Bricout et al., (2008) evaluating catecholamine's kinetics during and after exercise. These authors showed that the plasma concentrations of epinephrine and norepinephrine after an exercise on bicycle or on treadmill were lower in subjects with DS than in control subjects, and could partly explain the relatively low elevation of HR during exercise, named "chronotropic incompetence".

However, some others factors may explain the reduced aerobic capacity and the possible incapacity to long physical exercise in DS. If endocrine dysfunction, cardiovascular pathologies, obesity, and musculoskeletal disorders are now well established as limiting to do prolonged physical exercise, DS individuals were also not highly motivating to repeat exercise, which contributes to more easily adopt a sedentary lifestyle, because the effort can be quickly perceived as painful, difficult and without sense for them.

The mechanisms of exercise intolerance in trisomy 21 require further consideration and in particular the relationship between the sympathetic nervous system, hormonal system which its importance in the adaptation effort is crucial.

Thus, many studies confirm that DS subjects present some endocrine diseases, such as diabetes, hypothyroidism, and insulin resistance ... (Murdoch, 1977; Murdoch et al. 1978; Sharav et al., 1991; Sasagawa et al., 1993; Konings et al., 2001). In a study conducted at the University Hospital of Grenoble between 2003 and 2005, on 14 young adults with trisomy 21, some of these endocrine disorders at rest (hypothyroidism and hypogonadism) were confirmed.

During muscular effort, it was shown that the responses of the adrenal axis (cortisol and catecholamine) and gonadal axis (testosterone) especially are the most affected when exercise is prolonged. Indeed, with exercise, the elevated catecholamine response, classically described in healthy subjects (Galbo, 1985) is lower in DS patients, and it can be suggested that the decreased response of catecholamine during effort in DS subjects explains the lesser capacity of these subjects to perform a muscular exercise which intensity and duration rise (Nagaoka et al., 1996; Fernhall & Otterstetter, 2003,).

In addition, some studies show that in patients with Down syndrome without adrenal insufficiency, basal cortisol is always lower (Murdoch, 1977; Murdoch et al. 1978). The pathogenesis of this observation remains difficult to explain, although it may have metabolic and physiological implications. During muscular exercise, the elevation of plasma cortisol, classically described in healthy subjects does not occur in DS subjects (Eberhard et al., 1993; 1996). Several hypotheses may be advanced to explain this fact:

- insufficient effort in intensity and / or duration, for subjects with trisomy are very reluctant to make long efforts,
- a possible adrenal dysfunction, which yet, remains unlikely (Konings et al., 2001). A more general dysfunction of the hypothalamic-pituitary-adrenal could exist, but the lack of studies on the regulation of secretion of CRF and ACTH in Down syndrome does not allow us to reverse or confirm this hypothesis. If dys-regulation of the HPA axis to stress in DS individuals partly explains the difficulty to use free fatty acids as energy substrates, there may be other endocrine factors directly related to adipose tissue, such as leptin, or in connection with the gonadotropic through testosterone, and its lipolytic action (Galbo, 1985).

Moreover, Bricout et al., (2008) show that DS subjects are characterised by an absence of elevated glycaemia during prolonged exercise, contrary to what is observed in healthy controls (Galbo, 1985). In addition, the concentration of lactatemia rises less than in controls suggesting that the peripheral utilisation of glucose is impaired. Therefore, it seems highly relevant to examine whether the gluco-regulation during exercise is impaired by a dysfunction of the autonomic nervous system response and / or impaired secretion of catecholamines and / or balance insulin / glucagon imbalance; and to know its impact on exercise capacity.

Furthermore, results of maximal exercise test show that 4 in 14 subjects presented chronotropic incompetence, and that these patients have an altered metabolic profile (increased fat mass, alterations in leptin, insulin, cortisol and plasma catecholamine at rest and during exercise) suggesting the close link between chronotropic incompetence, abnormal metabolic profile and endocrine regulation. These points deserve to be confirmed by future studies.

Recently, Fernhall et al., (2009) have conducted a study on catecholamine response to maximal exercise in persons with Down syndrome. This work reported an adrenergic drive largely absent in DS group, even though a sharp increase in catecholamine at high exercise intensities is largely responsible for increase in HR above the anaerobic threshold. In conclusion, the authors showed significant differences in baroreceptor sensitivity between individuals with and without DS, but not between DS compared with controls, suggesting that altered baroreceptor sensitivity does not fully explain the blunted HR response in DS population.

3. Exercise limitations and chronotropic incompetence

Meanwhile, investigation methods of the sympathetic nervous system are now well known and described in literature to be applied in this context (Nagaoka et al., 1996; Grote et al., 2004; Gouloupoulou et al., 2006). The measurement of heart rate variability is a non invasive method to assess both parasympathetic and sympathetic nervous activities (Task Force, 1996). The application of this method has revealed abnormalities associated with abnormal fatigue in athletes (Furlan et al., 1993). It has recently been used in trisomy 21 at rest, exercise and orthostatic tests (Baynard et al., 2004; Fernhall et al., 2005; Iellamo et al., 2005; Figueroa et al., 2005).

The common hypothesis found in literature is that the individual with Down syndrome, has a reduced exercise capacity associated with chronotropic incompetence, expressed by maximum heart rate values (HRmax) decreased in response to a standardised exercise (Fernhall et al., 2001). Because peak exercise HR is correlated with age, the traditional approach has been to consider a patient as chronotropically incompetent when 85% of the age-predicted HR is achieved (Lauer, 2004). This measure is still confounded (Lauer et al., 1996) by resting HR and functional capacity, and Wilkoff & Miller, (1992) proposed the concept of HR reserve which is the difference between maximal predicted HR (or 220 beats /min minus the patient's age) and resting HR. Failure to use 80% of HR reserve constitutes chronotropic incompetence (Lauer et al., 1996).

In DS population, reduced HR response to prolonged exercise has been identified as the primary contributor to the low physical work capacity and cardiorespiratory fitness (Fernhall et al., 1996; 2001), but chronotropic incompetence is also an independent predictive factor of sudden death even in adult DS population without underlying coronary heart disease. Although it is debated (Guerra et al., 2003); understand the chronotropic incompetence in DS may be clinically relevant because it could partially explain the higher incidence of premature cardiac death in this population (Day et al., 2005).

Nevertheless, the mechanism of this alteration of cardiac response remains unknown, although dysregulation of the ANS appears to be the most probable explanation, by a decrease in sympathetic stimulation during exercise, and vagal tone incompletely removed (Fernhall et al., 2000; 2001). The rise in heart rate, normally induced by the removal of vagal inhibition and a gradual increase in sympathetic activation, is lower in DS population during a muscular effort (Fernhall & Otterstetter, 2003). This autonomic dysfunction has been studied by Figueroa et al. (2005) who used the HR variability [HRV] to explore the autonomic modulation of the sinoatrial node at rest and during exercise. Spectral components of HRV analysis in the low frequency [LF] and high frequency [HF] bands reflect sympathetic activity [LF/HF ratio] and parasympathetic tone [HF spectrum] (Task Force, 1996). These authors report an attenuated HR in individuals with DS due to blunted vagal withdrawal.

The results of these studies show significant abnormalities of ANS, with an observed increase in parasympathetic tone at rest (Baynard et al., 2004) a decrease of sympathetic stimulation during stress and during the tilt test, evoke a possible recall impaired baroreflex (Fernhall et al., 2005).

So, the mechanism responsible for the impairment of the autonomic cardiac regulation in DS population remains unclear. Even if the dysfunction of the ANS and /or the hormonal system is the main areas of research, we can also suggest that neurological damage are involved in the impairment of this cardiac regulation. The consistent findings of abnormalities in brain stem auditory evoked potentials, failure of growth and maturation in the brain from an early age, with loss of neurons and dentrites, and damage to the neurotransmitter system would provide the anatomic substrate for the autonomic dysfunction occurring at a central, brain stem site as a result of the genetic disorder (Yates et al., 1980; Mann et al., 1985; Wisniewski, 1990).

In the future, this dysfunction of the ANS must be supplemented by further investigations to better understand the possible mechanisms, especially through the involvement of hormonal factors.

4. Exercise limitations and obesity

One of the characteristics of the person with trisomy 21 is the propensity for becoming obese (Murray & Ryan-Krause, 2010). It affects between 15 and 20% of children and develops in most cases early in age; some studies have shown that nearly 10% of the children with Down syndrome were already located beyond the 95° percentile at 4 years old (Beange et al., 1995). The development of physical activity in the management of the obesity of young Down syndrome could play a major role. Indeed, the benefits of physical activity (combined with dietary measures) on cardiovascular risk have been clearly demonstrated in these populations, whether they live in special centers or in a family environment (Draheim et al., 2002; Montgomery et al., 1988).

Thus, in the general population, as in that of Down's syndrome, cardiovascular risk factors are associated with metabolic abnormalities, which are grouped under the generic common name 'metabolic syndrome' (Grundy et al., 2000). Among these metabolic abnormalities we can note a decrease in insulin resistance and excess body fat. Being overweight or obese can increase insulin resistance, which is characterised by a lack of insulin to stimulate glucose uptake by peripheral tissues and muscles, even though the plasma insulin concentration is abnormally high. The numerous endocrine studies showed that hyper-insulinemia stimulates the sympathetic nervous system, as is found in obese subjects (Monroe et al., 2000). This activation of the sympathetic nervous system is paradoxical, because it is part of a vicious circle in which there is a desensitisation of adrenergic signalling pathways (Lohse, 1996) hence a decrease in energy expenditure easing body fat storage. Simultaneously, this activation of the sympathetic nervous system adrenergic effects on the heart, blood vessels and kidneys promotes the development of hypertension. All these factors contribute highly to rise cardiovascular risk factors.

However, the factors restricting the effort in obesity are still insufficiently explored, especially for subjects with a mental disability. It seems that the place of regular physical activity in this population is highly relevant, especially since many studies have shown smaller performance in trisomy 21 (Pitetti & Tan, 1991a; Pitetti & Campbell, 1991b; Guerra et al., 2003; Fernhall & Otterstetter, 2003). The reasons for this disability to exercise are not clear and may reflect an insufficient stimulation (motivation problem) and / or the onset of fatigue induced by a limitation of use of energy substrates during prolonged exercise (Bricout et al., 2008) or to increased oxidative stress (Flore et al., 2008).

In adults, excess body fat may induce inflammation called 'low grade' and excessive oxidative stress (Wellen & Miller, 2005). Adipose tissue, then produce pro-inflammatory cytokines that alter insulin sensitivity. On the other hand, an inverse relationship between fitness level and markers of inflammation (high-sensitivity CRP) suggest a protective role of physical activity. Thus, the decrease in circulating CRP in regular physical activity suggests that it may limit this low-grade systemic inflammation (Oberbach et al., 2006). The effects of acute exercise have also been clearly demonstrated on the action of TNF-α (suppressive effect). Thus in young Down syndrome often over-weight and with a high percentage of body fat, the study of low-grade inflammation, its relationship with insulin sensitivity, biological markers of metabolic risk and cardiovascular inactivity and fitness need to be clarified. Several authors have demonstrated the positive impact of endurance exercise training on these markers. This reduced level of sensitivity CRP could reach 40% and was distinct from body composition and the level of initial CRP (Colbert et al., 2004). The checking of such a systemic effect in favour of a specific population "at risk" is therefore highly pertinent. This reduction in plasma levels of inflammatory markers may represent a relevant therapeutic target.

5. Hormonal results during physical exercise in people with Down syndrome and possible link with an exercise limitation?

Historically, people with intellectual disabilities have long been away from sports associations. Then gradually, with the development of adapted physical activities, awareness of the benefits of such control on health has raised, and attitudes to integrate these people have evolved (Eberhard, 2006). The first work that reports on the involvement of subjects with mental disabilities in sport is those of Bell and colleagues in 1977, demonstrating the feasibility of integrating these people into sport. In the following decade, many studies will have demonstrated that training and regular codified sports practices are not only possible but present real health benefits (Pitetti et al., 1989; 1991a; 1991b; 1993; Draheim et al., 2002). In this analysis, we must differentiate the effects of practice on health indicators (*e.g.* on body fat, the risk of obesity ...) from indicators of performance, not specifically looked for in this context.

Thus, for subjects with trisomy 21, regular physical activity can for example:

- promote fat loss, and positively influence lipid parameters (cholesterol, lipoproteins; (Eberhard et al., 1993))
- reduce the risk of developing diabetes (Marliss & Vranic, 2002; McGavock et al., 2004)
- reduce the risk of developing hypertension (Fernhall et al., 2001)
- help perform long-term efforts.

For twenty years, the department of Sports Medicine, at the hospital of Grenoble, has been focusing on hormonal adaptations during exercise in young trisomy 21. Early works attached in 1989 (Eberhard et al., 1989) tested the effects of a short physical exercise on a cycle ergometer to evaluate the physical abilities of young DS teenagers. These preliminary results showed that DS subjects had a less important physical ability to make efforts not only because of a lack of motivation or behavioural problems, but also a possible cardiovascular dysfunction. Two years later the major result led, to propose further investigations on the relationship between "the biochemical adaptations and catecholamine responses after a maximum incremental exercise in these young DS teenagers (Eberhard, et al., 1991). This study has highlighted that exercise performed by young DS individuals is reflected by elevated plasma catecholamine lower than that traditionally seen in control subjects, also correlated with a maximum heart rate always lower than control subjects at the end of exercise. The hypothesis of a blunted adrenergic response in this population therefore emerged. In 1993, a new study was proposed in the department with the aim to assess metabolic parameters at rest then an effort, but also and after 12 weeks of training, the idea was to make the possible link with adaptive responses to exercise (Eberhard, et al., 1993, 1996, 1997). The results obtained in these studies confirmed the previous ones results, but also demonstrated that endurance training over a period of three months led to a better balance of lipid profile frequently observed to be abnormal in a sedentary population with Down syndrome.

This promotion of physical activity has becomes a real concern for this specific population. Relayed by local associations, it has given rise to a major support of young Down syndrome, involving them more in physical activities. Over the last years, adaptive sports clubs which include a large population of mentally handicapped people, have regularly organized weekly training sessions that allow these young people to compete at a national level, and some of them achieve excellent results. These benefits had an immediate impact, improving measurable physiological parameters during exercise testing.

For example, in a last study proposed in 2002 in France (Grenoble), VO_{2max} values (gold index of aerobic fitness) obtained by a group of young DS adults, are excellent (44.2 ± 3.0 $ml.min^{-1}.kg^{-1}$ - Min = 39 Max = 60). For higher values, some young DS subjects get even better results than some control subjects of similar age. However, in this work, hormonal and metabolic investigations have shown that DS subjects present some alterations in adaptive response to maximal and sub-maximal exercise. Specific factors appear to be associated with result, such as obesity, a high percentage of body fat, hyper-insulinemia, and hyper-leptin levels (Bjorntrop & Rosmond, 2000). During the sub-maximal exercise, hormonal responses of young DS adults (cortisol, catecholamine) do not follow the observed rise in controls, whereas these adaptations allow glycolysis, gluconeogenesis and lipolysis when muscular exercise continues.

This result is expressed in a moderate elevation of blood glucose and HR, which could explain why people with Down syndrome can not continue muscular effort even at levels below maximum (Bjorntrop & Rosmond, 2000; McMurray & Hackney, 2005). This is also confirmed by low values of lipid oxidation in DS group and may be related to lower VO_{2max} for these subjects, and by free fatty acids values that remain high, suggesting that peripheral utilisation of lipids is insufficient when intensity and duration of the effort increases.

Compared with controls, hormonal responses to exercise in young adults with trisomy 21 were thus attenuated, which could explain cardiovascular and metabolic limitation of these subjects to continue muscular exercise (Bricout et al., 2008; Flore et al., 2008). The aim of these two studies was to analyse if hormonal responses could explain an exercise limitation in DS, and if it exist an oxidative stress in this population. DS is a risk factor for metabolic syndrome and cardiovascular disease. The greater oxidative stress described in DS can increase this risk owing to its potential deleterious effects on insulin sensitivity. We hypothesised that metabolic syndrome or its markers, at rest and during exercise, are more pronounced in young adults with DS.

Fourteen young men with DS (mean age 22.5 ± 0.7 years) took part to the study. During a treadmill sub-maximal incremental test, blood samples were collected for determination of hormonal and metabolic variables.

Compared to controls, DS individuals showed lower VO_{2max} (60.8 ± 2.4 *versus* 44.4 ± 3.3 $ml.min^{-1}.kg^{-1}$respectively; $P < 0.05$) but it was close to the predicted value (95 ± 6%). They presented a lower duration of sub-maximal incremental exercise ($P<0.001$).

At rest, DS individuals showed greater catecholamine, insulin and leptin values ($P<0.05$), but lower testosteronemia and cortisolemia ($P<0.05$) compared to controls. During sub-maximal incremental tests, catecholamine and cortisol did not increased, whereas the insulin concentration of DS individuals was significantly higher ($P<0.01$) compared to controls. Glycaemia increased significantly at the end of sub-maximal incremental test for controls but not for DS individuals ($P<0.01$). In DS participants, as expected, oxidative stress was greater than in controls (+ 15%; $P<0.001$) at rest and throughout the exercise protocol. Although a greater fat mass (DS: 19.9 ± 1.3%; controls: 13.5 ± 0.9%; $P<0.001$), and a lower insulin sensitivity (HOMA-IR DS: 1.09 ± 0.16; HOMA controls: 0.64 ± 0.13; $P<0.05$) was observed for DS participants, a metabolic syndrome could not be shown. Maximal fat-oxidation rate was lower in DS participants (DS = 394.2 ± 69.9 *versus* controls = 486.1± 134.8 $mg.min^{-1}$; $P <0.01$) but it was in the normal range.

These endocrine and metabolic profiles at rest and during exercise may limit endurance performance in DS individuals.

So now, the aim of our research team is to assess chronotropic adaptation to exercise in non obese young physically active adult males with DS and its relationships with exercise tolerance and catecholamine response. In a preliminary study, fourteen DS and healthy age-matched controls initially performed a graded maximal exercise test. Chronotropic incompetence (CI) was characterised if less than 80% of the chronotropic reserve was achieved.

Only four DS subjects (28%) had CI whereas none in controls. DS with CI showed exercise intolerance with HR peak and peak oxygen uptake lower than those without CI. Conversely, DS with CI had impaired epinephrine and norepinephrine responses to exercise. The association between CI, exercise intolerance and impaired catecholamine response in a subgroup of DS, indicate that biological effects of catecholamine are necessary for optimising acute exercise adaptations. Nevertheless, the results suggest that reduced chronotropic response and aerobic power in DS without CI are likely to be due to the metabolic consequences of fat mass excess and inherited oxidative stress rather than to impaired catecholamine drive.

However, the results of that work are still being acquired and it will be necessary to obtain results on a more important number of subjects to confirm our current results.

6. Interest of the promotion and guidance of an active lifestyle in populations with specific needs such as Down Syndrome

Direct assessment of health

There is no pharmacological treatment for trisomy 21. Nevertheless, the knowledge of physiological and biological parameters of trisomy 21 by means of studies based on protocols of effort is an original path that could bring: ***(1)*** load response adapted to the daily lives of subjects with trisomy 21, ***(2)*** results directly applicable to the health of these subjects (treatment of endocrine diseases, nutritional advice, and rehabilitation training ...).

By promoting a physically active life, as it has been shown in various reports across the Atlantic (A Report of the Surgeon General. U.S. Department of Health & Human Services, 1996) a reduction in health costs is logically expected for all categories of "persons with special needs", usually victims of the adverse effects of inactivity. The qualitative accompanying aging people with disabilities, is an important goal for our wealthy societies. The basic criteria for this support which actually extends from childhood to old age, is provided by professionals who educate, guide and look after these populations. These professionals should benefit from the results of this completed investigation on the effects of physical activity. Indeed, while renewing their knowledge and professional practices, they should be able to provide better care, better quality of life and even better end of life for all the elderly, disabled or not.

In addition, regular physical activity is widely recognised as a means of improving the health and the quality of life of people with disabilities. These benefits have already been demonstrated, at least temporarily. Over the last decade, the advanced educational media have helped give these people a more active lifestyle that has immediately impacted on their recognition and social integration. But as physical exercise is considered as a stress, questions remain as to the metabolic and hormonal adaptations of these DS subjects.

Similarly, long-term benefits of an active lifestyle, with a perspective of delaying the ageing of the person to maintain a certain level of mental and physical well-being, must be better identified.

Propositions could be considered, and should aim at finding the best conditions (nature, intensity, frequency) of an intervention based on physical activity among this specific population. It seems likely that the physical training of people with trisomy 21 should be scheduled, monitored and controlled in order to derive benefits for their health and quality of life.

In this context, Rimmer et al., (2004) have shown that a combined resistance and aerobic training program can improve physical fitness in this population; however, it remains unclear whether this transfers to improved performance on functional tasks of daily living.

Persons with DS have also reduced muscle strength and muscular endurance compared with their peers without disability and also compared with their peers with an intellectual disability but without DS (Croce & Horvat, 1992). Muscle weakness can also impact the ability of DS subjects to perform everyday activities, such as walking, maintaining balance while standing, and achieving all the movements of daily life. Further, because their workplace activities typically emphasize physical rather than cognitive skills, decreased strength can negatively impact the vocational and social development of adults with DS in the workforce. It has been shown that resistance training can improve work productivity in individuals with intellectual disability (Croce & Horvat, 1992). It might be expected that adults with DS have difficulty taking part in or being motivated to continue with a progressive resistance exercise program. Compliance with a training program can be very variable depending on the intellectual disabilities. To obtain a positive impact, it is necessary that the training program appeared to be a safe intervention for people with DS. No major adverse events should be reported by the participants, their families, or the fitness trainers involved in the program, during or after the training sessions.

To support the opinion that the activity is required in DS population, Heyne et al. (1997) have shown that the absence of a meaningful leisure program will foster maladaptive or aggressive behaviours. These authors point out the significance of leisure programs but also the importance of physical activities which will expand the social network, promote friendships and, introduce a sense of autonomy. Songster et al. (1997) reinforce this argument and emphasise that consistent training and sports competition in Special Olympics are essential to the physical, mental and social developments of young person with Down syndrome.

7. Conclusion

Children and young adults with Down syndrome have the opportunities to learn the different aspects of physical education and thus the means to become a physically educated person. They are capable of learning sports techniques, can progress, and participate in sports competition.

Nevertheless, physical activities need to be carefully taught and chosen for their fitness benefit. It is necessary to encourage enough recreational activities to maintain a sufficient motivation, so physical educational programs for this specific population should include all activities to learn, to understand both kinaesthetically and cognitively movements and abilities. Finally, the physical activity becomes enjoyable, social, repeatable, valued for its own sake, and we contribute to the formation of autonomous adults, physically active and educated.

CARDIOVASCULARA DATA Authors	Review	age years	FC rest bpm	FC peak bpm	VO2 peak ml/min/kg	SBP mmHg
Baynard et al., (2004)	Arch. Phys. Med Rehabil.	20,8 +/- 0,9	71 +/- 3,4	161 +/- 5,3	27,4 +/- 1,8	nd
Baynard et al., (2008)	M.S.S.E	25 +/- 2	nd	167 +/- nd	24 +/- nd	nd
Bricout et al., (2008)	J. NeuroEndocrinol.	22,5 +/- 0,7	57,7 +/- 3,7	180 +/- 2	44,2 +/- 3,04	116,0 +/- 2,8
Draheim et al., (2002)	Mental Retard.	34,5 +/- 10,0	nd	nd	nd	111,4 +/- 13,6
Eberhard et al., (1989)	J. Ment. Defic. Res.	14,8 +/- 2,2	67,1 +/- 12,6	123,6 +/- 19,7	47,6 +/- 8,1	107 +/- 14,6
Eberhard et al., (1997)	Adapt. Phys. Activ. Quater.	17,5 +/- 1,7	nd	162,2 +/- 18,9	48 +/- 1	nd
Fernhall et al., (1996)	M.S.S.E	26,7 +/- 5,9	nd	164 +/- 14,4	27,6 +/- 6,4	nd
Fernhall et al., (2003)	J.A.P	23,8 +/- 1,8	66,4 +/- 4,6	154, +/- 4,2	18,1 +/- 1,6	112,2 +/- 6,6
Fernhall et al., (2005)	Arch. Phys. Med Rehabil.	25,1 +/- 7,3	72,5	159 +/- 16,8	19,7 +/- 6,4	117,5 +/- nd
Fernhall et al., (2009)	Am. J Cardiol.	24 +/- 7	nd	170 +/- 10	27,3 +/- 5,6	nd
Figueroa et al., (2005)	Clin. Auton. Res.	27,8 +/- 8,1	76 +/- 3	nd	nd	115 +/- 4
Guerra et al., (2003)	Arch. Phys. Med Rehabil.	24,3 +/- 3,5	69,0 +/- 11,2	165,0 +/- 14,7	31,9 +/- 6,6	nd
Gouloupoulou et al. (2006)	Am. J. Ment. Retard.	24 +/- 0,9	70 +/- 1,5	162 +/- 2,4	24,5 ++/- 1,0	nd
Hefferman et al., (2005)	M.S.S.E	25 +/- 2,4	72 +/- nd	nd	nd	106,1 +/- 2,9
Iellamo et al., (2005)	Am. J. Physiol.	26,3 +/- 2,3	nd	nd	nd	116,1 +/- 2,7
Mendonca et al., (2011)	Arch. Phys. Med Rehabil.	36,5 +/- 5,5	69,6 +/- 12,2	167,6 +/- 19,1	31,7 +/- 7,9	nd
Mendonca et al., (2011)	Res. Dev. Disabilities	34,9 +/- 1,1	71 +/- nd	171,5 +/- 4,9	30,4 +/- 2,1	nd
Millar et al., (1993)	M.S.S.E	18,4 +/- 2,9	nd	172,8 +/- 15,1	26,95 +/- 7,92	nd
Rimmer et al., (2004)	Am. J. Ment. Retard.	40,6 +/- 6,5	nd	133 +/- 21	14,7 +/- 4,5	nd
Tsimaras et al., (2003)	Percept. Motor Skills	24,7 +/- 2,7	nd	181,0 +/- 3,8	30,5 +/- 4,3	nd

nd : not determined, SBP : systolic blood pressure.

Table 1. Cardiovascular data.

A.N.S DATA Authors	Review	age (years)	LF	HF	LF/HF
Baynard et al., (2004)	Arch. Phys. Med Rehabil.	20,8 +/- 0,9	1264,1 +/- 226,2 ms^2	1418,1 +/- 268,6 ms^2	1,81 +/- 0,42
Figueroa et al., (2005)	Clin. Auton. Res.	27,8 +/- 8,1	5,4 +/- 0,2 $ln.ms^2$	6,3 +/- 0,2 $ln.ms^2$	1,18 +/- 0,06
Iellamo et al., (2005)	Am. J. Physiol.	26,3 +/- 2,3	51,3 (35,5 to 59,4) n.u	34,6 (27,4 to 49,9) n.u	nd
Gouloupoulou et al. (2006)	Am. J. Ment. Retard.	24 +/- 0,9	6,93 +/- 0,12 $ln.ms^2$	6,57 +/- 0,16 $ln.ms^2$	0,35 +/- 0,11 $ln.ms^2$
Mendonca et al., (2011)	Res. Dev. Disabilities	34,9 +/- 1,1	6,8 ln ms^2	5,8 ln ms^2	1,1

LF: low frequency power expressed in ms^2 or ln ms^2 or n.u (normalised units)

HF: high frequency power; LF/HF ratio reflected the Autonomic Nervous System balance (sympathetic/parasympathetic).

Table 2. Autonomic Nervous System Data.

ENDOCRINE DATA Authors	Review	age (years)	Testosterone	TSH	T3	T4
Sakadamis et al., (2002)	Eur. J. Obstetr. Gynecol	26.4 +/- 3.9	31.26 +/- 14.1nmol/L	nd	nd	nd
Suzuki et al., (2010)	Int. J. Urol.	28 (15 - 54)	3.68 +/- 1.34 ng/mL	nd	nd	nd
Bricout et al., (2008)	J. NeuroEndocrinol.	22.5 +/- 0.7	15.45 +/- 1.63 nmol/L	6.33 +/- 0.93 mUI/L	4.35 +/- 0.11 pmol/L	16.22 +/- 0.60 pmol/L
Oliveira et al., (2002)	J. Pediatr (Rio J)	3.4 +/- 1.8	nd	7.2 ± 4.2 µU/mL	9.8 ± 2.1 ng/dL	1.7 ± 0.4 ng/dL
Murdoch et al., (1977)	J. Clin. Endocrinol. Metab	adults	nd	7.6 +/- 10.7 mU/L	1.61 +/- 0.47 nmol/L	69.1 +/- 22.2 nmol/L
Konings et al., (2001)	Eur. J. Endocrinol.	1.5 to 13	nd	6.5 +/- 1.3 mU/L		14.3 to 18.5 pmol/L

TSH: thyroid stimulating hormone; T3: tri-iodothyronine; T4: thyroxine; nd : not determined,

Table 3. Endocrine data.

ENDOCRINE DATA Authors	Review	age years	cortisol (rest) nmol/L	Epinephrine rest (pmol/mL)	NorEpinephrine rest (pmol/mL)	Epinephrine post ex (pmol/mL)	NorEpinephrine post ex (pmol/mL)
Murdoch et al., (1979)	J. Ment. Defic. Res.	39 (22 - 57)	476.6 +/- nd				
Bricout et al., (2008)	J. NeuroEndocrinol.	22.5 +/- 0.7	365.1 +/- 14.7	0.67 +/- 0.14	3.62 +/- 0.53	1.19 +/- 0.22	10.21 +/- 2.64
Eberhard et al., (1991)	J. Ment. Defic. Res.	17.5 +/- 1.7	nd	0.38 +/- 0.23	1.08 +/- 0.78	0.92 +/- 0.41	6.32 +/- 3.41
Eberhard et al., (1997)	Adapt. Phys. Activ. Quater.	Boys: 18 +/- 1.7	nd	0.45 +/- 0.3	1.3 +/- 0.9	1 +/- 0.45	6.4 +/- 4.4
Eberhard et al., (1997)	Adapt. Phys. Activ. Quater.	Girls: 16.7 +/- 1.5	nd	0.4 +/- 0.3	0.63 +/- 0.25	0.78 +/- 0.3	6.9 +/- 1.6

TSH: thyroid stimulating hormone; T3: tri-iodothyronine; T4: thyroxine; nd : not determined,

Table 4. Endocrine data.

8. References

Baynard, T.; Pitetti, KH.; Guerra, M. & Fernhall, B. (2004). Heart rate variability at rest and during exercise in persons with Down syndrome. *Archives of* Physical *Medicine and* Rehabilitation. *Vol.*85, n°.8, pp. 1285-1290.

Baynard, T.; Pitetti, KH.; Guerra, M.; Unnithan, VB & Fernhall, B. (2008). Age-related changes in aerobic capacity in individuals with mental retardation: A 20-yr review. *Medicine & Science in Sports & Exercise*. Vol.40, N°.11, pp. 1984–1989.

Beange, H.; Mc Elduff, A. & Baker, W. (1995). Medical disorders of adults with mental retardation: a population study. *American Journal of Mental Retardation*. Vol.99, pp. 595-604.

Bell, NJ.; Kozar, W. & Martin, AW. (1977). The impact of Special Olympics on participants, parents and the community. Lubbock, TX Technical University.

Bjorntrop, P. & Rosmond, R. (2000). Neuroendocrine abnormalities in visceral obesity. International Journal of Obesity *and related metabolic* disorders. Vol.24, pp. S80–S85.

Bricout, V-A.; Guinot, M.; Faure, P.; Flore, P.; Eberharrd, Y.; Garnier, P. & Favre-Juvin, A. (2008). Are hormonal responses to exercise in young men with Down's Syndrome related to reduced endurance performance? *Journal of Neuroendocrinology*. Vol.20, pp. 558-565.

Colbert, LH.; Visser, M. & Simonsick, EM. (2004). Physical activity, exercise and inflammatory markers in older adults: findings from the Health, Aging and Body composition Study. *Journal of American Geriatrics Society*. Vol.52, pp. 1098-1104.

Croce, RV. & Horvat, M. (1992). Effects of reinforcement based exercise on fitness and work productivity in adults with mental retardation. *Adapted Physical Activity Quaterly*. Vol.9, pp. 148-178.

Day, SM.; Strauss, DJ.; Shavelle, RM. & Reynolds, RJ. Mortality and causes of death in persons with Down syndrome in California. (2005). *Developmental Medicine and Child Neurology*. Vol.47, pp. 171-176.

Draheim, CC.; Williams, DP. & Mc Cubbin, JA. (2002). Prevalence of physical inactivity and recommended physical activity in community-based adults with mental retardation. *Mental Retardation*. Vol.40, n°.6, pp. 436-444.

Eberhard, Y.; Eterradossi, J. & Rappachi, B. (1989). Physical aptitudes to exertion in children with Down's syndrome. *Journal of Mental Deficiency Research*. Vol.33, pp. 167-174.

Eberhard, Y.; Eterradossi, J. & Therminarias, A. (1991). Biochemical changes and catecholamine responses in Down's syndrome adolescents in relation to incremental maximal exercise. *Journal of Mental Deficiency Research.* Vol.35, n°.2, pp. 140-146.

Eberhard, Y.; Eterradossi, J.; Foulon, T. & Groslambert, P. (1993). Variations des lipoprotéines plasmatiques chez les adolescents trisomiques 21 en réponse à un test d'endurance physique. *Pathologie & Biologie.* Vol.41, n°.5, pp. 482-486.

Eberhard, Y.; Eterradossi, J.; Foulon, T. & Groslambert, P. (1996). Influence conjuguée de conseils alimentaires et de l'activité physique d'endurance sur les lipoprotéines plasmatiques chez les adolescents trisomiques 21. *Sciences & Sports.* Vol.11, pp. 145-151.

Eberhard, Y.; Eterradossi, J. & Debû, B. (1997). Biological Changes induced by Physical Activity in Individuals with Down's Syndrome. *Adapted Physical Activity Quaterly.* Vol.14, pp. 166-175.

Eberhard, Y. (2006). A better living and a better ageing thanks to sport for persons with intellectual deficits. *Sciences & Sports.* Vol.21, pp. 236–242.

Fernhall, B.; Pitetti, KH.; Rimmer, JH.; Mc Cubbin, JA.; Rintala, P.; Millar, AL.; Kittredge, J. & Burkett, LN. (1996). Cardiorespiratory capacity of individuals with mental retardation including Down syndrome. *Medicine & Science in Sports & Exercise.* Vol.28, n°.3, pp. 366-371.

Fernhall, B.; McCubbin, JA.; Pitetti, KH.; Rintala, P.; Rimmer, JH.; Millar, AL. & De Silva, A. (2001). Prediction of maximal heart rate in individuals with mental retardation. *Medicine Sciences & Sports Exercise.* Vol.33, n°.10, pp. 1655-1660.

Fernhall, B. & Otterstetter, M. (2003). Attenuated responses to sympathoexcitation in individuals with Down syndrome. *Journal of Applied Physiology.* Vol.94, n°.6, pp. 2158-2165.

Fernhall, B.; Figueroa, A.; Collier, S.; Baynard, T.; Giannopoulou, I.; Gouloupoulou, S. (2005). Blunted Heart Rate Response to Upright Tilt in People With Down Syndrome. *Archives of* Physical *Medicine and* Rehabilitation. *Vol.*86, pp. 813-818.

Fernhall, B.; Baynard, T.; Collier, SR.; Figueroa, A.; Gouloupoulou, S.; Kamimori, GH. & Pitetti, KH. (2009). Catecholamine response to maximal exercise in persons with Down syndrome. *American Journal of Cardiology.* Vol. 103, pp. 724-726.

Figueroa, A.; Collier, S.; Baynard, T.; Giannopoulou, I.; Gouloupoulou, S. & Fernhall, B. (2005). Impaired vagal modulation of heart rate in individuals with Down syndrome. *Clinical Autonomic Research.* Vol.15, n°.1, pp. 45-50.

Finesilver, C. (2002). A new age for childhood diseases: Down syndrome. *RN.* Vol.65, pp. 43–48.

Flore, P.; Bricout, V-A.; Van Biesen, D.; Guinot, M.; Laporte, F.; Pépin, J-L.; Eberhard, Y.; Favre-Juvin, A. & Faure, P. (2008). Oxidative stress and metabolism at rest and during exercise in persons with Down Syndrome. *European Journal of Cardiovascular Prevention & Rehabilitation.* Vol. 15, N°.1, pp. 35-42.

Furlan, R.; Pagani. & M, Malliani, A. (1993). Effects of exercise and training on control of heart rate. *Cardiovascular Research.* Vol.27, pp. 2286-2287.

Galbo, H. (1985). The hormonal response to exercise. *Proceedings of the* Nutrition Society. Vol. 44, pp. 257-266.

Gouloupoulou, S.; Baynard, T.; Collier, S.; Giannopoulou, I.; Figueroa, A.; Beets, M.; Pitetti, K. & Fernhall, B. (2006). Cardiac autonomic control in individuals with Down syndrome. *American Journal of Mental Retardation.* Vol.111, n°.1, pp. 27-34.

Grote, L.; Hedner, J. & Peter, JH. (2004). The heart rate response to exercise is blunted in patients with sleep-related breathing disorder. *Cardiology*. Vol.102, n°.2, pp. 93-99.

Grundy, S.; Bazzarre, T. & Cleeman, J. (2000). Prevention conference V. Beyond secondary prevention: identifying the high risk patient for primary prevention, medical office assessment. *Circulation*. Vol.101, pp. e3-e11.

Guerra, M.; Llorens, N. & Fernhall, B. (2003). Chronotropic incompetence in persons with Down Syndrome. *Archives of* Physical *Medicine and* Rehabilitation. *Vol.84, pp.* 1604-1608.

Horvat, M. & Croce, R. (1995). Physical rehabilitation of individuals with mental retardation: physical fitness and information processing. *Critical Reviews in Physical and Rehabilitation Medicine. Vol.* 7, pp. 233–252.

Hefferman, KS.; Baynard, T.; Gouloupoulou, S.; Giannopoulou, I.; Collier, SR.; Figueroa, A. & Fernhall B. (2005). Baroreflex sensitivity during static exercise in individuals with Down syndrome. *Medicine & Science in Sports & Exercise*. Vol.37, n°.12, pp. 2026–2031.

Heyne, LA.; Schleien, SJ. & Rynders, JE. (1997). Promoting quality of life through recreation participation. In Pueschel, SM. & Sustrova, M. (Eds.). Adolescents with Down Syndrome. pp. 317-340. Baltimore: Paul H Brookes Publishing Co.

Iellamo, F.; Galante, A.; Legarante, JM.; Lipp, ME.; Condoluci, C.; Albertini, G. & Volterrani, M. (2005). Altered autonomic cardiac regulation in individuals with Down syndrome. American Journal *of* Physiology - Heart *and Circulatory Physiology*. Vol.289, n°.6, pp. H2387-2391.

Konings, CH.; Van Trotsenburg, AS.; Ris-Stalpers, C.; Vulsma, T.; Wiedijk, BM. & De Vijlder, JJ. (2001). Plasma thyrotropin bioactivity in Down's syndrome children with subclinical hypothyroidism. *European Journal of Endocrinology*. Vol.144, pp. 1-4

Lauer, MS.; Okin, PM.; Larson, MG.; Evans, JC. & Levy, D. (1996). Impaired heart rate response to graded exercise. Prognostic implications of chronotropic incompetence in the Framingham Heart Study. *Circulation*. Vol.93, pp. 1520–1526.

Lauer, MS. (2004). Chronotropic incompetence: ready for prime time. *The Journal of American College of Cardiology*. Vol.44, pp. 431-432.

Lohse, MJ. (1996). Mechanisms of the regulation of adrenergic beta-receptors. *Zeitschrift für kardiologie*. Vol.85, n°.7S, pp. 1-3.

Mann, DM.; Yates, PO.; Marcyniuk, B. & Ravindra CR. (1985). Pathological evidence for neurotransmitter deficits in Down's syndrome of middle age. *Journal of Mental Deficiency Research*. Vol.29, pp. 125-135.

Marliss, EB. & Vranic, M. (2002). Intense exercise as a unique effect on both insulin release and its role in glucoregulation: implications for diabetes. *Diabetes*. Vol.51, n°.1, pp. S271-283.

McMurray, RG. & Hackney, AC. (2005). Interactions of metabolic hormones, adipose tissue and exercise. *Sports Medicine*. Vol.35, pp. 393–412.

McGavock, JM.; Eves, ND.; Mandic, S.; Glenn, NM.; Quinney, HA. & Haykowsky, MJ. (2004). The role of exercise in the treatment of cardiovascular disease associated with type 2 diabetes mellitus. *Sports Medicine.* Vol.34, n°.1, pp. 27-48.

Monroe, M.; Van Pelt, R.; Schiller, B.; Seals, D. & Jones, P. (2000). Relation of leptin and insulin to adiposity-associated elevations in sympathtic activity with age in humans. International Journal of Obesity. Vol.24, pp. 1183-1187.

Mendonca, GV.; Pereira, FD. & Fernhall, B. (2011). Cardiac autonomic function during submaximal treadmill exercise in adults with Down syndrome. *Research in Developmental Disabilities.* Vol.32, pp. 532–539.

Mendonca, GV.; Pereira, FD. & Fernhall, B. (2011). Effects of combined aerobic and resistance exercise training in adults with and without Down syndrome. *Archives of* Physical *Medicine and* Rehabilitation. *Vol. 92, pp. 37-45.*

Millar, A.; Fernhall, B. & Burkett L. (1993). Effects of aerobic training in adolescents with Down syndrome. *Medicine & Science in Sports & Exercise.* Vol. 5, pp. 270-274.

Montgomery, D.; Reid, G. & Seidl, C. (1988). The effects of two physical fitness programs designed for mentally retarded adults. *Canadian* Journal of Sports *Sciences.* Vol.13, pp. 73-78.

Murray, J. & Ryan-Krause, P. (2010). Obesity in children with Down syndrome: background and recommendations for management. Pediatric Nursing. *Vol. 36, n°.6, pp. 314-319.*

Murdoch, JC. (1977). Thyroid function in adults with Down's syndrome. Journal *of Clinical Endocrinology & Metabolism.* Vol.44, n°.3, pp. 453-458.

Murdoch, JC.; Gray, CA.; McCarty, DG. & Ratcliffe, JG. (1978). Pituitary function in Down's syndrome. *Journal of Mental Deficiency Research.* Vol.22, n°.4, pp. 273-275.

Murdoch, JC.; Giles, CA.; Grant, JK. & Ratcliffe, JG. (1979). Hypothalamic-pituitary-adrenocortical function in adults Down's syndrome. *Journal of Mental Deficiency Research.* Vol.23, pp. 157-162.

Nagaoka, H.; Sachio, S.; Lizuka, T.; Imai, S. & Nagai R. (1996). Relation between depressed cardiac response to exercise and autonomic nervous activity in mildly symptomatic patients with idiopathic dilated cardiomyopathy. *Chest.* Vol.109, n°.4, pp. 925-932.

Oberbach, A.; Tonjes, A.; Kloting, N.; Fasshauer, M.; Kratzsch J. & Busse, MW. (2006). Effect of 4 week physical training program on plasma concentrations of inflammatory markers in patients with abnormal glucose tolerance. *European Journal of Endocrinology.*Vol.154, pp. 577-585.

Oliveira, ATA.; Longui, CA.; Calliari, LEP.; Ferone, EA.; Kawaguti, FS. & Monte, O. (2002). Evaluation of the hypothalamic–pituitary–thyroid axis in children with Down syndrome. *Jornal de Pediatria. (Rio J).* Vol.8, n°.4, pp. 295-300.

Pitetti, K.; Jackson, J.; Stubbs, B.; Campbell, K. & Battar, S. (1989). Fitness levels of adult Special Olympics participants. *Adapted Physical Activity Quaterly.* Vol.6, pp. 354-370.

Pitetti, K. & Tan, DM. (1991a). Effects of a minimally supervised exercise program for mentally retarded adults. *Medicine Sciences & Sports Exercise.* Vol.23, n°.5, pp. 594-601.

Pitetti, KH. & Campbell, KD. (1991b). Mentally retarded individuals: a population at risk? *Medicine Sciences & Sports Exercise.* Vol;23, n°.5, pp. 586-593.

Pitetti, K.; Rimmer, J. & Fernhall, B. (1993). Physical fitness and adults with mental retardation. An overview of current research and future directions. *Sports Medicine.* Vol.16, n°.1, pp. 23-56.

Prasher, VP. & Krishnan, VHR. (1993). Age of onset and duration of dementia in people with Down syndrome. A study of 98 reported cases. International Journal of Geriatric Psychiatry. Vol. 8, pp. 915-922.

Rimmer, JH.; Heller, T.; Wang, E. & Valerio, I. (2004). Improvements in physical fitness in adults with Down syndrome. *American Journal of Mental Retardation.* Vol.109, n°.2, pp. 165-174.

Sakadamis, A.; Angelopoulou, N.; Matziarib, C.; Papameletiouc, V. & Souftas V. (2002) Bone mass, gonadal function and biochemical assessment in young men with trisomy 21. *European Journal of Obstetrics & Gynecology and Reproductive Biology.* Vol.100, pp. 208–212.

Sasagawa, I.; Nakada, T.; Hashimoto, T.; Ishigooka, M.; Izumiya, K.; Kubota, H. & Tomaru, M. (1993). Hormone profiles and contralateral testicular histology in Down's syndrome with unilateral testicular tumor. *Archives of Andrology.*Vol.30, pp. 93–98.

Sharav, T.; Landau, H.; Zadik, Z. & Einarson, TR. (1991). Age-related patterns of thyroid-stimulating hormone response to thyrotropin-releasing hormone stimulation in Down syndrome. *American Journal of Diseases of Children.* Vol.145, pp. 172-175.

Songster, TH.; Smith, G.; Evans, M.; Munson, D. & Behen, D. (1997). Special Olympics and athletes with Down syndrome. In Pueschel, SM. & Sustrova, M. (Eds.). Adolescents with Down Syndrome. pp. 341-357. Baltimore: Paul H Brookes Publishing Co.

Sutherland, G.; Couch, M. & Iacono, T. (2002). Health issues for adults with developmental disability. *Research in Developmental Disabilities.* Vol.23, pp. 422–445.

Suzuki, K.; Nakajima, K.; Kamimura, S.; Takasugi, K.; Suzuki, Y.; Sekine, H. & Ishii, N. (2010). Eight case reports on sex-hormone profiles in sexually mature male Down syndrome. *International Journal of Urology.* Vol.17, pp. 1008–1010.

Task force of the European society of cardiology and the North American society of pacing and electrophysiology. Heart rate variability: guidelines. (1996). *European Heart Journal.* Vol.17, pp. 354-381.

Thompson, SB. (1999). Examining dementia in Down syndrome (DS): decline in social abilities in DS compared to other learning disabilities. *Topics in Clinical Gerontology.* Vol.20, pp. 3–44.

Tsimaras, V.; Giagazoglou, P. & Fotiadou, E. (2003). Jog-walk training in cardio-respiratory fitness of adults with Down syndrome. *Perceptual and* Motor Skills. Vol.96, pp. 1239–1251.

Wellen, KE. & Hotamisligil, GS. (2005). Inflammation, stress, and diabetes. Journal *of Clinical Investigation.* Vol.115, n°.5, pp. 1111-1119

Wilkoff, BL. & Miller, RE. (1992). Exercise testing for chronotropic assessment. *Cardiology Clinics.* Vol.10, pp. 705-717.

Wisniewski, KE. (1990). Down's syndrome children often have brain with maturation delay, retardation of growth, and cortical dysgenesis. *American Journal of Medical Genetics.* Vol. 7 suppl, pp. 274-290.

Yates, CM.; Simpson, J.; Maloney, AFJ.; Gordon, A. and Reid, AH. (1980). Alzheimer-like cholinergic deficiency in Down's syndrome. Lancet. Vol.2, pp. 979.

15

Language and Visuospatial Abilities in Down Syndrome Phenotype: A Cognitive Neuroscience Perspective

George Grouios and Antonia Ypsilanti
Department of Physical Education and Sport Sciences
Laboratory of Motor Control and Learning
Aristotle University of Thessaloniki
Greece

1. Introduction

Down syndrome (DS) is the most common genetic disorder with a prevalence that ranges from 1:700 to 1:100 live births and accounts for 25–30% of people with intellectual disability (Nadel, 1999; Rogers, Roizen, & Capone, 1996; Rondal, 1988, 1998; Rondal, Perera, & Nadel, 1999). Trisomy 21, one of the three forms of DS, is caused by the presence of a third chromosome at band 21q22 of the long arm. The other two forms, namely translocation 21 and mosaicism, account for only 6% of children with DS (Rogers et al., 1996). Recent medical advances suggest that over 300 genes are affected, making the genetic etiology of DS a complex mechanism that implicates gene interactions that are not clearly understood (Pennington, Moon, Edgin, Stedron, & Nadel, 2003; Antonarakis et al., 2004). The syndrome is characterized by specific phenotypic characteristics, health related problems, cognitive and language impairments, neuromotor dysfunction and early aging, often associated with increased prevalence of Alzheimer's disease.

Interest in the cognitive profile of DS has been robust during the past decades, with a large number of published studies discussing the atypical and unique profile of cognitive abilities in this population. Yet, there is no clear understanding of the cognitive profile of individuals with DS and how this differentiates from other forms of intellectual disability. The uniqueness of the cognitive make-up of individuals with DS will contribute to a better understanding of the specific strengths and impairments of this population, as well as to the development of more effective educational programs suitable for them. This chapter will focus on language and visuo-spatial abilities of individuals with DS from a cognitive neuroscience perspective. The chapter is organized in four parts. The first part discusses language abilities in individuals with DS, with particular emphasis on expressive and receptive vocabulary and grammar. In the second part, research in visuospatial abilities in individuals with DS is reviewed. The third part deals with the concept of atypical cerebral laterality (ACL) in DS individuals and, in particular, how ACL may affect their language and visuospatial abilities. Finally, the last part discusses the contribution of laterality research in understanding the unique pattern of cognitive abilities in DS.

2. Neurobiology of DS

At birth, the total brain volume of individuals with DS is close to normal, although microscopically some changes have been observed as early as 22 weeks of gestation that become more obvious by 6 months of age (Nadel, 2003). This condition has been linked to neural density reduction in the cerebral cortex (Florez, 1992). Indeed, the most affected area of the brain of individuals with DS is the cortex, both in neural density and in weaker neural synapses, caused by fewer dendritic spines. (Florez, 1992; also see Lubec & Engidawork, 2002 for a review). Although, the reduced brain volume cannot be directly associated with the observed intellectual disability of this group, it is suspected that these abnormalities in the neural density of the cortex may contribute to the weak cognitive deficits associated with the syndrome (e.g., memory and attention). Shapiro and colleagues (1992) reported abnormal neuronal interactions between the frontal and parietal lobes of individuals with DS, suggesting the involvement of Broca's area. More specific differences in the brain's neuroanatomy of individuals with DS include reduced growth of the frontal lobes (Kesslak et al. 1994), narrowing of the superior temporal gyrus, smaller brain stem and cerebellum (Cole et al., 1993).

Research using magnetic resonance imaging (MRI), comparing demented and non-demented individuals with DS, indicates the presence of reduced volume of left hippocampus and amygdala in the former group (Pearlson et al., 1998). In a different MRI study, measuring hippocampal and amygdala volumes, non-demented individuals with DS exhibited smaller hippocampal size compared to age-matched typically developing controls, but there were no differences in amygdala volumes between the two groups (Pinter, Brown, Eliez, Schmitt, Capone, & Reiss, 2001). In their study, Pinter and colleagues (2001) confirmed that individuals with DS have smaller brain volumes, both in gray and white matter, smaller cerebellar volumes, and relatively larger subcortical gray matter volumes, both in parietal and temporal structures. Finally, Teipel and colleagues (2003) found decreased size of the corpus callosum in a group of non-demented individuals with DS, even when total brain volume was controlled for (Teipel et al., 2003). Thus, although the neuropathology of individuals with DS is widespread, particularly in older adults, it is also selectively affecting mainly cortical areas that are involved in higher cognitive processes.

3. Cognitive profile of individuals with DS

Individuals with DS demonstrate a unique cognitive profile of strengths and weaknesses that is characteristic to the syndrome. The general intellectual ability of individuals with DS ranges from mild to severe mental retardation, with a decline as they grow older (e.g., Hoddap & Zigler, 1990; Pennington, Moon, Edgin, Stedron, & Nadel, 2003). This decline, which begins early in adulthood, has been related to the gradual deterioration of several brain areas, such as the hippocampus and the cerebellum (Pennington et al., 2003). Alternatively, this decline has been linked to the increased prevalence of dementia in adults with DS (Takashima, Ieshima, Nakamura, & Becker, 1989).

Hippocampal function that supports tasks that tap short-term and long-term memory are severely affected in individuals with DS, as opposed to those supported by prefrontal areas (e.g., executive functions) (Pennington et al., 2003). Explicit memory (verbal and non-verbal) is particularly weak when compared both to typically developing (TD) individuals matched for mental age, and non-Down syndrome individuals with intellectual disability (ID)

(Carlesimo, Marlota, & Vicari, 1997). These findings suggest that memory is disproportionally affected in DS due to the specific neurological abnormalities mentioned earlier (i.e., hippocampal dysfunction, reduced brain volume) (Lubec & Engidawork, 2002).

Sustained attention has been also examined in infants with DS (Brown, Johnson, Paterson, Gilmore, Longhi, & Karmiloff-Smith, 2003). Results showed that infants with DS exhibit poor engagement and less duration in sustained attention than TD mental-age controls (Brown et al. 2003). These results are unlikely to reflect lack of motivation or task difficulty. In older individuals with DS, this condition has been associated with other dementia symptoms, such as lack of orientation (e.g., Granholm, Sanders, & Crnic, 2000).

Language is the most extensively studied domain within the cognitive system in individuals with DS. Most authors agree that language is severely affected in these individuals, with expressive vocabulary, grammar and syntax being the weakest areas of function. Indeed, individuals with DS document an unusual disparity in performance in expressive and receptive vocabulary tasks, with the latter being more affected than the former. Particular emphasis has been placed in identifying the specific nature of the expressive language difficulties, their neural substrates, as well as the developmental changes throughout the life span.

Grammar and syntax are disproportionally affected in individuals with DS as well. Spoken language is characterized by a systematic omission of tense-related grammatical morphemes that persists throughout development. Surprisingly, in most studies examining English-speaking children with DS, regular past tense formation is more affected than irregular past tense formation, suggesting a difficulty with understanding and applying grammatical and syntactic rules, as opposed vocabulary entry and retrieval.

Visuo-spatial abilities have been less extensively investigated in DS. Some authors propose that visuo-spatial working memory is relatively preserved compared to verbal working memory in DS individuals (e.g., Lanfranchi, Carretti, Spanò & Cornoldi, 2009). In fact, they have often been characterized with relative strengths in visuo-spatial processing and poor verbal processing skills (Jarrold, Baddeley & Hewes, 1999; Klein & Mervis, 1999; Wang & Bellugi, 1994). The relative strength of visuo-spatial skills is supported by strong fine motor skills documented through the use of gestures in early development (Bilovsky & Share, 1965). More specifically, it has been reported that children with DS are better at the construction subtests of the Stanford-Binet (e.g., block building, drawing line, copying, folding), compared to mental age controls, due to their strong visuo-motor abilities (Silverstein, Legutski, Friedman, and Takayama, 1982). Pueschel and collegues (1987) documented that young children with DS were better at figure closure and hand movement tasks, compared to verbal tasks (using the Kaufman Assessment Battery for Children), while TD children exhibited the reverse pattern of performance and children with IDs without DS exhibited equally weak performance in both tasks.

Bellugi and colleagues (1994) proposed that individuals with DS are better at sustaining the global configuration of objects, as opposed to local forms, a pattern that is reversed in individuals with intellectual disability of different genetic origin. Similar findings have been reported in drawing, where individuals with DS tend to reproduce the global features of a stimulus and omit the local details of the object. This pattern of performance is often encountered in patients with left hemisphere damage, suggesting lateralized brain lesions in individuals with DS. However, MRI data do not exhibit asymmetrical damage in individuals with DS. This evidence supports the existence of an atypical functional lateralization in this clinical group (Jernigan & Bellugi, 1990).

4. Language of individuals with DS

One of the earlier studies on language of individuals with DS explored speech reproduction and observed weak expressive skills in this population (Dodd, 1975). During the same decade Gibson (1978) discussed the language production of individuals with DS during the first two years of life. He suggested that some aspects of language, particularly expression, fall behind their chronological age. Almost a decade later, Cardosa- Martins and colleagues (1985) found weaknesses in speech production in individuals with DS. Since then, it has been repeatedly documented that children with DS exhibit an unusual disparity between expressive and receptive language, compared to what would be expected, based on their mental age, with the latter being less affected than the former (e.g., Jenkins, 1993; Chapman, 1997). This delay in expressive performance is evident from infancy, even prior to development of formal vocal speech.

Likewise, it has been found that infant gesture development in DS population is delayed, compared to TD infants (e.g., Miller, 1992). Longitudinal studies examining one-to-two word formations, found that individuals with DS exhibit a delay in speech production up to 18 months, with large individual variation that reached 19 months (e.g., Oliver and Buckley, 1994). The "vocabulary spurt", typically observed in TD 24-month old infants, was commonly absent in individuals with DS. As the syntax becomes more complex and the vocabulary for speech production more demanding, the discrepancies between DS and TD individuals become more pronounced (Miller, 1992).

Receptive language and comprehension appear to be more advanced than expressive speech in DS adolescents (Chapman, Schwartz, & Kay-Raining Bird, 1991). However, some evidence suggests that comprehension declines with age in non-demented individuals with DS (Chapman, Hesketh, & Kistler, 2002). In our study, receptive and expressive vocabulary was investigated in DS and TD individuals matched for mental age (Ypsilanti, Grouios, Alevriadou & Tsapkini, 2005). Four subtests of the Test of Word Knowledge (TOWK) (Wiig & Secord, 1992) were used to assess naming pictures (expressive vocabulary), matching a spoken word to a picture among four semantically related detractors (receptive vocabulary), relational word knowledge and ability to provide definitions to orally presented words. We found no differences between the two groups in three of the four tasks of expressive and receptive vocabulary. The only reliable weakness of individuals with DS was evidenced in the word definitions subtest that demands complex syntactic constructions, requirement which is challenging for these individuals.

Surprisingly, narrative production, which is closely related to expressive language and syntax, seems to be less affected in individuals with DS. Chapman, and colleagues (1998) compared the performance of 33 individuals with DS with two TD control groups matched for syntactic comprehension and for mean length of utterance (MLU), respectively, and failed to find reliable differences in number of episodes (stories) described by the three groups. Individuals with DS documented syntactic errors that included verb omissions, suggesting that narrative production may be weak due to syntactic deficits and not vocabulary restrictions.

Grammatical word formation, particularly the omission of tense-related morphemes, is another area of difficulty for individuals with DS (e.g., Laws & Bishop, 2003). Regular past tense formation is more affected than irregular in individuals with DS (Laws & Bishop; Eadie, Fey, Douglas, & Parsons, 2002). This peculiar finding suggests that irregular past tense formation resembles accessing vocabulary entries, which does not rely on understanding and applying grammatical rules (Pinter, 1991). This theorization has been subsequently supported by evidence indicating significant correlation between irregular past formation and vocabulary level in individuals with DS (Laws and Bishop, 2003).

In summary, most published studies agree that expression is more affected than reception in individuals with DS (for a review see Ypsilanti & Grouios, 2008) and that phonological short-term memory may be mediating the performance on such tasks. This hypothesis is supported by research findings indicating that auditory short-term memory predicts early vocabulary entry in individuals with DS (Chapman & Hesketh, 2001). Several investigators have proposed that children with DS may exhibit difficulties in naming and sentence repetition tasks due to strong anatomical and functional deficiencies in the corpus callosum (e.g., Wang, Hesselink, Jernigan, Doherty, & Bellugi, 1992). Bunn et al. (2002) argued that if interhemispheric communication is necessary for picture naming before speech production, then deficiencies in the corpus callosum, such as those observed in individuals with DS, would influence performance on naming, but not on reading tasks.

5. Visuospatial abilities in DS

Studies on visuospatial abilities of individuals with DS reveal the existence of strengths and weaknesses within this domain. In particular, individuals with DS are stronger in visuomotor integration and visual memory, compared to spatial memory and spatial construction (Fidler, 2005). Visuospatial short-term memory was found to be relatively unaffected in individuals with DS (e.g., Jarrold & Baddeley, 1997). Bellugi and colleagues (1999) found a unique dissociation in the visuospatial abilities of individuals with DS and Williams Syndrome (WS) (a genetically linked disorder associated with intellectual disability). Individuals with DS tended to maintain a holistic strategy in drawing tasks, while those with WS matched for mental age, reproduced local features of the drawing objects (Bellugi, Lichtenberger, Mills, Galaburda, & Korenberg, 1999). Moreover, individuals with DS exhibited increased difficulty in depicting internal details of objects in block construction and integrating simple shapes. In the same study, a clear dissociation in global/local features of individuals with DS was illustrated using the Navon task, in which participants were asked to maintain the global or local form of letter stimuli. Individuals with DS were unable to reproduce the local details of the stimuli, maintaining only the global aspect of the presented letter.

In another study, Bellugi and colleagues (2000) presented comparative data from drawings of individuals with DS and WS demonstrating that individuals with DS produce drawings conforming with gestalt rules (such as, closure and continuation) that lack detail, but are easily recognizable (Bellugi, Lichtenberger, Jones, Lai, & St. George 2000). Interestingly, the two groups were equally weak in the block design subtest of the WISC-R (Wechsler, 1974). However, further analysis of the process of block design indicated that although erroneously, individuals with DS maintained the global configuration of the block arrangements, while individuals with WS exhibited a more local perspective in their arrangements (Bellugi et al., 1999). The characteristic profile of the visuospatial abilities of individuals with DS implicates the neural substrates supporting these processes that are ultimately linked to the chromosomal abnormality of the disorder and its unique phenotype. This profile may also indicate variations in neuronal plasticity in different disorders with intellectual disability (Bellugi et al., 2000).

6. Atypical cerebral laterality in individuals with DS

Atypical cerebral laterality (ACL) has been associated with the cognitive deficits of individuals with intellectual disability since the early 1920s (Gordon, 1921). ACL refers to the reverse or weak or bilateral representation of language in the two cerebral hemispheres (Geschwind & Galaburda, 1985). The majority of right-handed individuals (97%) exhibit left-hemisphere lateralization for language. Only about 60% of left-handed individuals exhibit left-hemisphere lateralization for language, 30% bilateral lateralization and 10% right-hemisphere lateralization for language (Bishop, 1990). Geschwind & Behan (1982) termed atypical laterality any laterality pattern that differed from the "standard dominance pattern" (pp. 70). According to Geschwind & Galaburda (1985a; 1985b), atypical dominance may involve the inverse or weak dominance of three features; hand dominance, language dominance and visuospatial dominance.

Several accounts have been put forward to explain the increased incidence of atypical laterality in individuals with neurodevelopmental disorders, which fall into four main categories: hormonal, genetic, pathological, and developmental. According to hormonal theories a number of exogenous and endogenous factors increase the secretion of prenatal testosterone in the fetus (Geschwind & Galaburda, 1987). This increment enhances the growth of the right cerebral hemisphere and inhibits that of the left cerebral hemisphere. In particular, their posterior regions, cortical areas tightly linked to intellectual disability and poor language development (Geschiwind & Galaburda, 1985a, 1985b, 1985c). This speculation has been repeatedly challenged during the past decades for its complexity (e.g., McManus & Bryden, 1991; McManus, Bryden & Bulman-Fleming, 1994; Annett, 1994; Previc, 1994), although the implication of testosterone levels in the establishment of cerebral lateralization remains well supported (e.g. Witleslon, 1985). For example, Witelson (1985, 1989) suggested that larger callosal isthmus is related to increased left-handedness in TD individuals, resulting from less axonal loss in the corpus callosum during foetal development, which is influenced by prenatal testosterone levels. Specifically, decreased levels of prenatal testosterone may cause decreased axonal loss in the corpus callosum, causing increased bilateral representation of cognitive functions and enhanced prevalence of non-right-handedness (Witelson, 1989, 1991).

Genetic theories argue that ACL results from genetic variation determined by a single gene (Annett, 1985; McManus & Bryden,1982). Individuals who are not carriers of this gene will exhibit random hand preference (right or left). Any pathology during development may inhibit the expression of the right-hand gene causing ACL (Annett & Alexander, 1996). Alternatively, Satz (1973) proposed that ACL may be the result of early brain damage in the left hemisphere, causing a mild dysfunction of the contralateral hand for motor activities, which in turn, forces a genetically right handed person to switch to non-right handedness. According to this account, individuals with ACL are "pathological" left handers, genetically programmed to become right handers, but brain pathology altered this biological expression. From a developmental perspective, ACL may be caused by an atypical maturational process in motor development that initiates from the trunk, followed by the shoulders and then the hands. If this maturational process is arrested, or lagged, it could cause increased randomness which would be documented by lack of hand preference (i.e., ambiguous handedness) (Palmer, 1964). Bishop (1983; 1990) speculated that non right handedness is an indicator of an immature development of the motor system, caused by diffuse brain abnormalities in individuals with intellectual disability.

The characteristic dissociation of language being disproportionately affected to visuospatial abilities in individuals with DS that cannot be accounted by the hearing impairments (Laws, 2004) provides suspicion for the link between ACL and language problems in DS population. Indeed, an extensive review of the literature indicates that individuals with DS document an ACL pattern in speech perception and oral motor movements (e.g., Elliott & Weeks, 1993; Elliott, Weeks, & Chua, 1994; Heath & Elliott, 1999).

In a typical dichotic listening paradigm, two different auditory verbal stimuli are simultaneously presented in each ear using headphones. The participant is asked to repeat the stimulus that was best heard. TD right-handed individuals document a right-ear advantage (REA) for speech stimuli, which is indicative of left hemisphere lateralization for speech perception. According to the original account, auditory information incoming from the right ear is predominately represented in the opposite hemisphere (i.e., the left hemisphere) due to anatomical contralateral auditory pathways and, thus, closer to the language centers of the same hemisphere (Kimura, 1961). In order for verbal stimuli incoming from the left ear to reach the left-hemisphere's language centers, information crosses from the right to the left cerebral hemisphere via the corpus callosum, causing significant delays. In individuals with DS, a left-ear/right-cerebral hemisphere preference for speech sounds (Hartley, 1981; Pipe, 1988), or no ear advantage (Sommer and Starkey, 1977; Tannock et al., 1984) has been observed, instead of the typical right-ear/left-cerebral hemisphere preference found in TD controls. Using dichotic listening tasks, Welsh, Elliot, and Simon (2003) verified this hypothesis with right-handed individuals with DS exhibiting a left-ear/right-cerebral hemisphere advantage for speech perception, unlike the right-ear/left-cerebral hemisphere laterality for speech perception typically observed in TD adults. Similar results were obtained in a Japanese study with individuals with DS (Shoji, Koizumi & Ozaki, 2008).

Recently, Groen, Alku and Bishop (2008) used T-complex auditory event-related potentials to investigate whether individuals with DS show ACL, as reflected by atypical patterns of brain activity elicited by verbal and tone sounds presented in each ear. The relationship between atypical lateralization, language deficits and handedness was further explored. The laterality patterns of individuals with DS were significantly different, compared to TD individuals, confirming the existence of ACL for auditory processing in this population. However, this atypicality was not specific to verbal stimuli, but also to non-verbal stimuli, suggesting a more "generalized abnormality in auditory processing in individuals with DS" (Groen et al., 2008, p. 155).

Overall, in line with behavioral studies of language lateralization in individual with DS, there is reasonable evidence for the existence of ACL in this group.

Laterality studies indicate that individuals with DS exhibit increased non-right handedness, and inconsistent hand preference compared to healthy adults (Groen, Yasin, Laws, Barry & Bishop, 2008). This finding is in accordance with laterality studies examining handedness in other populations with intellectual disability of different etiology (e.g., Grouios, Sakadami, Poderi & Alevriadou, 1999).

7. Discussion

An overview of studies examining language and visuospatial abilities in individuals with DS suggests that there is a unique profile of cognitive abilities characteristic to the syndrome that cannot be explained by intellectual disability. Individuals with DS exhibit diverse levels of strengths and weaknesses in both cognitive domains. Namely, the deficits in language abilities usually exceed impairments in visualspatial abilities. Recent studies demonstrate a more complex neuropsychological profile in this population, suggesting that the dissociation between language and visuospatial abilities is too simplistic. Indeed, we presented research that indicates that there are strengths and weaknesses in the visuospatial domain and the level of performance rarely exceed that of TD individuals matched for mental age. Moreover, the strength in visuospatial ability may be an artifact of comparisons with another genetic syndrome with intellectual disability, namely WS.

The brain abnormalities of individuals with DS result in a complex pattern of a behavioral phenotype that involves a number of interacting cognitive systems. It also implicates atypical lateralization of function reflected in the abnormal auditory perception for speech stimuli and increased incidence of non-right handedness. According to the neuronal network hypothesis, the cognitive deficits of individuals with intellectual disability are the result of weak connectivity of different areas of the cerebral cortex (Ramakers, 2002). If this holds true, then processing difficulties are not limited to cognitive systems, but also perceptual systems such as auditory pathways. Indeed, difficulties in perceptual organization have been correlated with severity of intellectual disability, which is consistent with the hypothesis of a more general deficit in information processing (Ramakers, 2002). Future research should investigate the development of language and visuospatial abilities longitudinally to provide information on when the divergence of these cognitive domains becomes apparent.

8. References

Annett, M. (1985). Left, right hand and brain: The right shift theory. London: Erlbaum.

Annett, M. (1994). Commentary Geschwind's legacy. *Brain and Cognition, 26,* 236-242. Annett, M. & Alexander, M.P. (1996). Atypical cerebral dominance: Predictions and tests of the right shift theory. *Neuropsychologia, 34,* 1215-1227.

Antonarakis, S., Lyle, R., Dermitzakis, E., Reymond, A., & Deutsch, S. (2004). Chromosome 21 and Down syndrome: from genomics to pathophysiology. *Nature Reviews Genetics 5*, 725-738.

Bellugi, U., Lichtenberger, L., Jones, W., Lai, Z., & St. George, M. (2000). The neurocognitive profile of Williams syndrome: A complex pattern of strengths and weaknesses. *Journal of Cognitive Neuroscience 12*, 7-29.

Bellugi, U., Lichtenberger, L., Mills, D., Galaburda, & A., Korenberg, J.R. (1999). Bridging cognition, brain and molecular genetics: Evidence from Williams syndrome. *Trends in Neurosciences, 5,* 197-208.

Bellugi, U., Wang, P. P., & Jernigan, T. L. (1994). Williams syndrome: An unusual neuropsychological profile. In S. H. Broman & J. Grafman (Eds), *Atypical cognitive profile in developmental disorders. Implications for brain function* (pp. 23–56). London: Lawrence Erlbaum.

Bilovsky, D., & Share, S. (1965) The ITPA and Down syndrome: an exploratory study. *American Journal of Mental Deficiency, 70, 78*-82.

Bishop, D. V. M. (1990). *Handedness and developmental disorders*. Hillsdale: Erlbaum.

Brown, J. H., Johnson, M. H., Paterson, S. J., Gilmore, R., Longhi, E., & Karmiloff-Smith, A. (2003). Spatial representation and attention in toddlers with Williams syndrome and Down syndrome. *Neuropsychologia, 41,* 1037–1046.

Bryden, M. P., McManus, I. C., & Bulman-Fleming, M. B. (1994). Evaluating the empirical support for the Geschwind-Behan-Galaburda model of cerebral lateralization. *Brain and Cognition, 26,* 103-167.

Bunn, L., Simon, D. A., Welsh, T. N., Watson, C., & Elliott, D. (2002). Speech production errors in adults with and without Down syndrome following verbal, written and pictorial cues. *Developmental Neuropsychology, 21,* 157–17.

Cardosa-Martins, C., Mervis, C. B., & Mervis, C. A. (1985). Early vocabulary acquisition by children with Down syndrome. *American Journal of Mental Deficiency, 90,* 177–184.

Carlesimo, G. A., Marotta, L., & Vicari, S. (1997). Long-term memory in mental retardation: Evidence for a specific impairment in subjects with Down's syndrome. *Neuropsychologia, 35,* 71–79.

Chapman, R. (1997). Language development in children and adolescents with Down syndrome. *Mental Retardation and Developmental Disabilities Research Reviews, 3,* 307–312.

Chapman, R. S., & Hesketh, L. J. (2001). Language, cognition and short-term memory in individu als with Down syndrome. Down Syndrome Research and Practice, 7, 1–7.

Chapman, R. S., Hesketh, L. J., & Kistler, D. J. (2002). Predicting longitudinal change in language production and comprehension in individuals with Down syndrome: Hierarchical linear model. *Journal of Speech Language and Hearing Research, 45,* 902–915.

Chapman, R. S., Schwartz, S. E., & Kay-Raining Bird, E. (1991). Language skills of children and adolescents with Down syndrome: I. Comprehension. *Journal of Speech and Hearing Research, 34,* 1106–1120.

Cole, L., Kardana, A., Park, S. & Braunstein, G. (1993). The deactivation of hCG by nicking and dissociation. *Journal of Clinical Endocrinology And Metabolism, 76,* 704-710.

Dodd, B. (1975). Recognition and reproduction of words by Down's syndrome and non-Down's syndrome retarded children. *American Journal of Mental Deficiency, 80,* 306–311.

Eadie, P. A., Fey, M. E., Douglas, J. M., & Parsons, C. L. (2002). Profiles of grammatical morphol- ogy and sentence imitation in children with specific language impairment and Down syndrome. *Journal of Speech, Language, and Hearing Research, 45,* 720–732.

Elliott, D., & Weeks, D. J. (1993). Cerebral specialization for speech perception and movement organization in adults with Down's syndrome. *Cortex, 29,* 103-113.

Elliott, T. K., & Watkins, M. J. (1998). Indices of Laterality in Turner syndrome. *Child Neuropsychology, 4,* 131-143.

Fildler, D. (2005). The Emerging Down Syndrome Behavioral Phenotype in Early Childhood Implications for Practice. *Infants and Young Children, 18,* 86-103.

Flórez, J. (1992). Neurologic abnormalities. In S. M. Pueschel & J. K, Pueschel (Eds.), *Biomedical concerns in persons with Down syndrome* (pp. 159-173). Baltimore: Paul H. Brookes Publishing Co.

Geschwind, N., & Behan, E. (1982). Left-handedness: Association with immune disease, migraine, and developmental learning disorder. *Proceedings of the National Academy of Science, 79,* 5097-5100.

Geschwind, N., & Galaburda, A. M. (1985a). Cerebral lateralization: Biological mechanisms, associations, and pathology: I. A hypothesis and a program for research. *Archives of Neurology, 42,* 428-459.

Geschwind, N., & Galaburda, A. M. (1985b). Cerebral lateralization: Biological mechanisms, associations, and pathology: II. A hypothesis and a program for research. *Archives of Neurology, 42,* 521-552.

Geschwind, N., & Galaburda, A. M. (1985c). Cerebral lateralization: Biological mechanisms, associations, and pathology: III. A hypothesis and a program for research. *Archives of Neurology, 42,* 634-654.

Geschwind, N., & Galaburda, A. S. (1987). Cerebral lateralization. Cambridge: MIT Press.

Gibson, D. (1978). *Down's syndrome: The psychology of mongolism.* Cambridge: Cambridge University Press.

Gordon, H. (1921). Left-handedness and mirror writing, especially among defective children. *Brain, 43,* 313-368.

Granholm, A. C., Sanders, L. A., & Crnic, L. S. (2000). Loss of cholinergic phenotype in basal fore- brain coincides with cognitive decline in a mouse model of Down's syndrome. *Experimental Neurology, 161,* 647–663.

Groen, M. A., Alku, P., & Bishop, D.V.M. (2008). Lateralisation of auditory processing in Down syndrome: a study of T-complex peaks Ta and Tb. *Biological Psychology, 79,* 148-157.

Grouios, G., Sakadami, N., Poderi, A. & Alevriadou, A. (1999). Excess of non-right handedness among individuals with intellectual disability: Experimental evidence and possible explanations. *Journal of Intellectual Disability Research, 43,* 306–313.

Hartley, X. Y. (1981). Lateralization of speech stimuli in young Down's syndrome children. *Cortex, 17,* 241-248.

Heath, M., & Elliott, D. (1999). The cerebral specialization for speech production in persons with Down syndrome. *Brain and Language, 69,* 193-211.

Hoddap, R. M., & Zigler, E. (1990). Applying the developmental perspective to individuals with Down syndrome. In D. M. Cicchetti & M. Beeghly (Eds.), *Children with Down syndrome* (pp. 1–28). New York: University Press.

Jarrold, C., & Baddeley, A. D. (1997) Short-term memory for verbal and visuospatial information in Down's syndrome. *Cognitive Neuropsychiatry, 2,* 101-122.

Jenkins, C. (1993). Expressive language delay in children with Down syndrome: A specific cause for concern. *Down Syndrome Research and Practice, 1, 10*–14.

Jernigan, T., & Bellugi, U. (1990). Anomalous brain morphology on magnetic resonance images in Williams syndrome and Down syndrome. *Archives of Neurology, 47,* 529-533.

Kesslak, J. P., Nagata, S. F., Lott, I. & Nalcioglu, O., (1994). Magnetic resonance imaging analysis of age-related changes in the brains of individuals with Down's syndrome. *Neurology 44,* 1039–1045.

Kimura D. (1961). Cerebral dominance and the perception of verbal stimuli. *Canadian Journal o Psychology,15,* 166–171.

Klein, B. P., & Mervis, C. B. (1999). Contrasting patterns of cognitive abilities of 9- and 10-year-olds with Williams syndrome or Down syndrome. *Developmental Neuropsychology, 16,* 177–196.

Lanfranchi, S., Carretti, B., Spanò, G. & Cornoldi, C. (2009). A specific deficit in visuo-spatial simultaneous working memory in Down Syndrome. *Journal of Intellectual Disability Research, 53,* 474-483.

Laws, G., & Bishop, D. V. M. (2003). A comparison of language abilities in adolescents with Down syndrome and children with specific language impairment. *Journal of Speech, Language, and Hearing Research, 46,* 1324–1339.

Lubek, G., & Engidawork, E. (2002). The brain in Down syndrome. *Journal of Neurology, 249,* 1347–1356.

McManus, I. C., & Bryden, M. P. (1992). The genetics of handedness, cerebral dominance and lateralization. In I. Rapin & S. Segalowitz, (Eds.), Handbook of Neuropsyhcology Vol.6: Section 10 Child Neuropsychology Part 1.pp. 115-145. Amsterdam: Elsevier.

McManus, I. C., & Bryden, M. P. (1991). Geschwind's theory of cerebral lateralization: Developing a formal, causal model. Psychological Bulletin, 110, 237-253.

Miller, J. F. (1992). Development of speech and language in children with Down syndrome. In I. T. Lott & E. E. McCoy (Eds.), *Down syndrome: Advances in medical care* (pp. 39–50). New York: Wiley-Liss Inc.

Nadel, L. (1999). Down syndrome in Cognitive Neuroscience perspective. In H. Tager-Flusberg (Ed.), *Neurodevelopmental disorders* (pp. 197–221). Cambridge, MA: MIT Press.

Palmer, R. D. (1964). Development of differentiated handedness. *Psychological Bulletin, 62,* 257-272.

Pennington, B. F., Moon, J., Edgin, J., Stedron, J., & Nadel, L. (2003). The Neuropsychology of Down syndrome: Evidence for hippocampal dysfunction. *Child Development, 74,* 75–93.

Pennington, B. F., Moon, J., Edgin, J., Stedron, J., & Nadel, L. (2003). The Neuropsychology of Down syndrome: Evidence for hippocampal dysfunction. *Child Development, 74,* 75–93.

Pinker, S. (1991). Rules of language. *Science, 253,* 530–535.

Pinter, J. D., Brown, W. E., Eliez, S., Schmitt, J. E., Capone, G. T., & Reiss, A. L. (2001). Amygdala and hippocampal volumes in children with Down syndrome: A high resolution MRI study. *Neurology, 56,* 972–974.

Pipe, M. E. (1988). Atypical laterality and retardation. *Psychological Bulletin, 104,* 343-347.

Previc, F. H. (1994). Assessing the legacy of the GBG model. *Brain & Cognition, 26,* 174-180.

Pueschel, S., Gallangher, P., Zaltler, A., & Pezzullo, J. (1987). Cognitive and learning processes in children with Down syndrome. *Research in Developmental Disabilities, 8,* 21-37.

Rogers, P. T., Roizen, N. J., & Capone, G. T. (1996). Down syndrome. In A. J. Capute & P. J. Accardo (Eds.), *Developmental disabilities in infancy and childhood: Volume II The spectrum of developmental disabilities* (2nd ed., pp. 221–244). New York: Paul H. Brookes.

Rondal, J. A. (1988). Down's Syndrome. In D. Bishop & K. Magrad (Eds.), *Language development in exceptional circumstances* (pp. 21–36). Edinburgh: Churchill Livingstone.

Rondal, J., Perera, J., & Nadel, L. (1999). *Down Syndrome: A review of current knowledge.* London: Whurr.

Satz, P. (1973). Left-handedness and early brain insult: An explanation, *Neuropsychologia, 11,* 115-117.

Shoji, H., Koizumi, N., & Ozaki, H. (2009).Linguistic lateralization in adolescents with Down syndrome revealed by a dichotic monitoring test. *Research in Developmental Disability, 30,* 219-228.

Sommer R. K., Starkey K. L. (1977). Dichotic verbal processing in Down's syndrome children having qualitatively different speech and language skills. *American Journal of Mental Deficiency, 82,* 44–53.

Takashima, S., Ieshima, A., Nakamura, H., & Becker, L. E. (1989). Dendrites, dementia and the Down syndrome. *Brain Development, 2,* 131–143.

Tannock R. Kershner J. R. & Oliver J. (1984). Do individuals with Down's syndrome possess right hemisphere language dominance? *Cortex, 20,* 221- 231.

Teipel, S. J., Schapiro, M. B., Alexander, G. E., Krasuski, J. S., Horwitz, B., Hoehne, C., Möller, H., Rapoport, S. I., & Hampel, H. (2003). Relation of corpus callosum and hippocampal size to age in nondemented adults with Down's syndrome. *American Journal of Psychiatry, 160,* 1870–1878.

Wang, P. P., & Bellugi, U. (1994). Evidence from two genetic syndromes for a dissociation between verbal and visual-spatial short-term memory. *Journal of Clinical and Experimental Neuropsychology, 16,* 317–322.

Wang, P. P., Hesselink, J. R., Jernigan, T. L., Doherty, S., & Bellugi, U. (1992). *Neocerebellar preservation is associated with a specific neurobehavioral profile in Williams syndrome.* American Academy of Neurology, San Diego, CA.

Welsh, T. N., Elliott, D., & Simon, D. A. (2003). Cerebral specialization and verbal-motor integration in adults with and without Down syndrome. *Brain and Language, 84,* 152-169.

Wiig, E. H., & Secord, W. (1992). *Test of word knowledge.* San Antonio, TX: The Psychological Corporation.

Witelson, S. F. (1985). The brain connection: The corpus callosum is larger in left-handers. *Science, 229,* 665-668.

Witelson, S. F. (1989). Hand and sex differences in the isthmus and genu of the human corpus callosum: A post-mortem morphological study. *Brain, 112,* 799-835.

Witelson, S. F. (1991). Neural sexual mosaicism: Sexual differentiation of the human temporoparietal region for functional asymmetry. *Psychoneuroendocrinology, 16,* 131-153.

Ypsilanti, A., Grouios, G., Alevriadou, A., & Tsapkini, K. (2005). Expressive and receptive vocabulary in children with Williams and Down syndromes. *Journal of Intellectual Disability Research, 49,* 353–364.

Ypsilanti, A., & Grouios, G. (2008). Linguistic Profile of Individuals with Down Syndrome: Comparing the Linguistic Performance of Three Developmental Disorders. *Child Neuropsychology, 14,* 148-170.

Part 4

Prenatal Diagnosis and Screening

16

Prenatal Diagnosis of Down Syndrome

Myungshin Kim, Jong Chul Shin and In Yang Park
The Catholic University of Korea, Seoul, Korea

1. Introduction

Chromosomal aberration is a phenomenon occurring relatively commonly in the development process. Chromosomal aberration is known to have various causes, and its frequency has been reported to vary particularly according to maternal age. Though different among reports, the frequency was around 0.6-0.8% in analysis with all childbirths[1] and around 2-3% in case childbirths were reclassified based on maternal age of 35.[2] In addition, the frequency increased when the maternal age was relatively young, artificial insemination was used, etc.[3] Spontaneous abortion related to such chromosomal aberrations occurs usually in the first trimester, and consequently, the prevalence of trisomy 21, 18 and 13 decreases with the advance of gestational age.[4] Chromosomal aberrations that can be found in prenatal diagnosis are largely divided into aneuploidy, structural aberration, mosaicism, uniparental disomy, small defect, etc., and additionally, there can be marker chromosomes. Marker chromosomes are observed in around one out of 1000 cases of chromosomal analysis, and are known to be related to old maternal age.[5] It is reported that around 80% of marker chromosomes detected are new ones, and 13% of marker chromosomes are associated with physical abnormalities or cognitive disorders.[6]
The frequency and type of chromosomal aberration are known to be different depending on the time of evaluation, population group under the analysis of structural chromosomal aberration, and the banding level of the laboratory performing cytogenetic evaluation.[7] Thus, it is increasingly important to conduct adequate prenatal genetic screening and analyze its results properly. Among chromosomal aberrations detected in pregnant women who received amniocentesis because of their age, 64% were trisomy (21% trisomy 21), 11% translocation, 17% sex chromosomal aberration, and 8% other types of chromosomal aberration.[2] Thus, considering the increasing number of old age pregnancies in Korea, careful attention should to paid in analyzing the results of prenatal genetic tests. Thus, this study purposed to discuss how to analyze the results of maternal serum marker tests and sonography used in prenatal genetic evaluation.

2. Maternal serum screening

2.1 Alpha fetoprotein

Brock and Sutcliffe [2] found in 1972 that the level of alpha fetoprotein in amniotic fluid increased when the fetus had a neural tube defect, and from the 1980s, the maternal serum alpha fetoprotein test began to be used for screening fetal anomalies in pregnant women.

Alpha fetoprotein, which is glycoprotein, is produced in the yolk sac in the early stage, and later in the fetal gastrointestinal tract and liver. A small portion of alpha fetoprotein in fetal serum may be discharged to urine and amniotic fluid, and it may diffuse through the fetal membrane and the placenta and enter maternal serum. Whereas the alpha fetoprotein level in fetal serum and amniotic fluid increases until 13 week and then decreases thereafter, the level in maternal serum increases continuously until 32 week because the size of the fetus keeps growing.[8] Between 16-20 week of gestational age, the level of alpha fetoprotein in maternal serum is only around 1/100,000 of that in fetal serum.

2.1.1 Analysis of serum alpha fetoprotein data

As is known, the concentration of alpha fetoprotein in maternal serum or amniotic fluid is measured as a test for screening fetal neural tube defects. When the measurements of alpha fetoprotein are analyzed, we should be careful not to attach clinical importance to absolute values. It is because the test method of each laboratory or company may seem to have been stabilized by itself, but absolute values from the method are often different from those obtained by other laboratories or test methods. For this reason, the measurements of alpha fetoprotein are often reported as the multiples of the median (MoM). A median is the value in the middle when result values are put in order of size, so it can reduce errors and allow the comparative analysis of result values without being influenced by laboratory or test method.

On the other hand, the measurements of alpha fetoprotein in maternal serum can be affected not only by multiple pregnancy and gestational age but also by maternal weight, diabetes, race, etc.[9,10], so these factors should be confirmed before the analysis of such measurements. Because the absolute level of serum alpha fetoprotein rises along with gestational age[8], underestimated gestational age is the most common cause of increased alpha fetoprotein concentration. In such a case, we can avoid unnecessary additional tests by correcting gestational age and recalculating the median.

2.1.2 Causes of increased alpha fetoprotein in maternal serum

Fetal anomalies

The rise of the alpha fetoprotein level in maternal serum is often accompanied by fetal anomalies. This is not because of a special function of alpha fetoprotein but because fetal tissue leaks to amniotic fluid due to neural tube defect, abdominal wall defect, sacrococcygeal teratoma, cystic hygroma, skin defect, etc. and, as a result, an increasing amount of alpha fetoprotein flows into amniotic fluid and maternal serum[11] or because alpha fetoprotein is not reabsorbed but discharged to urine due to fetal kidney anomaly.[12]

In fetal neural tube defect, alpha fetoprotein exudes through exposed nervous tissue, so the level of alpha fetoprotein in maternal serum is relatively higher in spina bifida aperta or anencephaly than in spina bifida occulta. In most laboratories, those whose median alpha fetoprotein level in maternal serum is over 2.0-2.5 are classified into a high-risk group of fetal neural tube defect. When median 2.5 was used, spina bifida aperta was detected at a detection rate of 80% and the false positive rate was 3-4%.[13]

The anomaly found second most commonly to neural tube defect in alpha-fetoprotein screening is abdominal wall defect. Particularly in case of gastroschisis, organs removed out of the abdominal cavity contact amniotic fluid directly, and therefore, the alpha fetoprotein level tends to be higher than that in omphalocele.[11] Maternal serum alpha fetoprotein screening detects around 85% of gastroschisis and around 50 % of omphalocele.[11]

Placental abnormalities

Because the concentration of alpha fetoprotein in fetal serum is 100,000 times higher than that in maternal serum[8], even a small inflow of fetal blood increases the fetoprotein level in maternal serum rapidly. In case of chorioangioma in the placenta and hemangioma in the umbilical cord, fetal serum exudes into amniotic fluid and the maternal body due to mass bleeding[14], and in case of placenta accreta, placental infarct, etc. as well, alpha fetoprotein increases in the same way.[16]

2.2 Maternal serum test for aneuploidy screening

2.2.1 Second trimester multiple marker screening test

In 1984, Merkatz et al.[16] found that the risk of Down syndrome was high when the level of serum alpha fetoprotein was low during the second trimester, but this finding alone was not sufficient for using alpha fetoprotein as an accurate Down syndrome marker.[16] Later, double marker test that added human chorionic gonadotropin (hCG) test, and triple test that added also estriol (E3) to the double test were introduced as Down syndrome screening tests in the second trimester.[18] Recently, quad test that added inhibin A was developed[18] for higher accuracy of screening. The mean median (MoM) of each marker in trisomy 21 and 18 is presented in Table 1. There were large-scale prospective studies that compared accuracy among a number of multiple markers in the U.K. (Serum, Urine and Ultrasound Screening Study; SURUSS)[19] and the U.S. (First and Second Trimester Evaluation of Risk for Fetal Anueploidy; FASTER),[20] and in both studies the detection rate of quad markers was reported to be 81 %. Table 2 summarized the Down syndrome detection rates of multiple markers from the two studies.

Aneuploidy	AFP	hCG	uE3	Inhibin A
Trisomy 21	0.74 * (↓)	2.05 * (↑)	0.70 * (↓)	2.548 * (↑)
Trisomy 18	0.65** (↓)	0.32** (↓)	0.42** (↓)	-

AFP, α-fetoprotein; hCG, human chorionic gonadotropin; uE3, unconjugated estriol
* Modified from the results of the FASTER trial
** Modified from the results of Benn PA et al. Obstet Gyenecol 1999;93:707-11.

Table 1. The mean MoM (multiples of the median) values for the second trimester maternal serum quad markers.

		Detection rate at a 5% false-positive rate	
		SURUSS[19]	FASTER[20]
Double markers	AFP + hCG	66%	-
Triple markers	AFP + hCG + uE3	74%	70%
Quad markers	AFP + hCG + uE3 + inhibin A	81%	81%

AFP, α-fetoprotein; hCG, human chorionic gonadotropin; uE3, unconjugated estriol

Table 2. The detection rate of second trimester serum markers for Down syndrome.

2.2.2 First trimester screening test

Maternal serum triple marker test

Among first trimester serum markers, pregnancy-associated plasma protein A (PAPP-A) and free β-hCG are known to have the highest discrimination for haploidy. In Down syndrome, the MoM of maternal serum PAPP-A is 0.38, decreasing by 60%, and that of free β-hCG is 1.83, increasing by around two times.[21] Accordingly, both of the two markers are used in first trimester screening, and with this test, the Down syndrome detection rate is 60-74% and the false positive rate is 5%.[19,20] The detection rate is lower than that of the quad test in the second trimester but similar to that of the triple test.

Nuchal translucency measuring

The thickness of nuchal translucency in the first trimester is related to fetal haploidy, in particular, to Down syndrome, apart from maternal serum markers.[22] Accordingly, the accuracy of screening can be enhanced through the first trimester combined test that measures the thickness of nuchal translucency in addition to serologic tests that measure PAPPA-A and free β-hCG.[22] In the results of a meta-analysis with 209,603 subjects, the combined screening test showed a detection rate of 86% (84-88 95%, CI) with a false positive rate of 5.1% and Down syndrome was detected in 785 subjects.[23] When only nuchal translucency was measured without serologic tests, the Down syndrome detection rate was 77% with a false positive rate of 6.0%, so it was less accurate than the combined test. The positive predictive value of the combined screening test was 16.8 (16.3-17.4, 95% CI), which means that one out of 17 pregnancies with a positive result of the combined screening test is found to have a Down syndrome fetus.[23] On the other hand, because PAPP-A decreases but free β-hCG increases for 11-14 weeks of pregnancy, the detection rate varies significantly according to gestational age.[23] In the results of FASTER, the Down syndrome detection rate was 73% and the false positive rate was 1% in 11 weeks of pregnancy, but 67% and 5%, respectively, in 13 weeks, and based on this result the research reported that the accuracy of the combined test was highest at the gestational age of 11 weeks.[20] However, it was reported that if second trimester screening would be performed additionally, it would be more efficient to have the combined test in 10 weeks of pregnancy.[23]

2.2.3 First and second trimester integrated test

Wald et al.[24] proposed integrated test, which uses information on first and second trimester markers in sequence. They expected that if nuchal translucency and serum PAPP-A are measured in 10-13 weeks, and alpha fetoprotein, total hCG, estriol and inhibin A in 15-18 weeks, Down syndrome can be detected at a rate of 94% with a false positive rate of 5%, or 85% with a false positive rate of 1%.[25] Accordingly, because Down syndrome can be screened with a false positive rate of 1%, it reduces the need of additional diagnoses such as amniocentesis, and prevents fetal death resulting from invasive examination. In the results of SURUSS[19] and FASTER,[20] the integrated test was most accurate as a Down syndrome screening test (Table 3).

However, the integrated test has a number of shortcomings to be an alternative general screening test in prenatal examination. First, most of pregnant women who receive a screening test in the first trimester want the termination of pregnancy immediately if abnormalities are found in the fetus, and it is safer to terminate pregnancy in the first trimester. Second, it is hard to distinguish pregnant women who cannot be followed up after first trimester serologic tests. In SURUSS [19] as well, 20% of pregnant women who had a first trimester test did not appear in the second trimester test. In such a case, there could be the legal risk of not telling the results of the first trimester test, so it was not an adequate alternative at present. Third, if the risk is unusually high in the results of the first trimester test the results are not provided until the second trimester, and this may raise an ethical issue. Thus, the integrated test can be the method of highest sensitivity and specificity if a pregnant woman receives prenatal examination from the beginning of pregnancy and takes both the first and second trimester screening tests, but is not adequate for those who want to get invasive chorionic villus sampling immediately based on the results of the first trimester screening test.

	FASTER[20]					SURUSS[19]				
	FPR(%) for DR of			DR(%) for FPR of		FPR(%) for DR of			DR(%) for FPR of :	
	75%	85%	95%	1%	5%	75%	85%	95%	1%	5%
1st trimester										
NT only	8.1	20	55	54	68	12.9	25	55	33	60
PAPP-A + f-βhCG	7.1	16	42	46	67	5.5	12.1	33	52	74
Combined†	1.2	3.8	18	72	85	2.3	6.1	22	66	83
1st + 2nd trimester:										
Serum integrated‡§	1.2	3.6	15	70	86	0.8	2.7	12.5	77	90
Full integrated§	0.2	0.6	4.0	87	95	0.3	1.2	7.2	84	95
2nd trimester										
Triple (AFP+hCG+E3)	7.0	14	32	45	69	2.9	7.1	22	51	74
Quad (Triple+inhibin A)	3.1	7.3	22	60	81	2.6	6.1	18	63	83

DR, detection rate; FPR, false positive rate; NT, nuchal translucency; PAPP-A, pregnancy associated plasma protein-A; f-βhCG free beta subunit of human chorionic gonadotropin; Quad, second trimester quadruple screen; AFP, alphafetoprotein; uE3, unconjugated estriol
† Combined: NT, PAPP-A, and f-βhCG in the first trimester
‡ Serum integrated: PAPP-A in the first trimester and quad screen in the second trimester
§ Full integrated: NT and PAPP-A in the first trimester with quad screen in the second trimester
Data from Rosen T et al. Semin Perinatol 2005;29:367-75.

Table 3. Direct comparative data for the first and second trimester Down syndrome screens from the prospective FASTER and SURUSS trials.

2.2.4 Alternatives to the integrated test

Sequential screening

If the result of the first trimester screening test is positive, chromosomal analysis is performed immediately and if the result is negative, the second trimester screening test is performed and if the result is positive, chromosomal analysis is performed. A characteristic of this method is that the result of the first trimester screening test is provided to the pregnant woman and then the second trimester test is performed additionally. It can enhance the Down syndrome detection rate up to 98% but its false positive rate is also high as 17%.[26]

Contingency screening

If the first trimester screening test indicates high risk, chromosomal analysis is performed, and if the result indicates low risk no additional test is performed, but if it indicates moderate risk integrating screening is performed.[27]

3. Genetic sonographic markers of aneuploidy

Most of fetuses with chromosomal aberration have organs whose appearance is anomalous or abnormal, and such defects can be detected through prenatal sonography. A fetal structural anomaly may be caused by multiple factors, but it can be the result of chromosomal aberration. Therefore, if a fetal anomaly has been found, we should determine whether to perform cytogenetic analysis through amniocentesis after checking if other abnormalities accompany. Using genetic sonographic findings, we can detect pregnancies with high risk of aneuploidy at a sensitivity of 50-93%[28], and the absence of genetic sonographic findings may be regarded as sure evidence for the low risk of haploidy. Genetic sonographic findings can be divided into major structural anomalies and minor anomalies. In particular, anomalies that are observed frequently also in normal fetuses and occasionally disappear with the advance of gestational age are called sonographic markers. It is generally accepted that a major anomaly is a sign of high risk of chromosomal aberration and thus chromosomal analysis is required, but it is still controversial whether additional tests are required when only a minor anomaly has been found. It is important to determine in consideration of the likelihood of chromosomal aberration on a case basis rather than applying a uniform rule to every case, and for this, we need to be familiar with the risk of chromosomal aberration and representative types of haploidy in connection to each genetic sonographic marker (Table 4).

3.1 Major anomalies related to haploidy

The characteristic and frequency of sonographic findings in fetuses with chromosomal aberration are various according to gestational age, and the detection of abnormal findings is affected by the reason of sonography, criteria for positive finding, the level of sonographic equipment, etc. Structural major anomalies are detected mostly by sonography in trisomy 13 and 18, but are missed relatively often in trisomy 21. Table 5 summarized structural major anomalies detected commonly in pregnancies with trisomy 13, 18 and 21 and Turner syndrome.

3.2 Sonographic markers related to haploidy

The most common sonographic markers in the second trimester include nuchal thickening, hyperechoic bowel, short limbs, pyelectasia, echogenic intracardiac focus, and choroid plexus cysts. In general, the risk of chromosomal aberration is higher when the number of markers is large. Table 6 summarized the likelihood ratio of haploidy when each sonographic marker has occurred singly. The likelihood ratio was calculated by sensitivity / false positive rate, and if two or more sonographic markers have occurred together, the combined likelihood ratio is the product of their respective likelihood ratios.

Structural defect	Population incidence	Aneuploidy risk	Most common aneploidy (Trisomy)
Cystic hygroma	1/120 EU–1/6,000 B	60-75%	45X (80%),21,18,13,XXY
Hydrops	1/1,500–4,000 B	30-80%	13,21,18,45X
Hydrocephalus	3–8/10,000 LB	3-8%	13,18,triploidy
Hydranencephaly	2/1,000 IA	Minimal	
Holoprosencephaly	1/16,000 LB	40-60%	13,18,18p-
Cardiac defect	7-9/100 LB	5-30%	21,18,13,22,8,9
Diaphragmatic hernia	1/3,500–4,000 LB	20-25%	13,18,21,45X
Omphalocele	1/5,800 LB	30-40%	13,18
Gastroschisis	1/10,000–15,000 LB	Minimal	
Duodenal atresia	1/10,000 LB	20-30%	21
Bladder outlet obstruction	1-2/1,000 LB	20-25%	13,18
Facial cleft	1/700 LB	1%	13,18, deletions
Limb reduction	4-6/1,000 LB	8%	18
Clubfoot	1.2/1,000 LB	20-30%	13,18, 4p-, 18q-
Single umbilical artery	1%	Minimal	

B, birth; EU, early ultrasonography; LB, livebirth; IA, infant autopsy.

Data from Shipp TD, et al. Am J Obstet Gynecol 1998; 178: 600–2. and Nyberg DA and Crane JP. Chromosome abnormalities. In: Nyberg DA, et al. Diagnostic ultrasound of fetal anomalies: text and atlas. Chicago (IL): Year Book Medical; 1990. p. 676–724.

Table 4. Aneuploidy risk of major structural fetal malformation.

Aneuploidy	Sonographic finding	Aneuploidy	Sonographic finding
Trisomy 13	heart (VSD, dilated right ventricle) CNS (ventriculomegaly, holoprosencephaly) Face (midline defects, ocular abnormalities) Kidney(enlarged cystic kidneys) IUGR with polyhydramnios	Trisomy 21	Heart (septal defects) Abnormal fluid accumulation (thickened nuchal fold, cystic hygroma, fetal hydrops) Abdominal malformations IUGR with polyhydramnios
Trisomy 18	Heart (VSD) CNS (posterior fossa cyst, abnormal head shape, ventriculomegaly) Facial anomalies Choroid plexus cyst Abnormal fluid accumulation (thickened nuchal fold, cystic hygroma, fetal hydrops) Abdominal malformations IUGR with polyhydramnios	Turner syndrome	Heart (Coarctation of aorta) Abnormal fluid accumulation (increased nuchal translucency/ thickened nuchal fold, cystic hygroma, feta hydrops) Renal anomalies Short femur or humerus

CNS, central nervous system; IUGR, intrauterine growth restriction; VSD, ventricular septal defect

Table 5. Sonographic finding with high incidence in different fetal chromosomal abnormalities

	Likelihood ratio (95% confidence interval)	
Sonographic marker	Nyberg et al.	Smith-Bindman et al.
Nuchal thickening	11.0 (5.5-22.0)	17 (8-38)
Hyperechoic bowel	6.7 (2.7-16.8)	6.1 (3.0-12.6)
Short humerus	5.1 (1.6-16.5)	7.5 (4.7-12.0)
Short femur	1.5 (0.8-2.8)	2.7 (1.2-6.0)
Echogenic intracardiac focus	1.8 (1.0-3.0)	2.8 (1.5-5.5)
Pyelectasis	1.5 (0.6-3.6)	1.9 (0.7-5.1)
Normal ultrasound	0.36	-

Data from Nyberg DA, et al Ultrasound Obstet Gynecol 1998; 12: 8-14. and Smith-Bindman R et al. JAMA. 2001; 285: 1044-55.

Table 6. Likelihood ratio of sonographic soft marker for fetal aneuploidy

3.2.1 Choroid plexus cysts

Choroid plexus cyst is found relatively commonly during the second trimester, showing a prevalence of 0.3-3.6%.[29] This type of cyst is known to be benign, disappearing spontaneously at the later stage of pregnancy without affecting the development of the fetus. As a sonographic marker of haploidy, choroid plexus cyst is found in 50% of fetuses with trisomy 18[30] but most of the cases are accompanied by another anomaly, and it is reported that no particular prenatal care including chromosomal analysis is necessary if only isolated choroid plexus cysts are found.[29]

3.2.2 Mild cerebral ventricular dilatation

Mild cerebral ventricular dilatation, in which the diameter of the cerebral lateral ventricle is over 10-15 mm, is related to aneuploidy like trisomy 21.[32] Bromley et al.[32] reported that 12% of pregnancies with mild cerebral ventricular dilatation are related to abnormal karyotype (trisomy 18, 21). In addition, mild cerebral ventricular dilatation was observed in 4.3% of fetuses with trisomy 21[33] and all of them had accompanying anomalies. It is known that the presence of cerebral ventricular dilatation alone does not increase the risk of chromosomal aberration.

3.2.3 Nuchal thickening

Excessive skin on the back neck is a characteristic finding of trisomy 21. It is observed in 80% of neonates with trisomy 21 and can be found in other chromosomal aberrations (trisomy 13 and 18, 45X).[34] Although the sensitivity and the false positive rate vary according to gestational age and criteria for positive value are different among institutions, its sensitivity for detecting chromosomal aberrations is generally within the range of 20-40%.

3.2.4 Hyper-echoic bowel

Hyper-echoic bowel is found in 0.5% of normal fetuses, but in fetuses with aneuploidy like trisomy 21, it is known to be observed more frequently and increase the risk 6-7 times higher.[35] Assuming that the likelihood ratio of isolated hyper-echoic bowel is 6.7 and the total risk of Down syndrome in the entire population is one per 500, isolated echoic bowel is expected to be related to the risk of Down syndrome in around 1-2% of the general population. Hyper-echoic bowel is also known to be related to ileus, congenital infection, and rarely to secondary meconium ileus in cystic fibrosis.[36]

3.2.5 Skeletal abnormalities such as shortened limbs

Shortened limbs are a characteristic observed in fetuses with trisomy 21[37] and the length of shortened humerus seems to be a slightly more specific marker than the length of shortened femur. These results may be different according to gestational age, racial group, expected sex of the fetus, and used criteria.

3.2.6 Echogenic intracardiac focus

Echogenic intracardiac focus is a common finding in the second trimester. It is observed in 3-4% of normal fetuses and disappears spontaneously in the third trimester.[39] If the size of echogenic intracardiac focus is large or there are multiple of them, the risk of aneuploidy increases. Bromley et al.[40] reported that the risk of aneuploidy is 2 times higher when echogenic intracardiac focuses are in the right ventricle or bilateral than when they are only in the left ventricle.

4. Conclusions

Chromosomal aberration is closely related to the in intrauterine fetal death and perinatal prevalence. However, amniocentesis and chorionic villus sampling used for prenatal diagnosis of haploidy are invasive methods, and the reported fetal loss rate resulting just from the examinations is around 1-2%. Accordingly, it is very important to screen those with high risk of chromosomal aberration before such invasive examinations.

Serologic test of pregnant women for the screening of trisomy 18 and 21 is an important diagnostic process in prenatal care, and in particular, second trimester serum alpha fetoprotein is used as an important screening marker to detect anomalies such as fetal neural tube defect. If the concentration of alpha fetoprotein is over 2.5 MoM, sonography should be performed in order to detect neural tube defect and other problems. Recently, because sonography shows a high detection rate for neural tube defect, amniocentesis is used less frequently in diagnosing neural tube defect.

The preferred type of serum screening test is various among countries and institutions. In general, the first trimester screening test is increasingly preferred, but second trimester screening is still used frequently at hospitals that cannot measure fetal nuchal translucency or perform chorionic villus sampling. The triple test has been used commonly as second trimester screening, but recently the use of the quad test, which adds inhibin A, is increasing. If both first and second trimester tests are performed, they can increase the detection rate of fetal anomalies, but because the two tests have to be applied at an interval of 3-4 weeks, it is quite important to provide an adequate explanation to the patient. The serum screening test can be performed in various ways depending on the combination of serum factors. Thus, rather than using a uniform test for every case, we need to understand the characteristic, detection rate and false positive rate of each test, and individualize the test for each case according to maternal age, sonographic findings, and compliance.

In conclusion, in order to determine the risk of chromosomal aberration, we should analyze each case based on maternal age, nuchal fold thickness in the first trimester, the results of maternal serum screening in the first or second trimester, and sonographic findings in the second trimester. Through this approach, we may reduce the number of unnecessary chromosomal analyses, lower the fetal loss rate resulting from invasive examination, and enhance the accuracy of screening for fetal chromosomal aberrations.

5. References

[1] Nielsen J, Wohlert M. Chromosome abnormalities found among 34,910 newborn children: results from a 13-year incidence study in Arhus, Denmark. Hum Genet 1991; 87: 81-3.

[2] Ferguson-Smith MA, Yates JR. Maternal age specific rates for chromosome aberrations and factors influencing them: report of a collaborative european study on 52,965 amniocenteses. Prenat Diagn 1984; 4: 5-44.

[3] Munné S, Sultan KM, Weier HU, Grifo JA, Cohen J, Rosenwaks Z. Assessment of numeric abnormalities of X, Y, 18, and 16 chromosomes in preimplantation human embryos before transfer. Am J Obstet Gynecol 1995; 172(4 Pt 1): 1191-9.

[4] Snijders RJ, Sundberg K, Holzgreve W, Henry G, Nicolaides KH. Maternal age- and gestation-specific risk for trisomy 21. Ultrasound Obstet Gynecol 1999; 13: 167-70.

[5] Li MM, Howard-Peebles PN, Killos LD, Fallon L, Listgarten E, Stanley WS. Characterization and clinical implications of marker chromosomes identified at prenatal diagnosis. Prenat Diagn 2000; 20 : 138-43.

[6] Warburton D. De novo balanced chromosome rearrangements and extra marker chromosomes identified at prenatal diagnosis: clinical significance and distribution of breakpoints. Am J Hum Genet 1991; 49: 995-1013.

[7] American College of Obstetricians and Gynecologists. ACOG Practice Bulletin No. 88, December 2007. Invasive prenatal testing for aneuploidy. Obstet Gynecol 2007; 110: 1459-67.

[8] Haddow JE. Prenatal screening for open neural tube defects, Down's syndrome, and other major fetal disorders. Semin Perinatol 1990; 14: 488-503.

[9] Haddow JE, Kloza EM, Knight GJ, Smith DE. Relation between maternal weight and serum alpha-fetoprotein concentration during the second trimester. Clin Chem 1981; 27: 133-4.

[10] Wald NJ, Cuckle H, Boreham J, Stirrat GM, Turnbull AC. Maternal serum alpha-fetoprotein and diabetes mellitus. Br J Obstet Gynaecol 1979; 86: 101-5.

[11] Palomaki GE, Hill LE, Knight GJ, Haddow JE, Carpenter M. Second-trimester maternal serum alpha-fetoprotein levels in pregnancies associated with gastroschisis and omphalocele. Obstet Gynecol 1988; 71(6 Pt 1): 906-9.

[12] Albright SG, Warner AA, Seeds JW, Burton BK. Congenital nephrosis as a cause of elevated alpha-fetoprotein. Obstet Gynecol 1990; 76(5 Pt 2): 969-71.

[13] Wald NJ, Hackshaw AK, George LM. Assay precision of serum alpha fetoprotein in antenatal screening for neural tube defects and Down's syndrome. J Med Screen 2000; 7: 74-7.

[14] Bernstein IM, Barth RA, Miller R, Capeless EL. Elevated maternal serum alpha-fetoprotein: association with placental sonolucencies, fetomaternal hemorrhage, vaginal bleeding, and pregnancy outcome in the absence of fetal anomalies. Obstet Gynecol 1992; 79: 71-4.

[15] Butler EL, Dashe JS, Ramus RM. Association between maternal serum alpha-fetoprotein and adverse outcomes in pregnancies with placenta previa. Obstet Gynecol 2001; 97: 35-8.

[16] Merkatz IR, Nitowsky HM, Macri JN, Johnson WE. An association between low maternal serum alpha-fetoprotein and fetal chromosomal abnormalities. Am J Obstet Gynecol 1984; 148: 886-94.

[17] Wald NJ, Cuckle HS, Densem JW, Nanchahal K, Royston P, Chard T, et al. Maternal serum screening for Down's syndrome in early pregnancy. BMJ 1988; 297: 883-7.

[18] Wald NJ, Densem JW, George L, Muttukrishna S, Knight PG. Prenatal screening for Down's syndrome using inhibin-A as a serum marker. Prenat Diagn 1996; 16: 143-53.

[19] Wald NJ, Rodeck C, Hackshaw AK, Walters J, Chitty L, Mackinson AM. First and second trimester antenatal screening for Down's syndrome: the results of the Serum, Urine and Ultrasound Screening Study (SURUSS). J Med Screen 2003; 10: 56-104.

[20] Malone FD, Canick JA, Ball RH, Nyberg DA, Comstock CH, Bukowski R, et al. First- and Second-Trimester Evaluation of Risk (FASTER) Research Consortium. First-trimester or second-trimester screening, or both, for Down's syndrome. N Engl J Med 2005; 353: 2001-11.

[21] Benn PA, Leo MV, Rodis JF, Beazoglou T, Collins R, Horne D. Maternal serum screening for feta trisomy 18: a comparion of fixed cut off and patient-specific risk protocols. Obstet Gyenecol 1999; 93: 707-11.

[22] Brizot ML, Snijders RJ, Butler J, Bersinger NA, Nicolaides KH. Maternal serum hCG and fetal nuchal translucency thickness for the prediction of fetal trisomies in the first trimester of pregnancy.Br J Obstet Gynaecol 1995; 102: 127-32.

[23] Rosen T, D'Alton ME. Down syndrome screening in the first and second trimesters: what do the data show? Semin Perinatol 2005; 29: 367-75.

[24] Berry E, Aitken DA, Crossley JA, Macri JN, Connor JM. Screening for Down's syndrome: changes in marker levels and detection rates between first and second trimesters. Br J Obstet Gynaecol 1997; 104: 811-7.

[25] Spencer K, Souter V, Tul N, Snijders R, Nicolaides KH. A screening program for trisomy 21 at 10-14 weeks using fetal nuchal translucency, maternal serum free beta-human chorionic gonadotropin and pregnancy-associated plasma protein-A. Ultrasound Obstet Gynecol 1999; 13: 231-7.

[26] Wapner R, Thom E, Simpson JL, Pergament E, Silver R, Filkins K, et al. First Trimester Maternal Serum Biochemistry and Fetal Nuchal Translucency Screening (BUN) Study Group.First-trimester screening for trisomies 21 and 18. N Engl J Med 2003; 349: 1405-13.

[27] Cuckle H, Benn P, Wright D. Down syndrome screening in the first and/or second trimester: model predicted performance using meta-analysis parameters. Semin Perinatol 2005; 29: 252-7.

[28] Shipp TD, Benacerraf BR. Second trimester ultrasound screening for chromosomal abnormalities. Prenat Diagn 2002; 22: 296-307.

[29] Yoder PR, Sabbagha RE, Gross SJ, Zelop CM. The second-trimester fetus with isolated choroid plexus cysts: a meta-analysis of risk of trisomies 18 and 21.Obstet Gynecol 1999; 93(5 Pt 2): 869-72.

[30] Snijders RJ, Shawa L, Nicolaides KH. Fetal choroid plexus cysts and trisomy 18: assessment of risk based on ultrasound findings and maternal age. Prenat Diagn 1994; 14: 1119-27.

[31] Vintzileos AM, Ananth CV, Fisher AJ, Smulian JC, Day-Salvatore D, Beazoglou T, et al. An economic evaluation of prenatal strategies for detection of trisomy 18. Am J Obstet Gynecol 1998; 179: 1220-4.

[32] Bromley B, Frigoletto FD Jr, Benacerraf BR. Mild fetal lateral cerebral ventriculomegaly: clinical course and outcome. Am J Obstet Gynecol 1991; 164: 863-7.

[33] Nyberg DA, Souter VL, El-Bastawissi A, Young S, Luthhardt F, Luthy DA. Isolated sonographic markers for detection of fetal Down syndrome in the second trimester of pregnancy. J Ultrasound Med 2001; 20: 1053-63.

[34] Borrell A, Costa D, Martinez JM, Delgado RD, Casals E, Ojuel J, et al. Early midtrimester fetal nuchal thickness: effectiveness as a marker of Down syndrome. Am J Obstet Gynecol 1996; 175: 45-9.

[35] Nyberg DA, Resta RG, Luthy DA, Hickok DE, Mahony BS, Hirsch JH. Prenatal sonographic findings of Down syndrome: review of 94 cases. Obstet Gynecol 1990; 76(3 Pt 1): 370-7.

[36] Muller F, Dommergues M, Aubry MC, Simon-Bouy B, Gautier E, Oury JF, et al. Hyperechogenic fetal bowel: an ultrasonographic marker for adverse fetal and neonatal outcome. Am J Obstet Gynecol 1995; 173: 508-13.

[37] Benacerraf BR, Neuberg D, Frigoletto FD Jr. Humeral shortening in second-trimester fetuses with Down syndrome.Obstet Gynecol 1991; 77: 223-7.

[38] Petrikovsky BM, Challenger M, Wyse LJ. Natural history of echogenic foci within ventricles of the fetal heart. Ultrasound Obstet Gynecol 1995; 5: 92-4.

[39] Bromley B, Lieberman E, Shipp TD, Richardson M, Benacerraf BR. Significance of an echogenic intracardiac focus in fetuses at high and low risk for aneuploidy. J Ultrasound Med 1998; 17: 127-31.

17

First Trimester Screening for Trisomy 21 by Maternal Age, Nuchal Translucency and Fetal Nasal Bone in Unselected Pregnancies

Ksenija Gersak[1], Maja Pohar-Perme[2] and Darija M. Strah[3]
[1]*Department of Obstetrics and Gynecology, University Medical Center Ljubljana*
[2]*Institute for Biostatistics and Medical Informatics, Faculty of Medicine, University of Ljubljana*
[3]*Diagnostic Centre Strah, Domzale*
Slovenia

1. Introduction

Screening programs play a significant role in the assessment of fetal chromosomal defects and provide the appropriate prenatal counseling and diagnostic tests.

Every pregnant woman has a risk that her fetus might be affected by trisomy 21. At the beginning of the 1980's the screening based on a woman's age was introduced. With the cut-off age of 35 years, 5% of the pregnant women population were classified as "high-risk". However, only 30% of fetuses with trisomy 21 were detected in this group while the majority of trisomy 21 babies were born to mothers from the "low-risk" group.

Later, biochemical screening tests in the second trimester became widely used. The test is based on the concentration of various fetoplacental markers in the maternal circulation: alpha-fetoprotein (AFP), unconjugated estriol (uE3), human chorionic gonadotropin (hCG) and inhibin-A. This method of screening is proved to be more effective than maternal age alone and at the same rate of invasive testing (about 5%) it can identify about 50 to 70% of the fetuses with trisomy 21 (Nicolaides KH 2004).

In the 1990's screening tests were moved to the first trimester. The woman's age was first combined with sonographic measurement of fetal nuchal translucency and fetal heart rate. Later sonographic screening was upgraded by the measurement of maternal serum free β-human chorionic gonadotropin (β-hCG) and pregnancy-associated plasma protein-A (PAPP-A) (Wright D et al, 2008; Kagan KO et al, 2008). Fetal nuchal translucency screening identifies 75 to 80% of fetuses with trisomy 21 at a false positive rate of 5%.

In the last 10 years, several additional first trimester sonographic markers have been described (nasal bone, tricuspid flow, ductus venosus flow) which improve the detection rate of chromosomal abnormalities and reduce the false positive rate. At a risk cut-off of 1 in 100, the detection rate of trisomy 21 is about 95% at a false positive rate of 2.5%.

The ability to achieve reliable measurements and evaluation of sonographic markers depends on an appropriate training of sonographers, adherence to a standard ultrasound technique in order to achieve uniformity of results among different operators (Nicolaides KH 2011). Health professionals undertaking the first trimester scan have to be adequately trained and their results have to be subjected to an audit. The Fetal Medicine Foundation (FMF) has introduced a process of training and certification to help establish high standards of scanning on an international basis (www.fetalmedicine.com).

1.1 Nuchal translucency

Nuchal translucency (NT) is the assessment of the amount of fluid behind the neck of the fetus, also known as the nuchal fold. An anechoic space is visible and measurable sonographically in all fetuses between the 11th and 14th weeks of pregnancy (Figure 1). Underlying pathophysiological mechanisms for nuchal fluid collection include cardiac dysfunction, venous congestion in the head and neck, altered composition of the extracellular matrix, failure of lymphatic drainage, fetal anemia or hypoproteinemia and congenital infection (Nicolaides KH 2004). Accumulation of nuchal fluid decreases after the 14th week. Enlarged NT helps us to identify the high-risk fetuses for trisomy 21 and other chromosomal abnormalities (Nicolaides KH et al, 1992; Nicolaides KH et al, 1994).

NT is evaluated in fetuses with crown-rump length (CRL) range from 45 to 84 mm. The scan may be performed transabdominally but in some cases transvaginal approach may be beneficial. During the measurement, the fetus lies in a neutral position, with the head in line with the spine (www.fetalmedicine.com). The assessment of the NT is obtained in a mid-sagittal view of the fetal profile. The measurements are taken with the inner border of the horizontal line and callipers are placed on the line that defines the NT thickness. Normally, NT increases with the CRL.

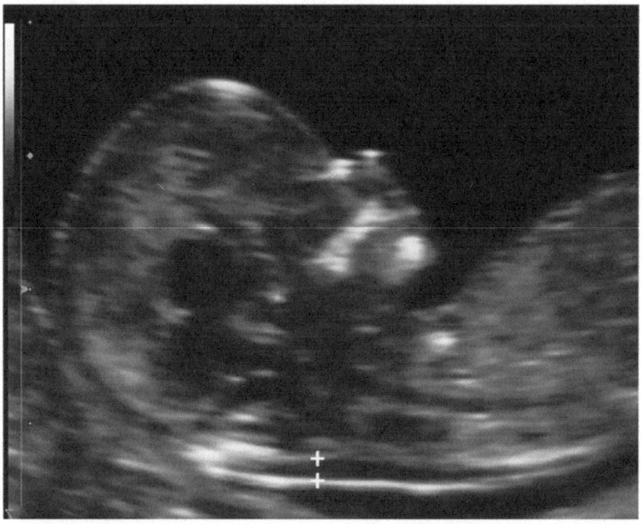

Fig. 1. Measurement of nuchal translucency behind the neck of the fetus.

1.2 Nasal bone

The nasal root depth is abnormally short in 50% of trisomy 21 cases (Cicero S et al, 2003). Sonographic studies at the 15th to 22nd weeks of gestation reported that about 65% of trisomy 21 fetuses had an absent or abnormally short nasal bone. The fetal nasal bone can be visualized between the 11th and 14th weeks of gestation, when CRL is between 45 and 84 mm. The assessment of the nasal bone should be obtained in a mid-sagittal view of the fetal profile (Figure 2). The image of the nose includes three lines. The top line represents the nasal skin, in continuity with the skin is the tip of the nose, and the bottom line represents the nasal bone which is thicker and more echogenic.

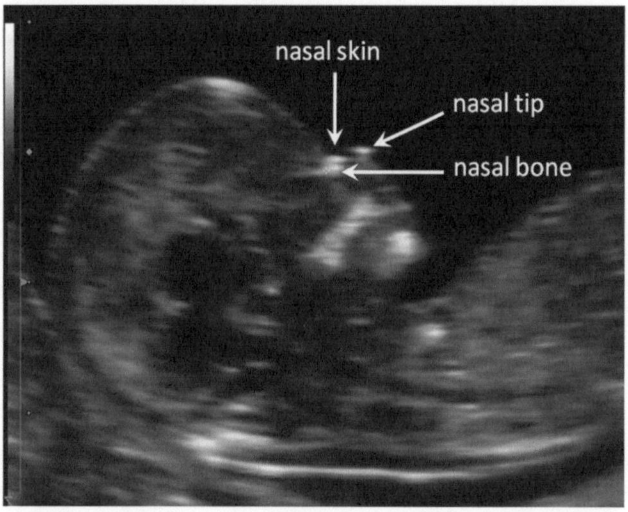

Fig. 2. Assessment of the nasal bone in a mid-sagittal view of the fetal profile.

2. Sonographic screening for trisomy 21 by maternal age, nuchal translucency and fetal nasal bone

The best performance of first trimester screening is achieved by a combination of maternal age, serum biochemical testing and multiple sonographic markers. But Doppler assessment of tricuspid and ductus venosus flow can be time consuming and it requires properly trained sonographers. As a first stage policy the assessment only by maternal age, nuchal translucency and fetal nasal bone, without biochemical testing, has some advantages (Nicolaides KH 2011). Beside the examination of fetal anatomy which leads to early diagnosis of many abnormalities in all pregnancies, the major advantage is the reduction in the cost of screening. The measurement of biochemical markers is undertaken only in the subgroup with positive first stage screening results.

Our study reports the results of the first trimester trisomy 21 risk assessment by a combination of maternal age, sonographic measurement of fetal NT thickness and assessment of fetal nasal bone in unselected pregnancies in Slovenia.

3. Subjects and methods

The study included all pregnant women appointed for the first trimester ultrasound screening examination at a single outpatient clinic between January 4, 2005 and April 30, 2010. Before the screening they all received counseling by their level one gynaecologists and an information leaflet about the ultrasound examination and the aim of screening.

At the time of the visit, they gave details about their demographic characteristics and medical history, which were entered into the computer database. The examinations were carried out by two experienced sonographers, certified by the Fetal Medicine Foundation Certificate of Competence in the 11th to 14th weeks scan.

In the majority of the cases the examination was performed transabdominally within 20 minutes. In less than 1% of the cases a transvaginal ultrasound examination had to be carried out.

In the fetal CRL less than 45 mm, the pregnant woman was given a new appointment, while in the fetal CRL more than 83 mm, only a detailed ultrasound scan was performed and the pregnant woman received further information about the possibility of the second trimester biochemical test.

For the examinations we used 2-5 MHz and 3.7-9.3 MHz transducers GE Healthcare Voluson 730 Pro, Milwaukee, USA, and 4-6 MHz, 4-7 MHz, 5-9 MHz and 7-9 MHz transducers Acuson S2000, Siemens Medical Solutions, Mountain View CA, USA.

Only singleton pregnancies with live fetus from the 11th to 14th weeks of gestation with the CRL of 45-83 mm were included in the further analysis. Pregnancy outcomes were obtained from the participating women, referred by level one gynecologists and paediatricians. Karyotype results were reported by the three cytogenetic laboratories.

3.2 Statistical methods

Risks were calculated according to the FMF program, following the FMF guidelines (Snijders RJM et al, 1999; www.fetalmedicine.com). The distribution of maternal age of the examined women was compared to the age distribution in the pregnant population in Slovenia for the time interval 2005-2010 (www.stat.si).

We calculated the sensitivity, false positive rate, positive predictive value and negative predictive value for a cut-off risk of 1 in 300. We accompanied the most important results with a 95% confidence interval. The balance between the false positive rate and the detection rate was studied and the trends were inspected graphically. The cut-off risk that would yield 5% false positives was calculated for trisomy 21.

Additionally, the expected numbers for the Slovene population were estimated by weighting the values of each woman according to the frequency of her age in the Slovene population.

4. Results

4.1 Study population

A total of 13,535 pregnant women were offered first trimester screening for detecting fetal chromosomal abnormalities at a single outpatient clinic between January 4, 2005 and April 30, 2010.

The sample represented unselected population of pregnant women of Caucasian ethnic origin. Twin pregnancies (3.6% of the cases, 486 of 13,535) were excluded. All further analyses included 13,049 women with singleton pregnancies.

4.2 Age distribution

The average maternal age (at the time of screening) was 29 years (range 11 to 47, SD=3.9) with a distribution as shown in the Figure 3 (black columns). When compared to the age distribution in the pregnant population in 2005-2010 in Slovenia, the average maternal age was the same - 28.9 years (Figure 3, red columns). The pregnant population however varied more, in particular there was a larger proportion of women aged 36 and more in the Slovene pregnant population (10.2%) as compared to only 3.6% in our sample. The sample on the other hand included a considerably larger percent of the women between 26 and 30 (47.9%

compared to 40.6%). Only 2.5% were 37 and older compared to the 7.2% in the population of Slovene pregnant women.

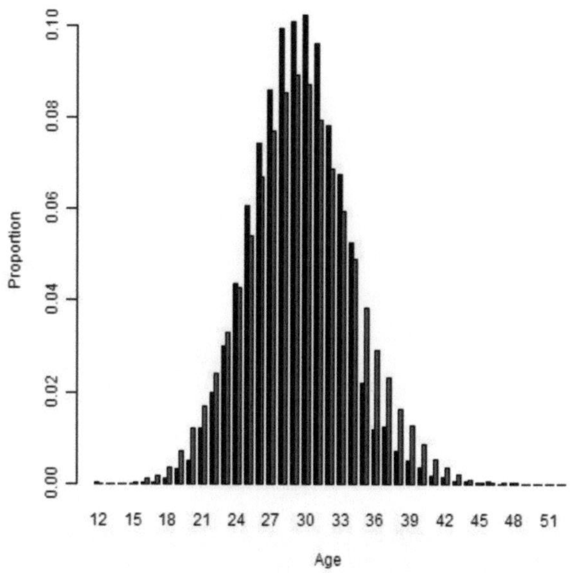

Fig. 3. Age distribution comparison at screening; Slovene population (red columns), our sample of unselected population of pregnant women (black columns).

4.3 The screening results

The average gestation was 12 weeks 4 days (range 11 weeks 1 day to 14 weeks 0 days). The average fetal CRL was 63.2 mm (range 45 to 83 mm). And the average NT thickness was 1.7 mm (range 0.9 to 13.4 mm).

The distribution of NT for fetal CRL in normal pregnancies and pregnancies with fetuses affected by chromosomal abnormalities is shown in Figure 4. The NT was above the 95th centile of the normal range for the CRL in 75% (15 of 20) of trisomy 21 pregnancies and in 64% (16 of 25) pregnancies with other chromosomal abnormalities.

At the time of testing in 3% of all pregnancies (394 of 13,049) the estimated risk for trisomy 21 was 1 in 300 or higher, considering the calculation based on FMF program. Three hundred and sixty cases (2.8%) turned out to be false positive. At the invasive testing, chromosomal abnormalities were identified in 8.6% of high risk cases (34 of 394), which represents one case of fetal chromosomal abnormality detected per 12 invasive diagnostic procedures.

4.4 Detection rate

We detected 34 out of 45 cases with chromosomal abnormalities (75.6%), diagnosed prenatally or postnatally.

Trisomy 21 was detected in 20 cases (Figure 4). Among women with an estimated risk of 1 in 300 or higher there were 17 cases of trisomy 21. The detection rate for trisomy 21 was 85% (17 out of 20), the 95% confidence interval for the detection rate was [69.4, 100]. The positive predictive value for the trisomy 21 was 4.3% (17 of 394); and the negative predictive value was 99.98% (12,652 of 12,655).

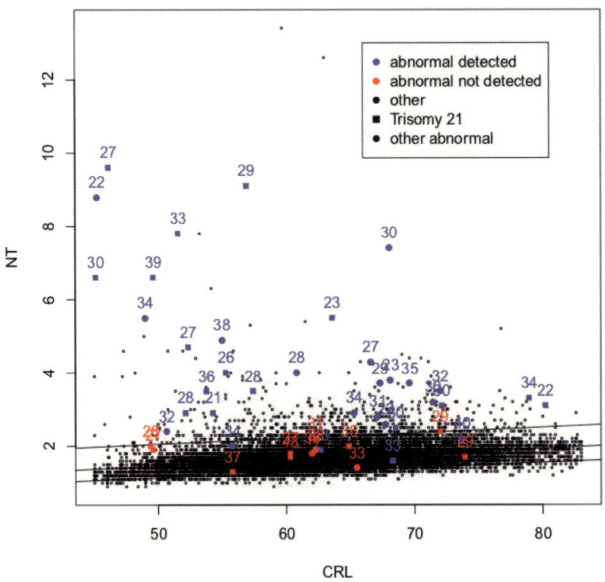

Fig. 4. Distribution of NT (in mm) with respect to CRL (in mm) in our sample. The curves present the 5th, 50th and 95th centiles.

Other chromosomal abnormalities were diagnosed in 25 cases (Figure 4). Among women with an estimated risk of 1 in 300 or higher there were 17 cases of other chromosomal abnormalities. The detection rate was 68% (17 out of 25). The 95% confidence interval for the detection rate was [49.7, 86.3]. The positive predictive value for the other chromosomal abnormalities was 4.3% (17 of 394); and the negative predictive value was 99.94% (12,647 of 12,655).

The diagnosed chromosomal abnormalities and their frequencies are presented in Table 1. The assessment of nasal bone was performed in 98.5%of the cases (12,847 out of 13,049). In 12 cases nasal bone was absent (0.1%), and in 3 out of those 12 cases (25%), the chromosomal abnormality was detected.

Karyotype	**No.**
Trisomy 21	20
Trisomy 18	10
Trisomy 13	2
45,X (Turner syndrome)	3
47,XXY	2
Mosaic structure	3
Unbalanced structural rearrangements	5
Total	**45**

Table 1. Chromosomal abnormalities in fetuses and newborns in our sample of 13,049 women with singleton pregnancies.

4.5 The risk threshold

The risk values of the undetected cases of trisomy 21 were as follows: 1 in 1979, 6365, 7435; for other chromosomal abnormalities they were 1 in 493, 872, 1102, 1279, 2016, 2180, 3816, 6731.

It was thus clear that a less conservative limit for probability threshold (for example 1 in 500) would not yield different detection rate in case of trisomy 21, but would rather improve the detection of other chromosomal abnormalities.

These changes are explored in Figure 5, which shows how detection rate would change by changing the risk threshold. The black curve shows how detection rate of trisomy 21 changes by changing the risk threshold (value 200 implies probability threshold set at 1/200). The red curve represents the same information for other chromosomal abnormalities. The numbers above the points indicate the percentage of false positives that would occur in our sample at that threshold.

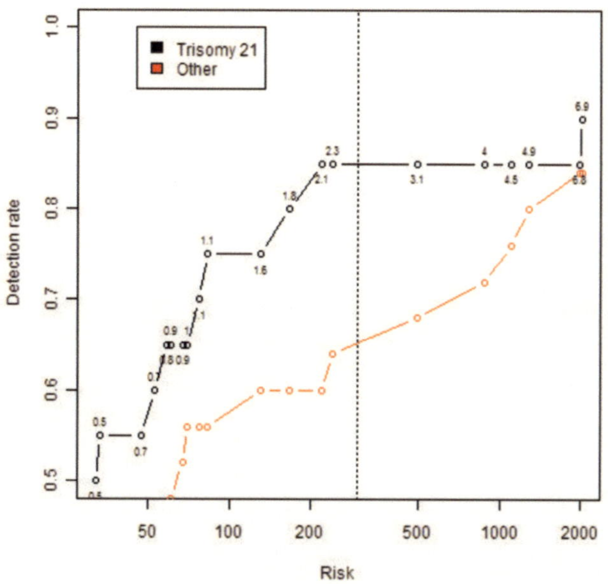

Fig. 5. Detection rate of trisomy 21 (black curve) and other chromosomal abnormalities (red curve) with respect to the risk threshold set (value 200 implies probability threshold set at 1/200). The numbers above the points give the false positive rate.

Inversely, Figure 6 shows the detection rate with respect to the percentage of false positives, the numbers above the points indicate the risk threshold (value 200 implies threshold 1/200).

4.6 Prediction for the Slovene population

Since the age distribution in our sample was different from the age distribution in the Slovene pregnant women population, we can expect all the above results to be slightly different. In particular, the rate of false positives can be expected to change. Figure 7 gives the false positive rate in our sample with respect to calendar year and compares it to the predicted false positive rate in the Slovene pregnant women population.

Inversely, Figure 8 gives the probability threshold that would result in the 5% false positives rate.

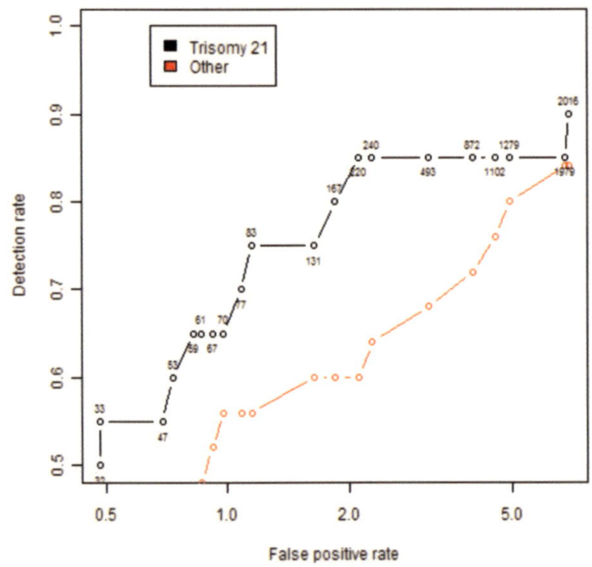

Fig. 6. Detection rate of trisomy 21 (black curve) and other chromosomal abnormalities (red curve) with respect to the false positive rate. The numbers above the points give the risk threshold (value 200 implies probability threshold set at 1/200).

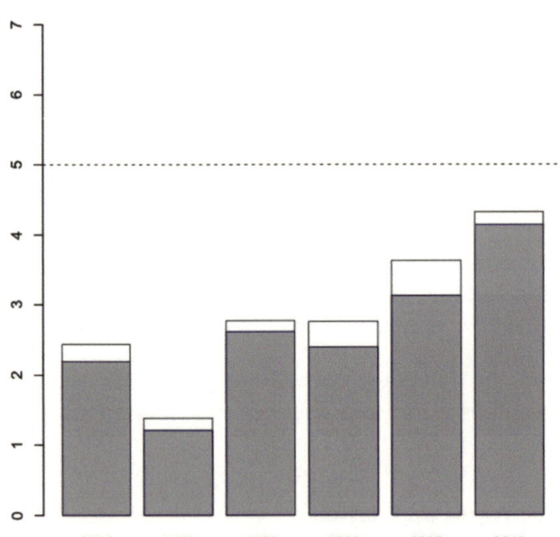

Fig. 7. The percentage of false positives in our sample (gray columns) and the predicted false positive rate in the Slovene pregnant women population (white columns) with respect to calendar year.

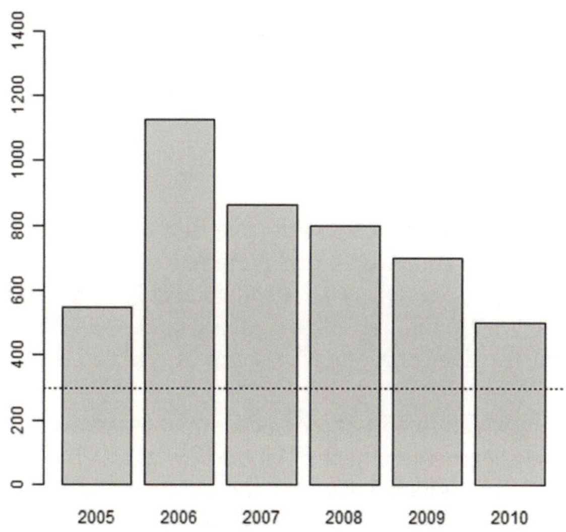

Fig. 8. The risk threshold that would result in a 5% false positive rate with respect to calendar year.

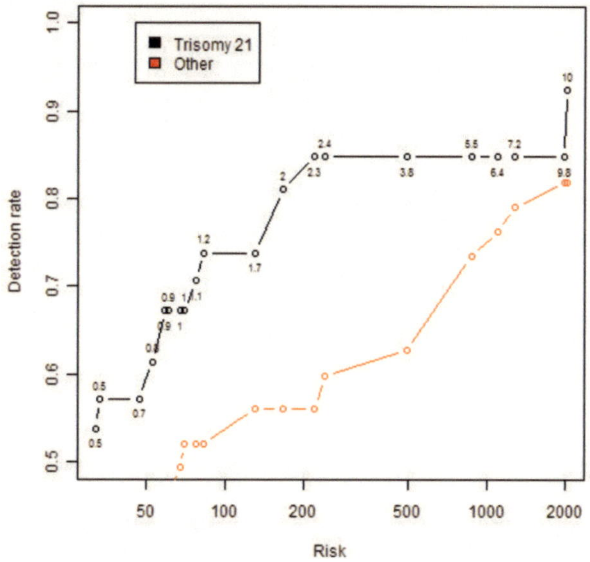

Fig. 9. Detection rate of trisomy 21 (black curve) and other chromosomal abnormalities (red curve) with respect to the risk threshold set (value 200 implies probability threshold set at 1/200) - prediction for the Slovene population. The numbers above the points give the false positive rate.

5. Discussion

The retrospective study of the first trimester screening for trisomy 21 in 5-year period from 2005 to 2010 by a combination of maternal age, sonographic measurement of fetal NT thickness and assessment of the fetal nasal bone represented a detection rate of 85% at a false positive rate of 2.8%.

5.1 Detection rate

The findings of many studies suggest that effective first trimester screening for trisomy 21 can be provided only by the combination of maternal age and measurement of fetal NT (Pajkrt E et al, 1998; Economides DL et al, 1998; Bindra R et al, 2002; Liu SS et al, 2004; Rozenberg P et al, 2006; Westin M et al, 2006; Czuba B et al., 2007; Kagan KO et al, 2010). At a risk cut-off of 1 in 100, the detection rate of trisomy 21 is about 75%, at a false positive rate of about 2%.

The detection can be improved to 85% by the additional assessment of the fetal nasal bone and even more by the Doppler assessment of blood flow across the tricuspid valve or blood flow in the ductus venosus, which increased the detection rate to about 95% at a false positive rate of 2.5% (Kagan KO et al, 2010). The disadvantage of the Doppler assessment of tricuspid and ductus venosus flow is that it is time consuming and it requires appropriately trained sonographers (Nicolaides KH 2011).

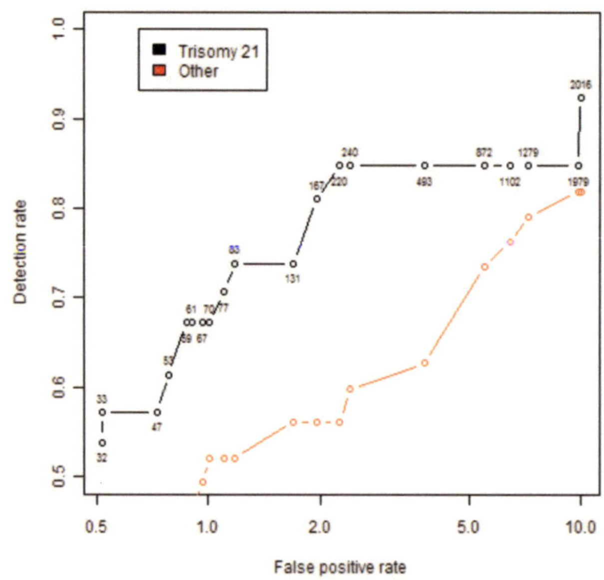

Fig. 10. Detection rate of trisomy 21 (black curve) and other abnormalities (red curve) with respect to the false positive rate - prediction for the Slovene population. The numbers above the points give the risk threshold (value 200 implies probability threshold set at 1/200).

By the measurement of fetal NT thickness and the assessment of the fetal nasal bone we were able to achieve the expected results at a risk cut-off of 1 in 300. In our sample the relationship between the false positive rate and the detection rate was proved to be in line

with the prediction from the Nicolaides study (Nicolaides KH 2011) and highly comparable to other reports (Prefumo F et al, 2006; Kagan KO et al, 2010).
Choosing sonographic assessment rather than biochemical testing as a first stage policy has a few advantages. In all sonographically screened pregnancies in addition to chromosomal markers, fetal anatomy is observed and both provide early diagnosis of many major abnormalities, not just in the subgroup with a positive first stage biochemical screening results (Nicolaides KH 2011). Further measurements of maternal serum free β-hCG and PAPP-A can be limited only to high risk subgroup.

5.2 Prediction for the Slovene population

But the trend of ageing the population of pregnant women is noticed and the false positive rate at the risk cut-off 1 in 300 is changing almost linearly with time (Figure 7).
Allowing ourselves 5% false positive rate in the population, we could lower the risk limit. But, as our detection rate is more than adequate according to FMF guidelines, at the moment we have no reason to actually change it, and we believe that any such change should also be weighted against the risk of pregnancy loss due to invasive testing.
Our calculations show that the FMF recommendations about the risk limit cannot be directly translated to our specific population distribution. We believe the limit that ensures a 5% false positive rate is constantly changing and could be adjusted within each country. To accurate the changing, the weighting could be performed using a large data set, preferably the data set on which the FMF algorithm was developed, using the respective population maternal age distribution. The only assumption needed for such estimation would be, that conditional on the maternal age, the NT and CRL distributions do not vary among the countries, which we believe is an assumption we can safely make.

6. Conclusion

The 11th to 14th weeks scan includes confirmation of the viability of the fetus, accurate dating of the pregnancy, and an early diagnosis of multiple pregnancies and identification of chorionicity.
Effective screening for trisomy 21 can be achieved in the first trimester of pregnancy by a combination of maternal age, sonographic measurement of fetal NT thickness and assessment of fetal nasal bone, with detection rate of 85% at a false positive rate of less than 3%.

7. References

Bindra, R., Heath, V., Liao, A., et al. (2002). One stop assessment of risk for trisomy 21 at 11–14 weeks a prospective study of 15030 pregnancies. Ultrasound Obstet Gynecol 20: 219–25.

Cicero, S., Sonek, J.D., McKenna, D.S., et al. (2003). Nasal bone hypoplasia in trisomy 21 at 15-22 weeks' gestation. Ultrasound Obstet Gynecol 21:15-8.

Czuba, B., Borowski, D., Cnota, W., et al. (2007). Ultrasonographic assessment of fetal nuchal translucency (NT) at 11th and 14th week of gestation - Polish multicentre study. Neuro Endocrinol Lett 28: 175–81.

Economides, D.L., Whitlow, B.J., Kadir, R., et al. (1998). First trimester sonographic detection of chromosomal abnormalities in an unselected population. Br J Obstet Gynaecol 105: 58–62.

Fetal Medicine Foundation. Online-education. Available from: http:// www.fetalmedicine.com/fmf/

Kagan, K.O., Wright, D., Spencer, K., Molina, F.S. & Nicolaides K.H. (2008). First-trimester screening for trisomy 21 by free beta-human chorionic gonadotropin and pregnancy-associated plasma protein-A: impact of maternal and pregnancy characteristics. Ultrasound Obstet Gynecol 31: 493–502.

Kagan, K.O., Staboulidou, I., Cruz, J., et al. (2010).Two-stage first-trimester screening for trisomy 21 by ultrasound assessment and biochemical testing. Ultrasound Obstet Gynecol 36: 542–7.

Liu, S.S., Lee, F.K., Lee, J.L., et al. (2004). Pregnancy outcomes in unselected singleton pregnant women with an increased risk of first-trimester Down's syndrome. Acta Obstet Gynecol Scand 83: 1130–4.

Nicolaides, K.H., Azar, G., Byrne, D., et al. (1992). Fetal nuchal translucency: ultrasound screening for chromosomal defects in the first trimester of pregnancy. BMJ 304(6831): 867-9.

Nicolaides, K.H., Brizot, M.L. & Snijders, R.J.M. (1994). Fetal nuchal translucency: ultrasound screening for fetal trisomy in the first trimester of pregnancy. BJOG 101:782-6.

Nicolaides K.H. (2004). Fetal Medicine Foundation. The 11-13+6 weeks scan, pp. 1–112, London, UK

Nicolaides, K.H. (2011). Screening for fetal aneuploidies at 11 to 13 weeks. Prenat Diagn 31: 7–15.

Pajkrt, E,, van Lith, J.M.M., Mol, B.W.J., et al. (1998). Screening for Down's syndrome by fetal nuchal translucency measurement in a general obstetric population. Ultrasound Obstet Gynecol 12: 163–9.

Prefumo, F., Sairam, S., Bhide, A., et al. (2006). First-trimester nuchal translucency, nasal bones, and trisomy 21 in selected and unselected populations. Am J Obstet Gynecol 194: 828–33.

Rozenberg, P., Bussières, L., Chevret, S., et al. (2006). Screening for Down syndrome using first-trimester combined screening followed by second-trimester ultrasound examination in an unselected population. Am J Obstet Gynecol 195: 1379–87.

Statistical Office of the Republic of Slovenia. SI-STAT data portal. Available from: http://www.stat.si/pxweb/Database/Dem_soc/05_prebivalstvo/10_rojeni_umrli /01_05544_rojeni/01_05544_rojeni.asp

Snijders, R.J.M., Noble, P., Sebire, N., et al. (1999). UK multicentre project on assessment of risk for trisomy 21 by maternal age and fetal nuchal translucency thickness at 10 – 14 weeks of gestation. Lancet 18: 519–21.

Westin, M., Saltvedt, S., Bergman, G., et al. (2006). Is measurement of nuchal translucency thickness a useful screening tool for heart defects? A study of 16,383 fetuses. Ultrasound Obstet Gynecol 27: 632–9.

Wright, D., Kagan, K.O., Molina, F.S., Gazzoni, A. & Nicolaides K.H. (2008). A mixture model of nuchal translucency thickness in screening for chromosomal defects. Ultrasound Obstet Gynecol 31:376–383.

18

Noninvasive Prenatal Nucleic Acid Diagnostics of Down Syndrome

Radek Vodicka, Radek Vrtel, Jana Böhmova, Romana Kratochvilova, Ladislav Dusek, Ishraq Dhaifalah and Jiri Santavy
Dept. of Medical Genetics and Fetal Medicine, University Hospital and Faculty of Medicine UP, Olomouc, Czech Republic

1. Introduction

Molecular composition of pregnant women blood plasma/serum is an indispensable tool for biochemists in the field of routine prenatal diagnostics aimed at the detection of the most common aneuploidies.

Predictive power of some biochemical markers respectively their sum is an important guide for the assessment of the status of the fetus and pregnancy.

But the diagnostic potential of maternal plasma is much broader.

Fragmented and apoptically degraded fetal cells and nucleic acid molecules, which overcame the placental (feto-maternal) barrier and got under the influence of the immune system of the mother, offer other options for molecular biologists.

Some of them will focus on the clarification of rules between the quantity of fetal molecules and pathology of the placenta and the fetus others are engaged in direct diagnostic potential.

In the maternal blood circulation can be detected fetal genetic material of a different integrity ranging from the nuclear DNA of living cells through fetal apoptically partially degraded molecules more or less packed in nucleoides to completely fragmented DNA molecules mostly of size between 100 - 400 bp. Cell free fetal (cff) mRNA molecules from trophoblast are also presented in detectable concentration in maternal plasma.

While the presence of fetal cells in maternal circulation is quite rare (1 fetal cell in 1 million maternal cells), the quantity of cffDNA molecules in plasma is considerably higher (typically 3 % - 6 %).

2. Source and transport of cff nucleic acid molecules into maternal plasma

The ways in which cffDNA forms and how gets into the maternal circulation, are not yet fully clarified. There are several hypotheses on the origin of cff DNA.

The main source of free DNA appears to be a placenta (Wataganara & Bianchi, 2004). Most likely the cff DNA forms by disintegration of placental cells and the direct transition to the maternal circulation.

Another possibility is that the placenta functions as an mediator of transition for DNA circulating in the fetal blood circuit into maternal tissues.

In this case, there should be a two-way traffic, however, the amount of analyzed fetal DNA in maternal plasma is much greater than the amount of free maternal DNA in umbilical plasma in childbirth (Sekizawa et al., 2003). It is indicative of an unequal transfer of free DNA from fetus to the mother. Another source of fetal molecules may be fetal hematopoietic cells which get into the maternal circulation (Bianchi, 2004). The fetal DNA is apoptically released into maternal plasma due to the effect of maternal immune system (Pertl et al., 2000). Apoptotic fetal cells were found in detectable concentrations also directly in the plasma (Van Wijk et al., 2000). Apoptosis proven in maternal plasma (Sekizawa et al., 2003) or in cord blood (Hristoskova et al., 2001) suggests that this mechanism could be an important source of fetal material. Another hypothesis assumes a simple diffusion of shorter DNA molecules from the amniotic fluid through placenta or membranes into maternal circulation. This DNA then comes from various fetal tissues.

Cff DNA was also demonstrated in the maternal plasma even before feto-maternal circulation establishment. This means that the DNA could be of the trofoblastic origin (Bianchi et al., 2004). In general, it could be assumed that cff DNA in maternal circulation is of different origin but its large portion likely comes from the trophoblastic placental tissue.

The transfer of fetal molecules through the feto-maternal barrier is continuous during pregnancy and after the delivery they are quickly eliminated from plasma (16 min halftime of degradation (Lo et al., 1999).

Free fetal RNA allows non-invasive prenatal profiling of gene expression and offers a number of research and diagnostic applications on the basis of easily detectable mRNA transcripts from placentally expressed genes in maternal plasma (Ng et al., 2003).

Considering serious degradation as a result of the activities of the ribonucleases, the stability of mRNA molecules in fetal free plasma is surprising. Plasma RNA molecules are much more stable than isolated and purified RNA molecules. Mechanisms that protect the circulating free fetal RNA are not fully clarified at present time. However their conjunction with the sub cellular particles could prevent their degradation (Hasselmann et al., 2001).

They can form complexes with proteins, lipids, lipoproteins, phospholipids bound to the DNA in nucleosomes or within protected apoptotic corpuscles or other vesicular structures (Halicka et al., 2000; Hasselmann et al., 2001; Tsui et al., 2002; Sisko et al., 2001).

The stability of placental mRNA molecules in maternal plasma is a promising assumption that fetal markers at the level of mRNA will be clinically useful.

It could be useful for prenatal detection of some pregnancy pathologies, including pre-eclampsia and certain chromosomal aneuploidies (Ng et al., 2004).

3. Placental trophoblast and trisomy 21

Trophoblast with chromosome 21 trisomy shows disturbed both cell fusion and formation of syncytiotrofoblast (ST) (Frendo et al., 2000b; Massin et al., 2001). An activation of caspases is necessary for formation of ST in early stage of differentiation (Huppertz and Kingdom, 2004). If ST is inadequate, the individual trophoblastic cells with trisomy 21 could continue on in the cascade of apoptic events and release more fragmented cff DNA than disomic trophoblastic cells. Another possible cause for the release of larger amounts of fetal molecules in pregnancy with trisomy 21 is a continuation of trophoblastic cells in the improper proliferation, without initiating events leading to the formation of ST. In this case maternal immune system would regulate the division by increased degradation of fetal cells.

4. Fragmentation profile of cffDNA

Publications, relating to the characterization of the DNA fragments in the plasma, are aimed to the level of fragmentation of fetal molecules related to the maternal ones in the course of pregnancy. For pregnant women were described in plasma longer fragments in comparison with non-pregnant women (Chan et al., 2004).

Real-time PCR is the most commonly used procedure for the analysis of fetal DNA fragments in present time (Alberry et al., 2009; Ariga et al., 2001; Lo et al., 1998). Honda et al. (2002) described the sensitivity of the detection of fetal DNA for this method and determined it at 5,38 copies/ml of the peripheral blood.

Molecules of fetal origin are more degraded and shorter than the maternal and their size is approximately in the range from 100 bp - to 700 bp. (Zhong et al., 2000; Koide et al., 2005). Fragments above 1 kb belong mostly to the mother (Li et al., 2004).

We have evaluated fragment analysis using three methods (capillary electrophoresis of STR loci, capillary electrophoresis and Real-time PCR of gonozomal sequences) from two different perspectives. The first relied on direct analysis of the size of fractions and the second assessed PCR efficiency with respect to the size of amplified DNA molecules (Vodicka et al., 2010).

Direct detection of fetal molecules has confirmed a large heterogeneity in the individual fractions both by capillary electrophoresis and Real-time PCR.

A direct dependency of fetal molecules on the week of pregnancy has been suggested only in the size fraction of 500 - 760 bp. Regression modeling at STR and gonozomal analyses was the most accurate in the pD system, where the size of molecules ranged from 395 bp to 440 bp. Statistical significance of regression declined towards the smaller molecules.

The fragment size was 200 bp to 223 bp in the D21S1446 system and 157-188 bp in D21S1435. Regression analysis was inconclusive in the AMELY (molecule size 109 bp).

If we compare analysis of the size of fractions to the results of the effectiveness of the STR and gonozomal analyses (Vodicka et al., 2008a), where was demonstrated statistically significant increase of fetal molecules in all 3 STR systems, we found out that it was confirmed an interesting trend, which indicates an increase in the larger fetal molecules during pregnancy while the number of smaller molecules of fetal origin does not change.

In the case of quantification using SRY probe, whose length is 64 bp it was observed even reverse trend and the number of amplified molecules in 150-300 bp fraction was in indirect relation to the week of gestation.

The tendency has decreased for larger fractions and in total plasma the trend has stopped even slightly reversed.

On the basis of these observations, we can therefore assume the most sensitive detection of fetal material using short probes. But these probes are not much suitable for quantitative analysis. Fractions from 400 bp above are the most appropriate for the assessment of the amount of fetal material, although in these fractions the relative amount of fetal DNA is less.

The importance of this study resides in decision-making, whether, from a diagnostic point of view, it is more important a detection of fetal molecules or their quantification (Vodicka et al., 2010).

5. The extraction of cffDNA/RNA from maternal peripheral blood

5.1 CffDNA isolation procedures

An essential precondition for the success of all subsequent procedures is a sufficient yield, reproducibility and the purity of the isolated plasma cffDNA. Isolation procedures are most often based on double centrifugation and subsequent binding (adsorption) of DNA molecules on a silica surface of membrane or magnetic particles.

5.1.1 Isolation by binding to a silica-gel membrane

The adsorption on silica surface is one of the most common techniques which is able to capture free fragmented DNA.

Silicate polymer in the presence of chaotropic salts (e.g. sodium iodide or guanidine thiocyanate) specifically binds to the DNA molecule on the surface of silicon dioxide (usually specially prepared glass) and in the presence of water or other elution reagent, which has a very low content of salt, this molecule releases from its surface.

High specificity of the link between DNA molecule and silicate material is useful in eliminating other extracellular substances.

5.1.2 Isolation by binding to the magnetic particles

Methods based on the (para) magnetic particles (MPs) are other approach to the cffDNA isolation. MPs are particles of size from 5 nm to 100 μm, consisting of a metal core, it is usually γ-Fe2O3 (maghemit) or Fe3O4 (magnetite) but could be also for example Au.

The core is coated with a layer that has specifically prepared surface for binding the molecules that we want to isolate.

The size of the MPs can be adapted according to the molecules which we are isolating: 5-50 nm proteins; 20-450 nm nucleic acids; 10-100 μm viruses.

MPs respond to the external magnetic field and are capable to bind different bioreaktive molecules, because of their affinity to the modified surface, directly from the biological material. The isolation is then as follows.

MPs are added to the sample where bind with the targeted molecule. Modified MPs are then attracted by magnet to the wall of the tube and the remaining solution with non-bind substances is removed.

The MPs with joined molecules are subsequently washed and released in added solution.

Bound molecules are separated from the MPs by some physical-chemical step (denaturing or change in pH).

This way we obtain targeted molecules which could be afterward analyzed (Húska et al., 2008).

5.1.3 Comparison of silica-gel to magentic particles methods

Both above mentioned isolation procedures were tested in our workplace.

For a comparison, cff DNA (male fetus) was measured and quantified both by Real-time PCR in SRY locus and by quantitative fluorescent (QF) PCR and capillary electrophoresis separation in AMELY locus in 38 samples from the 1st and 38 samples from the 2nd trimester. While the concentrations of total DNA measured spectrophotometrically were similar there were substantial differences in yield of cffDNA between tested DNA extraction methods (graph 1,2).

Isolation based on the separation of magnetic particles had significantly lower recovery compared with the amount of cffDNA extracted by binding on the silicate membrane.

According to our current findings "silica membrane" based method seemed to be clearly more suitable for isolation of cffDNA from the plasma of pregnant women.

DNA extraction using magnetic particles should present a simple way how relatively easily and without contamination obtained the cffDNA.

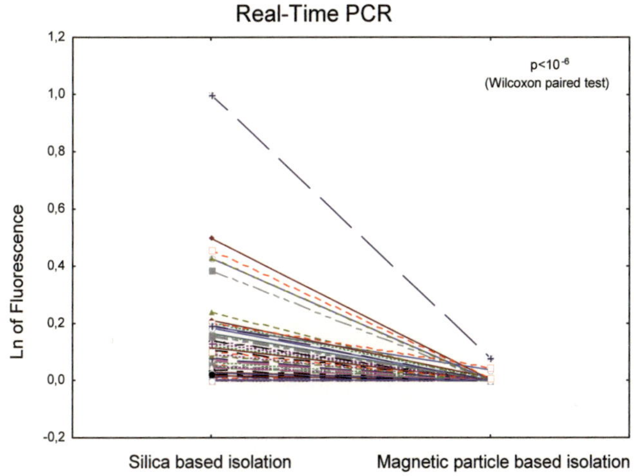

Graph 1. Comparison of silica gel and magnetic particles isolation effectiveness by Real-time PCR quantification.

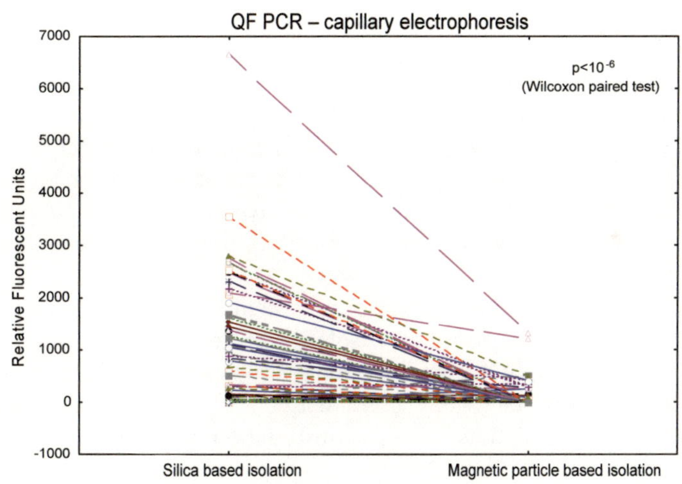

Graph 2. Comparison of silica gel and magnetic particles isolation effectiveness by capillary electrophoresis quantification

However, for the isolation of short fragments of cffDNA this method did not work, although the manufacturer declares, that it should be able to detect the DNA molecules of the size from 50 bp to 1,5 kb. Low efficiency of cffDNA capture can be caused by strong bond of free fragmented fetal DNA on magnetic particles, or by contraries, by weaker bond of these fragments on magnetic particles and their wash out during isolation.

To explain this, we re-isolated unbound DNA from supernatant. The subsequent quantification by capillary electrophoresis has demonstrated again only the maternal sequences, which suggests a stronger link of fragmented fetal DNA on magnetic particles.

If cffDNA was succsessfully detected by both methods, the amount of DNA has correlated to each other (Graph 3).

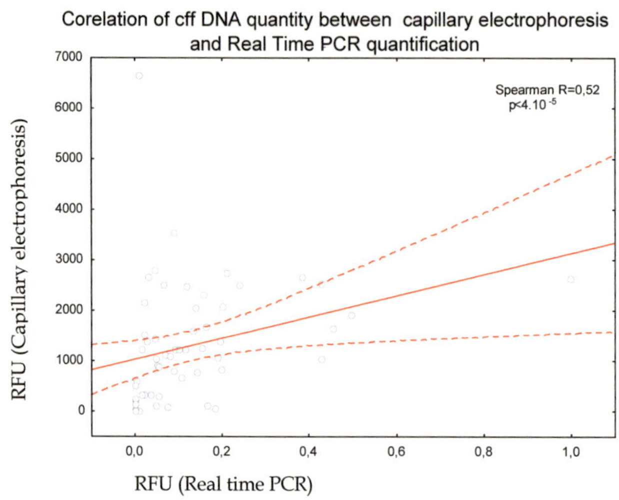

Graph 3. Correlation of the results of free fetal DNA quantification by capillary electrophoresis and real-time PCR (RT-PCR). The Y axis shows the Relative fluorescence units (RFU) obtained from capillary electrophoresis, X axis shows the fluorescence scanned in Real time system.

5.2 Cff mRNA isolation procedures

To maintain integrity of obtained free fetal RNA, it is important to use isolation techniques which have minimum isolation steps, are quick and contain RNA stabilizers.
Currently there are no commercially produced kits standardized for isolation of free fetal RNA directly from maternal plasma, but there are available kits specialized for isolation of viral RNA, which could be, with little modification, applied to the isolation of free fetal RNA.
Double centrifugation in cooled centrifuge or ultra centrifugation is necessary for separation of cellular component of blood prior to the isolation of free fetal RNA.
The combination of viral RNA Kit and vacuum pumps seems to be an optimal system for obtaining free fetal RNA in the highest possible quantity and the quality, with minimal risk of contamination during isolation, unlike centrifugation steps. Microfilters can be used to increase the concentration of free fetal RNA.

6. The use of cff DNA for diagnostic purposes

The resolution of the fetal genotype and precise quantification of cffDNA are crucial for diagnostic purposes.

6.1 Noninvasive fetal sex determination by cffDNA

So far, the most common and relatively simple for the analysis of fetal DNA was the use of Y specific sequences from male fetuses.
These sequences can be quantified by methods of Real-time PCR and QF PCR.
The methodology for fetal sex detection in maternal plasma is already relatively well developed and reliable (Lo et al., 1998; Honda et al., 2002; Wei et al., 2001; Zhong et al., 2000, Vodicka et al., 2008b).

Our quick and simplify fetal sex detection is based on refined QF PCR. We tested 475 DNA samples isolated from maternal plasma in different weeks of pregnancy ranging from 4th w.g. to 37th w.g. Y chromosomal sequences in AMELY were tested and quantify by comparison to AMELX using capillary electrophoresis.

The method is able to distinguish even less than 1 % of Y chromosomal sequences of artificial mixtures. Fetal sex was detected with 4.05 % of false positivity and 7.15 % of false negativity (Vodicka et al., 2008).

The methodology has very high detection sensitivity, which is comparable with a sensitivity of real-time PCR methodology (Sekizawa et al., 2001; Honda et al., 2002).

Possible contamination of the samples during collection and in the course of the isolation procedure is the main cause of false-positive detection of the male sex.

Minimization of any contamination is fundamental in sensitive DNA analyses in which it is necessary to capture the genotype in quantities of about 5%.

Mistakes in determination of male fetus (false-negative results) come mostly from early stages of pregnancy, when the concentration of cffDNA is still very low, so rather than non-compliance could be assessed these results as missing fetal DNA.

Capillary electrophoresis has proven to be uniquely able to capture even 1 % genotype artificial admixture.

The result of examinations of our group of pregnant women can be considered very satisfactory. The methodology is prepared for practical use, however, further improvement of isolation robustness and following laboratory procedures may increase specificity, sensitivity, and the yield of fetal DNA.

6.2 Noninvasive RHD genotyping by cffDNA

RHD genotype of the fetus can be identified from maternal plasma already at the beginning of pregnancy using molecular analysis of cffDNA.

Clinical significance of determination of fetal RhD status is dual:

1. Noninvasive fetal RHD determination from peripheral blood of Rh- alloimmunized pregnant women at the beginning of pregnancy allows to determine the fetuses which are really threatened by development of hemolytic disease of fetus and newborn.
2. If anti-D antibodies are not present at the beginning of pregnancy, RhD negative woman should be provided with anti-D immunoglobulin during pregnancy in sufficient dosage for each potentially sensitizing events including completion of antepartal prophylaxis at 28th week of gestation. Potentially sensitizing event means any situation in which may occur intersection of RhD positive fetal erythrocytes to the mother's blood, and subsequent development of the RhD alloimmunization (chorionic villus sampling, amniocentesis, cordocentesis, another intervention of the prenatal diagnosis and fetal therapy, obstetric hemorrhage in the 2nd and 3rd trimester, intrauterine death of fetus). Prevention of RhD alloimmunization should be provided to RhD negative pregnant woman by delivery of anti-D immunoglobulin in sufficient dosage in all above-mentioned cases. The administration of anti-d immunoglobulin is necessary if the fetus is RhD-positive, on the contrary, if the fetus is RhD negative, the pregnant woman is not threatened by the development of the RhD alloimmunization and administration of anti-D immunoglobulin is not necessary.

RHD genotyping of cffDNA is most often done using Taq man Real time PCR with probes from exone 7, 10, 4 or 5. System of negative and positive PCR control in addition to internal control of PCR amplification is necessary for the reliability of detection considering great sensitivity of the method. At the same time, you must have created calibration quantitative profile for exact specification of detection limit of RhD positivity.

6.3 Noninvasive cffDNA analysis of monogenic inherited diseases

CffDNA can be also used for examination of monogenic inherited diseases.

Many genetic abnormalities, for example autosomal dominant myotonic dystrophy (Amicucci et al., 2000), Huntington's disease (Gonzalez-Gonzalez et al., 2003) or gene mutations such as achondroplasia (Saito et al., 2000) has already been examined from cffDNA. Furthermore, it is possible to detect some autosomal recessive diseases, such as cystic fibrosis (Gonzalez-Gonzalez et al., 2002) or β-talasemia (Chiu et al., 2002).

7. Cff nucleic acid quantitation for noninvasive Down syndrome diagnostics

Targeted molecular analysis of fetal aneuploidy with maternal plasma utilization is more complicated and applicable differentiation of maternal and fetal genotypes within the desired chromosome brings with it many challenges.

Considering differences between the quantity of total cffDNA and cfDNA, in the fetuses with Down syndrome (DS) pathology can be observed a greater quantity of cffDNA compared to the physiological pregnancies (Vodicka et al, 2008a).

The total amount of cffDNA cannot be considered as unambiguous marker due to large variation in the amount of cffDNA in physiological pregnancies and, rather, it is possible to include it to the system of ultrasound and biochemical markers.

Direct examination of the loci responsible for the DS brings a substantial improvement of the diagnosis. Currently, there are several approaches or their combinations respectively, aimed to unambiguous resolution of pathological fetus with the DS.

7.1 Noninvasive cffDNA diagnostics of Down syndrome using genotype differences between paternal and maternal genotypes

DS analyses and quantifications of cffDNA are based on the resolution of paternal from maternal genotypes. The fetus must be always heterozygous for the monitored loci. Previous genotyping of the parents is therefore important for the selection of appropriate markers.

Targeted resolution assumes a sufficient number of reliable analyzable markers of paternal (fetal) origin on chromosome 21 and at the same time a sufficient number of reliable markers outside the chromosome 21.

The genotype of the fetus can be distinguished by means of DNA sequence variation using male specific sequences for male fetus, short tandem repeats (STR) or single nucleotide polymorphisms (SNP).

For the estimation of the relative amounts of cffDNA originating in chromosome 21 it is necessary to choose a strategy that combines the creation of sensitive and accurate calibration standards for each marker and reciprocal measuring of cffDNA amount from the locus on chromosome 21 and cffDNA quantity from autosomal locus or locus on chromosome Y respectively.

If the measurement is accurate enough, then the amount of cffDNA of chromosome 21 related to the quantity of the cffDNA locus outside the chromosome 21 should differ in the case of trisomy 21 from disomy 21. It is clearly distinguishable in the case of trisomy of paternal origin, where the extra chromosome comes from the father.

The methodology of quantitative calculations for STR loci on chromosome 21, where was mainly taken into account the relative length of alleles and preferential amplification of the shorter alleles has been developed at our department.

In pregnancies with trisomy 21, it was found statistically more cffDNA for systems in which the length of PCR products ranged mostly between 200 bp - 400 bp (Vodicka et al., 2008).

In total six genes that are specifically expressed in trofoblastic tissues (placenta) has been selected for quantification and genotyping on the DNA level in loci responsible for Down syndrome and for reference SNP genotyping (Böhmova et al. 2010).

These genes are DSCR4, KRTAP26-1, PLAC4, PLAC1, PAPPA and PSG11 of them DSCR4, KRTAP26-1 and PLAC4 are localized on chromosome 21 in the area responsible for Down syndrome. In total 12 SNPs were selected for genotyping in these genes.

Balanced allelic frequency for particular SNP alleles reported in the database of the NCBI website was the criterion for the SNP selection. For individual SNP variants have been defined TaqMan probes. Individual genotypes were identified initially by sequencing of the SNP regions for 30 randomly selected maternal DNA samples. Subsequently TaqMan Real Time PCR optimization and calibration was carried out.

Quantifiler kit (Applied Biosystems) has been used for verification of the quality of the dilutive series of calibration standards. The quantification itself was carried out on 240 DNA samples isolated from plasma of pregnant women in the 1st and 2nd trimester.

Heterozygozity in particular SNP ranged from 14 % to 55 % and the probability of appropriate genotypes capture for each SNP was stated in the range from 12 % to 28 %. Sensitivity of minor genotype capture depends on fluorescence background of non-specifically hybridized probe.

Taqman SNP probes were able to capture as low as 1 percent of artificial genotypic mixture and by the most sensitive systems we have detected 0,22 % artificial genotypic mixture.

R^2 values were in the range of 0,995 to 0,999 and the inclination (angular coefficient) assessing the effectiveness of the PCR (tendency around the values of -3.3 shows the optimum, 100% PCR amplification) from -3.2 to -3.6. All standard calibration curves were appropriate for the cffDNA quantification (Picture 1).

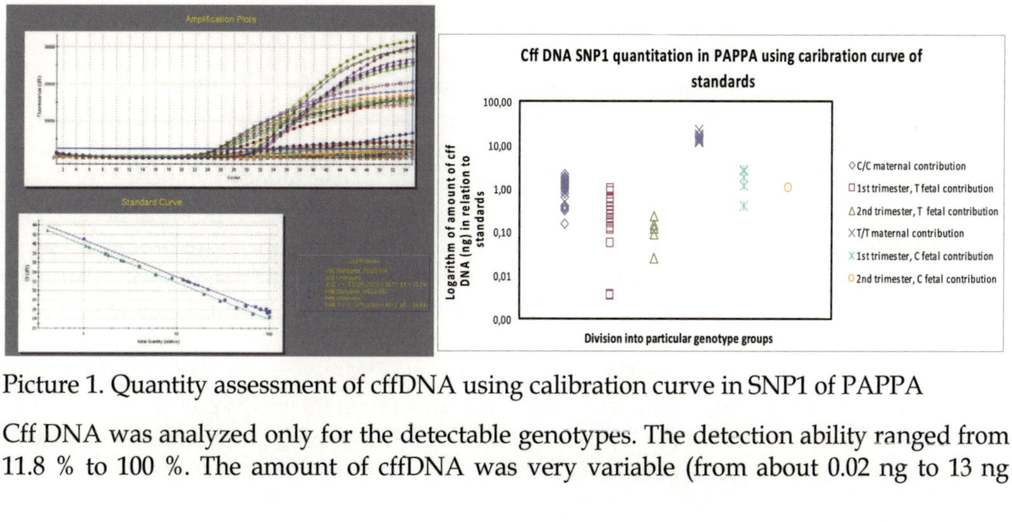

Picture 1. Quantity assessment of cffDNA using calibration curve in SNP1 of PAPPA

Cff DNA was analyzed only for the detectable genotypes. The detection ability ranged from 11.8 % to 100 %. The amount of cffDNA was very variable (from about 0.02 ng to 13 ng cffDNA in 200 ul of the plasma). All 12 selected SNP are able to detect cffDNA with the desired probability. Parameters of the calibration curve are suitable for the precise quantification of cffDNA (Picture 1) (Böhmova et al., 2010).

7.2 Noninvasive cff mRNA analysis for Down syndrome diagnostics

Placental tissue is ontogenetically much unrelated to blood cells and may express other genes whose expression is missing in maternal blood cells. The first work, which confirmed the RNA of fetal origin, was published in 2000 (Poon et al., 2000).

Using microarray technology in the maternal plasma have been detected RNA markers whose expression is specific to the placenta (Tsui et al., 2004). The same approach was used in the study, which described the cff mRNA transcribed from gene PLAC4 (placenta-specific 4), which is located on chromosome 21.

On the basis of the assumption of uniform batch theory (3 alleles of PLAC4 gene, without allele-specific preferential transcription, express 1/3 more mRNA than 2 alleles) quantitative detection of disomic and trizomic dose was developed. With the use of the SNP in the heterozygous state in the gene coding for the PLAC4 there were detected disomic fetus ratio 1: 1 and trizomic ratio 2: 1 with 90% of the diagnostic sensitivity and 96.5% specificity of trisomy 21 capture by mass spectrometry technique (Lo et al., 2007a).

The disadvantage of this method is relatively labour-intensive preparation of high-quality and reproducible matrix for mass spectrophotometry RNA analysis. Another limiting factor is the real amount of cff mRNA molecules in the isolate from plasma, which could affect the evenness of distribution of mRNA molecules transcribed from individual alleles. Only sufficient number of SNPs can assure desired heterozygozity. Therefore it is necessary to test and introduce new mRNA SNP markers (Go et al., 2007; Yang et al., 2008).

Another approach of measuring allelic SNP ratios in cff mRNA has been tested using digital PCR. It is based on the assumption that, in the PCR reaction is either 1 or no molecule of cDNA. PCR is carried out in parallel in many hundreds to thousands of mixtures. According to the number of positive responses, you can estimate an initial number of cff RNA molecules with a particular SNP and by measuring of the ratios between the SNP from RNA derived from chromosome 21 and another autosome, you can detect chromosome 21 trisomy with high sensitivity (Lo et al., 2007b).

7.3 Noninvasive Down syndrome diagnostics by cffDNA epigenetic detection and quantification

Methodology relies on different methylation of maternal and fetal or placental sequence. Sequences, which are subject to methylation are on principle situated in CpG islands of promoter areas. These islets may regulate the transcription of the gene by variable degree of methylation. In different tissues there are promoters of genes whose expression is tissue specific, and which are methylated differently, and specifically for the type of tissue.

Different fetal (placental) and maternal methylation of regions on chromosome 21 were tracked for the purposes of Down Syndrome non-invasive prenatal diagnostics. Different methylation showed 22 out of 114 assessed genomic regions on this chromosome (Chim et al., 2008).

This relatively large number of methylation specific fetal DNA sequences offers a promising source of prenatal biomarkers independent on maternal and fetal genotype.

Large loss of genetic material (90 %) in the course of DNA modification, based on cytosine deamination using bisulphite, is a disadvantage of this epigenetic way of examination.

The modification procedure, somewhat laborious, in addition increases the risk of contamination. Additional distortion of results could be due to heterogeneous methylation of CpG islands.

Some laboratories are trying to test methods that would eliminate the a forementioned shortcomings (Chan et al., 2006; Tong et al., 2007).

Digital methyl sensitive PCR, methyl sensitive HRM and, probably, massive parallel DNA sequencing are the most promising prospective technologies for precise quantification of epialleles.

7.4 Combination of genetic/epigenetic/cff mRNA methods

To increase the diagnostic sensitivity it is possible to combine methodological approaches, based on cffDNA, cff mRNA and hyper/hypomethylated placental DNA.

Tong et al (2010) published the epigenetic quantification of hypermethylated placental DNA from chromosome 21 (locus HLCS) using digital PCR and compared it to the male specific genetic marker of the Y chromosome.

The relative quantities of the epigenetic marker were shown to be increased for fetus with trisomy 21 compared to disomic fetus. This approach is very sensitive even for the DS diagnosis in the first trimester.

It will be appropriate to use different paternal genetic polymorphic markers at the level of the SNP or STR instead of male specific genetic marker.

To increase the reliability of resolution of trisomy 21 from disomy 21 is also possible to perform relative quantification of cffDNA/cff mRNA using exonal SNP of chromosome 21 and exonal SNP from the reference autosome.

8. Tasks for future

For the successful development of high accurate detection of DS and other frequent trisomies it is necessary to attend to the following tasks:

- Choice of isolation procedures for plasmatic DNA fragments length of which corresponds to the fetal molecules.
- Protection of plasmatic molecules from the disintegration of maternal lymphocytes.
- Prevention of free plasmatic fetal RNA degradation.
- Loss minimization during modification of hyper/hypomethylated DNA.
- Provision of sufficient number of reliable genetic and epigenetic fetal markers.
- More sensitive optimization of calibration and quantification for HRM, Real time PCR and QF PCR.
- Introduction of automation of digital PCR and digital HRM for quantification of CffDNA/cff mRNA/modified cffDNA.

9. Conclusion

Almost 15 years have passed since the first work, which pointed to the presence of the cff DNA in maternal plasma of pregnant women (Lo et al., 1997).

Since then many authors gradually contributed more and more theoretical and methodological knowledge.

Nowadays, also thanks to introduction of new and more robust technologies we can boldly predict that direct clinical outcome of this multi-year effort of noninvasive prenatal diagnostics of Down Syndrome will be feasible in very near future.

10. Acknowledgment

This work was supported by Grant agency IGA MZ CR: NS/9624-3

11. References

Alberry, M.S., Maddocks, D.G., Hadi, M.A., Metawi, H., Hunt, L.P., Abdel-Fattah, S.A., Avent, N.D. & Soothill, P.W. (2009). Quantification of cell free fetal DNA in maternal plasma in normal pregnancies and pregnancies with placental dysfunction. *American Journal of Obstetrics and Gynecology*, Vol. 200, No. 1, (January 2009), pp. 98. e1-6, ISSN 0002-9378

Amicucci, P., Gennarelli, M., Novelli, G. & Dallapiccola, B. (2000). Prenatal diagnosis of myotonic dystrophy using fetal DNA obtained from maternal plasma, *Clinical Chemistry*, Vol. 46, No. 2, (February 2000), pp. 301-302, ISSN 0009-914

Ariga, H., Ohto, H., Busch, M.P., Imamura, S., Watson, R., Reed, W. & Lee, T.H. (2001). Kinetics of fetal cellular and cell-free DNA in the maternal circulation during and after pregnancy: implications for noninvasive prenatal diagnosis. *Transfusion*, Vol. 41, No. 12, (December 2001), pp. 1524-1530, ISSN 0041-1132

Bianchi, D.W. Fetomaternal cell traffic, pregnancy-associated progenitor cells, and autoimmune disease. (2004). *Best Practice & Research Clinical Obstetrics & Gynaecology*, Vol. 18, No .6, (December 2004), pp. 959-975, ISSN 1521-6934

Bohmova, J., Vodicka, R., Dhaifalah, I., Vrtel, R., Kratochvilova, R., Prochazka, M., Kvapilova, M., Krejcirikova, E., Dusek, L., Santavy, J. (2010). Cell free fetal nucleic acid SNP quantitative analysis for potential noninvasive prenatal diagnosis purposes. *European Journal of Human Genetic*, Vol. 18, Suppl. 1, (June 2010), pp. 147, ISSN 1018-4813

Boom, R., Sol, C. J., Salimans, M. M. M., Jansen, C. L., Wertheim - van Dillen, P. M. E. & van der Noordaa, J. (1990). Rapid and simple method for purification of nucleic acid. *Journal of Clinical Microbiology*, Vol. 28, No. 3, (March 1990), pp. 495-503, ISSN 0095-1137

Fan, H.C. & Quake, S.R. (2007). Detection of aneuploidy with digital polymerase chain reaction. *Analytical Chemistry*, Vol. 79, No. 19, (October 2007), pp. 7576–7579

Frendo, J.L., Vidaud, M., Guibourdenche, J., Luton, D., Muller, F., Bellet, D., Giovagrandi, Y., Tarrade, A., Porquet, D., Blot, P. & Evain-Brion, D. (2000). Defect of villous cytotrophoblast differentiation into syncytiotrophoblast in Down syndrome. *Journal of Clinical Endocrinology & Metabolism*, Vol. 85, No. 10, (October 2000), pp. 3700-3707, ISSN 0021-972X

Go, A.T., Visser, A., Mulders, M.A., Blankenstein, M.A., van Vugt, J.M. & Oudejans, C.B. (2007). 44 single-nucleotide polymorphisms expressed by placental RNA: assessment for use in noninvasive prenatal diagnosis of trisomy 21. *Clinical Chemistry*, Vol. 53, No. 12, (December 2007), pp. 2223-2224, ISSN 0009-914

González-González, M.C., García-Hoyos, M., Trujillo, M.J., Rodríguez de Alba, M., Lorda-Sánchez, I., Díaz-Recasens, J., Gallardo, E., Ayuso, C. & Ramos, C. (2002). Prenatal detection of a cystic fibrosis mutation in fetal DNA from maternal plasma. *Prenatal Diagnosis,* Vol. 22, No. 10, (October 2002), pp. 946-948, ISSN 0197-3851

Gonzalez-Gonzalez, M.C., Trujillo, M.J., Rodriguez de Alba, M. & Ramos, C. (2003). Early Huntington disease prenatal diagnosis by maternal semiquantitative fluorescent-PCR. *Neurology,* Vol. 60, No. 7, (April 2003), pp. 1214-1215

Halicka, H.D., Bedner, E. & Darzynkiewicz, Z. (2000). Seregation of RNA and separate packaging of DNA and RNA in apoptotic bodies during apoptosis. *Experimental Cell Research,* Vol. 260, No. 2, (November 2000), pp. 248–256, ISSN 0014-4827

Hasselmann, D.O., Rappl, G., Tilgen, W. & Reinhold, U. (2001). Extracellular tyrosinase mRNA within apoptotic bodies is protected from degradation in human serum. *Clinical Chemistry,* Vol. 44, No. 8, (August 2001), pp. 1488–1489, ISSN 0009-914

Honda, H., Miharu, N., Ohashi, Y., Samura, O., Kinutani, M., Hara, T. & Ohama, K. (2002). Fetal gender determination in early pregnancy through qualitative and quantitative analysis of fetal DNA in maternal serum. *Human Genetics,* Vol. 110, No. 1, (January 2002), pp. 75-79, ISSN 0340-6717

Höss, M. & Pääbo, S. (1993). DNA extraction from Pleistocene bones by a silica-based purification method. *Nucleic Acids Research,* Vol. 21, No. 16, (August 1993), pp. 3913-3914, ISSN 0305-1048

Hristoskova, S., Holzgreve, W. & Hahn, S. (2001). More than one-half of the erythroblasts in the fetal circulation and cord blood are TUNEL positive. *Clinical Chemistry,* Vol. 47, No. 10, (October 2001), pp. 1870-1871, ISSN 0009-914

Huppertz, B. & Kingdom, J.C. (2004). Apoptosis in the trophoblast—role of apoptosis in placental morphogenesis. *Journal of the Society for Gynecologic Investigation,* Vol. 11, No. 6, (September 2004), pp. 353-362, ISSN 1071-5576

Húska, D., Baloun, J., Trnková, L., Adam, V. & Kizek, R. (2008). Využití paramagnetických částic pro izolaci mRNA. *CHEMagazín,* Vol. 18, No. 3, (2008), pp. 14-15, ISSN 1210-7409

Chan, K.C., Zhang, J., Hui, A.B., Wong, N., Lau, T.K., Leung, T.N., Lo, K.W., Huang, D.W. & Lo, Y.M. (2004). Size distributions of maternal and fetal DNA in maternal plasma. *Clinical Chemistry,* Vol. 50, No. 1, (January 2004), pp. 88–92, ISSN 0009-914

Chan, K.C., Ding, C., Gerovassili, A., Yeung, S.W., Chiu, R.W., Leung, T.N., Lau, T.K., Chim, S.S., Chung, G.T., Nicolaides, K.H. & Lo, Y.M. (2006). Hypermethylated RASSF1A in maternal plasma: a universal fetal DNA marker that improves the reliability of noninvasive prenatal diagnosis. *Clinical Chemistry,* Vol. 52, No. 12, (December 2006), pp. 2211–2218, ISSN 0009-914

Chim, S.S., Jin, S., Lee, T.Y., Lun, F.M., Lee, W.S., Chan, L.Y., Jin, Y., Yang, N., Tong, Y.K., Leung, T.Y., Lau, T.K., Ding, C., Chiu, R.W. & Lo, Y.M. (2008). Systematic search for placental epigenetic markers on chromosome 21: towards noninvasive prenatal diagnosis of fetal trisomy 21. *Clinical Chemistry,* Vol. 54, No. 3, (March 2008), pp. 500–511, ISSN 0009-914

Chiu, R.W., Lau, T.K., Leung, T.N., Chow, K.C., Chui, D.H. & Lo, Y.M. (2002). Prenatal exclusion of beta thalassaemia major by examination of maternal plasma. *Lancet,* Vol. 360, No. 9339, (September 2002), pp. 998-1000, ISSN 0023-7507

Johnson, L., McCracken, S.A., Morris, J.M., Woodland, N.B. & Flower, R.L. (2003). Variation in the reliability of RHD antenatal genotyping using the polymerase chain reaction and targeting multiple exons of the RHD gene. *Vox Sanguinis*, Vol. 85, No. 3, (October 2003), pp. 222–223, ISSN 0042-9007

Koide, K., Sekizawa, A., Iwasaki, M., Matsuoka, R., Honma, S., Farina, A., Saito, H. & Okai, T. (2005). Fragmentation of cell-free fetal DNA in plasma and urine of pregnant women. *Prenatal Diagnosis*, Vol. 25, No. 7, (July 2005), pp. 604–607, ISSN 0197-3851

Li, Y., Zimmermann, B., Rusterholz, C., Kang, A., Holzgreve, W. & Hahn, S. (2004). Size separation of Circulatory DNA in maternal plasma permits ready detection of fetal DNA polymorphisms. *Clinical Chemistry*, Vol. 50, No. 6, (June 2004), pp. 1002-1011, ISSN 0009-914

Lo, Y.M., Corbetta, N., Chamberlain, P.F., Rai, V., Sargent, I.L., Redman, C.W. & Wainscoat, J.S. (1997). Presence of fetal DNA in maternal plasma and serum. *Lancet*, Vol. 350, No. 9076, (August 1997), pp. 485–487, ISSN 0023-7507

Lo, Y.M., Tein, M.S., Lau, T.K., Haines, C.J., Leung, T.N., Poon, P.M., Wainscoat, J.S., Johnson, P.J., Chang, A.M. & Hjelm, N.M. (1999). Quantitative analysis of fetal DNA in maternal plasma and serum: implications for noninvasive prenatal diagnosis. *American Journal of Human Genetics*, Vol. 62, No. 4, (April 1998), pp. 768-775, ISSN 0002-9297

Lo, Y.M., Zhang, J., Leung, T.N., Lau, T.K., Chang, A.M. & Hjelm, N.M. (1999). Rapid clearance of fetal DNA from maternal plasma. *American Journal of Human Genetics*, Vol. 64, No. 1, (June 1999), pp. 218–224, ISSN 0002-9297

Lo, Y.M. & Chiu, R.W. (2007). Non-invasive prenatal diagnosis of Down's syndrome. *Lancet*, Vol. 369, No. 9578, (June 2007a), pp. 1997, ISSN 0023-7507

Lo, Y.M., Tsui, N.B., Chiu, R.W., Lau, T.K., Leung, T.N., Heung, M.M., Gerovassili, A., Jin, Y., Nicolaides, K.H., Cantor, C.R. & Ding, C. (2007b). Plasma placental RNA allelic ratio permits noninvasive prenatal chromosomal aneuploidy detection. *Nature Medicine*, Vol. 13, No. 2, (February 2007), pp. 218–223, ISSN 1078-8956

Massin, N., Frendo, J.L., Guibourdenche, J., Luton, D., Giovangrandi, Y., Muller, F., Vidaud, M. & Evain-Brion, D. (2001). Defect of syncytiotrophoblast formation and hCG expression in Down syndrome. *Placenta*, Vol. 22, Suppl. A, (April 2001), pp. 93-97, ISSN 0265-7023

Nelson, M., Eagle, C., Langshaw, M., Popp, H. & Kroneberg, H. (2001). Genotyping fetal DNA by non-invasive means: extraction from maternal plasma. *Vox Sanguinis*, Vol. 80, No. 2, (February 2001), pp. 112–116, ISSN 0042-9007

Ng, E.K., Tsui, N.B., Lau, T.K., Leung, T.N., Chiu, R.W., Panesar, N.S., Lit, L.C., Chan, K.W. & Lo, Y.M. (2003). mRNA of placental origin is readily detectable in maternal plasma. *Proceedings of the National Academy of Sciences of the United States of America*, Vol. 100, No. 8, (April 2003), pp. 4748-4753, ISSN 0027-8424

Ng, E.K., El-Sheikhah, A., Chiu, R.W., Chan, K.C., Hogg, M., Bindra, R., Leung, T.N., Lau, T.K., Nicolaides, K.H. & Lo, Y.M. (2004). Human chorionic gonadotropin beta-subunit mRNA concentrations in maternal serum in aneuploid pregnancies. *Clinical Chemistry*, Vol. 50, No. 6, (June 2004), pp. 1055–1057, ISSN 0009-914

Pertl, B., Sekizawa, A., Samura, O., Orescovic, I., Rahaim, P.T. & Bianchi, D.W. (2000). Detection of male and female fetal DNA in maternal plasma by multiplex fluorescent polymerase chain reaction amplification of short tandem repeats. *Human Genetics*, Vol. 106, No. 1, (January 2000), pp. 45-49, ISSN 0340-6717

Poon, L.L., Leung, T.N., Lau, T.K. & Lo, Y.M. (2000). Presence of fetal RNA in maternal plasma. *Clinical Chemistry*, Vol. 46, No. 11, (November 2000), pp. 1832–1834, ISSN 0009-914

Randen, I., Hauge, R., Kjeldsen-Kragh, J. & Fagerhol, M.K. (2003). Prenatal genotyping of RHD and SRY using maternal blood. *Vox Sanguinis*, Vol. 85, No. 4, (November 2003), pp. 300–306, ISSN 0042-9007

Saito, H., Sekizawa, A., Morimoto, T., Suzuki, M. & Yanaihara, T. (2000). Prenatal DNA diagnosis of a single-gene disorder from maternal plasma. *Lancet*, Vol. 356, No. 9236, (September 2000), pp. 1170, ISSN 0023-7507

Sekizawa, A., Kondo, T., Iwasaki, M., Watanabe, A., Jimbo, M., Saito, H. & Okai, T. (2001). Accuracy of fetal gender determination by analysis of DNA in maternal plasma. *Clinical Chemistry*, Vol. 47, No. 10, (October 2001), pp. 1856-1858, ISSN 0009-914

Sekizawa, A., Yokokawa, K., Sugito, Y., Iwasaki, M., Yukimoto, Y., Ichizuka, K., Saito, H. & Okai, T. (2003). Evaluation of bidirectional transfer of plasma DNA through placenta. *Human Genetics*, Vol. 113, No. 4, (September 2003), pp. 307-310, ISSN 0340-6717

Sisco, K.L. (2001). Is RNA in serum bound to nucleoprotein complexes? *Clinical Chemistry*, Vol. 47, No. 9, (September 2001), pp. 1744–1745, ISSN 0009-914

Siva, S.C., Johnson, S.I., McCracken, S.A. & Morris, J.M. (2003). Evaluation of the clinical usefulness of isolation of fetal DNA from the maternal circulation, *Australian and New Zealand Journal of Obstetrics and Gynaecology*, Vol. 43, No. 1, (February 2003), pp. 10–15, ISSN 0004-8666

Tong, Y.K., Chiu, R.W., Leung, T.Y., Ding, C., Lau, T.K., Leung, T.N. & Lo, Y.M. (2007). Detection of restriction enzyme-digested target DNA by PCR amplification using a stem-loop primer: application to the detection of hypomethylated fetal DNA in maternal plasma. *Clinical Chemistry*, Vol. 53, No. 11, (November 2007), pp. 1906–1914, ISSN 0009-914

Tong, Y.K., Jin, S., Chiu, R.W., Ding, C., Chan, K.C., Leung, T.Y., Yu, L., Lau, T.K. & Lo, Y.M. (2010). Noninvasive prenatal detection of trisomy 21 by an epigenetic-genetic chromosome-dosage approach. *Clinical Chemistry*, Vol. 56, No. 1, (January 2010), pp. 90-98, ISSN 0009-914

Tsui, N.B., Ng, E.K. & Lo, Y.M. (2002). Stability of Endogenous and Added RNA in Blood Specimens, Serum, and Plasma. *Clinical Chemistry*, Vol. 48, No. 10, (October 2002), pp. 1647-1653, ISSN 0009-914

Tsui, N.B., Chim, S.S., Chiu, R.W., Lau, T.K., Ng, E.K., Leung, T.N., Tong, Y.K., Chan, K.C. & Lo, Y.M. (2004). Systematic microarray-based identification of placental mRNA in maternal plasma: towards non-invasive prenatal gene expression profiling. *Journal of Medical Genetics*, Vol. 41, No. 6, (June 2004), pp. 461–467, ISSN 0022-2593

van Wijk, I.J., de Hoon, A.C., Jurhawan, R., Tjoa, M.L., Griffioen, S., Mulders, M.A., van Vugt, J.M. & Oudejans, C.B. (2000). Detection of apoptotic fetal cells in plasma of pregnant women. *Clinical Chemistry*, Vol. 46, No. 5, (May 2000), pp. 729-731, ISSN 0009-914

Vodicka, R., Vrtel, R., Dusek, L., Prochazka, M., Schneiderova, E., Vrbicka, D., Krejcirikova, E., Dhaifalah, I., Santava, A. & Santavy, J. (2008a). Refined fluorescent STR quantification of cell-free fetal DNA during pregnancy in physiological and Down syndrome fetuses. *Prenatal Diagnosis*, Vol. 28, No. 5, (May 2008a), pp. 425-433, ISSN 0197-3851

Vodička, R., Vrtěl, R., Schneiderová, E., Vrbická, D., Dhaifalah, I., Šantavá, A. & Šantavý J. (2008b). Neinvazivní detekce gonozomálních DNA sekvencí v plazmě gravidních žen s využitím kapilární elektroforézy. *Česká Gynekologie*, Vol. 73, No. 3, (2008b), pp. 150-153, ISSN 1210-7832

Vodicka, R., Böhmová, J., Dhaifalah, I., Blumenthalová, J., Kratochvílová, R., Procházka, M. & Vrtěl, R. (2010). Analysis of cell free fetal DNA fragmentation rate in pregnant women during the course of gravidit. *Ceská gynekologie*, Vol. 75, No. 4, (August 2010), pp. 312-316, ISSN 1210-7832

Wataganara, T. & Bianch, D.W. (2004). Fetal cell-free nucleic acids in the maternal circulation: new clinical applications. *Annals of the New York Academy of Sciences*, Vol. 1022, (January 2004), pp. 90-99

Wei, C., Sailer, D.N. & Sutherland, J.W. (2001). Detection and quantification by homogeneous PCR of cell-free fetal DNA in maternal plasma. *Clinical Chemistry*, Vol. 47, No. 2, (February 2001), pp. 336-338, ISSN 0009-914

Yang ,Y., Ding, J.H., Lee, M.S., Loria, O., Mohsenian, F., Tang, M., *et al.* (2008). Identification of mRNA-SNP markers for a noninvasive prenatal trisomy 21 (T21) test. *Prenatal Diagnosis*, Vol. 28, (2008), pp. S12, ISSN 0197-3851

Zhang, J., Fidler, C., Murphy, M.F., Chamberlain, P.F., Sargent, I.L., Redman, C.W.G., Hjelm, N.M., Wainscoat, J.S. & Lo, Y.M.D. (2000). Determination of fetal RhD status by maternal plasma DNA analysis. *Annals of the New York Academy of Sciences*, Vol. 906, (April 2000), pp. 153–155

Zhong, X.Y., Burk, M.R., Troeger, C., Jackson, L.R., Holzgreve, W. & Hahn, S. (2000). Fetal DNA in maternal plasma is elevated in pregnancies with aneuploid fetuses. *Prenatal Diagnosis*, Vol. 20, No. 10, (October 2000), pp. 795-798, ISSN 0197-3851

MEMBRANE-BOUND ATP-DEPENDENT ENERGY SYSTEMS AND THE GASTROINTESTINAL MUCOSAL DAMAGE AND PROTECTION

Authored by **Gyula Mozsik** and **Imre Szabó**

Membrane-bound Atp-dependent Energy Systems and the Gastrointestinal Mucosal Damage and Protection

http://dx.doi.org/10.5772/60095
Authored by Gyula Mozsik and Imre Szabó

Contributors

Gyula Mozsik, Imre Szabó

Published by InTech

Janeza Trdine 9, 51000 Rijeka, Croatia

Publishing Process Manager Danijela Duric

Technical Editor InTech DTP team

Cover InTech Design team

First published March, 2016

Printed in Croatia

Additional hard copies can be obtained from orders@intechopen.com

Membrane-bound Atp-dependent Energy Systems and the Gastrointestinal Mucosal Damage and Protection, Authored by Gyula Mozsik and Imre Szabó
p. cm.
ISBN 978-953-51-2251-7

Meet the authors

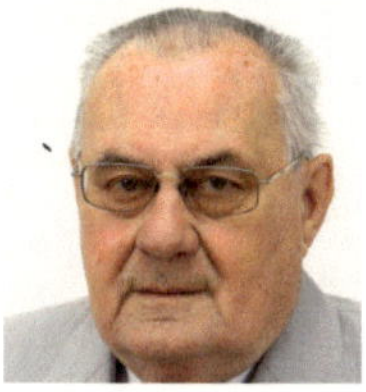

Gyula Mozsik, MD, PhD, ScD (med):professor emeritus of medicine at First Department of Medicine, University of Pécs, Hungary. He was head of this Department from 1993 to 2003. His specialization: internist, gastroenterologists, clinical pharmacologists. His research fields are biochemical pharmacological studies in the gastrointestinal tract, and the role of capsaicin-sensitive afferention in human gastrointestinal tract. He published more 350 papers in peer-revieved journal ,19 monographs and edited 30 books.He received André Robert award from International Union of Pharmacology ,Gastrointestinal Section (2014).From his students, fourtheen full University Professors were appointed in Cuba, Egypt and Hungary.

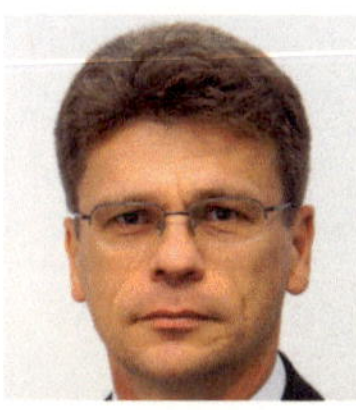

Dr. Imre Szabó is a medical doctor holding Ph.D. (2004) and habilitation (2012) degrees in Gastroenterology from the University of Pécs (Hungary, 2004), where he studied the mechanisms of cytoprotection and mucosal healing processes in different regions of human gastrointestinal system. He currently works as an Associate Professor at the First Department of Medicine, University of Pécs and has 12 years of experience in teaching Internal Medicine and Gastroenterology at graduate and postgraduate level. His research in the United States included the study of ulcer healing, nonsteroidal gastroenteropathy in animal models and their molecular mechanisms in isolated cells. He has published his work in several peer reviewed journals and given oral and poster presentations at national and international conferences. In addition he has authored Hungarian grants and participated in grants from U.S. Veteran's Administration. His fields of special experience include gastrointestinal mucosal injury, defense and healing mechanisms.

Contents

Preface

This monograph deals with various aspects of peptic ulcer disease, like clinical pharmacology, nutrition, molecular biochemical pharmacology as well as clinical aspects, and especially with the evaluation of certain biochemical mechanisms in human gastric mucosa and in animal gastric tissues obtained from different ulcer models.

The authors have been working from the 1960s up till now in the fields of basic research involving molecular pharmacological studies, to understand the bases of gastrointestinal mucosa damage in animal models and in human gastrointestinal tissues, and of clinical research involving clinical pharmacology of prospective, randomized, multiclinical studies, biochemical molecular pharmacology and nutrition.

The authors reported first that duodenal ulcer can heal without any decrease of gastric acid secretion in patients with duodenal ulcer (1965), then prepared the Na^+–K^+-dependent ATPase and adenylate cyclase from the human gastric mucosa (1969–1970), and finally discovered the key role of intact vagal nerve in the development of prostacyclin-induced gastric cytoprotection (1982).

The mitochondrial ATP is the common substrate for both membrane-bound Na^+–K^+-dependent ATPase and adenylate cyclase in the presence of Mg^{2+}. The actual level of mitochondrial ATP is the consequence of the equilibrium between the ATP breakdown and ATP resynthesis (by oxidative phosphorylation).

The membrane-bound ATP-dependent energy systems are common meeting points for different physiological and pathological phenomena (gastric acid secretion, tissue hypoxia, tissue damage and gastrointestinal ulceration) as well as drug-induced intracellular targets.

The authors have focused on feedback mechanisms existing between the different drugs, hormones, and mediator-induced extra- and intracellular regulatory pathways in the human gastrointestinal resecates obtained from surgical interventions performed for treating peptic ulcer in patients and from various ulcer experimental animal models at the time of the development of gastrointestinal mucosal damage and prevention. It was clear that no hypoxemic damage can be proven biochemically in the ulcerated gastric mucosa and that a very complex intracellular feedback mechanism system exists between the Na^+–K^+-ATPase and adenylate cyclase enzymes under normal and ulcerated gastrointestinal mucosa regulated by different mediators, hormones and drugs. The results of biochemical examinations clearly indicated that several generally and internationally stated theories cannot be further accepted in the light of results obtained from human and animal gastric mucosal biochemistry described in this book. *Helicobacter pylori* bacteria (given in doses of 10^6–10^8 germs/mL) can-

not produce cellular damage at the levels of cell membrane, mitochondrion and nucleic acids on freshly isolated rat gastric mucosal cells.

This book can be useful to physiologists; biochemists; pharmacologists, particularly molecular and biochemical pharmacologists; internists; gastroenterologists; biologists; surgeons and pharmacists.

Gyula Mozsik, MD, PhD, ScD (med): professor emeritus,
First Department of Medicine,
University of Pécs, Hungary

Dr. Imre Szabó,
Associate Professor,
First Department of Medicine,
University of Pécs, Hungary

Chapter 1

General Medical Backgrounds

Gyula Mozsik and Imre Szabó

Additional information is available at the end of the chapter

http://dx.doi.org/10.5772/60096

1.1. General medical introduction

The characteristics and epidemiology of the gastrointestinal diseases, including the peptic ulcer disease, have significantly changed during the past 40–50 years. Previously, physicians' diagnostic possibilities were limited to the patients' complaints, performance in physical examinations and basic X-ray examinations. Diagnosis was based mainly on the subjective (patients' complaints) and objective (physical observations) data obtained from the patients. However, the diagnostic modalities of the everyday medical practice have changed significantly during the past decades resulting in the usage of modern medical diagnostic instruments.

Peptic ulcers and gastrointestinal mucosal damage were accepted as the result of the unbalanced equilibrium between the aggressive (HCl and pepsin) and defensive (blood supply, mucus, bicarbonate, prostaglandins, biochemistry of target organs, etc.) factors. Consequently, the principal role of overproduction of gastric acid secretion and pepsin secretion or decreased defense against gastrointestinal damage (gastric, duodenal and jejunal ulcers) has been accepted as possible causes for the development of gastrointestinal mucosal damage. However, the details of these mechanisms and their key factors have changed over the past decades. The correction of unbalanced equilibrium between the aggressive and defensive factors in the gastrointestinal mucosa gave the basis of therapeutic possibilities in patients with peptic ulcers before the discovery of "gastric cytoprotection" by André Robert (1979). He indicated that prostaglandins prevent the gastric mucosal damage without the presence of gastric inhibitory actions in rats. Earlier, we observed that the duodenal ulcer in patients healed; however, the gastric secretory responses did not change during a prolonged atropine treatment (Mózsik et al., 1965 a, b). We observed this phenomenon in patients with duodenal ulcer, and we gave a clinical pharmacological explanation for the existence of this phenomenon (for details, see Chapter 2).

Conversely, we had very limited treatment options for patients, such as the application of alkaline mineral water, strict diets (which were not known in detail) and a small number of drugs to be applied in medical practice. Many changes have emerged in medical knowledge,

history of patients, civilization, life styles, working and living conditions, nutrition, drug research and the introduction of various medications. We have gained new insight from the physiology, pathology and etiology of diseases and from drug development, nutrition, immunology, biochemistry and other instrumental studies. The genetic code of living cells led to a significant increase in molecular genetics research in medical sciences. Therefore, the correct diagnosis is increasingly becoming the key point of successful therapy.

1.2. Problem- orientated medicine

Since the plat 40–50 years, there has been a significant increase (advantage) in the diagnostic panel for bedside medical practice (endoscopy, ultrasonography, computer tomography, positive emission tomography, angiography, scintigraphy, special immunologically based scintigraphy, etc.). During the same time period, extremely significant advances were observed in the laboratory, such as immunological, histological, immunohistological and genetic diagnostic examinations in everyday medical practices. During this period (mainly during 1970–1980), the different diseases (and our medical activities) were approached by the citation of "problem-orientated medicine," keeping in mind that primary and correct diagnosis was the main aim of everyday medical practice.

The medical treatments including the medical (pharmacological), dietetic, psychological, surgical and others were offered to patients based on the correct diagnosis.

1.3. Evidence-based medicine

We have to note that the evaluation of applied medical therapy was based on the changes in patients' complaints, physicians' opinion, better general health conditions (appearance of the appetite, increase of body weight, better laboratory results, etc). During the past 50 years, the correct methodologies (clinical pharmacology, clinical dietetics, etc.) for critical and objective evaluation of the performed medical treatments were not available.

During the period 1960–1970, we only had the parasympatholytics (atropine, scopolamine and other quaternary ammonium compounds) and different antacids to be used in the medical treatment of peptic ulcer in patients. Furthermore, the new generation of various drugs (for inhibition of gastric acid secretion) – as histamine receptor-blocking agents (from the first to fourth generation), gastrin antagonists, proton pump inhibitors (PPI) and other compounds (prostaglandins, sucralfate, scavengers, etc.) – appeared in the field of medical treatment of patients with classical peptic ulcer disease. The increased gastrointestinal pharmacology led us to learn – in the clinical practice – the terminology of "evidence-based therapy." This terminology still exists; however, the applicability of this medical practice went over a significant change in the plast dcades. The "evidence-based therapy" suggested the existence of its development of human clinical pharmacology by the increase in the emergence of new families of drug compounds. The established clinical pharmacology (form human phase I to human phase IV) during 1960–1970 is given an objective method to crease the "evidence-based medicine." During the first period of clinical pharmacology, the experts analyzed the absorption, metabolization and excretion of different drugs from the gastrointestinal tract; thereafter, the identification of oral/parenteral dose rates was calculated in the case of same drugs, and following these observations, the efficiencies of therapeutic values of drug treatments were

http://dx.doi.org/10.5772/60096

identified in small groups of patients, which extended many thousand patients in multiclinical, multicentric, multinational, randomized and prospective studies all over the world. The organizations of these large-scale studies, involvement (participation) of special patients, special clinical units and using the services of health experts (sisters, laboratory experts and physicians) represented extremely expensive financial requirements, which were covered by the involvement of other large pharmaceutical firms. The small countries (like Hungary) participated in these studies, however, together with others countries.

1.4. Changes in the etiologies and therapies in patients with peptic ulcer

During the past 50 years, the suggested etiological factors for the development of peptic ulcer diseases changed significantly and the medical terminology of peptic ulcer diseases changed as well ["genuine ulcer," secondary ulcer diseases that are associated with the presence of other chronic diseases (such as chronic pulmonary, liver diseases, stress, burn and stroke in the brain), and recently the increased drug consumption for reasons other than the gastrointestinal tract; however, these drugs cause gastrointestinal mucosal damage (e.g., nonsteroidal anti-inflammatory drugs (NSAIDs)) or overconsumption of alcohol]. In the 1980s, the terminology of "non-ulcer dyspepsia (NUD)" was introduced by Scandinavian researchers, which represented those patients who had typical complaints of peptic ulcer, but there was no possibility to detect any alterations (histology, endoscopy) in this group of patients. The gastric mucosal damage caused by different drugs was also introduced in the everyday medical practice.

The number of patients suffering from peptic ulcer diseases also changes over time, and the number of patients suffering from peptic ulcer diseases differs in different countries over the world. In our country (Hungary), the number of patients with peptic ulcer is about 10% of the total Hungarian population (inhabitants) since the 1960s.

We have to accept the changes in the terminology of "peptic ulcer disease." In the 1960s, only the "primary (or genuine)" and "secondary" peptic ulcer diseases were accepted in our medical practice. The patients with secondary peptic ulcer associated with other diseases (stress, sepsis, stroke, pulmonary and liver diseases, burn and trauma), whereas the presence of these factors in the cases of patients with "primary (or genuine)" peptic ulcer diseases was not detected. The "acid-related diseases" also came into medical practice (as diagnosis of patients).

The diagnosis of peptic ulcer disease is based on different objective factors, such as X-ray examination (only in the early period), endoscopic examination and histology.

The classical definition of peptic ulcer disease can be histologically accepted only by the presence of tissue mucosal damage that reaches the muscular mucosal layer. The correct histological definition is necessary for the diagnosis of patients with peptic ulcer diseases. Consequently, the presence of mucosal erosion cannot be considered as a "peptic ulcer disease" (independently from that, the treatment and prevention of these gastrointestinal mucosal injuries represent essential medical problems). After receiving the Nobel Prize in physiology (medicine) by Warren and Marshall (2005), the *Helicobacter pylori*-positive and -negative characterization appeared in patients with the above-mentioned clinical entities.

We have to note that various drugs (including the nonsteroidal anti-inflammatory drugs and others) can cause gastrointestinal diseases (increased complaints of pyrosis in the epigastric

region of the abdomen, vomiting, bleeding, etc.). The correct number of patients with these complaints is not known; however, the number of patients consuming NSAIDs is extremely high. These problems are very important in the our medical practices (looking for the etiology and later the treatment of disease) of medical practices; however, we have to emphasize very well and clearly that these patients are out from the patients with really peptic ulcer disease (because these mucosal damages are in present form out from the classical histological criterion of peptic ulcer disease in patients). These above-mentioned basic criteria of the histological events produced many offered (and gave) many misunderstanding information (results) to know and critically to evaluate thre of the different etiological factors, mechanisms and efficiencies of different medical treatments in patients with classical peptic ulcer diseases.

We have the details of the development of different gastrointestinal mucosal damages (injuries) and the possibilities to prevent these gastric (gastrointestinal) mucosal damages (injuries) through different experimental models in different animal spices.

1.5. Main lines of our research activities in field of peptic ulcer research in peptic ulcer in patients with peptic ulcer and in different animal models

The focus of our research is in accordance with the peptic ulcer research from the 1960s; in the beginning, we had many unresolved and unknown points to be addressed.

We started our research with the patients' problems, and later to other fields such as clinical pharmacology, general biochemistry, molecular pharmacology and biochemistry, oxygen free radicals and antioxidants, specific immunohistochemistry, clinical nutrition, experimental and clinical gastroenterology and nutrition as well as innovative drug research.

Our principal strategy was to understand the problems of patients. As we were not able to understand these problems, we started with animal observations (hoping that we receive correct answers to our questions). We tried answering different and concrete questions in the medical practice.

The research lines in our practice changed over time in the past decades (we started with patients' problems, followed by experimental observations and then back to patients' problems). This research philosophy has been kept in our life. We tried answering different and concrete questions of medical practice and followed this methodology later.

In the pertinent literature, the peptic ulcer disease appeared because of the unbalanced equilibrium between the aggressive and defensive factors in the gastrointestinal mucosa; however, the details of these factors remain to be unknown.

Recently, the possible mechanisms of gastric acid secretory responses have been widely studied in clinical gastroenterology. The extent of gastric basal acid secretory responses (basal acid output, BAO) and acid secretory responses (maximal acid output, MAO) produced by different doses of histamine (given subcutaneously in superliminal but submaximal or superliminal and supermaximal doses) was measured in different groups (gastric, duodenal and jejunal ulcers) of patients with peptic ulcer disease (PUD) (Semb and Myren, 1968). The real reason to study these gastric secretory responses in patients with PUD is that the increased gastric acid secretion has been suggested as one of the different factors, which is responsible for the increased aggressive factors in the gastrointestinal tract. The possible role of pepsin

http://dx.doi.org/10.5772/60096

secretion in the stomach has been suggested to be another aggressive factor for the development of PUD. The increased role of cholinergic dominance (by the increased activity of vagal nerve) is closely associated with the increased gastric acid secretory responses and pepsin production.

In these years, we have no concrete knowledge of the details of defensive factors. The presence of tissue hypoxia of gastroduodenal mucosa of patients with peptic ulcer has been indicated since many years in the ulcer development. Clinically, the presence of tissue hypoxia could be accepted in patients with massive bleeding, whereas no exact observations of gastric mucosal blood flow were carried out in patients during the development of ulcer. Many observations were carried out in animals under different conditions; however, it is interesting to note that the decreased gastric mucosal blood flow was not associated with the presence of tissue hypoxia in terms of biochemistry (increased level of lactate and decreased level of oxidative phosphorylation in the gastrointestinal mucosa).

After a careful survey of the pertinent literature, the research on the evaluation of the details of decreasing activity of vagal nerve in the everyday medical practice in patients with PUD (by parasympatholytic drugs at the beginning of our studies) was started.

During that time, only atropine and scopolamine (the only tertiary ammonium compounds) were used in the everyday medical practice.

Our primary aims of observations were as follows:

1. To establish the clinical pharmacological basis of anticholinergic agents in patients with PUD;
2. To measure the gastric secretory responses of patients with duodenal ulcer before and after (2–4 weeks treatment with atropine) healing of clinically detectable ulcer and
3. To detect the changes in complaints of patients during the medical treatment (especially at the beginning and at the end) (as in complaints of patients originated from the diseases and in the drug-induced side effects – tachycardia, mouth dryness and problems in visual functions).

These studies were carried out in patients with classical duodenal ulcer and were admitted to Second Department of Medicine, University of Debrecen, Hungary.

Author details

Gyula Mozsik[1*] and Imre Szabó[2]

*Address all correspondence to: gyula.mozsik@aok.pte.hu

1 First Department of Medicine, Medical and Health Centre, University of Pécs, Hungary

2 Associate Professor at the First Department of Medicine, University of Pécs, Hungary

Chapter 2

Clinical Pharmacology of Drugs Used in the Treatment of Patients with Peptic Ulcer

Gyula Mozsik and Imre Szabó

Additional information is available at the end of the chapter

http://dx.doi.org/10.5772/60097

2.1. Primary (genuine) and secondary (associated with stress, sepsis, stroke, pulmonary and liver diseases, burn, trauma) Peptic Ulcer Diseases (PUD)

The criteria of diagnosis and treatment of peptic ulcer disease (PUD) have been changed significantly in the past 40–50 years. At the beginning of this period, peptic ulcer disease was only diagnosed by X-ray examination. Currently, gastrofiberoscopy has also become a common practice in medical diagnosis.

Clinically, the PUD was divided into two groups: "primary" and "secondary". The diseases in the "secondary group" associated with a chronic liver, lung, brain damage or burn; however, no obvious reasons for the PUD could be provided as the etiological factor and these forms of the diseases were named as "genuine diseases."

The presence of two main factors was emphasized in the development of gastroduodenal ulceration: the hyperacidity and hypoxemic damage of gastroduodenal mucosa.

There was a significant contradiction between these mentioned factors, namely the gastric hyperacidity associated with the increased gastric mucosal blood flow (GMBF) and ulcer development, and it was practically impossible to understand the development of gastroduodenal mucosal damage based on the increased gastroduodenal mucosal blood flow (Bowen and Fairchild., 1984).

2.2. Medical treatment with anticholinergic agents in patients with gastric and duodenal ulcers

Our scientific attention focused on the medical treatment of patients with peptic ulcer diseases from 1960 onwards.

Our original aim was to create a complete scientific methodology for the evaluation of efficiencies of different drugs (previously, parasympatholytic agents, antacids) in the field of gastroenterology. We have to emphasize that during 1960–1970, no clinical pharmacology existed.

We wanted to introduce into the conventional human clinical pharmacological approaches using that we were established in our group at Debrecen, Hungary, in the field of gastroenterology (in the period of 1962–1970).

Our interest focused on changes of gastric secretory responses in patients with duodenal ulcer (DU) during chronic atropine treatment. In the earlier days, only atropine and scopolamine were used for treating DU patients in whom we studied the presence of DU using X-ray examination (fiberoptic endoscopy did not exist earlier).

We studied (at present) the changes of gastric acid secretory responses in patients with duodenal ulcer before and after a classical medical treatment. We measured the gastric basal acid output (BAO) and secretory responses to superluminal (but submaximal) dose of histamine.

We were surprised to find that the patients with DU were cured by a chronic (2–4 weeks) treatment with atropine. However, the gastric secretory responses in patients were not decreased (Mózsik et al., 1965c; Mózsik and Jávor, 1966 a, b; Mózsik et al., 2011) (see Table 1).

Examined Parameters	Before		After	
	A chronic atropine treatment			
	A	B	A	B
Volume of gastric juice (mL/h)	180±32	175±37	178±44	181±28
H^+ output (mEq/h)	0.97±0.02	1.49±0.2	0.8±0.02	1.61±0.11

Table 1. Gastric secretory responses before and after (3 × 0.3 mg orally given for 2–4 weeks) a chronic atropine treatment without and with histamine (A and B, respectively) (0.5 mg subcutaneously injected). The results were expressed as means ± SEM in ten patients. *P*-values between the identical parameters before and after chronic atropine treatments are not significant. [Mózsik et al., 1965c; 1966b (with kind permission).]

These results showed that duodenal protection could be obtained by independent effects on acid secretion: a phenomenon that defied the earlier well-established view, "no acid, no ulcer" originally pioneered by Lester Dragstedt in 1943 (Gustafson and Welling, 2010).

Following these observations, the acute inhibitory effect of atropine was tested on the gastric acid secretion before and after a chronic atropine treatment. Here, we observed that the extent of acute inhibitory effect of atropine on patients' acid secretion decreased significantly after a chronic treatment (Mózsik et al., 1965c; Mózsik and Jávor 1966b; Mózsik et al., 2011).

http://dx.doi.org/10.5772/60097

Examined Parameters	Before		After	
	A chronic atropine treatment			
	A	B	A	B
Volume of gastric juice (mL/h)	125±10	137±10	189±8	109±10
H^+ output (mEq/h)	0.25±0.08	0.4±0.1	0.49±0.08	0.68±0.09

Table 2. Changes in the gastric secretory responses before and after (3×0.3 mg orally given for 2–weeks) a chronic atropine treatment without and with histamine (A and B, respectively) (0.5 mg subcutaneously injected) administration in eight patients. The results were expressed as means ± SEM. *P*-values between the identical parameters before and after a chronic atropine treatment: $P < 0.05$. [Mózsik et al., 1965c; 1966b (with kind permission).]

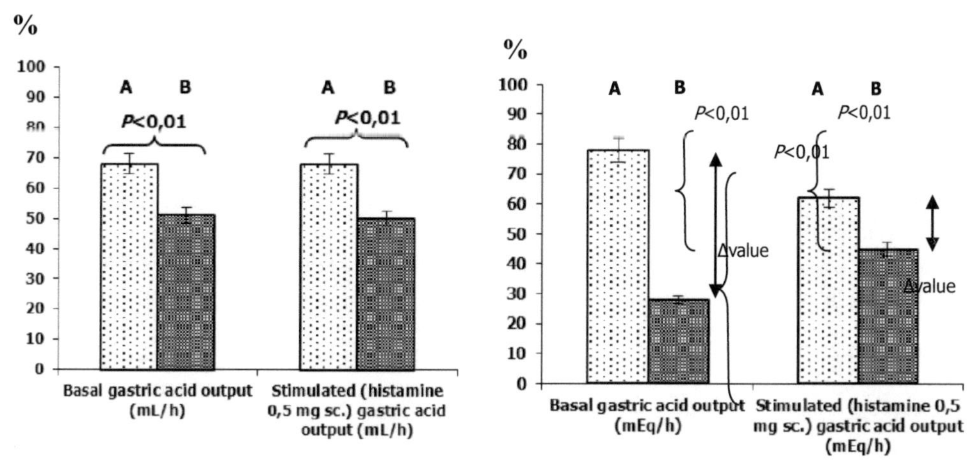

Figure 1. Decreased inhibitory effect of atropine (1 mg sc.) before (A) and after (B) chronic atropine treatment in patients with peptic ulcer disease ($n = 8$; means ± SEM).The results are expressed in percentage of their control. [Mózsik, Szabó, Czimmer: Curr. Pharm. Des. 17: 1556–1572, 2011 (with kind permission).]

2.3. Clinical Pharmacology of anticholinergic agents in patients with peptic ulcer disease (measurements of anticholinergic agents in the sera, urine in patients with duodenal ulcer)

It was hard to understand our previously demonstrated results obtained with application of atropine treatment in patients with duodenal ulcer because these results contradict the international experts' opinions. We assumed that:

1. The atropine will not absorb from the gastrointestinal tract owing to some reasons (e.g., some pharmaceutical industrial problem(s) appeared during the drug pharmaceutical production);
2. Even if the atropine absorbs well, some other unknown pharmacological event (such as tolerance) will appear during a chronic (classical) atropine treatment.

To evaluate these questions, we have to establish the real basis of clinical pharmacology. Therefore, we have to provide a good and scientific possibility to bring about different answers for our questions.

In the first step, the concentration of anticholinergic agents was measured by sera and urine bioassay (using isolated guinea-pig ileum for biological titration of parasympatholytic drugs in Magnus vessel) of patients. The absorption, metabolism and urinary excretion of parasympatholytics were studied after chronically applied parasympatholytic treatments (Győrffy et al., 1964; Jávor et al., 1965; 1967; Mozsik, 1969a; Mózsik et al., 1965 a, b; 1967d; Mozsik and Jávor, 1966 a, b, c; 1968a).

The atropine absorbed well from the gastrointestinal tract (during 4–5 hours), and it was proved by titration of atropine in the sera and urine of patients. These observations were carried out in the same patients when the same doses of atropine were given orally or subcutaneously injected. It was clear that the absorbed quantities of atropine were the same (given in the same doses), indicating that the oral/parenteral ration of atropine absorption is equal to 1.0. Furthermore, when we carried out these observations, we found the same results (with respect to the absorption and excretion of atropine) in the treated patients.

Since we had classical clinical pharmacological methods (e.g., detection of small doses of atropine in the serum and urine of treated patients), we were able to exclude any changes of absorption in gastrointestinal tract, metabolism and urinary excretion of atropine as a consequence of the effects of chronic atropine treatment (Mózsik et al., 1966 a, b, c; 1968; 1969 a, b, c, d, e, f; Mózsik, 1969a).

Later, we observed the development of tolerance along with the development of "pharmacological denervation supersensitivity" (e.g., the efficiencies of drugs used in the treatment of patients decreased significantly). These phenomena exist together (Mózsik et al., 1967a; Mózsik and Jávor, 1968 a, b) in the background of unchanged gastric acid secretion during a chronic atropine treatment in DU patients. It was also interesting to note the development of tolerance to atropine and the disappearance of pharmacological denervation phenomena in 6–10 days after cessation of atropine treatment (Mózsik et al., 1965b; Mózsik and Jávor, 1968b; 1969; Mózsik, 1969a). The development of tolerance to atropine does not represent a specific phenomenon related to atropine (during a chronic atropine treatment) because the development of tolerance was found with other parasympatholytics, which were not used in the medical treatment (Mózsik and Jávor, 1969).

The results of the clinical pharmacological studies proved the following main points:

1. No change was obtained in the gastric acid secretion during a chronic anticholinergic treatment;

2. The gastroduodenal ulceration healed during this time period;

3. The results of the clinical pharmacology could not provide an obvious explanation of how the gastroduodenal ulceration was healed without any changes in gastric secretory responses (Mózsik et al., 1965b; 1967a; Mózsik and Jávor, 1966b; 1968 a, b; 1969; Mózsik, 1969a).

http://dx.doi.org/10.5772/60097

This clinical pharmacological methodology was applied in the medical evaluation of different anticholinergic agents (drugs) before their clinical applications.

Recently, the pharmacological basic research offered a possibility to introduce new anticholinergic agents into the medical practice. The experts working in the field of experimental pharmacology showed that the actions of these anticholinergic agents can be enhanced on the autonomic nervous system by the changes in their chemical structures (perhaps by the production of quaternary ammonium compounds instead of only tertiary quaternary ammonium compounds) (Gyermek, 1951; 1953; Gyermek and Nádor, 1952; 1953 a, b; György et al., 1961).

The Gastropin® is one of the most representative quaternary ammonium compounds, which was introduced into the medical treatment in the 1960s. We were clearly able to prove that the Gastropin® does not absorb from the gastrointestinal tract. We were not able to detect any drug levels in the serum and urine of patients when the patients were orally given 1000 pills; however, these parameters were well detectable after it was injected in the same patients.

The established clinical pharmacological methods were widely used in the evaluation of different anticholinergic agents (Mózsik, 1969a).

Many clinical pharmacological studies (from human phase I to III) were carried out by our work team who were working on different drugs [(tertiary amine, oxyphen cylamine), muscarinic receptor blocking (gastrozepin), histamine$_2$ receptor blocking (first to fourth generation), proton pump inhibitors and other components] for patients with peptic ulcer (Mózsik et al., 1965b; Mózsik, 1969a; Jávor et al., 1967; Garamszegi et al., 1997; Nagy et al., 1997; Tárnok et al., 1979, 1997).

2.4. Comparative clinical pharmacology of anticholinergic drugs

Different clinical pharmacological studies were carried out in patients with peptic ulcer to compare the detectable concentrations in the sera, excretion in the urine and bile, inhibitory actions on the salivary secretion, gastric acid secretion, necessary dose rate to decrease glandular secretion and gastric motility, detectability of drug to proteins and the excretion time. The results are summarized in Table 3.

	Atropine	Novatropine	Isopropamide
Oral – parenteral dose rate	1 : 1	6-8 : 1	4-6 : 1
Detectable in serum	+	+	-
Detectable in urine	+	+	+
Detectable in saliva	-	-	+
Detectable in bile	-	-	+
Necessary dose rate to decreased glandular secretion and the gastric motility	1 : 2	1 : 2	1 : 2

	Atropine	Novatropine	Isopropamide
Ihibitory effect on salivary secretition	+	++	-
Inhibitory effect of gastric secretion	+	++	++
Inhibitory effect of gastric emtying in decreasing dose of glandular secretion	-	-	+
Duration of inhibitory effect on the salivary secretion	3-4 hours	6-8 hours	10-15 hours
Excretion in urine up	3-4 hours	6-8 hours	10-15 hours
detectable protein binding of the drug in serum			

Table 3. Comparative demonstration of the clinical pharmacological properties of parasympatholytics. [Mózsik, Vizi, Jávor, Recent Advances in Gastroenterology. The 3rd World Congress of Gastroenterology, Tokyo, 1967, 681–683 (with kind permission).]

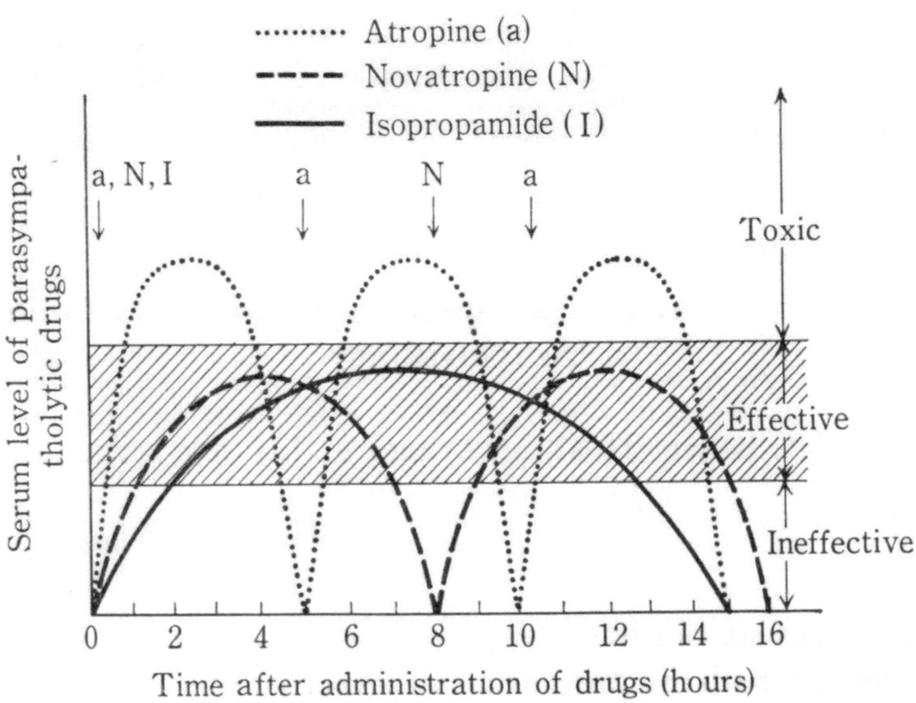

Figure 2. The schematic presentation of the measured serum levels of different parasympatholytic drugs in peptic ulcer patients. The ordinate shows the level of parasympatholytic drugs (toxic, effective and ineffective); the abscisse demonstrates the time after administration of these drugs. a: atropine; N: Novatropine; I: isopropamide. [Mózsik, Vizi, Jávor: Recent Advances in Gastroenterology. The 3rd World Congress of Gastroenterology, Tokyo, 1967, 681–683 (with kind permission).]

http://dx.doi.org/10.5772/60097

2.5. Clinical evidence of the existence of gastrointestinal protection differs from the decrease of gastric acid secretion (Gastric cytoprotection)

The results of our observation of chronic atropine treatment in DU patients were given in detail previously.

In 1978, we found that the GI anti-ulcer effects of atropine, cimetidine and carbenoxolone were superior to placebo in a multiclinical, randomized, prospective and comparative study in DU patients. However, no significant difference was obtained in the beneficial effects of atropine versus cimetidine versus carbenoxolone (Tárnok et al., 1979). Since carbenoxolone has no inhibitory action on the gastric acid secretion in DU patients, the ulcer-healing effects (due to stimulation of mucus) could be considered independent of any effects on gastric acid secretion.

Thus, these clinical observations during 1960–1970 were performed before the classical concept of "gastric cytoprotection" was formulated and published by André Robert (Robert et al., 1979).

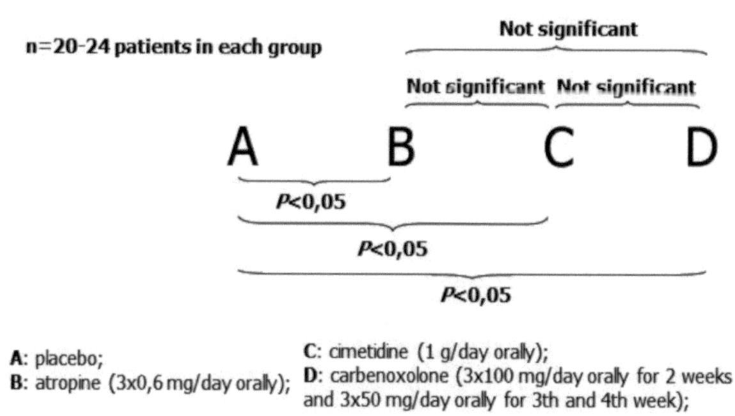

Figure 3. A prospective multiclinical study comparing the effects of placebo, carbenoxolone, atropine and cimetidine in patients with duodenal ulcer (4 weeks' study). [Tárnok et al., Drugs Exp. Clin. Res. 5: 157–166, 1979 and Mózsik, Szabó, Czimmer, Curr. Pharm. Des. 17: 1556–1572, 2011 (with kind permission).]

Our clinical pharmacological studies (1965) (Mózsik et al., 1965b; 1967 a, b, c, d; Mózsik and Jávor, 1968 a, b; Mózsik, 1969a; Tárnok et al., 1979) as well as randomized, prospective, multiclinical and comparative studies (1978) are clear even now in retrospect that we had been observing acid-independent gastroduodenal protection with atropine and other drugs before André Robert had defined the existence of "gastric cytoprotection" (Mózsik, 2010; Mózsik et al., 2011).

During 1965–1970, the existence of "gastric cytoprotection" was not reported; conversely, the clinical importance of gastric acid secretion had only been emphasized. Chaudhury and Jacobson (1978) were the first to indicate that the gastric mucosal damage could be prevented without inhibition of gastric secretion.

The existence of "gastric cytoprotection" has been widely accepted after the work of Robert et al. (1979) in animal experiments. The clinical applicability of gastric cytoprotection was later

accepted for patients with gastroduodenal ulcer (with the exception of our previously carried out observations in DU patients).

2.6. Randomized, multiclinical, prospective and multicentric study of treatment of chronic gastric ulcer patients with vitamin A

Later, we demonstrated in multiclinical, multicentric, prospective and randomized study the ulcer-healing effect of vitamin A (as scavenger component) in patients with gastric ulcer (Patty et al., 1982; 1983). However, no gastric acid inhibitory action of the vitamin A exists in humans (Jávor et al., 1983 a, b; Mózsik et al., 1986; 2001; 2005; 2007; Rumi et al., 2001 a, b).

EVALUATION OF THE DIFFERENT TREAT-
MENTS IN PATIENTS WITH GASTRIC ULCERS

1. ENDOSCOPIC MEASUREMENTS
   1.1 PLANIMETRIC MEASUREMENTS
   1.2 ENDOSCOPIC EVALUATION OF ULCER STATE
2. CLINICAL CONTROLS
   2.1 CHANGES IN COMPLAINTS OF PATIENTS
   2.2 CONSUMPTION OF ANTACIDS
3. LABORATORY CONTROLS
   3.1 BLOOD PICTURE
   3.2 URINE
   3.3 RENAL AND LIVER FUNCTIONS
   3.4 ELECTROLYTES
   3.5 pH-STATE

Figure 4. Evaluation of the different treatments of efficiency of vitamin A in patients with chronic gastric ulcer (4 weeks of study). The endoscopic and laboratory parameters were carried out at the beginning and during 2 and 4 weeks after the beginning of the treatment; meanwhile, the changes of complaints and consumption of antacids in patients were registered every day and these values were summarized with the similar points in this clinical study. [Patty et al., Lancet II, 872, 1982; Int. J. Tiss. React. 5: 301–307, 1983 (with kind permission).]

Fifty-six patients with chronic gastric ulcer were examined for this multiclinical, multicentric, randomized and prospective study (Patty et al., 1982; 1983).

The patients were divided into three groups: group A (16 patients) received only antacids; group B (18 patients) were treated with antacids plus vitamin A (3 × 50,000 IU orally) and group C (22 patients) received antacids, vitamin A (3 × 50,000 IU orally) and cyproheptadine (Peritol®).The observations were carried out in 4 weeks' time.

Endoscopic measurements, and clinical and laboratory parameters were carried out at the beginning and at the end (2nd and 4th week) of the treatment of these patients (Figure 4).

The parameters in Figure 4 help us to evaluate the different objective (planimetric measurement of ulcer sizes, presence or absence of gastric ulcer – at the beginning and end of different treatments – and states of ulcer) and subjective (changes in complaints of patients and

http://dx.doi.org/10.5772/60097

consumption of antacids) events of the process of ulcer healing (including the possible roles of drug actions). The obtained results are summarized in Figures 5–8.

The dynamism of the ulcer healing can be scientifically studied by the changes of ulcer sizes at 2 and 4 weeks after beginning the treatment (Figure 8). It was surprising to note that the healing rate differed significantly at 2 weeks; however, this value was the same at 4 weeks.

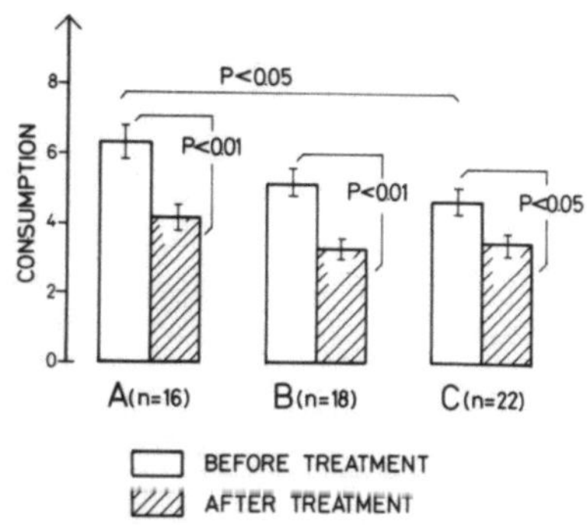

Figure 5. Changes in the antacid consumption in the different groups of patients with chronic gastric ulcer. [Patty et al., Lancet II, 872, 1982; Int. J. Tiss. React. 5: 301–307, 1983 (with kind permission).]

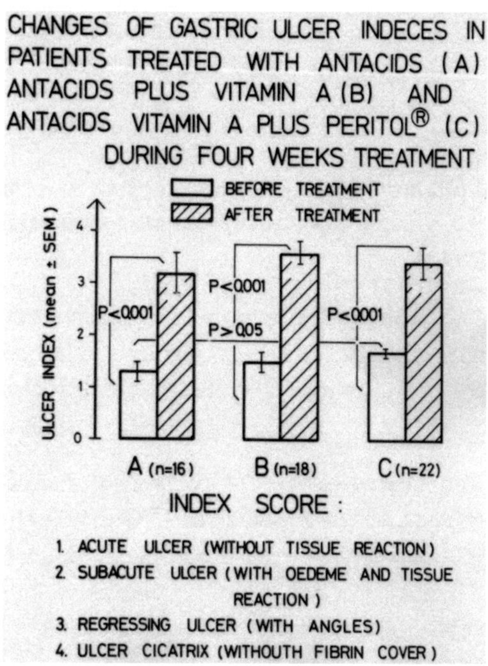

Figure 6. Changes of gastric ulcer indices in patients treated with antacids (A); antacids plus vitamin A (B) and antacids, vitamin A and Peritol® (C) during 4 weeks of treatment. [Patty et al., Lancet II, 872, 1982; Patty et al., Int. J. Tiss. React. 5: 301–307, 1983 (with kind permission).]

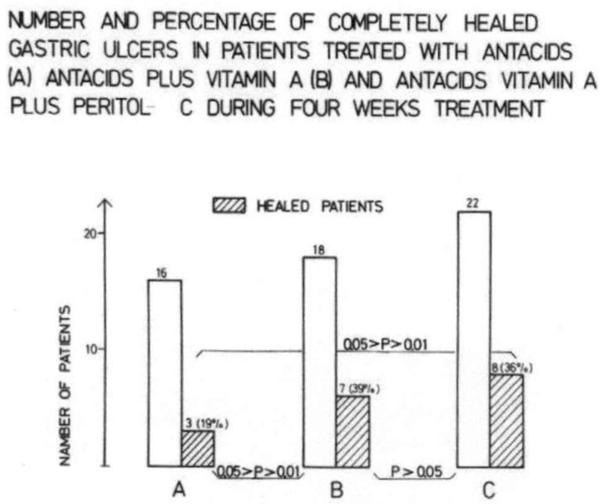

(A)

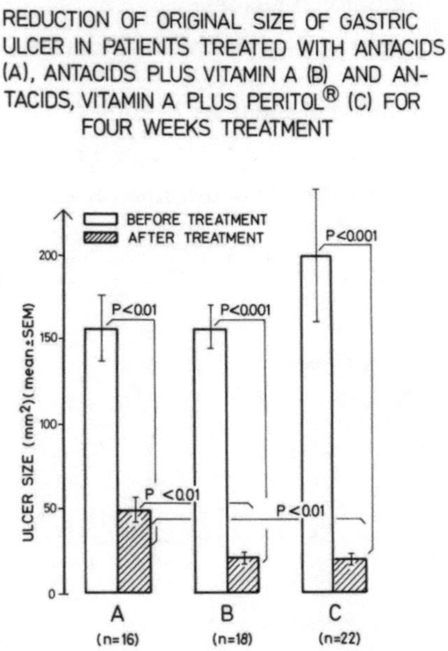

(B)

Figure 7. A. Changes in number (and percentage) of completely healed gastric ulcers in patients treated with antacids (A); antacid plus vitamin A (B) and antacid, vitamin A and Peritol® (C) during 4 weeks of treatment (with kind permission). B. Reduction of original planimetric size of gastric ulcers in patients treated with antacids (A); antacids plus vitamin A (B) and antacids, vitamin A plus Peritol® (C) before and after 4 weeks of treatment. [Patty et al., Lancet II, 872, 1982; Patty et al., Int. J. Tiss. React. 5: 301–307, 1983 (with kind permission).]

2.7. Comparative clinical pharmacology of "cytoprotective" and "anti-secretory" drugs (multiclinical, randomized, prospective and multicentric studies) in patients with chronic gastric and duodenal ulcers

Our work team participated in the clinical pharmacological studies of peptic ulcer patients (including different international studies as well as ours). After our previously performed studies, our attention focused on the results of clinical pharmacological studies with "cytoprotective" and "anti-secretory" drugs in patients with chronic gastric and duodenal ulcers.

In this subchapter, we summarized the results of clinical pharmacological studies of 441 chronic gastric and duodenal ulcers. The patients treated with nonsteroidal, anti-inflammatory drugs, steroids, antihypertensive drugs (e.g., Reserpine) and those who underwent some stress, burns or trauma were excluded from this comparative study. These patients were divided into different groups and were treated with different drugs: placebo (calcium carbonicum, magnesium trisilicate and sodium bicarbonate in equal portion), atropine (1.0 mg/os), cimetidine (1000 mg/day orally), ranitidine (300 mg/day orally), famotidine (80 mg/day orally), pirenzepine (150 mg/day orally), sucralfate (1000 mg/day orally), vitamin A (3 × 50,000 IU/day orally) alone or in combination with cyproheptadinum chloratum (3 × 4 mg/

http://dx.doi.org/10.5772/60097

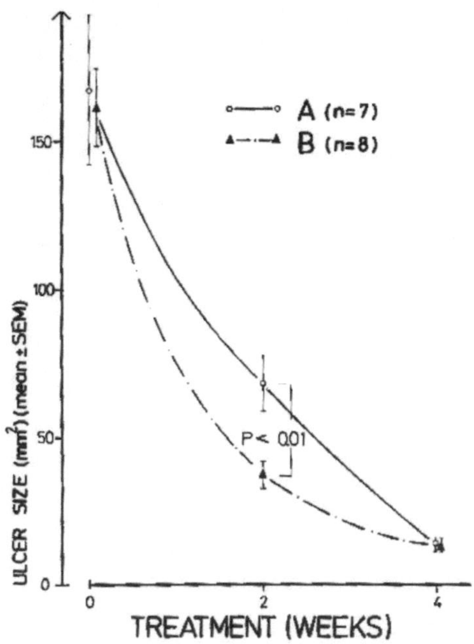

Figure 8. Dynamism of ulcer-healing effect of vitamin A in patients with chronic gastric ulcer, indicating the changes of ulcer size in unhealed patients (in 4 weeks of treatment). [Patty et al., Lancet II, 872, 1982; Patty et al., Int. J. Tiss. React. 5: 301–307, 1983 (with kind permission).]

day orally), DE-NOL (3 × 5 mL/day orally) and Tisacid® (Al–Mg–antacidum 3 × 1 g/day orally). The antacids in composition mentioned above were applied with the so-called active compounds. Twenty patients were allocated into each group. The treatments were carried out for 4 or 6 weeks. (These results are reused with the permission of Wiley publisher.)

Endoscopy (estimation of ulcer size), laboratory measurements (blood count, urine, kidney and liver functions), pH status, medical examinations, summed pain score (expressed in percentage of original values) and antacid consumption were evaluated at the beginning, during 2nd, 4th and 6th week (if the treatment extends) and after the treatment.

The aims of this study are as follows:

1. To compare the efficiencies of ulcer treatments by cytoprotective (Tisacid®, sucralfate, DE-NOL and vitamin A) and anti-secretory (atropine, pirenzepine, cimetidine, ranitidine, famotidine) drugs in a short-term study (4–6 weeks);

2. To evaluate the dynamism of ulcer healing in unhealed gastric and duodenal patients;

3. To evaluate the summed pain score and antacid consumption in GU and DU patients;

4. To compare the different results (ulcer healing, laboratory parameters, summed pain score and antacids) obtained in healed and unhealed GU and DU patients.

Treatment	Number of Patients	Number of Unhealed Patients (%)	P-value
Antacid	40	30(75)	-
Al-Mg-hydroxy- Carbonate (Tisacid®)	15	10(66.7)	NS
Vitamin A	18	11(61.1)	<0.05
Vitamin A and cyproheptadine	22	14(63.9)	<0.05
DE-NOL	16	5 (31.2)	<0.01
Sucralfate	19	14(73.7)	NS
Gastrozepine	16	9 (56.2)	< 0.0.5
Cimetidine	30	8 (26.7)	< 0.01

Table 4. Changes in the incidence of gastric ulcer (GU) healing during 4 weeks of treatment with different groups of patients compared with antacid. The numbers in parentheses are calculated in percentage. NS: not significant [Mózsik et al., J. Gastroenterol. Hepatol 9: S88–S92, 1994 (with kind permission).]

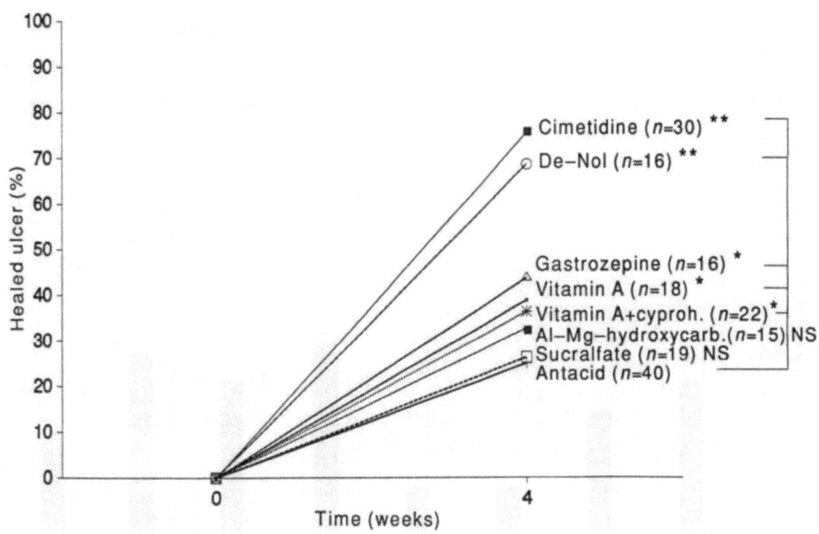

Figure 9. Changes in ulcer-healing rate during the different therapies in patients with chronic gastric ulcer (4 weeks). The results are expressed as means; *n* indicates the number of patients. *P*-values between the groups treated with antacids (placebo) and different groups. +: $P < 00.5$; ++: $P < 00.1$; NS: not significant. [Mózsik et al., J. Gastroenterol. Hepatol 9: S88–S92, 1994 (with kind permission).]

http://dx.doi.org/10.5772/60097

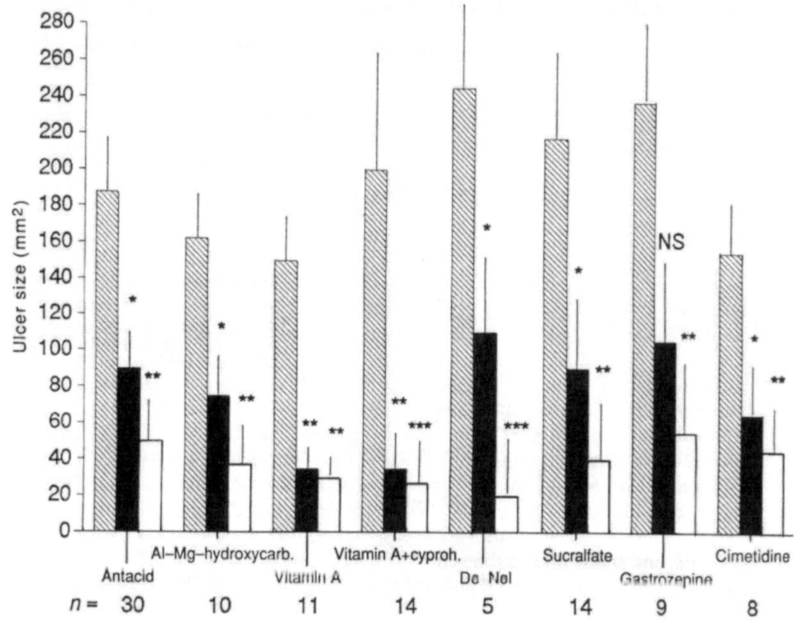

Figure 10. Changes in the ulcer size of patients with incompletely healed gastric ulcer during 4 weeks of treatment. The ulcer size was perceived at the beginning (first bar), 2 weeks (middle bar) and 4 weeks (right bar) of the treatment (*n*, the number of incompletely healed patients). *P*-values are based on the ulcer size at the beginning and at 2 and 4 weeks; *: $P < 0.0.5$; **: $P < 0.01$; ***: $P < 0.00.1$; NS: not significant. [Mózsik et al., J. Gastroenterol. Hepatol 9: S88–S92, 1994 (with kind permission).]

Treatment	Number of Patients	Unhealed Patients (%)	P values
Antacid	22	14 (63.6)	
Al-Mghydroxy- carbonate (Tisacid®)	39	13 (33.3)	< 0.0.5
Atropine and Cyproheptadine	22	5 (22.7)	< 0.0.1
Atropine and Cimetidine	25	9 (36)	< 0.0.5
Cimetidine	25	9 (36)	< 0.0.5
Ranitidine	25	9 (36)	< 0.0.5
Famotidine	33	9 (27.3)	< 0.0.1
Carbenoxolone	19	8 (42.1)	< 0.0.5
Sucralfate	31	15 (45.4)	< 0.0.5
Gastroozepine	24	10 (41.7)	< 0.0.5

Table 5. Changes in the incidence of duodenal ulcer healing during 4 weeks of treatment in different groups of patients compared with antacid. The numbers in parentheses are calculated in percentage. [Mózsik et al., J. Gastroenterol. Hepatol 9: S88–S92, 1994 (with kind permission).]

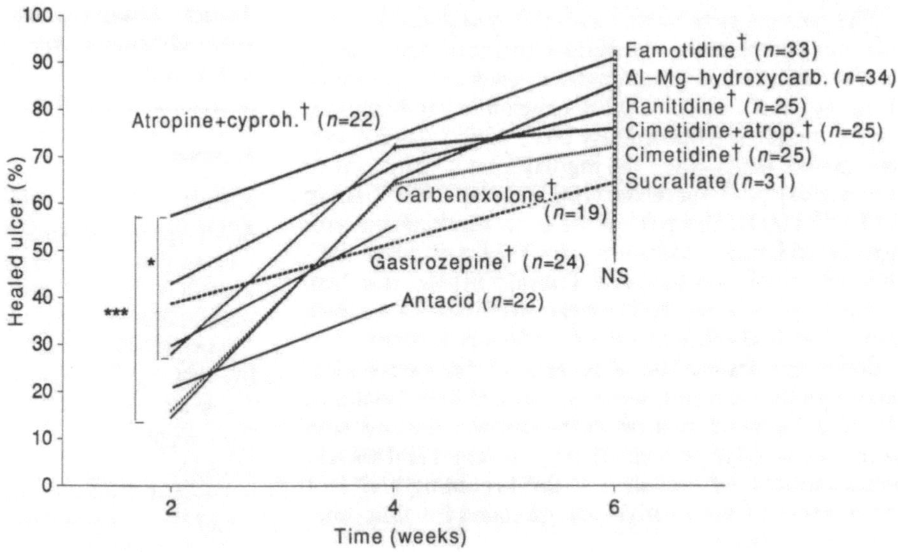

Figure 11. Changes in ulcer-healing rate in chronic duodenal ulcer patients treated with different drugs. *P*-values are between antacid (placebo) and treated groups at 4 and 6 weeks. *: $P < 0.05$; ***: $P < 0.001$; NS: not significant. [Mózsik et al., J. Gastroenterol. Hepatol 9: S88–S92, 1994 (with kind permission).]

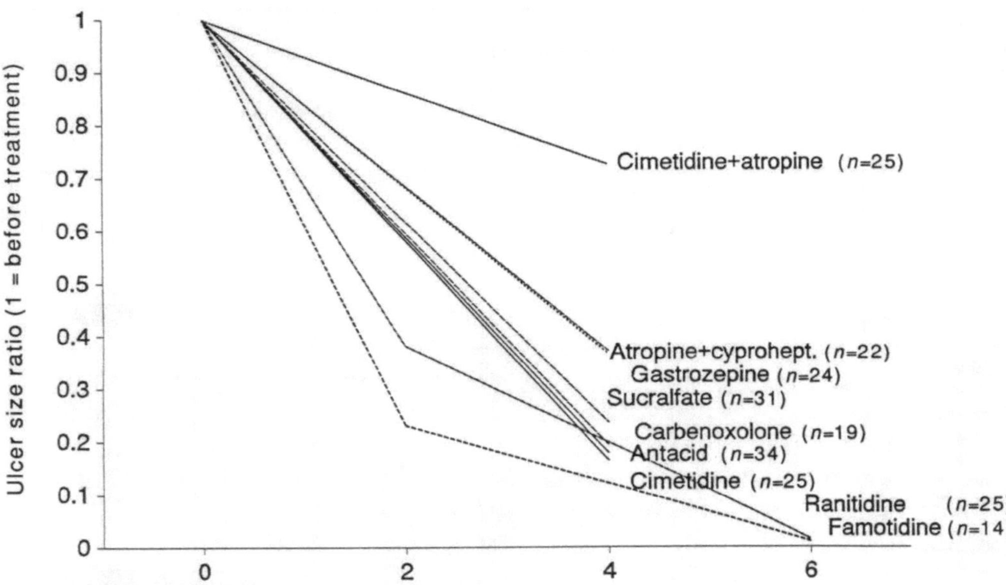

Figure 12. Changes in ulcer size in patients with incompletely healed duodenal ulcer after 4 weeks of treatment. Ulcer size before treatment = 1. [Mózsik et al., J. Gastroenterol. Hepatol 9: S88–S92, 1994 (with kind permission).]

http://dx.doi.org/10.5772/60097

2.8. General conclusion(s) of clinical pharmacological studies in patients with peptic ulcer

Returning the results of our earlier clinical pharmacological studies in patients with duodenal ulcer (see before), our final conclusion was that we have no any correct knowledge on the principle biochemical cellular and extracellular changes (mechanisms) are present in the keeping the normal homeostasis of the GI mucosa, and in time of development of GI mucosal damage and protection neither in animal experiments nor in humans (patients).

In addition to these, the discovery of "gastric cytoprotection" represented a new challenge to us in answer to the scientific problem mentioned above.

The results of these observations helped us to start a new scale of examinations in the field of peptic ulcer disease. We wanted to start with biochemical examinations in this field, but, unfortunately, nobody worked on it. Consequently, we have to learn the principal points of the general biochemical research to introduce it into the field of peptic ulcer research.

We have to emphasize that scientific problems and their knowledge have been changing over the past few decades, and many new scientific results are published.

Four well-known scientists were awarded the Nobel Prize [Jens Christian Skou (Department of Physiology, Aarhus University, Denmark) in chemistry, 1997; Earl W. Sutherland (Department of Physiology, Vanderbilt University, Nashville, TN, USA) in physiology (medicine), 1971; and Barry James Marshall and J. Robin Warren (Royal Perth Hospital, Australia) in physiology (medicine), 2005]. Their results inspired es to ttudy these fields in our peptic ulcer research in animals and humans.

Author details

Gyula Mozsik[1*] and Imre Szabó[2]

*Address all correspondence to: gyula.mozsik@aok.pte.hu

1 First Department of Medicine, Medical and Health Centre, University of Pécs, Hungary

2 Associate Professor at the First Department of Medicine, University of Pécs, Hungary

Chapter 3

Theoretical Backgrounds of the Necessarity for the Changes of Paradigm in Our Ulcer Research

Gyula Mozsik and Imre Szabó

Additional information is available at the end of the chapter

http://dx.doi.org/10.5772/60098

After the active participation in the human clinical pharmacology of patients with peptic ulcer, we were not able to understand how the ulcer actually heals in the patients. Our problems pointed out the following results:

1. The gastric acid secretion [as basal secretion and stimulated secretion produced (provoked) by superluminal – but submaximal – dose of histamine] was unchanged during the medical treatment; however, the ulcer healed. We were not able to explain these contradictory results;

2. The results of clinical pharmacological studies (wide scale of anticholinergic agents) gave us a lot of new insight from the clinical pharmacological parameters (e.g., their absorption, metabolism, excretion) of clinically used drugs. We learned well that different therapeutically applied drugs a priori (e.g., Troparin, Gastropin®) will not absorb from the GI tract during the treatment; consequently, we were not able to find the beneficial effects of these drugs during the medical treatment;

3. The development of tolerance to atropine together with development of "pharmacological denervation phenomenon" has been proven in the background of unchanged gastric acid secretion in patients with duodenal ulcer, during a chronic atropine treatment (see chapter 2.2.). This newer clinical pharmacological explanation has been applied for "existence of gastric cytoprotection." It is true that this phenomenon was observed in patients with duodenal ulcer in terms of the existence of "cytoprotection phenomenon" (not in animal experiments but in patients with duodenal ulcer);

4. When the existence of gastric mucosal protective effect was proved in animal experiments (Jávor et al., 1983), it was clear that vitamin A does not inhibit the gastric acid secretion.

Similar results were obtained in patients with vitamin A, for example, it does not inhibit the gastric basal acid (BAO) and maximal (MAO) acid outputs in healthy subjects (Morón et al.,

1984); however, it prevented the indomethacin-induced gastric mucosal damage in healthy human subjects (Mózsik et al., 1986).

The results of our randomized, prospective, multiclinical and multicentered studies in patients with chronic gastric ulcer clearly proved that the chronic gastric ulcer really heals without any decrease of gastric acid secretion (Patty et al., 1982; 1983). In other words, we also proved the existence of gastric "cytoprotection" in patients with chronic gastric ulcer.

The vitamin A is a typical scavenger and nutritional molecule, and we used the name of "nutritional gastrointestinal cytoprotection" for animals, healthy human subjects and in patients with different gastrointestinal disorders (Mózsik et al., 2013). These results are absolutely offered to exclude the privileged role of gastric acid secretion in the development of peptic ulcer disease in patients with gastric and duodenal ulcers;

5. To give a correct explanation for the together and simultaneously presence of ulcer with hyperacidity. It was clear at that time that the gastric acid secretion is a result of the very active metabolism; meanwhile, the development of ulcer was suggested as a consequence of impaired metabolism in the gastrointestinal mucosa. It was absolutely an unexplainable fact that both the gastric acid secretion (as an increased metabolic process) and the gastric ulcer (as a consequence of the impaired tissue metabolism) occur together and at the same time in the same organ;

6. In these years, we applied only anticholinergic drugs (together antacids) in the everyday medical treatment. If we suggest that these drugs are able to decrease the gastric acid secretion and if we apply the anticholinergic agent in the medical treatment, we can find a decrease in the metabolic process in the fundus of stomach. If we accept the presence of these decreased metabolic processes in the gastrointestinal tract, we can explain the healing process of ulcerated tissue and that really no hypoxemic presence exists in the ulcerated tissues around the gastric or duodenal ulcer in patients. If the last suggestion is true, than we contradict the generally suggested etiological theories published by the international experts;

7. We had no concrete information (knowledge) on the metabolism of gastrointestinal mucosa produced therapeutically (especially we had no information in this regard to humans).

We discussed very deeply our clinical pharmacological results obtained in patients with classical peptic ulcer disease. Our conclusion is that we do something (treatment) in the medical treatment; however, we have no concrete knowledge on the presence of the different biological events existing in the gastrointestinal tract.

We have to emphasize that we are in the second part of the 1960s–1970s. We had no knowledge of histamine-2 receptor antagonists, gastrin antagonist and, of course, proton pump inhibitors. The established clinical pharmacology helps us to select different compounds (from the medical practices), which were failures both clinically and pharmacologically (e.g., these agents are not absorbed from the gastrointestinal tract). These results offered clear pharmacological evidence to explain that the tertiary ammonium compounds absorb well from the

http://dx.doi.org/10.5772/60098

human GI tract, meanwhile the absorptions of the quaternary ammonium compounds failed. The aims of pharmacologists were the production of new quaternary ammonium compounds:

1. To produce new compounds with longer and stronger inhibitory actions on the gastric acid secretion in comparison to actions of tertiary ammonium compounds (and these were proved clearly in animal experiments);

2. The tertiary ammonium compounds are able to enter into the circulation of brain (going through the hemato-encephalic barrier), with the quaternary ammonium compounds not entering into thain circulation (through hemato-encephalic barrier).

The results of the established clinical pharmacology clearly indicated that the results of animal experiments can be accepted only with a significant criticism in the application of medical practice. It was also indicated clearly that the existence of clinical pharmacology is absolutely necessary in the pathways of new drug productions versus their clinical applications. The clinical pharmacology was established by us (Jávor et. al., 1965; Mózsik et al., 1965 a, b;,1967 a, b;,1969a;,Mózsik and Jávor, 1965 a, b;,1966 a, b, c;,1968 a, b; Mózsik, 1969a; Jávor, 1968) at Debrecen, Hungary (iuring tie period of 1—197 year.

Of course, there was a heated debate between the basic researchers and clinical pharmacologists, and the clinical pharmacologists prevailed over the basic researchers.

The classical pharmacology has been studied at our Department of Medicine of Universities (in Debrecen and Pécs, Hungary) up to now (2014) (Hunyady, 1997; Garamszegi et al., 1997; Mózsik et al., 1984d; Mózsik et al., 1985; 1986; 1997a; 1979c; 1981g; 1985; 1992e; Nagy et al., 1997; Patty et al., 1982; 1983; 1987; Tárnok et al., 1979; 1997).

Independently from the establishment of clinical pharmacology in patients with peptic ulcer, we wanted to know more and more on the nature of peptic ulcer disease. We tried to investigate and to know the most important possibilities of ulcer research:

1. The possibilities to approaches of neural effects in human patients with peptic ulcer were very complicated and their methodologies of clinicians were very limited. The increased activity of vagus nerve has been emphasized in the development of peptic ulcer disease. Clinically, our therapeutic possibility was only to apply the anticholinergic agents, which was the reason for starting with the clinical pharmacological evaluation of atropine treatment in patients with peptic ulcer;

2. The surgical intervention, as medical treatment, was frequently used in the 1970s. If the indication of surgery was based on the common consultations between the internists (later gastroenterologists) and surgeons (later gastrointestinal surgeons), then the "medical treatment" (generally for 4 weeks) was carried out as a primary therapeutic possibility, and this treatment was accepted as failed therapeutic process (the clinical pharmacology significantly decreased the number of patients with peptic ulcer disease who had to go over the surgical intervention).

The surgical tradition of Hungarian surgeons was based on the classical German surgical schools, and Billroth II surgical method was generally accepted by them. Only in the 1980s

surgical vagotomy appeared in the practice of Hungarian surgeons (Ihász, 1980). Consequently, we had no possibility to study and to follow these patients;

3. The possibility of the new therapeutic compounds was zero to clinicians;

4. There was little experimental ulcer research conducted in that time all over the world. Furthermore, experimental ulcer research was not effective in Hungary (these types of observations were done at First Department of Medicine, University of Szeged, Hungary, and were followed at Second Department of Medicine, University of Debrecen, Hungary, up to 1968 and thereafter at First Department of Medicine, University of Pécs, Hungary).

After a critical evaluation of our results obtained from our clinical pharmacology, we started in an absolutely onsure direction, namely the establishment of the biochemical approaches to gastrointestinal mucosa in the field of peptic ulcer research. (One of the authors, GyM, was the esy person.). Ths established biochemical research line was the first trend in peptic ulcer research inalover the World. We have to tethat the applicatin of biochemistry in the ulcer research wasgave a hard scientillaenginge to us (becauseno simends were existed in the Worwhere).

Of course, we tried to do some animal experiments (observations) to receive some practice in this field. Besides, we have to emphasize clearly that we wanted to study the different biochemical mechanisms in the gastrointestinal tract (obtained from the preparations at surgical intervention of patients with peptic ulcer).

Our principal aims were to obtain and to understand the reasons behind biochemical events in the gastrointestinal tract (during the ulcer development and at the time of gastric surgical interventions).

Author details

Gyula Mozsik[1*] and Imre Szabó[2]

*Address all correspondence to: gyula.mozsik@aok.pte.hu

1 First Department of Medicine, Medical and Health Centre, University of Pécs, Hungary

2 Associate Professor at the First Department of Medicine, University of Pécs, Hungary

http://dx.doi.org/10.5772/60098

Chapter 4

General Biochemical Methods to be Used in Gastrointestinal Mucosa in Animal Experiments and in Human Observations Done on Gastrointestinal Resecates (after Surgical Interventions)

Gyula Mozsik and Imre Szabó

Additional information is available at the end of the chapter

http://dx.doi.org/10.5772/60099

4.1. Introduction

General aims of these observations were to biochemically examine all the gastrointestinal tissues in both animals and humans. The outstanding point was that from 1965 to date, we have been unable to know the exact details of different regulatory mechanisms (by neural, hormonal, pharmacological, immunological and nutritional pathways) under normal (non-ulcerated) and damaged conditions. When we undertook clinical pharmacological studies, we had to face different hard-to-understand medical facts:

1. We had no scientific knowledge on the possible correlation between drug actions and biochemisms in the GI mucosa of animals and humans;
2. We only had different suggestions for the development of hypoxia-induced mucosal damage in the GI mucosa at the time of ulcer development; however, we had no evidence for the existence of this situation;
3. The regulatory mechanisms at the levels of out of gastrointestinal tract and of only in the gastrointestinal tract are absolutely indicated a gap between them;
4. Though the classical, histological definition of peptic ulcer is unchanged, many contradictory "actual discoveries" (new hormones, new growth factors, many chemical compounds, new trends in the medical and surgical treatments, *Helicobacter pylori*, etc.) appeared in the etiology of ulcer disease;
5. Our principal scientific question was in the period 1965–1970: How was the peptic ulcer healed in the human gastrointestinal tract without any decrease of gastric acid secretion?

> We suggested an answer to this question by applying different and precise biochemical methods in the study of human gastrointestinal tract (with and without the presence of the classical ulcer). Unfortunately, we had no methodology to answer this question.

These observations maintained the main trends of clinical pharmacology (e.g., time period with drugs, to keep the time period after cessation of treatment); however, we introduced the biochemical methodology to the pharmacology.

We tried to approach the biochemical events in the whole tissue by simultaneously using more parallel biochemical measurements (using the same tissue samples, with the measurements carried out at the same time).

Before the human biochemical examinations, we learned the biochemical methodology in animal experiments.

4.2. Methodologies of experimental models and clinical studies

The observations were carried out in CFY (Sprague-Dawley) (Gödöllő, Hungary) strain rats, weighing 180–210 g, and on the resecates of stomach and small intestine of patients who underwent gastric surgery because of unhealed ulcer disease (during 1970–1980).

The patients suffered from classical peptic ulcer diseases (PUD) with clinical symptoms (decreased appetite, feeling of dullness and pain in the epigastric region of the abdomen, pyrosis, impaired gastric emptying and retention syndrome). These patients presented one month before the surgical intervention. The presence of gastroduodenal ulcers was endoscopically diagnosed, and thereafter these patients received medical treatments (anticholinergic agents, late H_2 receptor antagonist and antacids for one month). A possibility of surgical interventions was evaluated for those patients who were not healed after the treatment.

The indication of gastric surgery was done by physicians [consultations between internists (gastroenterologists) and surgeons] independently from us]. The resecates of stomach and small intestine (according to the method of Billroth II). A small group of patients underwent classical partial gastrectomy (according to the method of Billroth II), and jejunal ulcer was developed. These patients were also medically (pharmacologically) treated during 1970–1980.

During surgical intervention, the stomach and small intestine were removed immediately and these were cut into two parts. One part was given for histological evaluation of resected tissues and the other part was immersed (after separation of mucosa and muscular layer) in liquid nitrogen and used for biochemical examinations. The mucosa specimens were also separated from each other (depending on the distance of ulcer edge). Both the biochemical measurements from the mucosa specimens and muscular layers (independently from the number of tissue specimens), obtained from one patient, and the surgical intervention were carried out at the same time.

The animal observations were carried out in both sexes of CFY-strain rats.

The following experimental models were used:

http://dx.doi.org/10.5772/60099

1. Pylorus ligation was carried out according to the method of Shay et al., (1945) (using different experimental time periods after pyloric ligation: 1, 4, 7, 24 hours);
2. Pylorus ligation plus surgical vagotomy (using different experimental time periods after surgical intervention);
3. Gastric mucosal damage was caused by aspirin given intragastrically according to the method of Guth et al., (1979);
4. Gastric mucosal preventive actions of atropine, vitamin A and β-carotene in 4-hour pylorus-ligated, aspirin-treated rats;
5. Indomethacin model (4 hours);
6. Gastric mucosal preventive effects of atropine, cimetidine, vitamin A and β-carotene in 4-hour indomethacin-treated rats;
7. Stress ulcer in rats was caused by 4 hours of immobilization (Nagy et al., 1982; 1983);
8. The stress ulcer in rats was caused due to 5 hours of swimming. In some animals, the stress ulcer provocation (swimming) was combined with pyloric ligation during the beginning of stress (Nagy et al., 1982; 1983);
9. Reserpine was subcutaneously injected in animals (Mózsik et al., 1983a);
10. Gastric fundic mucosal damage was caused by topical application of 1 mL from 25 v/v 0.2 M NaOH, 0.6 M HCl and 96 v/v ethanol (Robert et al., 1979);
11. Epinephrine model was completed according to Sethbakdi et al., (1970 a, b, and Pfeiffer, 1971; Pfeiffer and Sethbakdi, 1971). The epinephrine (Tonogén, Budapest) was injected in different doses at different times after pyloric ligation;
12. All biochemical examinations were carried out in the control (non-ulcerated) in the ulcerated (mucosa up to 2 cm around the ulcer) antral, duodenal, jejunal mucosa or from the corpus (fundic), antral, duodenal and jejunal mucosa and from the tissues located below the mucosa (muscular layer). All patients with jejunal ulcers previously underwent a gastric partial resection because of duodenal ulcer. No direct provocative agents such as drugs or primary diseases (renal, endocrine, hematological, liver, pulmonary diseases) could be detected in the background of peptic ulceration ("genuine ulcer"). The tissue specimens were obtained during the surgery.

The following measurements were carried out in different observations:

1. Determination of gastric acid output. The gastric basal acid output (BAO) and maximal acid output (MAO) were determined in patients;
2. The extent of experimental gastric ulcer (except in Shay rats) was scored in the following way: score 0: no ulceration; score 1: the erosions were less than 1 mm; score 2: the erosions were between 2 and 4 mm; score 4: the erosions were greater than 4 mm; and score 5: represents the mucosal damage in all part of fundus. The values of scores were summarized for every stomach, and the average ± SEM was given (Mózsik et al., 1983 a, b);

3. The number of ulcers was calculated;

4. The tissue levels of adenosine triphosphate (ATP), adenosine diphosphate (ADP) and adenosine monophosphate (AMP) were measured enzymatically (Boehringer, Ingelheim; Germany);

5. The tissue level of cyclic 3′,5′-adenosine monophosphate (cAMP) was measured by RIA (Beckton Dikinson, Orengeburg; USA) (Mózsik et al., 1970 a, b);

6. The tissue level of lactate was enzymatically measured (Ingelheim, Boehringer; Germany);

7. The separation and measurements of ribonucleic acid (RNA) and deoxyribonucleic acid (DNA) were completed according to the methods published earlier (Mózsik et al., 1967 b, c; 1969 c; 1976 a, b, c, d; 1978 a, b; 1979 a, b, c, d, e; Mózsik and Vizi, 1976 a, b);

8. The separation of membrane ATPase was carried out by the treatment with NaJ and differential centrifugation (Mózsik and Øye, 1969; Mózsik et al., 1974 a, b, c, d; 1979 a, b, c, d, g, e; Schmidt and Tannhauser, 1945);

9. The ATPase activity was measured *in vitro* system by liberation of inorganic phosphorus, followed by the ATP transformation into ADP in the presence of Mg^{2+} (Mg dependent) and Mg^{2+}, Na^{+} and K^{+} (total) or Mg^{2+}-, Na^{+}-, K^{+}-dependent ATPase. The Na^{+}- and K^{+}-dependent ATPase were calculated by the difference between the ATPase activities obtained in the presence of Mg^{2+}, Na^{+} and K^{+} and Mg^{2+} (Mg^{2+}-dependent part) (Mózsik and Øye, 1969; Mózsik, 1969 a, b; Mózsik et al., 1974 a, b, c, d);

10. The tissue levels of ATP, ADP, AMP, cAMP and lactate were calculated in accordance with 1.0 mg protein, as per the method of Lowry et al. (1951), or with 1.0 mg DNA (in human observations).

The enzyme activity was expressed as micromoles of Pi/mg membrane protein/hour. The results were given as means ± SEM (Mozsik and Øye, 1969; Mózsik, 1969 a, b).The Student "t" test was used for the statistical analysis of the parametric results and by Mann and Whitney's method for the severity of erosions.

We used the rats as experimental animals in these observations to approach the changes in the cellular energy systems and their regulation in different experimental conditions.

The rat's stomach is divided into two parts, namely glandular (fundic) and membranous (rumen). These parts can be separated well and clearly.

The following biochemical measurements were carried out from both parts of the rat's stomach: acid-soluble inorganic phosphates, acid-soluble organic phosphates, lipids, ribonucleic acids (RNA) and deoxyribonucleic acid (DNA) (see the scheme of these measurements in Table 6).

The measurements of these biochemical parameters generally represented the main components of the cells: lipids (as cell membrane), acid-soluble inorganic and organic phosphates (mitochondrion), RNA (partly the cytoplasm as well as nucleus) and DNA (nucleus). In other

http://dx.doi.org/10.5772/60099

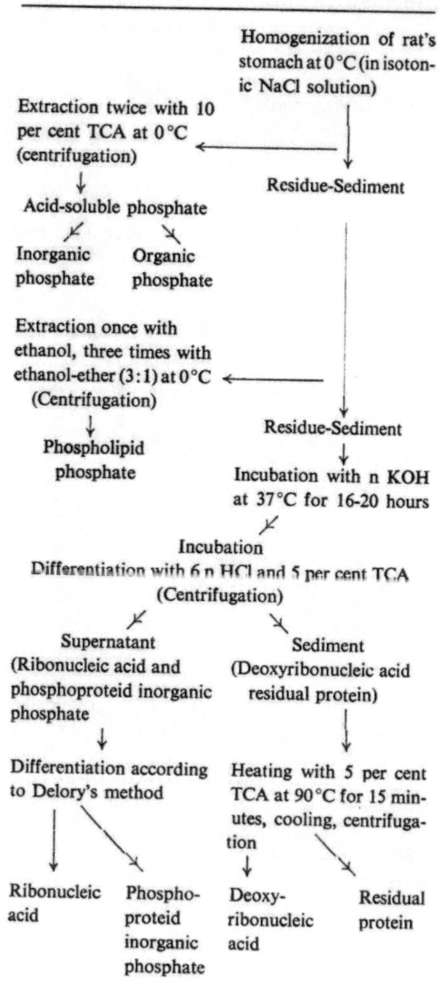

Table 6. Summarizing steps of the biochemical procedures for separation of phosphate fractions and nucleic acids of the rat's stomach and of resecates of human gastrointestinal tracts of patients with chronic gastric, duodenal and jejunal ulcer, who underwent surgical intervention because of peptic ulcer diseases. [Mózsik, Szabó, Krausz, Jávor: Scand. J. Gastroenterol. 2: 321–325, 1967 (with kind permission).]

words, we tried to observe different compartments of cells. The measurements of amounts of acid-soluble inorganic phosphates in the different tissues are widely used to approach the dephosphorylation [i.e., these compounds originated from the splitting of adenosine triphosphate (ATP) independently from its different pathways]. The components of the acid-soluble organic phosphates were not known at that time; meanwhile, the presence of adenosine triphosphate (ATP), adenosine diphosphate (ADP), cyclic 3′,5′-adenosine monophosphate (cAMP), adenosine monophosphate (AMP) and adenine and adenosine were incorporated in this tissue extract. Naturally, these methodologies were updated later by direct measurements of these compounds using thin-layer chromatographic and enzymatic methods.

4.3. The pharmacological–biochemical studies of animals in acute and chronic experimental conditions

4.3.1. General biochemistry of glandular (fundic) part and of forestomach (rumen) in 24-hour pylorus-ligated rats

The necessity of the biochemical analysis of the stomach (gastroduodenal) mucosa was suggested for a better understanding. The underline mechanisms involved in development of mucosal damage and prevention (1962–1964) (Gheorghui, 1975; Mózsik et al., 1967 a, b; 1969 a, b, c, d; Mózsik et al., 1970 a, b).

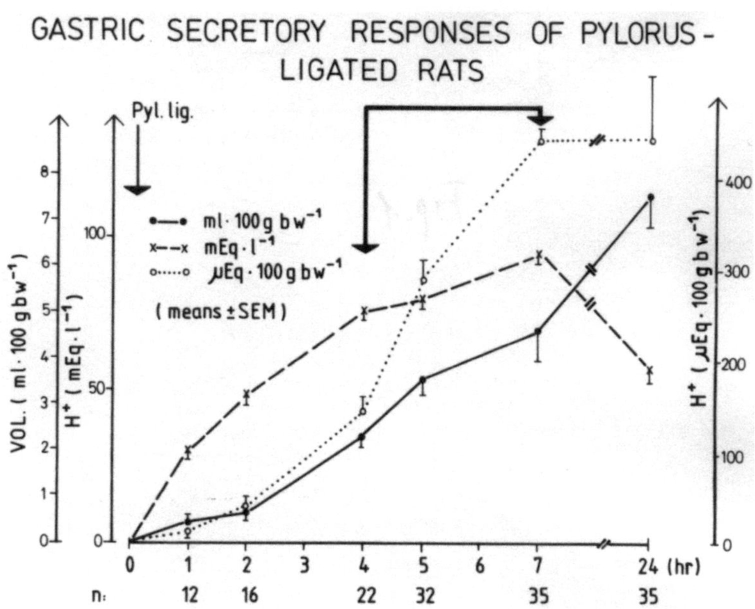

Figure 13. The pattern of gastric secretory responses in 24-hour pylorus-ligated rats. The volume of gastric secretory responses (mL/100 body weight), H^+ concentration (mEq/L) and H^+ output (μEq/100 b.w.) were measured and their results were expressed as means ± SEM, indicating the number of animals. The time period between 4 and 7 hours after pyloric ligation represents the optimal time period to study the actions of drugs and hormones and their biochemical changes in the different parts of the stomach. The peak of maximal acid output can be obtained in 7 hours; meanwhile, the gastric ulceration appears after 7 hours in pylorus-ligated rats (means ± SEM). [Mózsik et al., Scand. J. Gastroenterol 4:633–640; 1969 and Acta Physiol. Scand. Spec. Suppl. 1978a (with kind permission).]

In the first period, the acid-soluble organic and inorganic phosphates and phospholipids, ribonucleic acid (RNA) and deoxyribonucleic acid (DNA) were extracted from the gastric mucosa, and their quantities were measured with (Mózsik et al., 1969 a, b, c, d) and without surgical vagotomy (Mózsik et al., 1967 a, b) (Figures 13–17). Later adenosine triphosphate (ATP) and adenosine diphosphate (ADP) were measured during atropine treatment (Mózsik et al., 1970 a, b). The biochemical parameters were chosen as a suitable methodology to give a "biochemical cross-section" of gastroduodenal mucosa under different experimental conditions.

http://dx.doi.org/10.5772/60099

These results stimulated us for doing further biochemical observations in the animal stomach on dependence of increased and decreased vagal activity.

GENERAL BIOCHEMICAL MECHANISMS OF DEVELOPMENT OF GASTRIC HYPERSECRETION AND ULCER DEVELOPMENT IN PYLORUS-LIGATED RATS

	GLANDULAR STOMACH			FORESTOMACH		
	SHAM-OPERATED	7 HR	24 HR	SHAM-OPERATED	7HR	24HR
secretory vol. (ml)	-	5.85±0.06	15.76±0.8	-	-	-
H^+ output (μEq)	-	1145±35 +++	1260±64+++	-	-	-
ulcer number	-	-	-	-	-	60/10
wet weight (g)	0.68±0.02	0.81±0.02+++	0.80±0.04++	0.36±0.01	0.48±0.01+++	0.56±0.02+++
Acid soluble inorg. P (μg)	241±11	184±17+++	260±13++	115±18	87±16NS	214±22+++
org. P (μg)	156±18	245±18++	49±22+++	32±10	131±14+++	0±0+++
Lipid-P (μg)	255±22	365±42+++	749±123+++	178±28	291±30+	611±111+++
RNA (μg)	2886±237	3147±137NS	2766±78NS	905±71	1104±58+	1932±264++
DNA (μg)	4400±131	5335±336NS	5610±215++	650±48	1720±392+	1825±208

NS=not significant +=0.05>P>0.01 ++=0.01>P>0.001 +++=P<0.001
(means ± SEM) (n=10)

Figure 14. The changes in the chemical composition of glandular stomach (fundus) and forestomach (rumen) in pylorus-ligated rats. The following parameters were measured: gastric secretory volume (mL), H^+ output, number of ulcers, wet tissue (g), acid-soluble inorganic (P_i) and organic (P_i) phosphates, lipid phosphates (μg), ribonucleic acid (RNA) (μg) and deoxyribonucleic (DNA) (μg) acids. The results were expressed as percentage values of sham-operated (=100%) animals. The statistical analysis was carried out between the sham-operated rats and 7- and 24-hour pylorus-ligated rats (means ± SEM). [Mózsik et al., Scand J Gastroenterol 4: 633–640; 1969 (with kind permission).]

There were many criticisms for this experimental ulcer model because the ulceration appeared in the forestomach (not in the glandular part of the animal stomach); however, different typical events of experimentally developed ulcer can be detected using this model:

a. The gastric hypersecretion can be obtained before the ulcer development in accordance with the time (after surgical intervention);

b. The peak of gastric acid hypersecretion can be obtained in this model in 7 hours after the surgical intervention (see Figure 2), and its value does not change from 7 to 24 hours after pyloric ligation;

c. The time period between 4 and 7 hours offers excellent good possibility to study the stimulatory or inhibitory actions of different compounds on the gastric acid secretion in rats;

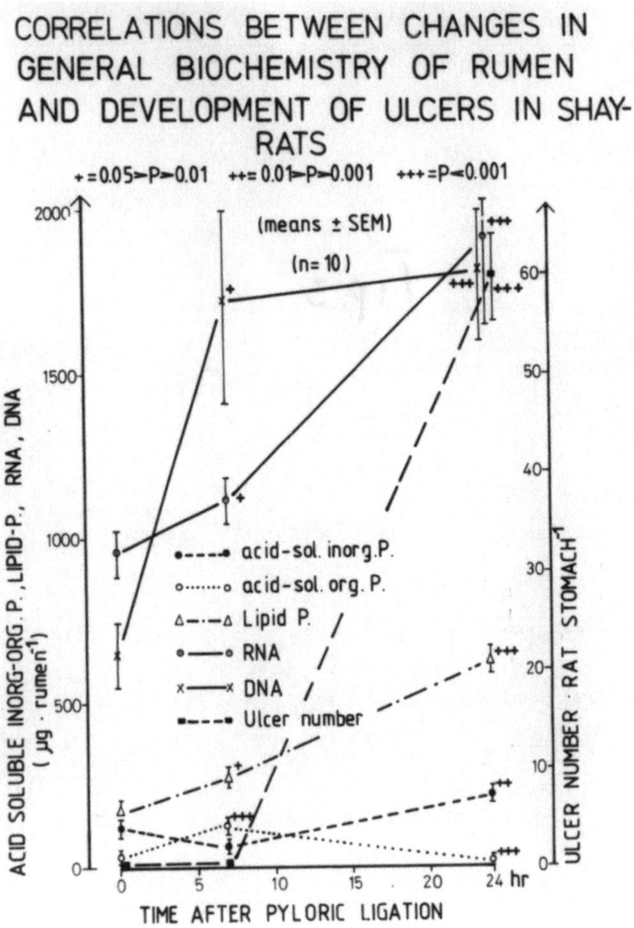

Figure 15. Correlation between the changes in the general biochemistry of ulcer development in forestomach (rumen) of the 24-hour pylorus-ligated rats depending on time after pyloric ligation. [Mózsik et al., Scand. J. Gastroenterol. 4: 633–640; 1969 (with kind permission).]

d. We can very well study the possible correlations between gastric acid secretory responses and development of gastric ulcer.

Bearing these conclusions in mind, we started with the "general biochemical" approach – the main biochemical events during the development of gastric acid hypersecretion and ulcer (of course, respecting the actual level of international research). We have to emphasize that no general biochemical examinations were given in the gastrointestinal research for animals and patients earlier. So, these types of observations internationally opened a new avenue ("biochemistry") in the gastrointestinal research.

We tried to select the different biochemically measured parameters for providing nearest approach to the cell functions (e.g., membrane, mitochondrion, ribonucleic acid and deoxyribonucleic acid).

http://dx.doi.org/10.5772/60099

BIOCHEMISMS OF GASTRIC FUNDIC MUCOSA FORE-STOMACH AND DEVELOPMENT OF GASTRIC HYPER-SECRETION AND ULCER IN PYLORUS-LIGATED RATS

	GLANDULAR STOMACH			FORESTOMACH (RUMEN)		
	0	7	24 HR	0	7	24 HR
H output	-	↑↑↑	↑↑↑	-	-	-
ULCER	-	-	-	-	-	↑↑↑
ACID-SOL. INORG. P		↓↓↓	↑↑↑		NS	↑↑↑
ACID-SOL. ORG. P		↑↑↑	↓↓↓		↑↑↑	↓↓↓
LIPID P		↑↑↑	↑↑↑		↑	↑↑↑
RNA		NS	NS		↑	↑↑
DNA		NS	↑↑		↑	↑↑↑

NS = NOT SIGNIFICANT ↑ = 0.05 > P > 0.01 ↑↑ = 0.01 > P > 0.001 ↑↑↑ = P < 0.001

↑ = INCREASE ↓ = DECREASE

Figure 16. Comparative changes in the biochemistry (acid-soluble inorganic and organic phosphates, lipid phosphates, RNA and DNA) of glandular stomach and forestomach of 24-hour pylorus-ligated rats. The means ± SEM values of sham-operated rats (=100%) are expressed in percentage. *P* values: $P < 0.05$; $P < 0.01$; $P < 0.001$. [Mózsik et al., Scand. J. Gastroenterol. 4: 633–640; 1969 (with kind permission).]

The functions of the organs are specific events (gastric secretion, ulcer development); meanwhile, the biochemical mechanisms obtained in the target organs are extremely complicated. The biochemical extractums (e.g., acid-soluble inorganic and organic phosphates, lipids, ribonucleic acid and deoxyribonucleic acid) from the gastric tissues dominantly represent the cell membranes (lipids), mitochondrion (lipid-soluble organic and inorganic phosphates, partly ribonucleic acid) and nucleus (deoxyribonucleic acid).

At that time, the measurements of acid-soluble inorganic phosphate represent the cumulative effect of breakdown of adenosine triphosphate (ATP) (by different pathways) from the effector organs; meanwhile, the compounds of the acid-soluble organic phosphates (when these observations were carried out) were unknown. Now, we know that the acid-soluble organic phosphates contain the adenosine triphosphate (ATP), adenosine diphosphate (ADP), adenosine monophosphate (AMP), cyclic 3′,5′-adenosine monophosphate (cAMP) and adenosines and adenines.

We have to emphasize that we tried to approach only the main biochemical lines in the stomach during the development of gastric acid hypersecretion and ulcer after surgical intervention.

The obtained results of our present observations clearly indicated to us:

a. All biochemical changes (in acid-soluble inorganic and organic phosphates, lipids, RNA and DNA) – depending on time – are similar to each other;

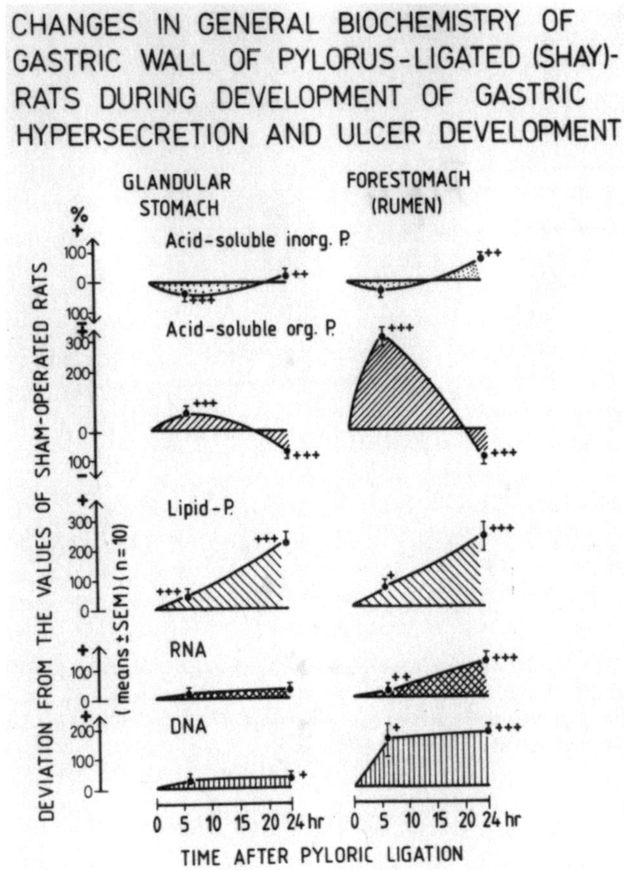

Figure 17. Schematic summary of the changes in gastric hypersecretion, ulcer development (forestomach) and biochemical compositions (acid-soluble inorganic and organic phosphates, lipid phosphates, RNA and DNA) observed in 24-hour pylorus-ligated rats. [Mózsik et al., Scand. J. Gastroenterol. 4:633–640; 1969 (with kind permission).]

b. The biochemical changes in both parts of stomach (glandular stomach and forestomach) appeared before the development of gastric acid hypersecretion and ulcer development;

c. Because gastric acid hypersecretion is the result of a consequence of very active metabolic processes in the glandular part of stomach and because the same biochemical changes were obtained from the forestomach, it can be concluded that the gastric ulceration appears after increased biochemism in the forestomach;

d. The decrease of acid-soluble inorganic phosphates (earlier) along with the increase of acid-soluble organic phosphates clearly indicates the increased biochemical metabolism in both parts of the stomach;

e. The mentioned changes in the acid-soluble inorganic and organic phosphates led to the significant changes of ATP breakdown and ATP resynthesis [in other words changes in the dephosphorylation and oxidative phosphorylation pATP synthesis)].

The critical evaluation of these experimental results called our attention to reconsider our previously created knowledge on the development of gastric acid hypersecretion and ulcer development in pylorus-ligated rats.

4.3.2. General biochemistry of glandular (fundic) part and forestomach (rumen) after acute "chemical" and "surgical" vagotomy in rats (using different anticholinergic compounds)

The effects of acute administrations of parasympatholytics [(atropine, isopropamide 2,2-diphenyl-4-diisopropylamino-methyl iodide) and Gastrixon (methyl-tropinium-bromide-xanthene-9-carboxylate)] and bilateral surgical vagotomy on the biochemism of stomach [glandular part and membranaceous (forestomach, rumen)] in 7-hour pyloric-ligation rats were studied.

Atropine is a tertiary ammonium amine, while the isopropamide and Gastrixon are quaternary ammonium components. The chemical diameter of quaternary ammonium structure of Gastrixon is greater than isopropamide (Gyermek, 1951, 1953; Gyermek and Nádor, 1952, 1953 a, b; György et al., 1961; De Jongh et al.,J1955; Proosdij-Harzeme,et al., J955). The blocking effects of parasympatholytics increase with the increasing diameter of tertiary and quaternary ammonium molecules on the autonomic nerve systems (Fehér, 1960; Grenell and Mullins, 1956).

Our aims were (1) to study the effects of different parasympatholytics and surgical vagotomy on the biochemical parameters of stomach and (2) to compare the changes in the gastric mucosal biochemical parameters produced by "chemical" and "surgical" vagotomy.

	Glandular stomach wall		Membranaceous stomach wall	
Experimental groups	n	quantities (*g*)	n	quantities (*g*)
7 hours after laparotomy + pyloric ligation	10	0.81±0.02 (1)	10	0.48±0.01 (2)
7 hours after laparotomy + pyloric ligation + atropine (1.0 mg s. c.)	13	0.89±0.04 (3)	10	0.61±0.03 (4)
7 hours after laparotomy + pyloric ligation + Isopropamide (1.0 mg s. c)	8	0.85±0.04 (5)	8	0.56±0.03 (6)
7 hours after laparotomy + pyloric ligation + Gastrixone (1.0 mg s. c)	8	0.80±0.02 (7)	8	0.48±0.01 (8)
24 hours after laparotomy + pyloric ligation	10	0.80±0.04 (9)	10	0.56±0.01 (10)
24 hours after laparotomy + pyloric ligation + vagotomy	8	0.70±0.02 (11)	8	0.51±0.03 (12)

Significances :

1 – 3 : P = 0.05	3 – 5 : P > 0.05	2 – 4 : P < 0.001	4 – 6 : P > 0.05
1 – 5 : P > 0.05	5 – 9 : P > 0.05	2 – 6 : P = 0.02	6 – 8 : P = 0.02
1 – 7 : P > 0.05	3 – 9 : P > 0.05	2 – 8 : P > 0.05	4 – 8 : P < 0.001
9 – 11 : P = 0.02		10 – 12 : P > 0.05	

Table 7. Changes of stomach weight in Shay rats after administration of parasympatholytics and bilateral surgical vagotomy. The results are expressed as means ± standard error of means (*n* indicates the number of animals). [Mózsik et al., Scand. J. Gastroenterol. 4: 641–651 1969c (with kind permission).]

Experimental groups	n	Volume of gastric secretion (ml)	Acidity (free/total)	Frequency of ulcer (number of ulcers/examined animals) Glandular stomach wall	Membranaceous stomach wall
7 hours after laparotomy + pyloric ligation	10	5.85±0.06	59/89	0/10	0/10
7 hours after laparotomy + pyrolic lig. + Atropine (1.0 mg s. c.)	13	0.60±0.002	0/5	0/13	0/13
7 hours after laparotomy + pyrolic lig. + Isopropamide (1.0 mg s. c.)	8	0.30±0.001	0/10	0/8	0/8
7 hours after laparotomy + pyloric lig. + Gastrixone (1.0 mg s. c.)	8	0.60±0.002	0/8	0/8	0/8
24 hours after laparotomy + pyloric ligation	10	15.76±0.80	80/100	0/10	12/10
24 hours after laparotomy + pyloric lig. + bilateral surgical vagotomy	8	1.40±0.06	32/64	0/8	0/8

Table 8. Changes of gastric secretion, acidity and frequency of ulcer in Shay rats after administration of parasympatholytics and surgical vagotomy. The results are expressed as means ± standard error of means (mL, mEq/L), and total number of ulcers in one rat's stomach. (*n* indicates the number of animals). [Mózsik et al., Scand. J. Gastroenterol. 4: 641–651, 1969c (with kind permission).]

Experimental groups	Glandular stomach wall n	quantities (*g*)	Membranaceous stomach wall n	quantities (*g*)
7 hours after laparotomy + pyloric ligation	10	0.81±0.02 (1)	10	0.48±0.01 (2)
7 hours after laparotomy + pyloric ligation + atropine (1.0 mg s. c.)	13	0.89±0.04 (3)	10	0.61±0.03 (4)
7 hours after laparotomy + pyloric ligation + Isopropamide (1.0 mg s. c)	8	0.85±0.04 (5)	8	0.56±0.03 (6)
7 hours after laparotomy + pyloric ligation + Gastrixone (1.0 mg s. c)	8	0.80±0.02 (7)	8	0.48±0.01 (8)
24 hours after laparotomy + pyloric ligation	10	0.80±0.04 (9)	10	0.56±0.01 (10)
24 hours after laparotomy + pyloric ligation + vagotomy	8	0.70±0.02 (11)	8	0.51±0.03 (12)

Significances :

1 – 3 : P = 0.05	3 – 5 : P > 0.05	2 – 4 : P < 0.001	4 – 6 : P > 0.05
1 – 5 : P > 0.05	5 – 9 : P > 0.05	2 – 6 : P = 0.02	6 – 8 : P = 0.02
1 – 7 : P > 0.05	3 – 9 : P > 0.05	2 – 8 : P > 0.05	4 – 8 : P < 0.001
9 – 11 : P = 0.02		10 – 12 : P > 0.05	

Table 9. Changes of stomach weight in Shay rats after administration of parasympatholytics and bilateral surgical vagotomy. The results are expressed as means ± standard error of means (mL, mEq/L), and total number of ulcers in one rat's stomach (*n* indicates the number of animals). [Mózsik et al., Scand. J. Gastroenterol. 4: 641–651, 1969c (with kind permission).]

http://dx.doi.org/10.5772/60099

Experimental groups	n	Acid-soluble inorganic phosphates quantities	n	Acid-soluble organic phosphates quantities
7 hours after laparotomy + pyloric ligation	10	185 ± 17 (1)	10	245 ± 18 (2)
7 hours after laparotomy + pyloric ligation + atropine (1.0 mg s. c.)	13	405 ± 52 (3)	13	119 ± 34 (4)
7 hours after laparotomy + pyloric ligation + Isopropamide (1.0 mg s. c.)	8	232 ± 9 (5)	8	208 ± 20 (6)
7 hours after laparotomy + pyloric ligation + Gastrixone (1.0 mg s. c.)	8	219 ± 17 (7)	8	281 ± 17 (8)

Significances

1–3: $P < 0.001$	3–5: $0.01 > P > 0.001$	2–4: $0.01 > P > 0.001$	4–6: $P = 0.04$
1–5: $P = 0.02$	3–7: $0.01 > P > 0.001$	2–6: $P > 0.05$	4–8: $0.01 > P > 0.001$
1–7: $P > 0.05$ (=0.08)	5–7: $P > 0.05$	2–8: $P > 0.05$	6–8: $0.01 > P > 0.001$

Table 10. Changes of the acid-soluble phosphates in Shay rats' glandular stomach wall after administration of parasympatholytics. The results are expressed as means ± standard error of means in μg phosphate per total wet glandular stomach wall (*n* indicates the number of animals). [Mózsik et al., Scand. J. Gastroenterol. 4: 641–651, 1969c (with kind permission).]

Experimental groups	n	Acid-soluble inorganic phosphates quantities	n	Acid-soluble organic phosphates quantities
7 hours after laparotomy + pyloric ligation	10	87 ± 16 (1)	10	131 ± 14 (2)
7 hours after laparotomy + pyloric ligation + atropine (1.0 mg s. c.)	13	116 ± 6 (3)	13	26 ± 10 (4)
7 hours after laparotomy + pyloric ligation + Isopropamide (1.0 mg s. c.)	8	133 ± 6 (5)	8	81 ± 10 (6)
7 hours after laparotomy + pyloric ligation + Gastrixone (1.0 mg s. c.)	8	88 ± 4 (7)	8	87 ± 5 (8)

Significances

1–3: $P > 0.05$ (=0.06)	3–5: $P = 0.06$	2–4: $P < 0.001$	4–6: $P = 0.001$
1–5: $0.01 > P > 0.001$	3–7: $P < 0.001$	2–6: $0.01 > P > 0.001$	4–8: $P < 0.001$
1–7: $P > 0.05$	5–7: $P < 0.001$	2–8: $0.01 > P > 0.001$	6–8: $P < 0.05$

Table 11. Changes of the acid-soluble phosphates in Shay rats' membranaceous stomach (rumen) wall after administration parasympatholytics. The results are expressed as means ± standard error of means in μg phosphate per total wet membranaceous stomach wall (*n* indicates the number of animals). [Mózsik et al., Scand. J. Gastroenterol. 4: 641–651, 1969c (with kind permission).]

	Phospholipid phosphates			
	Glandular stomach wall		Membranaceous stomach wall	
Experimental groups	n	quantities	n	quantities
7 hours after laparotomy + pyloric ligation	10	365 ± 42 (1)	10	291 ± 30 (2)
7 hours after laparotomy + pyloric ligation + Atropine (1.0 mg s. c.)	13	229 ± 27 (3)	13	137 ± 18 (4)
7 hours after laparotomy + pyloric ligation + Isopropamide (1.0 mg s. c.)	8	168 ± 21 (5)	8	107 ± 13 (6)
7 hours after laparotomy + pyloric ligation + Gastrixone (1.0 mg s. c.)	8	265 ± 20 (7)	8	128 ± 9 (8)

Significances

1–3: $P = 0.02$	3–5: $P > 0.05$	2–4: $P < 0.001$	4–6: $P > 0.05$
1–5: $P < 0.001$	3–7: $P > 0.05$	2–6: $P < 0.001$	4–8: $P > 0.05$
1–7: $P = 0.05$	5–7: $0.01 > P > 0.001$	2–8: $P < 0.001$	6–8: $P > 0.05$

Table 12. Changes of phospholipids (phosphates) in Shay rats' glandular and membranaceous stomach wall after administration of parasympatholytics. The results are presented as means ± standard error of means in μg phosphate per total wet glandular and membranaceous stomach wall (*n* indicates the number of animals). [Mózsik et al., Scand. J. Gastroenterol. 4: 641–651, 1969c (with kind permission).]

	Ribonucleic acid			
	Glandular stomach wall		Membranaceous stomach wall	
Experimental groups	n	quantities	n	quantities
7 hours after laparotomy + pyloric ligation	10	3147 ± 157 (1)	10	1104 ± 58 (2)
7 hours after laparotomy + pyloric ligation + atropine (1.0 mg s. c.)	13	2818 ± 340 (3)	13	685 ± 66 (4)
7 hours after laparotomy + pyloric ligation + Isopropamide (1.0 mg s. c.)	8	3400 ± 198 (5)	8	1270 ± 95 (6)
7 hours after laparotomy + pyloric ligation + Gastrixone (1.0 mg s. c.)	8	3538 ± 189 (7)	8	1048 ± 53 (8)

Significances

1–3: $P > 0.05$	3–5: $P > 0.05$	2–4: $P < 0.001$	4–6: $P < 0.001$
1–5: $P > 0.05$	3–7: $P > 0.05$	2–6: $P > 0.05$	4–8: $P < 0.001$
1–7: $P > 0.05$	5–7: $P > 0.05$	2–8: $P > 0.05$	6–8: $P > 0.05$

Table 13. Changes of ribonucleic acids in Shay rats' glandular and membranaceous stomach wall after administration of parasympatholytics. The results are presented as means ± standard error of means in μg nucleic acid per total wet glandular and membranaceous stomach wall (*n* indicates the number of animals). [Mózsik et al., Scand. J. Gastroenterol. 4: 641–651, 1969c (with kind permission).]

http://dx.doi.org/10.5772/60099

	Deoxyribonucleic acid			
	Glandular stomach wall		Membranaceous stomach wall	
Experimental groups	n	quantities	n	quantities
7 hours after laparotomy + pyloric ligation	10	5335 ± 366 (1)	10	1720 ± 392 (2)
7 hours after laparotomy + pyloric ligation + atropine (1.0 mg s. c.)	13	3058 ± 394 (3)	13	1273 ± 237 (4)
7 hours after laparotomy + pyloric ligation + Isopropamide (1.0 mg s. c.)	8	5834 ± 458 (5)	8	1577 ± 119 (6)
7 hours after laparotomy + pyloric ligation + Gastrixone (1.0 mg s. c.)	8	5815 ± 263 (7)	8	1247 ± 103 (8)

Significances

1–3: $P < 0.001$	3–5: $P < 0.001$	2–4: $P > 0.05$	4–6: $P > 0.05$
1–5: $P > 0.05$	3–7: $P < 0.001$	2–6: $P > 0.05$	4–8: $P > 0.05$
1–7: $P > 0.05$	5–7: $P > 0.05$	2–8: $P > 0.05$	6–8: $P = 0.02$

Table 14. Changes of deoxyribonucleic acids in Shay rats' glandular and membranaceous stomach wall after administration of parasympatholytics. The results are presented as means ± standard error of means in µg deoxyribonucleic acid per total wet glandular and membranaceous stomach wall (*n* indicates the number of animals). [Mózsik et al., Scand. J. Gastroenterol. 4: 641–651, 1969c (with kind permission).]

	Parts of stomach wall							
	Glandular stomach wall				Membranaceous stomach wall			
	Experimental groups				Experimental groups			
Examined experimental parameters	Control	After Atropine	After Isopropamide	After Gastrixone	Control	After Atropine	After Isopropamide	After Gastrixone
Gastric secretion	100.0	12.0	6.0	12.0	–	–	–	–
Acidity (free/total)	100/100	0/5	0/12	0/10	–	–	–	–
Acid soluble inorganic phosphates	100.0	225.0	128.0	121.0	100.0	145.0	166.0	100.0
Acid-soluble organic phosphates	100.0	49.0	86.0	117.0	100.0	20.0	62.0	66.0
Phospholipid phosphates	100.0	63.0	46.0	73.0	100.0	47.0	36.0	44.0
Ribonucleic acid	100.0	90.0	109.0	114.0	100.0	66.0	115.0	91.0
Deoxyribonucleic acid	100.0	57.0	110.0	109.0	100.0	80.0	93.0	73.0

Table 15. The changes in the percentage of examined parameters of Shay rats' stomach wall induced by parasympatholytics in percentage of control ($n = 100$) values 7 hours after pyloric ligation. [Mózsik et al., Scand. J. Gastroenterol., 4: 641–651, 1969c (with kind permission).]

Increasing inhibitory effects of parasympatholytics – depending on the extent of chemical diameters – did not run closely parallel with increasing diameter of tertiary and quaternary ammonium molecules, and we also perceived biochemical changes of gastric mucosal biochemistry. After bilateral surgical vagotomy, the quantities of acid-soluble inorganic

	Parts of stomach wall			
	Glandular stomach wall		Membranaceous stomach wall	
Examined experimental	Experimental groups		Experimental groups	
parameters	Control	After vagotomy	Control	After vagotomy
Gastric secretion	100.0	9.3	–	–
Acidity (free/total)	100/100	40/65	–	–
Acid-soluble inorganic phosphates	100.0	85.0	100.0	55.0
Acid-soluble organic phosphates	100.0	278.0	0.0	
Phospholipid phosphates	100.0	31.0	100.0	19.0
Ribonucleic acid	100.0	57.0	100.0	29.0
Deoxyribonucleic acid	100.0	115.0	100.0	74.0

Table 16. The changes in percentage of examined parameters of Shay rats' stomach wall induced by surgical vagotomy of control ($n = 100$) values 24 hours after pyloric ligation. [Mózsik et al., Scand. J. Gastroenterol. 4: 641–651, 1969c (with kind permission).]

phosphates decreased significantly in both glandular and membranaceous (forestomach and rumen) stomach wall. The alterations of acid-soluble inorganic and organic phosphates in the stomach wall showed contradictory trends of surgical vagotomy to those after administration of parasympatholytics ("chemical" vagotomy), the effects of surgical vagotomy on the nucleic acid metabolism being greater than the effects of different parasympatholytics.

A biochemical–cellular–morphological explanation of parasympatholytics and surgical vagotomy has been suggested (Figure 18). According to this explanation, the nucleic acids are in the center of Figure 18, and phospholipids, acid-soluble inorganic and organic phosphates are in periphery of a "hypothetic cell." The products of cells (HCl secretion) are presented in an outer part of the figure. After a large alteration of periphery, the center will change to a small degree and *vice versa.*

GENERAL FUNCTIONS OF ORGANS
↓↑
BIOCHEMICAL REACTIONS OF TISSUES (acid-soluble phosphates, phospholipids)
↓↑
PROTEINS, ENZYMES
↓↑
RIBONUCLEIC ACIDS
↓↑
DEOXYRIBONUCLEIC ACIDS

Table 17. Main steps of regulatory levels of cells in the living organs. The most stable regulatory steps are located at the level of DNA and the most instable regulatory steps are at the level of functions of organs.

http://dx.doi.org/10.5772/60099

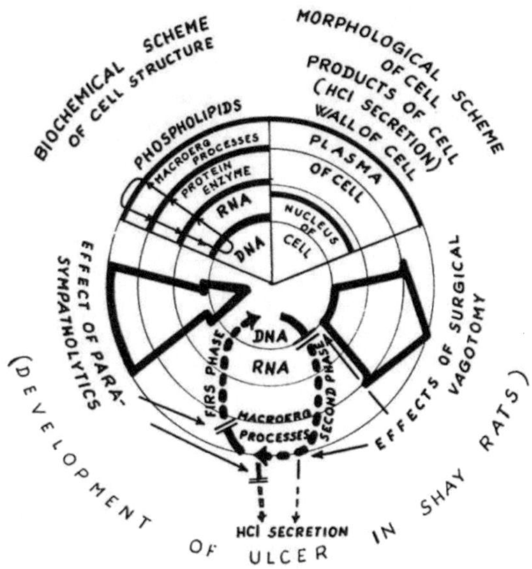

Figure 18. A schematic and possible biochemical–cellular–morphological explanation of parasympatholytics and surgical vagotomy. [Mózsik, Kiss, Krausz, Jávor: Scand. J. Gastroenterol. 4: 641–651, 1969c (with kind permission).]

4.3.3. Pharmacological and biochemical studies in rats after chronic "chemical" and "surgical" vagotomy and cholinesterase inhibitor treatment

Biochemical observations were carried out to study the changes in these biochemical parameters of rat's stomach after chronic "chemical vagotomy" (2 × 1.0 mg i.p. atropine for 25 days) and cholinesterase inhibitor treatment (2 × 0.25 mg of neostigmine i.p for three weeks).

The biochemical examinations in the drug-treated groups of animals were also divided into two different groups. The biochemical observations of the first group were carried out immediately after the end of the drug treatment, whereas the observations of the second group were carried out after cessation of drug treatments (10 days after the cessation of atropine treatment and three weeks after cessation of cholinesterase inhibitor treatment).

To compare the changes in the stomach after a chronic "chemical" vagotomy (atropine treatment), the surgical vagotomy was carried out in a group of animals (without any other treatment), and the biochemical measurements were done one month after surgical vagotomy.

The control animals were treated with saline solution for 25 days. It has been suggested that the results of these animal observations will give a biochemical explanation for the effects of increased cholinergic activity (produced by cholinesterase inhibitor), for "chemical" vagotomy and "surgical" vagotomy ("use" vs. "disuse" of vagal nerve on the metabolism of gastric tissues). The results of the biochemical examinations are presented in cases of chronic atropine treatment and chronic neostigmine (see the forthcoming tables). The biochemical results after one month of surgical vagotomy are presented only in comparison with the changes in the biochemical parameters obtained in rats treated chronically with atropine and neostigmine.

	Controls (treated with physiological saline)		Animals treated with atropine for 25 days		10 days after cessation of atropine treatment	
	n	quantities	n	quantities	n	quantities
Body weight (g)	11	227 ± 10 (1)	10	189 ± 8 (2)	6	207 ± 4 (3)
Weight of the glandular (pyloric) part of the stomach (g)	11	0.99 ± 0.06 (4)	10	0.91 ± 0.05 (5)	6	0.88 ± 0.07 (6)
Weight of the membranous (rumenal) part of the stomach (g)	11	0.65 ± 0.001 (7)	10	0.71 ± 0.05 (8)	6	0.63 ± 0.01 (9)

Statistical values:
Between 1 and 2: $0.01 > P > 0.001$, between 2 and 3 : $P > 0.05$, between 1 and 3 : $P > 0.05$.
Between 4 and 5 : $P > 0.05$, between 5 and 6 : $P > 0.05$, between 4 and 6 : $P > 0.05$ (= 0.06).
Between 7 and 8 : $P > 0.05$, between 8 and 9 : $P > 0.05$, between 7 and 9 : $P > 0.05$.

Table 18. Changes of body weight and weight of the stomach wall in animals treated with atropine. The results are expressed as mean values ± standard error (n indicates the number of animals). [Mózsik et al., Eur. J. Pharmacol 7: 66–72, 1969c (with kind permission).]

	Controls (animals treated with physiological saline for 25 days)		Animals treated with atropine for 25 days		10 days after cessation of atropine treatment	
	n	quantities	n	quantities	n	quantities
Acid-soluble inorganic phosphates	11	308 ± 15 (1)	10	259 ± 12 (2)	6	257 ± 8 (3)
Acid-soluble organic phosphates	11	374 ± 21 (4)	10	169 ± 39 (5)	6	284 ± 10 (6)
Phospholipid phosphates	11	499 ± 61 (7)	10	219 ± 19 (8)	6	338 ± 6 (9)
Ribonucleic acid	11	4237 ± 467 (10)	10	3405 ± 217 (11)	6	3009 ± 81 (12)
Deoxyribonucleic acid	11	6181 ± 457 (13)	10	5504 ± 303 (14)	6	5228 ± 115 (15)

Statistical values:
between 1 and 2 : $P = 0.02$; between 2 and 3 : $P > 0.05$; between 1 and 3 : $0.01 > P > 0.001$
between 4 and 5 : $P < 0.001$; between 5 and 6 : $P = 0.02$; between 4 and 6 : $0.01 > P > 0.001$
between 7 and 8 : $P < 0.001$; between 8 and 9 : $P < 0.001$; between 7 and 9 : $P = 0.02$
between 10 and 11 : $P = 0.03$; between 11 and 12 : $P > 0.05$; between 10 and 12 : $P < 0.001$
between 13 and 14 : $P > 0.05$; between 14 and 15 : $P > 0.05$; between 13 and 15 : $P > 0.05$ (= 0.06).

Table 19. Changes of phosphate and nucleic acid content in glandular (pyloric) part of the stomach wall in rats treated with atropine for 25 days. The results are expressed as means (μg per total body weight of the glandular part of the stomach wall) ± standard error (n indicates the number of animals). [Mózsik et al., Eur. J. Pharmacol 7: 66–72, 1969c (with kind permission).]

http://dx.doi.org/10.5772/60099

	Controls (animals treated with physiological saline for 25 days)		Animals treated with atropine for 25 days		10 days after cessation of atropine treatment	
	n	quantities	*n*	quantities	*n*	quantities
Acid-soluble inorganic phosphates	11	151 ± 5 (1)	10	169 ± 10 (2)	6	162 ± 15 (3)
Acid-soluble organic phosphates	11	158 ± 12 (4)	10	145 ± 19 (5)	6	98 ± 18 (6)
Phospholipid phosphates	11	236 ± 14 (7)	10	221 ± 23 (8)	6	160 ± 30 (9)
Ribonucleic acid	11	1611 ± 38 (10)	10	1788 ± 73 (11)	6	1301 ± 115 (12)
Deoxyribonucleic acid	11	1757 ± 147 (13)	10	915 ± 273 (14)	6	1415 ± 188 (15)

Statistical values:

between 1 and 2 : $P > 0.05$	between 2 and 3 : $P > 0.05$	between 1 and 3 : $P > 0.05$
between 4 and 5 : $P > 0.05$	between 5 and 6 : $P > 0.05$	between 4 and 6 : $0.01 > P > 0.001$
between 7 and 8 : $P > 0.05$	between 8 and 9 : $P > 0.05$	between 7 and 9 : $P = 0.04$
between 10 and 11 : $P > 0.05$	between 11 and 12 : $P = 0.02$	between 10 and 12 : $P = 0.02$
between 13 and 14 : $0.01 > P > 0.001$	between 14 and 15 : $P > 0.05$	between 13 and 15 : $P > 0.05$.

Table 20. Changes of phosphate and nucleic acid content in membranaceous (rumenal) part of the stomach wall in rats treated with atropine for 25 days. The results of mean values (µg per total body weight of the membranaceous part of the stomach wall) are calculated as means ± standard error (*n* indicates the number of animals). [Mózsik et al., Eur. J. Pharmacol 7: 66–72, 1969c (with kind permission).]

Parts of the stomach wall	Controls		At the end of neostigmine treatment		One month after cessation of neostigmine treatment	
	n	quantities	n	quantities	n	quantities
Glandular stomach wall	10	0.92±0.04 (1)	10	0.93±0.03 (2)	7	0.88±0.07 (3)
Membranaceous stomach wall	10	0.71±0.06 (4)	10	0.45±0.02 (5)	7	0.43±0.02 (6)
Whole stomach wall	10	1.63±0.06 (7)	10	1.37±0.05 (8)	7	1.31±0.08 (9)

Significance:

1–2: $P > 0.05$	2–3: $P > 0.05$	1–3: $P > 0.05$
4–5: $P < 0.001$	5–6: $P > 0.05$	4–6: $P < 0.001$
7–8: $P = 0.001$	8–9: $P > 0.05$	7–9: $0,01 > P > 0.001$

Table 21. Changes in the weight of the stomach wall in animals treated with high doses of neostigmine. The results are presented as means ± SEM in grams (*n* indicates the number of animals). [Mózsik, Kiss, Jávor, Krausz, Tóth, Pharmacology 2: 45–59, 1969d (with kind permission).]

The treatment's effects on the body weight and weight of the glandular and membranaceous (forestomach) parts are shown in Table 18: there was a significant decrease in body weight ($0.01 > P > 0.001$), but no significant change in the weight of the parts of the stomach.

Fractions	Controls		At the end of neostigmine treatment		One month after cessation of neostigmine treatment	
	n	quantities	n	quantities	n	quantities
Acid-soluble inorganic phosphates	10	305±16 (1)	10	217±15 (2)	7	223±21 (3)
Acid-soluble organic phosphates	10	284±19 (4)	10	355±20 (5)	7	264±22 (6)
Phospholipid phosphates	10	443±40 (7)	10	386±44 (8)	7	283±34 (9)
Total phosphates in incubate	10	747±24 (10)	10	720±20 (11)	7	651±21 (12)
RNA – P.	10	397±35 (13)	10	290±19 (14)	7	270±19 (15)
Ribonucleic acid (according to *Brown*)	10	3999±359 (16)	10	2884±195 (17)	7	2660±149 (18)
DNA – P.	10	395±26 (19)	10	430±20 (20)	7	395±13 (21)
Deoxyribonucleic acid (according to *Seibert*)	10	3812±278 (22)	10	4259±194 (23)	7	3915±272 (24)

Significance:

1–2 : $P<0.001$	2–3: $P>0.05$	1–3: $0.01>P>0.001$
4–5: $P = 0.03$	5–6: $0.01>P>0.001$	4–6: $P>0.05$
7–8: $P>0.05$	8–9: $P>0.05$	7–9: $0.01>P>0.001$
10–11: $P>0.05$	11–12: $P = 0.03$	10–12: $0.01>P>0.001$
13–14: $P = 0.04$	14–15: $P>0.05$	13–15: $0.01>P>0.001$
16–17: $0.01>P>0.001$	17–18: $P>0.05$	16–18: $0.01>P>0.001$
19–20: $P>0.05$	20–21: $P>0.05$	19–21: $P>0.05$
22–23: $P>0.05$	23–24: $P>0.05$	22–24: $P>0.05$

Table 22. Changes in quantities of phosphate fractions and nucleic acids in the glandular stomach wall of animals treated with high doses of neostigmine. The results are presented as means ± SEM in μg phosphate or nucleic acid per total weight (*n* indicates the number of animals). [Mózsik, Kiss, Jávor, Krausz, Tóth, Pharmacology 2:45–59, 1969d (with kind permission).]

After prolonged atropine, there was a decrease in acid-soluble inorganic phosphate ($P = 0.02$), acid-soluble organic phosphates ($P < 0.001$), phospholipids phosphates ($P < 0.001$), ribonucleic acid ($P = 0.03$) and deoxyribonucleic acid ($P < 0.05$) in the glandular part. Ten days after cessation of atropine treatment, levels of acid-soluble organic phosphates ($P = 0.02$) and phospholipid phosphates ($P < 0.001$) improved but levels of ribonucleic acid and deoxyribonucleic acid did not.

Fractions	Controls		At the end of neostigmine treatment		One month after cessation of neostigmine treatment	
	n	quantities	n	quantities	n	quantities
Acid-soluble inorganic phosphates	10	163±15 (1)	10	81±7 (2)	7	114±14 (3)
Acid-soluble organic phosphates	10	110±14 (4)	10	69±13 (5)	7	69±17 (6)
Phospholipid phosphates	10	190±13 (7)	10	91±14 (8)	7	59±16 (9)
Total phosphates in incubate	10	210±7 (10)	10	170±20 (11)	7	211±19 (12)
RNA – P.	10	136±15 (13)	10	110±25 (14)	7	81±17 (15)
Ribonucleic acid (according to *Brown*)	10	1382±151 (16)	10	1110±287 (17)	7	789±177 (18)
DNA – P.	10	71±9 (19)	10	55±10 (20)	7	126±21 (21)
Deoxyribonucleic acid (according to *Seibert*)	10	758±89 (22)	10	527±118 (23)	7	1260±264 (24)

Significance:

1–2: P<0.001	2–3: P = 0.04	1–3: P = 0.03
4–5: P = 0.04	5–6: P>0.05	4–6: P = 0.06
7–8: P<0.001	8–9: P>0.05	7–9: P>0.05
10–11: P>0.05	11–12: P>0.05	10–11: P>0.05
13–14: P>0.05	14–15: P>0.05	13–15: P = 0.02
16–17: P>0.05	17–18: P>0.05	16–18: P = 0.05
19–20: P>0.05	20–21: 0.01>P>0.001	19–21: P = 0.04
22–23: P>0.05	23–24: P = 0.02	22–24: P>0.05

Table 23. Changes in quantities of phosphate fractions and nucleic acids in the membranaceous stomach wall (forestomach) of animals treated with high doses of neostigmine. The results are presented as means ± SEM in µg phosphate or nucleic acid per total weight (*n* indicates the number of animals). [Mózsik, Kiss, Jávor, Krausz, Tóth, Pharmacology 2: 45–59, 1969d (with kind permission).]

Prolonged atropine treatment did not alter the acid-soluble inorganic and organic, phospholipids phosphate and ribonucleic acid, but there was a decrease in deoxyribonucleic acid (0.01 > P > 0.001). Ten days after cessation of atropine treatment, there was a further reduction of ribonucleic acid (P = 0.02) and increase of deoxyribonucleic acid (P > 0.05).

Fractions	Controls		At the end of neostigmine treatment		One month after cessation of neostigmine treatment	
	n	quantities	n	quantities	n	quantities
Acid-soluble inorganic phosphates	10	332±13 (1)	10	239±13 (2)	7	302±21 (3)
Acid-soluble organic phosphates	10	296±15 (4)	10	393±44 (5)	7	328±39 (6)
Phospholipid phosphates	10	461±44 (7)	10	430±47 (8)	7	382±39 (9)
Total phosphates in incubate	10	830±26 (10)	10	787±28 (11)	7	845±63 (12)
RNA – P.	10	409±17 (13)	10	315±26 (14)	7	320±8 (15)
Ribonucleic acid (according to *Brown*)	10	4333±349 (16)	10	3155±250 (17)	7	3228±96 (18)
DNA – P.	10	398±17 (19)	10	470±20 (20)	7	515±25 (21)
Deoxyribonucleic acid (according to *Seibert*)	10	4128±187 (22)	10	4777±252 (23)	7	5159±259 (24)

Significance:

1–2: P<0.001	2–3: P = 0.02	1–3: P>0.05
4–5: P = 0.06	5–6: P>0.05	4–6: P>0.05
7–8: P>0.05	8–9: P>0.05	7–9: P>0.05
10–11: P>0.05	11–12: P>0.05	10–12: P>0.05
13–14: 0.01>P>0.001	14–15: P>0.05	13–15: P<0.001
16–17: 0.01>P>0.001	17–18: P>0.05	16–18: P = 0.001
19–20: P = 0.02	20–21: P>0.05	19–21: P = 0.001
22–23: P = 0.05	23–24: P>0.05	22–24: 0.01>P>0.001

Table 24. Changes in quantities of phosphate fractions and nucleic acids in the glandular stomach wall of animals treated with high doses of neostigmine. The results are presented as means ± SEM in μg phosphate or nucleic acid per 1 gram of fresh gastric tissue (*n* indicates the number of animals). [Mózsik, Kiss, Jávor, Krausz, Tóth, Pharmacology 2: 45–59, 1969d (with kind permission).]

http://dx.doi.org/10.5772/60099

Fractions	Controls		At the end of neostigmine treatment		One month after cessation of neo-stigmine treatment	
	n	quantities	n	quantities	n	quantities
Acid-soluble inorganic phos-phates	10	224±31 (1)	10	177±14 (2)	7	261±14 (3)
Acid-soluble organic phos-phates	10	147±18 (4)	10	153±35 (5)	7	154±23 (6)
Phospholipid phosphates	10	270±22 (7)	10	207±35 (8)	7	161±23 (9)
Total phos-phates in incubate	10	320±7 (10)	10	330±26 (11)	7	390±28 (12)
RNA – P.	10	190±10 (13)	10	230±30 (14)	7	110±30 (15)
Ribonucleic acid (according to *Brown*)	10	1922±72 (16)	10	2390±350 (17)	7	1180±352 (18)
DNA – P.	10	101±10 (19)	10	110±21 (20)	7	290±40 (21)
Deoxyribonuc-leic acid (accor-ding to *Seibert*)	10	1073±113 (22)	10	1139±217 (23)	7	2880±492 (24)

Significance:

1–2: P×0.05	2–3: P<0.001	1–3: P>0.05
4–5: P>0.05	5–6: P>0.05	4–6: P>0.05
7–8: P>0.05	8–9: P>0.05	7–9: 0.01>P>0.001
10–11: P>0.05	11–12: P>0.05	10–12: P = 0.06
13–14: P>0.05	14–15: P = 0.02	13–15: P = 0.03
16–17: P>0.05	17–18: P = 0.03	16–18: P>0.05
19–20: P>0.05	20–21: P = 0.001	19–21: P<0.001
22–23: P>0.05	23–24: 0.01>P>0.001	22–24: 0.01>P>0.001

Table 25. Changes in quantities of phosphate fractions and nucleic acids in the membranaceous gastric wall (forestomach) of animals treated with high doses of neostigmine. The results are presented as means ± SEM in μg phosphate or nucleic acid per 1 gram of fresh gastric tissue (*n* indicates the number of animals). [Mózsik, Kiss, Jávor, Krausz, Tóth, Pharmacology 2: 45–59, 1969d (with kind permission).]

The results obtained from chronic neostigmine treatment provided the following conclusions:

1. The cholinergic dominance involves the decrease of the weight and biochemical constituents of the membranaceous (forestomach). This is the effect of cholinergic dominance on the membranaceous stomach wall.

2. Examined biochemical constituents of the glandular stomach behave differently during the existence of the cholinergic dominance due to the decrease of acid-soluble inorganic phosphates, phospholipid phosphates and ribonucleic acid and the increase of acid-soluble organic phosphates during neostigmine treatment.

3. We had observed "short-term" and "long-term" biochemical changes in the glandular stomach wall after neostigmine treatment. The "short-term" biochemical change (acid-soluble organic phosphates) was a reversible process lasting up to one month after cessation of neostigmine treatment. At the same time, the "long-term" biochemical changes (acid-soluble inorganic phosphate, phospholipids phosphate and ribonucleic acid) were observed as irreversible processes. It is interesting to note that the stomach can "remember" to the neostigmine treatment one month after cessation of treatment.

In the 1970s, there was a famous topic on physiology to approach the possible backgrounds of "use" and "disuse" of the neural regulation (especially after denervation of muscles) (Graff et al., 1965 a, b, c; Gregory, 1962). The surgical ablation of nerves was used extensively in these types of observations. There was a general note that the denervated organ became to b seniitive to mediators than that inavated organ. Emmelin and Rosenblueth (1951), Emmelin and Muren (1951 a, b; 1952), and Elin (1952, 1961) observed that the efficenciees of drugs and mediators changes after a prolonged reatment (including the atropine). In these observations, no surgical manipulation was done with the nerves of different organs, however, they dichronic drunt was done to inhibit the neural functions at the levels of synapses or at the levels of tra to organs. This phenomenon was named as "pharmacological denervation" and was associated with the supersensitivity (Emmelin, 1952, 1961). We were the first authors, who demonstrated the existence of supersensitivity of "pharmacologic denervation" phenomenon, together along with opment of tolerance to drugs used in the treatment and cross-tolerance to the pharmacologicallypharmarugs, but that are not used in the trea, under classical medical treatment with parasympatholytics in patients with peptic ulcer (see chapters of Sections 2.2-.2.3-– 2.4)

There was an important note that the efficacy of atropine decreased during a chronic atropine treatment in patients with peptic ulcer, however, the decrease effect of atropine returned in time 0 days after cessation of atropine treatment.

These human observations called our attention to carry out different biochemical observations in the rat's stomach after cessation of atropine and neostigmine treatment.

We tried to approach the biochemical backgrounds of the "use" and "disuse" of the gastric tissues in rats (under experimental conditions). The changes in gastric mucosal constituents were presented in percentage values of "sham treated" (with physiological saline solution) (=100%) after chronic "chemical" and "surgical" vagotomy and neostigmine treatments. The

http://dx.doi.org/10.5772/60099

comparative results are presented in the glandular stomach wall (Figure 19) and membranaceous stomach wall (forestomach) (Figure 20).

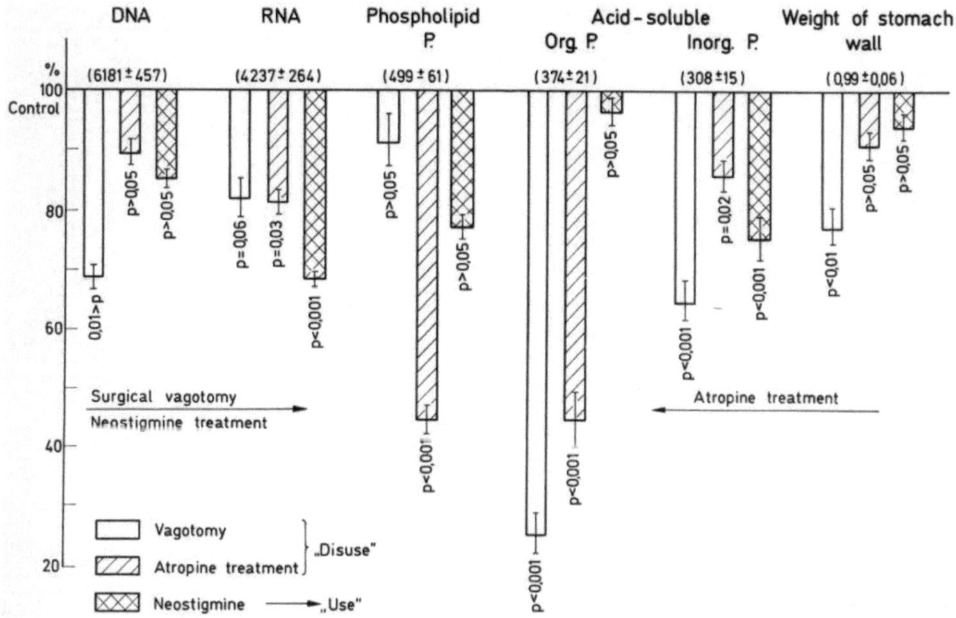

Figure 19. Biochemical backgrounds of "use" and "disuse" of cholinergic innervations on gastric tissue in the glandular stomach wall (in one month's treatment or surgical vagotomy). The results are expressed as means ± SEM in percentage values of control (sham-treated) rats. [Mózsik, Kiss, Jávor, Krausz, In: Gregor O., Riedl O. (eds) Modern Gastroenterology, Schattauer Verlag, Stuttgard, New York, 561–563, 1968 (with kind permission).]

The comparative biochemical results of "use" and "disuse" on cholinergic function of vagus nerve offered us the following conclusions:

1. The behavior of membranaceous and glandular stomach wall is not the same from the point of view of cholinergic innervation;

2. The "surgical," "chemical" vagotomy ("disuse") and neostigmine treatment ("use") can induce alterations in the stomach at the levels of general functions, biochemical reactions, ribonucleic and deoxyribonucleic acids;

3. The effects of "surgical" and "chemical" vagotomy are different at biochemical levels in the stomach wall. We assumed that the "surgical" vagotomy induces the alterations of DNA and RNA at first and that the alterations of other biochemical constituents follow these. On the contrary, DNA and RNA alternate only after the "chemical" vagotomy changes the metabolism of phosphorus components. The neostigmine can change the biochemism of the stomach wall similarly to the "surgical" vagotomy;

4. The "use" and "disuse" can involve the same biochemical alterations in the biochemism of the stomach in rats.

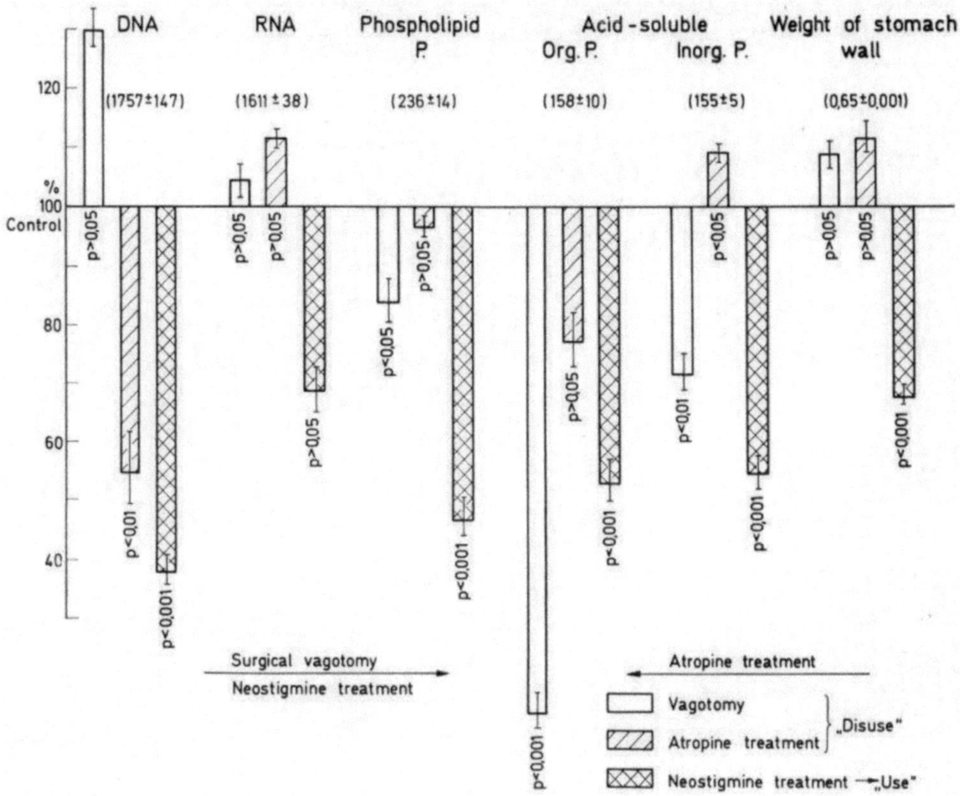

Figure 20. Biochemical backgrounds of "use" and "disuse" of cholinergic innervations at the biochemical level on gastric tissue in the membranaceous stomach wall (forestomach) (in one month's treatment or surgical vagotomy). The results are expressed as means ± SEM in percentage values of control (sham-treated) rats. [Mózsik, Kiss, Jávor, Krausz, In: Gregor O., Riedl O. (eds) Modern Gastroenterology, Schattauer Verlag, Stuttgard, New York, 561–563, 1968 (with kind permission).]

Author details

Gyula Mozsik[1*] and Imre Szabó[2]

*Address all correspondence to: gyula.mozsik@aok.pte.hu

1 First Department of Medicine, Medical and Health Centre, University of Pécs, Hungary

2 Associate Professor at the First Department of Medicine, University of Pécs, Hungary

Chapter 5

Membrane-Bound Atp-Dependent Energy System (A Short Historic View from Their Discoveries up to Now)

Gyula Mozsik and Imre Szabó

Additional information is available at the end of the chapter

http://dx.doi.org/10.5772/60100

This chapter is important and hence we felt that some general information has to be given globally on the physiological research, as we could not do a detailed study being interns in the medical department of the medical services.

We met the presentations of these new results at different times in our life, which modified our aims and possibilities in the research. On the other hand, our lifes gave to us a possibility to our scientific and methological konowledges to incorporate these new fields in our research field.

We have to learn the following:

1. Being clinicians, our main work is related to the medical service of patients' problems; however, we wanted to learn the main biochemical events in the gastrointestinal tract (in terms of development of mucosal damage and prevention);
2. We started with the biochemical examinations of gastric tissues from 1960s, and these new observations offered us to do the forthcoming steps in our research work;
3. We had time periods in our lifes when we had contamining (infecting) with basic and fruitful international research lines , when we had opportunities to participate and to work in research of different foreign countries (GyM in Norway in 1968–1969 and USA in 1985; IL Szabo in USA in 1999–2001);
4. We learned new research methods while working with foreign countries, and we tried to apply the new knowledge in researches that we did in our country (Hungary);
5. It was very clear that there is a big gap between the problems (results) of a basic research and clinical practice; however, we wanted to understand the main common problems in the basic research and in clinical science;

6. We had many ethical and medical problems in doing biochemical observations in the gastrointestinal resecates of human GI tract in patients with peptic ulcer who underwent surgical interventions owing to their primary disease;

7. We participated in the different international forums of GI research (as established persons, future leaders, organizers and responsible persons).

Our main lines of research series of international conferences are as follows:

a. An international series of international conferences [International Conference of Experimental Ulcer (from 1970 to 1994), International Conference on Ulcer Research (from 1994 to 2000) and International Conference on Gastrointestinal Research (from 2000)] has been internationally established at Copenhagen (Denmark) – in connection with Fourth World Congress of Gastroenterology – in 1970. Thereafter, different international conferences were organized in different countries of different continents (Copenhagen, Denmark, 1970; Cologne, Germany, 1972; Parádfürdő, Hungary, 1976; Tokyo, Japan, 1980; Boston, USA, 1985; Jerusalem, Israel, 1988; Berlin, Germany, 1991; Kyoto, Japan, 1994; Hong Kong, China, 1997; Budapest-Pécs, Hungary, 2000; Dubrovnik, Croatia, 2003; Osaka, Japan, 2006; Split, Croatia, 2009; Tokyo, Japan, 2012) (for details, see Mózsik, 2006b);

b. Another series of international symposiums was established in connection with main World Congresses of the International Union of Pharmacology (from 1984). The gastrointestinal section of International Union of Pharmacology was established at Montreal (Canada) in 1994 (IUPHAR GI Section); however, this series of the international symposiums started earlier (Pécs, Hungary, 1984; Pécs, Hungary, 1990; Pécs, Hungary, 1995; Sperlonga, Italy, 1996; Pécs, Hungary, 1998; Honolulu, USA, 2002; Kyoto, Japan, 2004; Osaka, Japan, 2006; Honolulu, Hawaii, USA, 2009; Tokyo, Japan, 2012) (for details, see Mózsik et al., 2006);

c. International Symposia on "Cell/Tissue Injury and Cytoprotection/Organoprotection" [Heidelberg, Germany, 1986; Boston, USA, 1989; Long Beach, CA, USA, 2000; 2006; Yalta (Crimea), Ukraine, 2008; Saint Petersburg, Russia, 2011; Honolulu, USA, 2012; Budapest, Hungary, 2014];

d. International Symposia on Gastrointestinal Cytoprotection (Pécs, Hungary, 1983; 1987; 1991; 1995, 2000);

e. International Symposia of the "International Brain-Gut Society" (Lake Arrowhead, Los Angeles, USA, 1988; Pécs, Hungary, 1990; Florence, Italy, 1993; Pécs, Hungary, 1995);

f. Interscience World Conferences on Inflammation [Antirheumatics, Analgesics, Immunomodulators (Venice, Italy, 1984; Monte Carlo, France, 1986; 1989; Geneva, Switzerland, 1995; 1998)].

8. This part of the book has been tried to give a short information on the different membrane-bound ATP-dependent energy systems with emphasizing the main problems in these

http://dx.doi.org/10.5772/60100

fields, however in briefly up to now (we had no these summaries of these studies in our mind during the time of our observations done in GI tract).

We have to emphasize that we have not done a very detailed study on the membrane-bound ATP-dependent energy systems; however, the results of our study (namely the study of the details of ATP splitting by different membrane-bound enzymes, Na^+–K^+-dependent ATPase and adenylate cyclase, represent different pathways of energy-liberating cellular events) offered us a very successful research possibility in our field. As ATP splitting results in energy liberation of cells, and the circumstances of the ATP resynthesis (by oxidative phosphorylation) confirmed the presence of tissue hypoxia in the GI mucosa under different (e.g., in the ulcerated or the damaged mucosal tissues) experimental and clinical circumstances.

The main lines of the studies on membrane-bound ATP-dependent energy systems were carried dominantly from GI tract, except for H^+–K^+-ATPase system (we did not participate in these studies), and hence we started with these studies in our field. Furthermore, these studies offered good possibility to understand the presence of tissue hypoxia (anoxia) during the development of mucosal damage, which was suggested as one of the main reasons (or consequences) of peptic ulcer.

Before the demonstrations of our biochemical results, we will give a very short summary of the main membrane-bound ATP-dependent energy systems (of course, not in the gastric mucosa).

5.1. Na^+-K^+dependent ATP-ase

This enzyme (other names: sodium–potassium adenosine triphosphatase, Na^+/K^+ pump, sodium–potassium pump, sodium pump) is located in the plasma membrane of all animal cells. The Na^{+-}–K^+-ATPase enzyme pumps sodium out of the cells, while pumping potassium into the cells.

Active transport is responsible for cells containing relatively high concentrations of potassium ions but low concentrations of sodium ions. The mechanism responsible for this sodium-potassium pump moves these two ions in opposite directions across the plasma membrane. This was investigated by following the passage of radioactive ions across the plasma membrane of certain cells. It was found that the concentrations of sodium and potassium ions on the two sides of the membrane are independent, which suggests that the same carrier transports both ions. It is now known that the carrier is an ATPase and it pumps three sodium ions of the cell for every two potassium ions pumped in.

The sodium–potassium pump was discovered in the 1950s (Skou, 1957) by Jens Christian Skou (Department of Physiology, Aarhus University, Denmark), who was awarded Nobel Prize in chemistry in 1997 (http://nobelprize.org/chemistry/laureates/1997/index.html). It marked an important step forward in our understanding of how ions get into and out of cells, and it is particularly significant for excitable cells such as nervous cells, which depend on this pump for responding to stimuli and transmitting impulses (Skou, 1965).

5.1.1. Schematic morphological bases of sodium-potassium pump (Na^+-K^+-dependent adenosine triphosphatase enzyme)

The Na^+–K^+-ATPases belong to the P_2 class and specifically to the P_{2c} subclass of ATPases. These ATPases are composed of two subunits (α and β). The α-subunit (about 113 kD) binds ATP and both Na^+ and K^+ ions and contains the phosphorylation sites typical of the P-type ATPases. The autophosphorylation site is the P domain. The P-type ATPases are also subject to additional phosphorylation events via other kinases. The smaller β-subunit (about 35-kD glycoprotein) is absolutely necessary for activity of the complex. It appears to be critical in facilitating the plasma membrane localization and activation of the α-subunit.

Several isoforms of both α- and β-subunits have been identified that exhibit different kinetic parameters and tissue distribution. There are four α-subunit genes and three β-subunit genes in humans. The α_1 isoform is the predominant form and is ubiquitously expressed. The α_2 isoform is primarily expressed in muscle tissues (skeletal, smooth and cardiac) as well as in adipose tissue, brain and lungs. The α_3 isoform is expressed primarily in the heart and neurons. The α_4 isoform is only expressed in the testes. The β_1 isoform is ubiquitously expressed and is associated with the α-subunit in the ubiquitously expressed α_1 β_1 Na^+–K^+-ATPase complex. There are many more detailed parts and interactions of Na^+–K^+-ATPase discovered and proved in the last decades (http://themedicalbiochemistrypage.org/membranes.php; Morth et al., www.nature.com/reviews/molcellbio 12:60–70, 2011).

5.1.2. Main functions of Na^+-K^+-ATPase

The Na^+–K^+-ATPases help to maintain resting potential and regulate cellular volume (Hall and Guyton, 2006). It also functions as signal transducer/integrator to regulate the mitogen-activated protein kinase (MARK) pathway, mitochondrial reactive oxygen species (ROS) as well as intracellular calcium. In most animal cells, the Na^+–K^+-ATPase is responsible for about 1/5 of the cell's energy expenditure, meanwhile, for neurons, the Na^+–K^+-ATPase can be responsible for up to 2/3 of the energy expenditure (Howard et al., 2012).

5.1.2.1. Resting potential

In order to maintain the cell membrane potential, cells keep a low concentration of sodium ions and high levels of potassium within the cell (intracellular). The sodium–potassium pump moves three sodium ions out and moves two potassium ions in, thus in total removing one positive-charge carrier from the intracellular space.

5.1.2.2. Transport

Export of sodium from the cell provides the driving force for several secondary active transporters, membrane transport proteins, which import glucose, amino acids and other nutrients into the cell by the use of sodium gradient.

Another important task of the Na^+–K^+-pump is to provide a Na^+ gradient that is used by certain carrier processes. In the gut, sodium is transported out of the reabsorbing cell on the blood

http://dx.doi.org/10.5772/60100

(intestinal fluid) side via the Na^+–K^+-pump, whereas, on the reabsorbing (luminal) side, the Na^+-glucose symporter uses the created Na^+ gradient as a source of energy to import both Na^+ and glucose, which is far more efficient than simple diffusion. Similar processes can be found and located in the renal tubular system.

5.1.2.3. Controlling cell volume

Failure of the Na^+–K^+ pumps can result in swelling of the cell. A cell's osmolarity is the sum of the concentrations of the various ion species and many proteins and other organic compounds inside the cell. When this is higher than the osmolarity outside of the cell, water flows into the cell through osmosis. This can cause the cell to swell up and lyze. The Na^+–K^+ pump helps to maintain the right concentrations of ions. Furthermore, when the cell begins to swell, this automatically activates the Na^+–K^+ pump.

Within the last decade, many independent laboratories have demonstrated that, in addition to classical ion transporting, this membrane protein can relay extracellular ouabain-binding signaling into the cell through regulation of protein tyrosine phosphorylation. The downstream signals through ouabain-triggered protein phosphorylation events include activation of the mitogen-activated protein kinase (MARK) signal cascades, mitochondrial reactive oxidative species (ROS) production, as well as activation of phospholipase C (PLC) and inositol triphosphate (IP3) receptor (IP3R) in different intracellular compartments (Yuan et al., 2005).

Protein–protein interactions play a very important role in Na^+–K^+ pump-mediated signal transduction (e.g., Na^+–K^+ pump interacts directly with Scr, a non-receptor tyrosine kinase) to form a signaling receptor complex (Tian et al., 2006). Scr kinase is inhibited by Na^+–K^+ pump, while, upon ouabain binding, the Scr kinase domain will be released and then activated. Based on this scenario, NaKtide, a peptide Scr inhibitor derived from the Na^+–K^+ pump, was developed as a functional ouabain-Na^+–K^+ pump-mediated signal transduction (Li et al., 2009; Forrest et al., 2012; Cannon, 2004; Calderon et al., 2011; Young et al., 2008).

5.1.3. Main steps of mechanism

The following main steps are involved in the mechanism:

- The pump, while binding ATP, binds three intracellular Na^+ ions (Hall and Guyton, 2006);
- ATP is hydrolyzed, leading to phosphorylation of the pump at a highly conserved aspartate residue and subsequent release of ADP;
- A conformational change in the pump exposes the Na^+ ions to the outside. The phosphorylated form of the pump has a low affinity for Na^+ ions, so they are released;
- The pump binds two extracellular K+ ions. This causes the phosphorylation of the pump, reverting it to its previous state, transporting the K+ ions into the cells;
- The unphosphorylated form of the pump has a higher affinity for Na^+ ions than K^+ ions, so two bound K^+ ions are released. ATP binds and the process starts again.

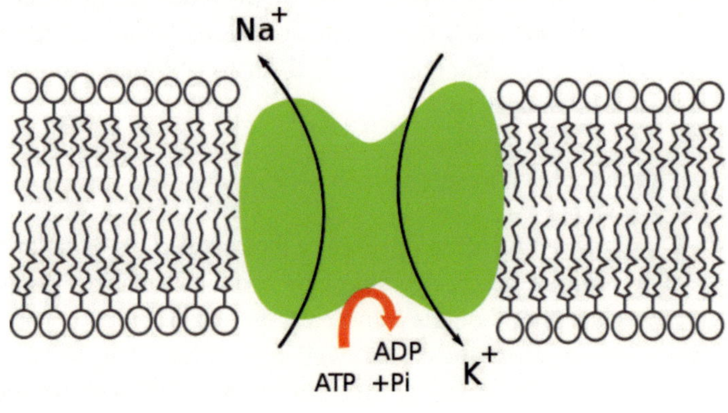

Figure 21. Schematic representation of the sodium pump (Na^+–K^+ ATPase): flow of ions (http://enzyme.expasy.org/EC/3.6.3.9).

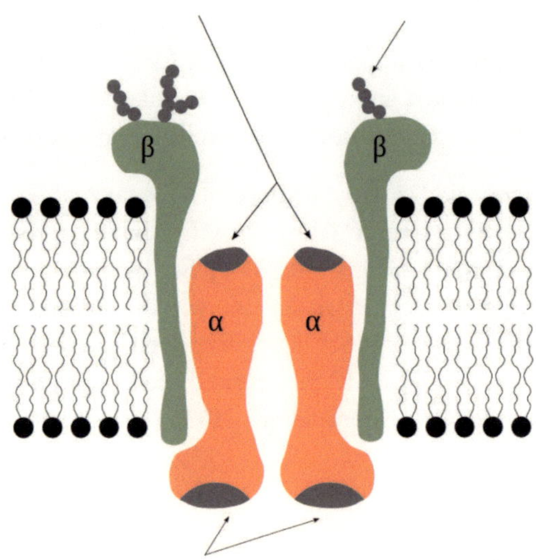

Figure 22. Schematic representation of the sodium pump (Na^+–K^+ ATPase): alpha and beta units (http://enzyme.expasy.org/EC/3.6.3.9).

The function of Na+–K+ pump can be regulated endogenously and exogenously.

The Na^+–K^+ pump is upregulated by cyclic adenosine monophosphate (cAMP) (Bunnier 2008). Thus, substances causing an increase in cAMP level upregulate the Na^+–K^+ ATPase. These include the ligands of the G_s-coupled GPCRs. In contrast, the substances causing a decrease in cAMP downregulate the Na^+–K^+-ase. These include the ligands of G_i-coupled GPCRs.

The ouabain (as cardiac glycoside) inhibits the Na^+–K^+ ATPase activity. The prove the presence of ouabain inhibition of different preparates of plasma membranes was one of the most criteria to indicate presence a good Na^+-K^+-dependent ATPase.

http://dx.doi.org/10.5772/60100

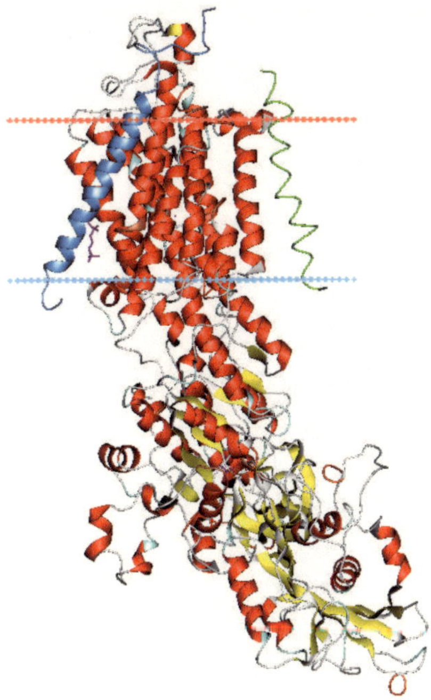

Figure 23. Schematic representation of the sodium pump (Na^+–K^+ ATPase), E2-P_i state. Calculated hydrocarbon boundaries of the lipid bilayer are shown as blue (intracellular) and red (extracellular) planes (http:// enzyme.expasy.org /EC/3.6.3.9).

5.2. The gastric H^+- K^+-ATP-ASE

The gastric hydrogen potassium ATPase or H^+/K^+-ATPase is the proton pump of the stomach and hence it is the enzyme primarily responsible for the acidification of the stomach (acid secretion) (Potassium Hydrogen ATPase (https://www.nlm.nih.gov/cgi/mesh/2011/MB_cgi? mode= &term=Potassium +Hydrogen+ ATPase).

The H^+–K^+- ATPase is found in the parietal cells, which are highly specialized epithelial cells located in the inner cell lining of the stomach called gastric mucosa. Parietal cells process an extensive secretory membrane system and the H^+–K^+-ATPase is the major protein constituent of these membranes.

The enzyme that keeps the stomach at pH 0.6:

- The parietal cells of the gastric mucosa (lining of the stomach) have an external pH of 7.4;
- H^+–K^+-ATPase pumps protons from these cells into the stomach (using energy of ATP) to maintain a pH difference across a single plasma membrane of 6.6;
- This is the largest known transmembrane gradient in eukaryotic cells.

5.2.1. The gastric H^+-K^+-ATPase can be characterized by the followings

- H^+–K^+-ATPase is similar in many respects to Na^+–K^+-ATPase and Ca^{2+}-ATPase;

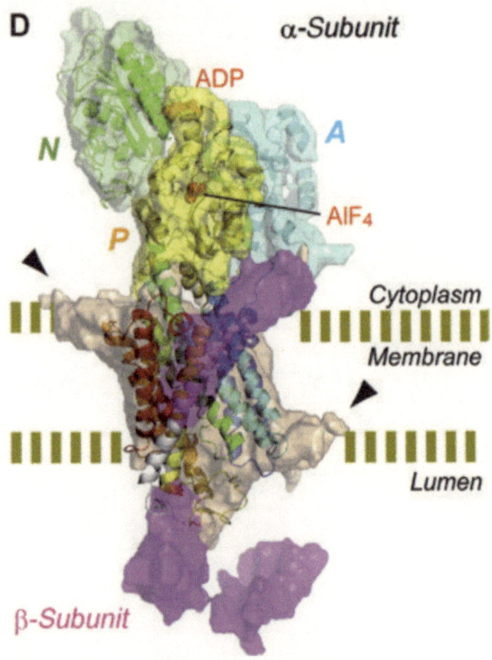

Figure 24. Schematic surface representation of gastric H^+–K^+-ATPase $\alpha\beta$-protomer with the fit homology model in ribbon representation. Color code of the density map: N domain, green; A domain, cyan; P domain, yellow; TM domain of the α-subunit, wheat; β-subunit, magenta. Color code of the homology model: N, A and P domains have the same color as the density map; TM helices M1–M10 of the α-subunit, gradual change from M1 (blue) to M10 (red); TM helix of β-subunit, white. The dotted lines indicate the probable position of the lipid head group and result in total thickness of approximately 35 Å, which is based on the densities protruding perpendicular from the TM domain (arrowheads). The bound ADP and AlF_4 molecules are shown as red sphere.

- All three enzymes form covalent E–P intermediates (P-type pumps);
- All three have similar sequences for the large (α) subunit;
- All three are involved in active transport.

The H^+–K^+-ATPase is a heterodimeric protein, the product of two genes. The gene ATP4A encodes the H^+–K^+-ATPase α-subunit and is about 1000 amino acid protein that contains the catalytic sites of enzyme and forms the pore through the cell membrane that allows the transport of ions.

The gene ATP4B encodes the β-subunit of the H^+–K^+-ATPase, which is about 300-amino acid protein with a 36 –amino acid N-terminal cytoplastic domain, a single transmembrane domain and a highly glycosylated extracellular domain. The H^+–K^+-ATPase β-subunit stabilizes the H $^+$–K^+-ATPase α-subunit and is required for function of the enzyme. It also appears to contain signals that direct the heterodimer to membrane destinations within the cell, although some of these signals are subordinate to signals found in H^+–K^+-ATPase α-subunit.

The H^+–K^+-ATPase is a member of the P-type ATPase superfamily, a large family of related proteins that transport ions, usually cations, across biological membranes of nearly all species.

http://dx.doi.org/10.5772/60100

The H^+–K^+-ATPase transports one hydrogen ion (H^+) from the cytoplasm of the parietal cell in exchange for potassium (K^+) retrieved from the gastric lumen. As an ion pump, the H^+–K^+-ATPase is able to transport ions against a concentration gradient using energy derived from the hydrolysis of ATP. Like all P-type ATPases, a phosphate group is transformed from adenosine triphosphate (ATP) to the H^+–K^+-ATPase during transport cycle. This phosphate transfer powers a conformational change in the enzyme that helps drive ion transport (Yao and Forte, 2003; Kühlbrandt, 2004; Dunbar and Caplan, 2001; Sachs et al., 1995) (http://www.mlm.nih.gov/cgi/mesh/2011/MB_cgi?mode=&term=Potassium+Hydrogen+ATPase).

The Na^+–K^+-ATPase and H^+–K^+-ATPase indicate some similarities in the structural building of these enzymes; however, they can be separated from each other by using immunological methods (Stoll and Berglinch, 1987; Sachs, 1987; Chang et al., 1977; Faller et al., 1982; Ganser and Forte, 1973; Lee et al., 1974; 2001; Maclennan et al., 1985; Saccomani et al., 1979 a, b; Sachs, 1977; Sachs et al., 1972; 1980; 1995; Shull et al., 1985; Koenderink et al., 1999; Asano et al., 2003).

5.3. Adenylate cyclase

5.3.1. Short historic background

Sutherland (1951) studied how the hormone epinephrine (adrenaline) signals to regulate the degradation of glycogen to glucose in the liver, thereby increasing glucose output into the blood, so that an organism can respond to stress. He worked alongside future Nobel Prize winners Edmond Fishers and Edwin Krebs, who demonstrated that adenosine triphosphate (ATP) and magnesium were required for phosphorylase activation. Sutherland (1953) agreed to be the chairman of the pharmacology department of Case Western Reserve University in Cleveland and was joined by Theodore R. Rall, "marking the beginning of a long and fruitful period of collaboration between us" [Sutherland EW. Studies on the mechanism of hormone. Science 177: 401–408, 1972 (Lecture delivered 11 December 1971 when he received the Nobel Prize in Physiology or Medicine)]. Sutherland and Rall discovered that epinephrine works by stimulating another chemical messenger, the enzyme glycogen phosphorylase, to begin the sugar-releasing process in the cells (Henion and Sutherland, 1955). This stimulation occurs by means of an intermediary that Sutherland called it the "second messenger," which he identified as a nucleotide and named cyclic AMP (Sutherland et al., 1957; Sutherland and Rall, 1957; Rall and Sutherland, 1957; 1958; Butcher and Sutherland, 1962; 1965; Klainer et al., 1962; Murad et al., 1962). As early as 1960, Sutherland suggested that cyclic AMP acts as a "second messenger" for other hormones as well (Sutherland and Rall, 1958) (for other summaries, see Butcher, 1966; Sutherland, 1962; Sutherland and Rall, 1960; Sutherland et al., 1962; Sutherland and Robison, 1966; Andrási, 1997).

Practically at the same time, the discovery of cyclic 3’-5’-AMP appeared in the organ pharmacology (Sutherland et al., 1965; 1968).

The adenylate cyclase is an enzyme with key regulatory roles in essentially all cells. It is the most polyphyletic known enzyme: six district classes have been described, all catalyzing the same reaction, but representing unrelated gene families with no known sequence or structural homology (Class I AC, Class II AC, Class III AC, Class IV AC, Class V AC and Class VI AC).

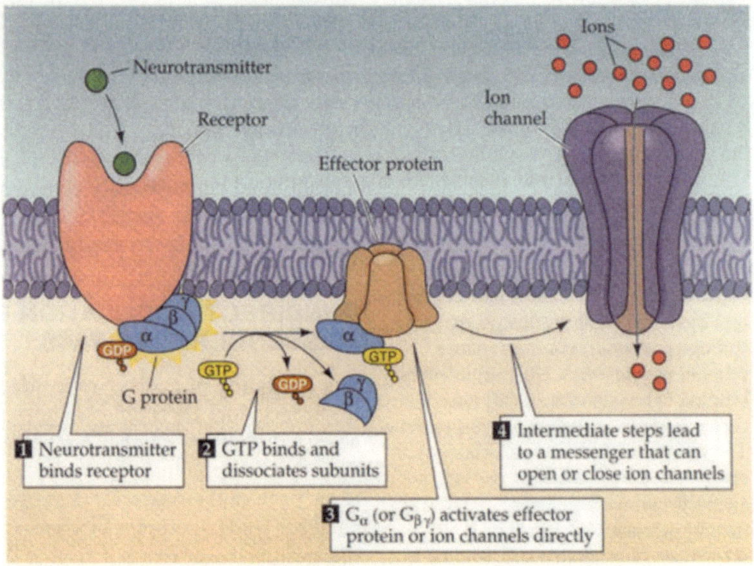

Figure 25. Schematic representation of adenylate cyclase location in the plasma membrane and main steps of intracellular regulatory pathways (http://www.cs.stedwards.edu/chem/Chemistry/ CHem43/).

The Classes AC I (*E. coli*), II (Bacillus anthracis and Bordetella pertussis), IV (Aeromonas hydrophyla, Yersinia pestis), V and VI (Prevotella ruminicola and Rhizobium etli) are present in different bacteria. The best-known AC class is class III or AC-III (Roman numerals are used for classes). The AC-III occurs widely in eukaryotes and has important roles in many human tissues.

All classes of AC catalyze the conversion of ATP to 3′,5′-cyclic adenosine monophosphate (cAMP) and pyrophosphate. Divalent cations (usually Mg^{2+}) are generally present in the enzymatic mechanism. The cAMP produced by AC then serves as regulatory signal via specific cAMP-binding proteins, either transcription factors or other enzymes (e.g., cAMP-dependent kinases).

Most AC-IIIs are integral membrane proteins involved in transducing extracellular signals into intracellular responses. A Nobel Prize in physiology (medicine) was awarded to Earl W. Sutherland (Department of Physiology, Vanderbilt University, Nashville, TN, USA) in 1971 for discovering the key role of AC-III in human liver, where adrenaline directly stimulates AC to mobilize stored energy in the "fight or flight" response (Robinson GA, Butcher RW, Sutherland EW: Cyclic AMP. Academic Press, New York and London, 1971) (two papers published by myself – Mozsik G.: Eur. J. Pharmacol 7: 319, 1969 and in 9: 107, 1970 – were cited by the authors in this book).

The effect of adrenaline is via a G protein-signaling cascade, which transmits chemical signals from outside the cell across the membrane to the inside of the cell (cytoplasm). The outside signal (in this case, adrenaline) binds to a receptor, which transmits a signal to the G protein,

http://dx.doi.org/10.5772/60100

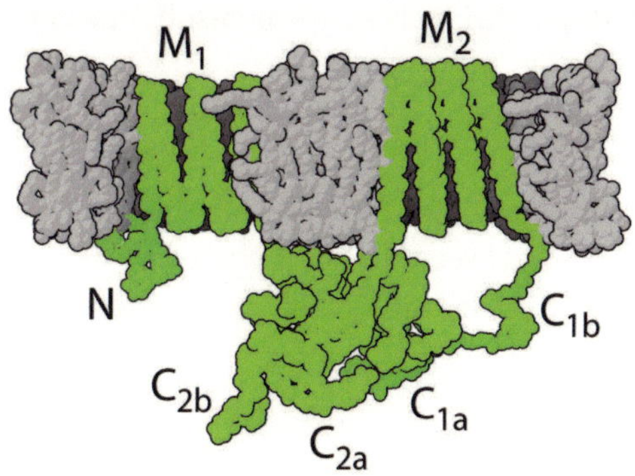

Figure 26. Schematic representation of the structure of adenylate cyclase enzyme (http://enzyme. expasy.org/EC/ 4.6.1.1).

which transmits a signal to adenylate cyclase, which transmits a signal by converting adenosine triphosphate (ATP) to cyclic adenosine monophosphate (cAMP). Cyclic AMP is known as the so-called "second messenger" (Reece and Campbell, 2002).

Adenylate cyclases are often activated or inhibited by G proteins, which are coupled to membrane receptors, and thus can respond to hormonal or other stimuli. Following the activation of adenylate cyclase, the resulting cAMP acts as a second messenger by interacting with and regulating other proteins, such as protein kinase A and cyclic nucleotide-gated ions channels.

AC-III structure:

Most class-III adenylate cyclases are transmembrane proteins with 12 transmembrane segments. The protein is organized with six transmembrane segments, the C1 cytoplasmic domain, another six membrane segments and then a second cytoplasmic domain called C1 and C2 regions.

The C1a and C2a sub-domains are homologous and form an intracellular "dimmer" that forms the active site.

There are ten known isoforms of adenylate cyclases in mammals: ADCY1, ADCY2, ADCY3, ADCY4, ADCY5, ADCY6, ADCY7, ADCY8, ADCY9 and ADCY10. These are sometimes called as AC1, AC2, etc., and sometimes Roman numerals are used for these isoforms that all belong to the overall AC class III. They differ mainly in how they are regulated, and are differentially expressed in various tissues throughout mammalian development.

Adenylate cyclase AC-III regulation:

Adenylate cyclase is dually regulated by G proteins (Gs stimulating activity and Gi inhibiting activity) and forskolin, as well as other isoform-specific effectors:

Isoforms III, V and VIII are also stimulated by Ca^{2+} /calmodulin;

Isoforms I and VI are inhibited by Ca2+ in a calmodulin-independent manner;

Isoforms II, IV and IX are stimulated by beta–gamma-subunits of the G protein;

Isoforms I, V and VI are most clearly inhibited by Gi, while other isoforms show less dual regulation by the inhibitory G protein.

Soluble AC (sAC) is not a transmembrane form and is not regulated by G proteins or forskolin, instead it acts as a bicarbonate/pH sensor. It is anchored at various locations within the cell and, with phosphodiesterases, forms local cAMP-signaling domain

[(http://www.nlm.nih.gov/cgi/mesh/2011/MB_cgi?mode=&term=Adenylate +cyclase) (http://proteopedia.org/wiki/index.php/Adenylyl_cyclase)].

5.4. Sodium-pump and second messenger system in the gastrointestinal mucosa

5.4.1. Short personal background

After taking short reviews on these biochemical problems in the nature of living cells, we faced a unique situation, when one of us (GyM) received a fellowship possibility in the Department of Pharmacology, University of Blindern, Oslo, in 1968–1969. We encountered these problems in this Department. Furthermore, I worked together with associate professor Ivar Øye, who spent 4 years in the Vanderbilt University (Department of Physiology) and worked together with Professor Sutherland on the problems of cyclic AMP.

After returning home (Norway) from USA, Ivar Øye wanted to do his research in the field of cardiac tissues. He wanted to obtain "plasma membrane" materials, and he wanted to use the "membrane materials" for the study of pharmacological regulation of cyclic AMP transformation in the heart muscles. I was moved to this Department at that time, and I had to receive the critically good evaluation of action of these drugs, all of those were able to inhibit the preparations of "membrane materials" from the heart.

I had some methodological knowledge gained from our earlier biochemical studies of the stomach. However, my new scientific work offered a new challenge in the gastrointestinal mucosal research.

Furthermore, I had some other affinities to enter into this research field, which are as follows:

a. We earlier mentioned that we were not able to understand and explain the results of clinical pharmacology in patients with peptic ulcer. This is because most of the researchers emphasized the key role of vagus nerve (by the increase of gastric acid secretion); thereby the application of various inhibitory drugs was thought to be reasonable in terms of decrease of gastric acid production. However, if we evaluated critically the actions of these drugs, we had to learn that these drugs are able to inhibit the active metabolism in the gastric tissues. Consequently, we can explain the beneficial effects of these drugs on the healing of peptic ulcer (which was explained by impaired tissue metabolism).

We concluded that we have to do some change in paradigm of the peptic ulcer research. These facts and suggestions led us to study the biochemisms in the gastrointestinal mucosa;

http://dx.doi.org/10.5772/60100

b. Many neural, hormonal (and pharmacological) factors, discovered absolutely new mechanisms; later, the immunological events could be collected in participation of peptic ulcer disease. Practically, the researchers studied the influences (action) of one or two factors (especially HCl and pepsin secretion, mucus secretion, bicarbonate secretion, prostaglandins, scavengers and antacids, and their different actions) on the stomach (gastrointestinal tract) in respect to development and protection (healing) of peptic ulcer disease. The results of these observations reflect only indirectly to the gastrointestinal tract.

Besides these results, we were uninformed on the biochemical changes in the gastrointestinal tract in time of gastric acid secretion and mucosal damage versus mucosal protection;

c. We wanted to study the biochemism of gastrointestinal tract, and we suggested that the final results (and summary) of different etiological factors can modify the functions of cells in the gastrointestinal tract. The blood supply was a remarkable extracellular factor; however, the changes in the blood flow also produce significant cellular biochemical changes in the target organ;

d. A general biochemical approach to study the biochemisms was built up in animal experiments from 1967. Our biochemical methodologies gave absolutely new insight into the biochemism of the gastrointestinal tract.

These biochemical observations were done dominantly on pylorus-ligated rats (as in an acute animal model). One of the most surprising results was to note that similar biochemical changes were detected in both the rumen and glandular parts (Mózsik et al., 1967 a, b). These results led us to study the changes in both the parts of the rat stomach after chronic "surgical vagotomy," chronic atropine treatment and cholinesterase (neostigmine) inhibitor treatments (for details, refer sections 4.3.1.–4.3.3 of Chapter 4). From the evaluation of the results of clinical pharmacological studies, we conducted biochemical observations in rats after cessation of drug (atropine, cholinesterase inhibitor) treatments.

The evaluation of these biochemical results in rats led us to understand some main lines of cellular biochemistry (cytoplasm, nucleic acids):

a. They were reversible in rat gastric tissues;

b. They were irreversible also.

The first one accepted the metabolic changes in biochemistry and the second one accepted the metabolic changes in genetic field (nucleic acids). These reversible and irreversible lines in the biochemical changes especially can be seen during the time of chronic "use" and "disuse" of vagus nerve. In some observations, we studied the changes of tissue levels of ATP, ADP (Mózsik et al., 1970a) and base alterations of nucleic acids in the stomach wall after a chronic atropine treatment (Mózsik et al., 1969b).

The results of these observations opened our eyes to start new observations with the main cellular functions of cells;

c. The international discoveries with membrane-bound ATP-dependent energy systems left a great impression and offered new possibilities to understand the regulations of ATP splitting and its resynthesis in the cells of the gastrointestinal tract;

d. There was no question that energy liberation exists in all of the functions of membrane-bound ATP-dependent enzymes (Na^+–K^+-dependent ATPase, H^+–K^+-ATPase, adenylate cyclase). However, the presence of these enzymes was not known in 1968;

e. In my works (in the Department of Pharmacology of Oslo University, Norway), the biochemical presence of Na^+–K^+-ATPase was used in my works to prove clearly that we really work with "membrane preparates," and these preparates were used to study the functions of adenylate cyclase. It's true that my boos wanted to see and to study these steps in cardiac muscles; however, I used parallelly the gastric mucosa (earlier obtained in rats, later in human gastric resecates) (Mózsik and Øye, 1969), and we wanted to study the actions of different drugs (epinephrine, ouabain, NaF) on the adenylate cyclase. The NaF was used as the most powerful compound to stimulate the adenylase cyclase, because it inhibits the activity of all membrane ATPase activity (this fact is well known in the pertinent literature).

Therefore, consequently, I realized two important things during my study tour in Oslo (Norway), namely to prepare the adenylate cyclase from the crude "membrane materials" (from heart muscles and gastric mucosa) and the presence of Na^+–K^+-ATPase was used as a chemical marker for the plasma membrane.

We have to emphasize that the presence of neither Na+–K+-ATPase nor adenylate cyclase was known in animals and especially in humans;

f. I suggested that the functions of these enzymes can be modified by different drugs (not by only hormones) under different experimental conditions (including the animal experiments and human medical problems).

Author details

Gyula Mozsik[1*] and Imre Szabó[2]

*Address all correspondence to: gyula.mozsik@aok.pte.hu

1 First Department of Medicine, Medical and Health Centre, University of Pécs, Hungary

2 Associate Professor at the First Department of Medicine, University of Pécs, Hungary

Chapter 6

Actual Positions in the Research of Membrane-bound ATP-dependent ATP-ase Systems in the World in the Different Tissues and Gastrointestinal Mucosa (in 1968-69)

Gyula Mozsik and Imre Szabó

Additional information is available at the end of the chapter

http://dx.doi.org/10.5772/60101

During the close of the 1960s, two different workgroups dealt with the problems of active movements of cations across the cell membrane:

a. Skou (Skou, 1965; Albers, 1967; Askari, 1974; Schwartz et al., 1975; Glynn, 1964) indicated the existence of sodium–potassium pump located in the plasma membrane, which is responsible for the active movements of sodium and potassium. He clearly stated that: (a). this enzyme is located in the plasma membrane; (b) the activity of the enzyme located in plasma membrane can be enhanced by the combined application of sodium and potassium; (c) this enzyme splits the ATP located in the mitochondria into ADP in the presence of magnesium ion and (d) the activity of this enzyme can be specifically inhibited by the application of ouabain (Skou, 1965). The preparation of the membrane enzyme (sodium–potassium-dependent ATPase) was tried to prepare from the amphibian; frog-, rat-, rabbit- gastric mucosa without any success (Kasbekar and Durbin, 1965; Post and Albright, 1961; Sachs et al., 1972).

We used a special treatment for the preparation of plasma membrane and separation or centrifugation, which resulted in a "typical" sodium–potassium-dependent ATPase from the rat and human gastric mucosa (Mózsik and Øye, 1969).

b. Practically at the same time as the years up to the preparation of sodium–potassium-dependent ATPase (Butcher and Sutherland, 1962; Øye et al., 1964; Øye and Sutherland, 1966; Øye and Butcher, 1967 a, b) discovered another enzyme located in the plasma membrane, which spilled the ATP into 3′, 5′-cyclic AMP in the presence of magnesium

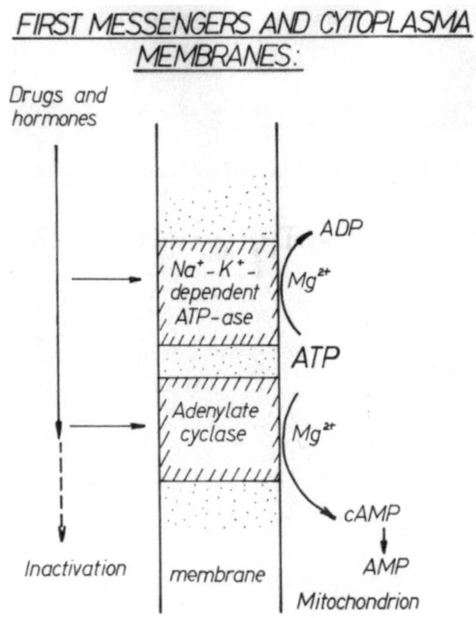

Figure 27. First (drugs, hormones) and second messenger systems located in the plasma membrane of cells. [Mózsik et al., Acta Medica Acad Sci Hung 36, 1–29, 1979 (with kind permission).]

ions (Butcher and Sutherland, 1962; Øye and Sutherland, 1966; Robinson et al., 1971; Sutherland and Rall, 1957; Butcher, 1966).

We were successful in preparing this enzyme from the human gastric mucosa (Mózsik and Øye, 1969).

It was exciting when we were able to detect the changes in different adenosine phosphates (adenosine triphosphate – ATP, adenosine diphosphate – ADP, adenosine monophosphate – AMP, cyclic 3′, 5′-adenosine monophosphate – cAMP) together with the changes in sodium–potassium-dependent ATPase and in adenylate cyclase activities (Figure 27).

We planned to carry out these types of observations under different experimental conditions (with and without drug administration, acute and chronic surgical and chemical vagotomy and with and without application of different necrotizing agents) in rats and patients with different gastric basal acid outputs (BAO) and maximal acid outputs (MAO), and the gastric antral, duodenal and jejunal mucosa around ulcer and the mucosal tissue samples without ulcer.

The energy liberation through the membrane-bound ATP-dependent energy systems (sodium–potassium pump and adenylate cyclase) can be detected well. The ATP–ADP transformation by sodium–potassium–ATPase enzyme releases 7.3 kcal/mol, while the ATP–cAMP transformation by adenylate cyclase results in 2 × 7.3 kcal/mL. Both the ADP–AMP and cAMP–AMP transformations release 7.3 kcal/mol (Figure 28).

http://dx.doi.org/10.5772/60101

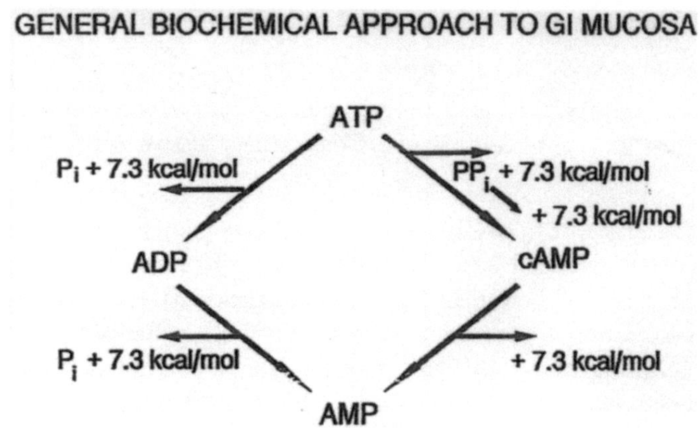

Figure 28. Pathways of energy liberation from ATP to ADP by membrane ATPase and from ATP to cAMP by adenylate cyclase located in the plasma membrane. The ATP–ADP transformation releases 7.3 kcal/mol, while ATP–cAMP transformation results in 2 × 7.3 kcal/mol. On the other hand, ADP–AMP and cAMP–AMP transformations produce 7.3 kcal/mol energy liberation. [Mózsik, Abdel Salam, Király, Morón, Nagy, Sütő, Tárnok, Jávor: in: Mózsik Gy., Nagy L., Király Á. (eds): Twenty Five Years of Peptic Ulcer Research in Hungary: From Basic Science to Clinical Practice.Akadémiai Kiadó, Budapest, pp. 159–170, 1997 (with kind permission).]

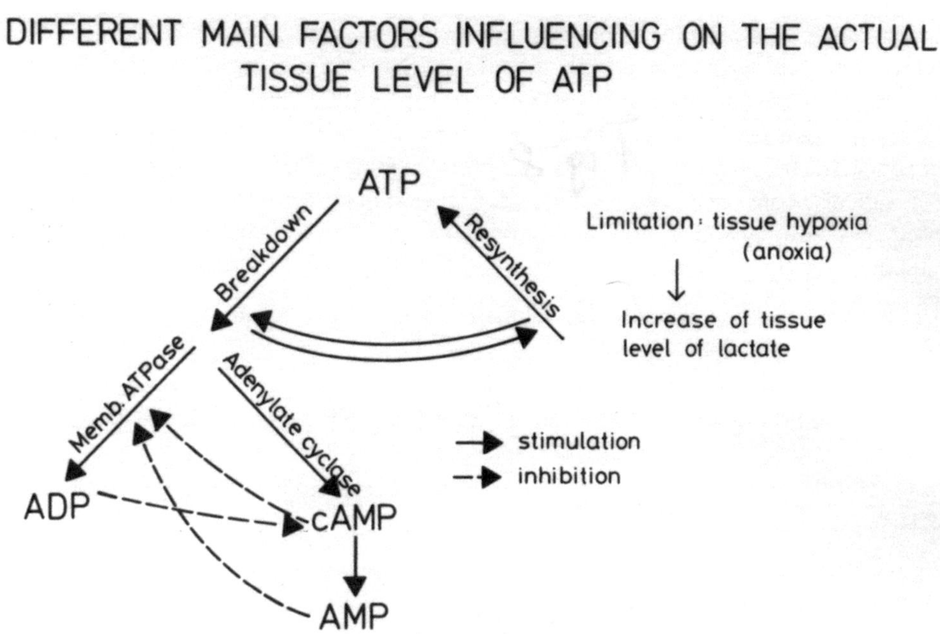

Figure 29. Different regulatory steps in the determination of actual levels of tissues of ATP. The tissue level of ATP is a consequence of ATP breakdown and ATP resynthesis. The limiting factor of ATP resynthesis by the pathway of oxidative phosphorylation is the presence of tissue hypoxia. The presence of tissue hypoxia can be proven biochemically by the increase of lactate levels in the tissue.

6.1. Materials and methods of experiments and human observations

The observations were carried out in CFY (Sprague-Dawley) (Gödöllő, Hungary) strain rats, weighing 180–210 g body weight and on the resecates of stomach and small intestine of patients who underwent gastric surgery because of unhealed ulcer disease (during 1970–1980).

The patients suffered from classical peptic ulcer disease (PUD) together with classical clinical symptoms (decreased appetite, feeling of dullness and pain in epigastrial region of the abdomen, pyrosis and impaired gastric emptying and retention syndrome). These patients presented in about one month before the surgical intervention. The presence of gastroduodenal ulcers were endoscopically diagnosed, and thereafter these patients received medical treatments (anticholinergic agents, later H_2 receptor antagonist and antacids for one month time period). The patients who did not heal during this time period were evaluated with the possibility of surgical interventions.

The indication of gastric surgery was given by physicians [with consultations between internists (gastroenterologists vs. surgeons) independently from us] on the resecates of stomach and small intestine (according to the method of Billroth II). A small group of patients underwent classical partial gastrectomy (according to the method of Billroth II) and jejunal ulcer was identified. The patients in this group were also treated medically (pharmacologically) for the same time period as mentioned earlier.

During the time of surgical intervention, the removals of stomach and small intestine were obtained immediately and these were cut into two parts from which one part was given for histological evaluation of resected tissues and the other part was immersed (after separation of mucosa and muscular layers) in liquid nitrogen and used for biochemical examinations. The mucosa specimens were also further separated from each other (depending on the distance of ulcer edge). The biochemical measurements from the mucosa specimens and muscular layers (independently from the number of tissue specimens) obtained from one patient were done (carried out) simultaneously dominantly on the same the as the surgical intervention was carried out.

The animal observations were carried out in both sexes of CFY-strain rats (the used methods are detailed in Section 4.2).

6.2. Membrane-bound ATP-dependent energy systems in the rat and human gastric mucosa

6.2.1. General characterization of membrane ATPase prepared from the rat and human gastric fundic mucosa

The method for preparation of membrane ATPase from the human gastric mucosa was published in 1969 (Mózsik and Øye, 1969; Mózsik et al., 1971 a, b; 1973 a, b; 1974 a, b, c, d; 1975 a, b; 1976 a, b). Figure 30 shows the typical characterization of membrane ATPase from the human gastric fundic mucosa. The membrane ATPase split the ATP into ADP *in vitro* incubation system in the presence of Mg^{2+} (Mg^{2+}-dependent), which can be enhanced by the combined application of Na^+ and K^+ (Mg^{2+}–Na^+–K^+-dependent ATPase), in liberation of inorganic phosphorus followed by the ATP splitting process. The total ATPase can be inhibited by the application of ouabain (g-strophanthin). The difference between the total (Mg^{2+}–Na^+–K

http://dx.doi.org/10.5772/60101

+-dependent) versus only Mg^{2+}-dependent ATPase is given as Na^+–K^+-dependent ATPase (Mózsik et al., 1978 a, b, c). This Na^+–K^+-dependent ATPase has been associated with the active movements of Na^+ and K^+ (Skou, 1967; Albers, 1967; Askari, 1974; Glynn, 1964).

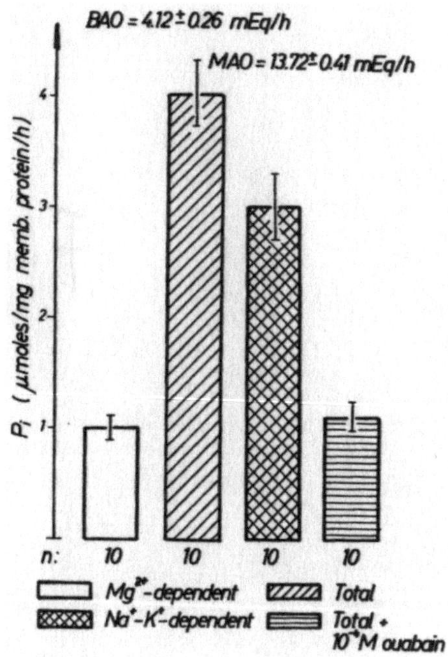

Figure 30. Biochemical characterization of membrane ATPase prepared from human gastric fundic mucosa. The membrane ATPase activity was measured by the liberation of inorganic phosphate from ATP produced by membrane ATPase *in vitro* incubation system in the presence of Mg^{2+}, Mg^{-2+}, Na^+ and K^+ (total ATPase). The difference between the total and only magnesium-dependent ATPase activity is equal to Na^+–K^+-dependent ATPase activity. The g-strophanthin (ouabain) is able to inhibit the Na^+–K^+-dependent ATPase (means ± SEM). [Mózsik et al.: Acta Physiol Scand Spec Suppl. 199–208; 1978 (with kind permission).]

There was a question whether there is any correlation between the neural regulation Andana +– K^+-dependent ATPase. A log-concentration dose–response curve for acetylcholine, prepared from the human gastric fundic mucosa, was identified (Csáky, 1969; Mózsik et al., 1978 a, b, c) (Figure 31).

6.2.2. Determination of affinity and intrinsic activity curves for the dugs modifying the Na^+-K^+-dependent ATPase activity obtained from rat and human gastrointestinal mucosa

The affinity and intrinsic activity curves were determined and calculated according to the method of Csáky (Csáky, 1969). The intrinsic activity (α) of ouabain was taken to be equal to 1.00. The values of pD_2 (dose necessary to produce 50% inhibition in affinity curves) and pA_2 (the dose necessary to produce 50% inhibition in the intrinsic curves) were calculated from affinity and intrinsic activity curves.

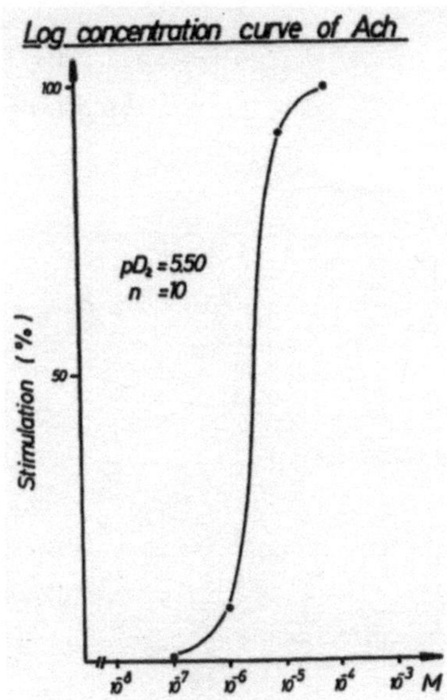

Figure 31. Log-concentration curve of acetylcholine (ACh) on the membrane ATPase prepared from the human gastric fundic mucosa. [Mózsik et al.: Acta Physiol Scand Spec Suppl 199–208; 1978 (with kind permission).]

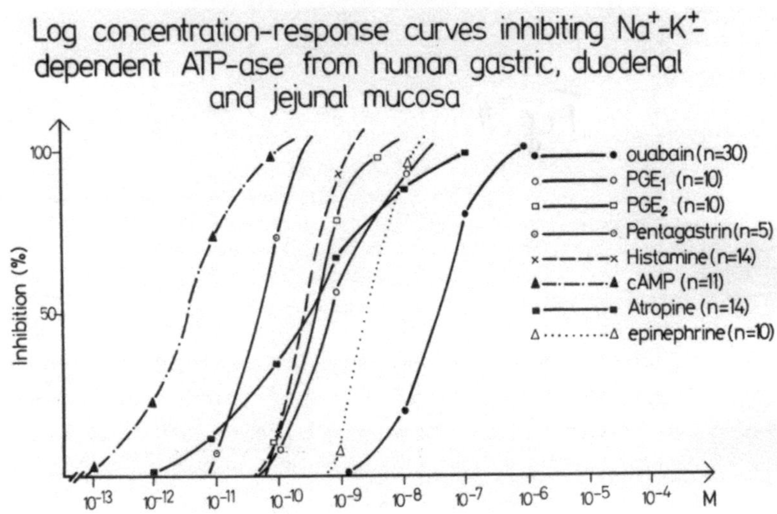

Figure 32. Dose–response curves for the drugs on the sodium–potassium-dependent ATPase prepared from human gastric, duodenal and jejunal mucosa (affinity curves). [Mózsik, Kutas, Nagy, Tárnok: Acta Medica Acad Sci Hung 36:459–466; 1979c (with kind permission).]

The dose–response curves (affinity curves) of the drugs were analyzed on the Na^+–K^+-dependent ATPase prepared from the human gastric fundic, duodenal and jejunal mucosa (Mózsik et al., 1979 a, b, c, d, e) (Figures 32–34).

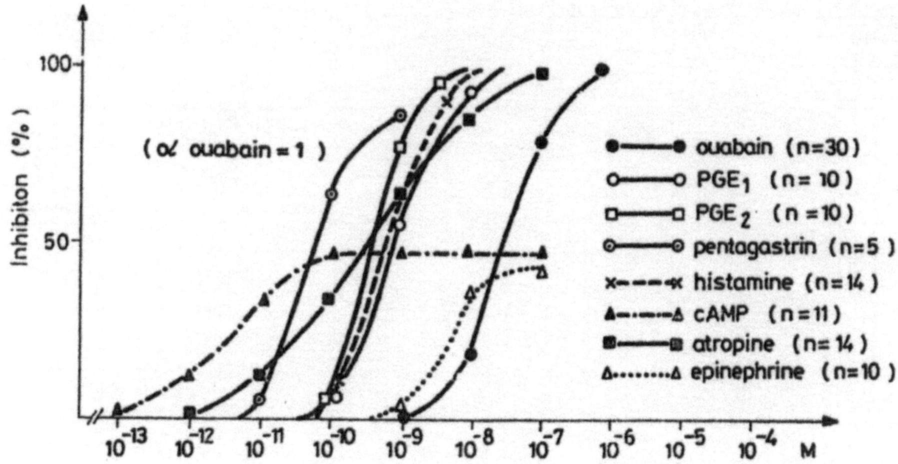

Figure 33. Dose–response curves for drugs inhibiting the Na^{+}–K^{+}-dependent ATPase prepared from the human gastric fundic mucosa. The intrinsic activity (α) of ouabain to Na^{+}–K^{+}-dependent ATPase system was taken to be equal to 1.00 and the effects of different drugs were compared with its effect; *n* indicates the number of patients. The values of intrinsic activities of drugs to Na^{+}–K^{+}-dependent ATPase system were calculated from the curves and presented in Table 3. [Mózsik, Kutas, Nagy, Tárnok: Acta Medica Acad Sci Hung 36:459–466, 1979c (with kind permission).]

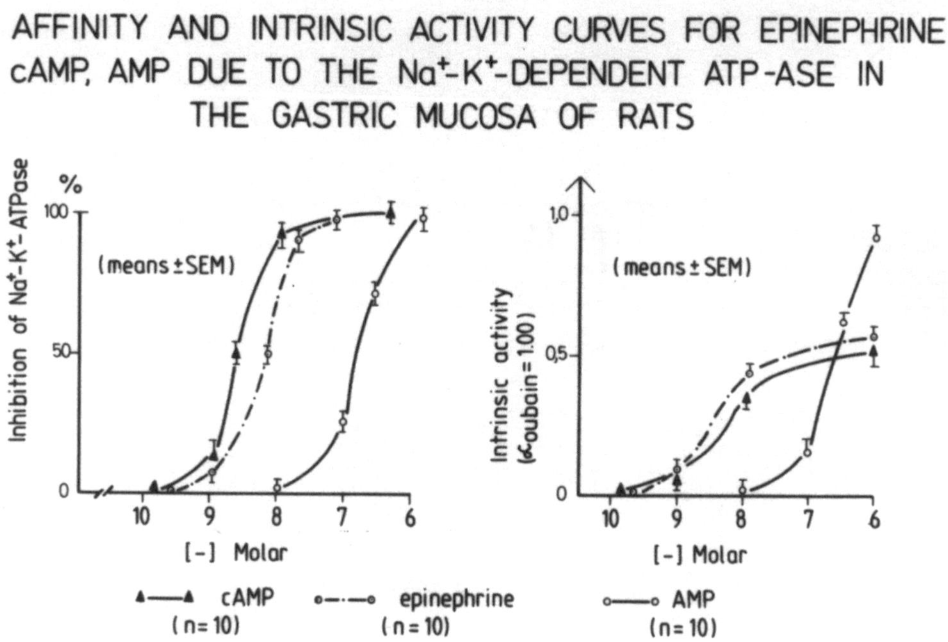

Figure 34. Affinity and intrinsic activity curves of epinephrine, cAMP and AMP on Na^{+}–K^{+}-dependent ATPase prepared from the rat gastric fundic mucosa. [Mózsik Gy, Garamszegi M, Jávor T, Nagy L, Patty I, Sütő G, Vincze Á: Ann N Y Acad Sci 597:264–281, 1990a (with kind permission).]

Drugs	Affinities	Intrinsic activities	
	(pD_2)	(α)**	(pA_2)
Atropine	9.50	1.00	9.50
Epinephrine	8.60	0.41	8.60
cAMP	11.30	0.48	11.30
PGE_1	9.30	1.00	8.30
PGE_2	9.45	1.00	9.45
Pentagastrin	10.55	0.87	10.55
Histamine	9.70	1.00	9.70
Ouabain	7.50	1.00	7.50

Table 26. Characterization of the actions of drugs inhibiting Na^+–K^+-dependent ATPases prepared from human fundic mucosa.* expressed in [-], ** α_{oubain}=1.00

The values of pD_2 and pA_2 were calculated from the measured affinity and calculated intrinsic activity curves (Table 26).

6.3. Adenylate cyclase preparation from the rat and human gastric fundic mucosa

The adenylate cyclase was originally and first prepared from the human gastric fundic mucosa (Mózsik, 1969b; Mózsik et al., 1970b). Similar observations and results were done and obtained from the rat fundic mucosa (Ruoff and Sewing, 1974; Salganik and Bersimbaev, 1976; Thompson et al.; 1977 a, b).

The fresh gastric mucosal tissues of rats and humans were put into 20 mL of ice-cold 0.25 M sucrose solution, and it was homogenized in the room temperature of 4°C, then centrifugation was done at 0°C with 2000 g for 20 minutes. The supernatant material was removed and the sediment was resuspended in 25 mL ice-cold glycil–glycin buffer solution (264 mg of glycil–glycin and 24.65 mg of $MgSO_4$ were immersed in 100 mL of distilled water, and its pH value was fixed at 7.8). The rehomogenization was done, and thereafter centrifugation was carried out with 2000 g value for 20 minutes at 0°C. The supernatant material was removed after centrifugation, and the sediment was resuspended in 20 mL glycil–glycin buffer solution. Two-milliliter samples from this sediment solution were put in other tubes and centrifuged with 2000 g for 10 minutes at 0°C. After this centrifugation, the supernatant material was removed and the sediment was resuspended in 150-μL glycin–glycin buffer solution and it was used for measurements of adenylate cyclase.

The incubation solution (150 μL of resuspended enzyme, 50 μL of tested compounds: H_2O, epinephrine, NaF, atropine, acetylcholine, 150 μL Tris–buffer, 50 μL C^{14}–ATP – 20–25 mC/mmol dissolved in Mg solution) was used for 10 minutes at 30°C temperature before the measurements of enzyme activity of adenylate cyclase. The enzyme activity was stopped after boiling for 3 minutes; however, before the heat treatment 20 μL H^3-cyclic 3′, 5′-adenosine monophosphate was added into incubated samples.

http://dx.doi.org/10.5772/60101

The ATP, ADP, cyclic AMP and AMP were separated from the 300 μL of incubated suspension by Dowex 50 ion exchange column (Krishna et al., 1968), and three peaks were obtained. The first peak contained the ATP and ADP, the second one the cyclic AMP and the third one the 5′-AMP. The other components (such as nucleotides, inorganic phosphate and cyclic 3′, 5′-AMP) were then precipitated by the treatment of $ZnSO_4$–$Ba(0H)_2$. After centrifugation of these samples, the supernatants were evaporated and thereafter the residue was immersed in 10 mLLof Bay's solution. The radioactivity of cyclic AMP was detected by liquid scintillation equicment (H. Pacard) of H^3 and C^{14} labelld cyclic 3′, 5′-AMP. The extent of the ATP—AMP transformation was given as ounts of C^{14} ounts of 100 H^3 (see Table 7) .

Examined compounds	Incubation time (min)	C^{14} / 100 H^3
1. H_20	0	12.36
2. H_20	10 (control)	23.96
2. Epinephrine (10^{-4} M)	10	28.43
4. NaF (10^{-2} M)	10	35.84
5. Atropine (10^{-4} M)	10	29.60
6. Acetylcholine (10^{-4} M)	10	21.52

Table 27. Testing of the effects of epinephrine, NaF, atropine and acetylcholine on the transformation of ATP into cyclic AMP by adenylate cyclase prepared from the human gastric mucosa (Mózsik, 1969a: PhD Dissertation of Pécs University, Hungary)

6.4. Feedback mechanism systems between the membrane-bound ATP-dependent energy systems in the gastrointestinal mucosa in rats and humans

6.4.1. Pharmacological regulatory mechanisms between the membrane ATPase (ATP – ADP transformation) and adenylate cyclase (ATP – cAMP transformation) prepared from the rat and human gastric fundic mucosa

The origin of the suggestion to existence of feedback system between the Na^+–K^+-dependent ATP and adenylate cyclase was created by me (GyM) based on the results of personal observations and after studying the actions of different drugs on these enzymes.

It was interesting to compare the effects of drugs on Na^+–K^+-dependent ATPase and adenylate cyclase activity from different "membrane fractions" under *in vitro* conditions (Table 28). The Na^+–K^+-dependent ATPase activity was inhibited by epinephrine, NaF and atropine (Mózsik,

Drugs	Na⁺-K⁺-dependent ATPase activity: Effects	Tissue specimens
Adrenaline	Inhibition (10^{-10} to 10^{-4} M)	rat heart rat gastric mucosa human gastric mucosa
NaF	Inhibition (10^{-3} to 10^{-2} M)	rat heart rat gastric mucosa human gastric mucosa
Atropine	Inhibiton (10^{-10} to 10^{-4} M)	rat heart rat gastric mucosa human gastric mucosa
Acetylcholine	No effect (10^{-10} to 10^{-4} M)	rat heart rat gastric mucosa human gastric mucosa

	Adenylate cyclase activity: Effecs	Tissue specimens	References to adenylate Cyclase
Adrenaline	Stimulation (10^{-7} to 10^{-4} M)	rat heart rat gastric mucosa human gastric mucosa	Murad et al., 1962 Mózsik, 1969a,b
NaF	Stimulation (10^{-3} to 10^{-2} M)	rat heart rat gastric mucosa human gastric mucosa erythrocyte	Sutherland et al., 1962 Mózsik, 1969a, b Øye and Sutherland, 1966
Atropine	Stimulation (10^{-5} to 10^{-4} M)	rat heart rat gastric mucosa human gastric mucosa	Murad et al., 1962a, b Mózsik, 1969
Acetylcholine	Inhibition (10^{-5} to 10^{-4} M) (30 %)	rat heart	Murad et al., 1962

Table 28. Effects of drugs used on Na^+–K^+-dependent ATPase and adenylate cyclase activity by different "membrane preparates" prepared from rat heart, rat and human gastric mucosa under *in vitro* conditions (Mózsik, 1969 a, b).

http://dx.doi.org/10.5772/60101

1969b), whereas the adenylate cyclase activity was stimulated by adrenaline (epinephrine) (Murad et al., 1962; KlainerCet al., 1962; Øye and Sutherland, 1966), NaF (Sutherland, t al., 1962; Øye and Sutherland, 1966) and by tropine (5 t 20 % aplied in 10^{-5} and 10^{-4} cocentrations) (Murd, Chal., 1962). The adenylate cyclase activity was inhibited by acetylcholine and acetyl-β-methylcholine (Murad, Chi, R 1962). Acetylcholine had no effect on Na^+—K^+-dependent APase activity (consequently, the ATP transformation into ADP is workeding wiout hinnceany trouble duringcholine's effect on Na^+—K^+-dependent ATPae).

When adenylate cyclase activity is studied in course particle preparations having high ATPase activity, the local concentration of ATP at the catalytic site of adenylate cyclase might be rate limiting for the reaction. An inhibition of Na^+–K^+-dependent ATPase by adrenaline, NaF and atropine might therefore apparently stimulate the adenylate cyclase activity (by the increase of ATP concentration). It was particularly interesting that NaF not only inhibited Na^+–K^+-ATPase activity, but also stimulated the adenylate cyclase activity more than other drugs. The inhibition of adenylate cyclase activity by acetylcholine is due to a decrease in local concentration of ATP caused by Na^+–K^+-dependent ATPase activity at the catalytic site of adenylate cyclase. The inhibitory effect of acetylcholine on adenylate cyclase activity was prevented by adding atropine in a concentration of 10^{-7} M leading to an inhibitory effect on Na^+–K^+-dependent ATPase; there was no effect of this concentration of atropine alone on the adenylate cyclase (Murad et al., 1962).

The inhibition caused by adrenaline and atropine was present in concentrations from 10^{-9} to 10^{-4} M (Mózsik, 1969 a, b), whereas the stimulation by adrenaline and atropine on adenylate cyclase activity was obtained by concentrations from 10^{-6} to 10^{-5} M (Klainer et al., 1962; Murad et al., 1962; Mózsik, 1969 a, b). Thus, *in vitro* Na^+–K^+-dependent (active transport) ATPase system was 100–1000 times more sensitive to drugs than the adenylate cyclase system.

The difference in sensitivity between the Na^+–K^+-dependent (transport) ATPase and adenylate cyclase activity, and the contradictory effects of drugs on them indicated the following:

1. The stimulatory effects by these drugs on adenylate cyclase activity is associated with blocking of Na^+–K^+-dependent ATPase activity;

2. The Na^+–K^+-dependent ATPase (transport) system and adenylate cyclase system can be separated.

A direct inhibitory effect of cyclic AMP and adenosine 5′-monophosphate (5′-AMP) of Na^+–K^+-dependent ATPase activity from human gastric mucosa was observed in a wide range of concentrations (Mózsik, 1970).The cyclic 3′, 5′-AMP and 5′-AMP are present in the cells as products of adenylate cyclase activity. The direct inhibition of Na^+–K^+-dependent (active transport) ATPase by cyclic 3′, 5′-AMP and 5′-AMP showed an antagonistic interrelationship between the adenylate cyclase system and the active transport ATPase system (Figure 35).

In the forthcoming years and thereafter, the tissue levels of ATP, ADP, cyclic AMP, AMP (adenine–adenosine) were measured *in vivo* conditions (in different human gastrointestinal diseases and under different animal experiments) directly from the gastrointestinal mucosal

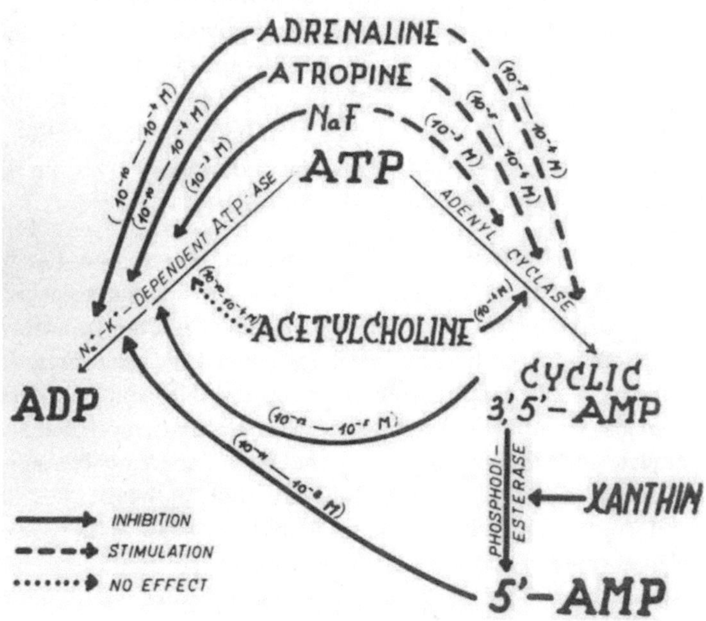

Figure 35. The summary of some feedback mechanisms of drugs with interrelationship between the active transport (Na^+–K^+-dependent ATPase) system and the adenylate cyclase prepared from rat and human gastric mucosa (Mózsik, 1969b). These types of observations were carried out under *in vitro* conditions (with kind permission).

tissues. However, the details of the above entioned hypothesis iere taken into account for the evaluation of the forthcoming observations.

These pharmacological regulatory functions were opposite ones on the Na^+–K^+-dependent ATPase and adenylate cyclase (Tables 28, 29). Generally, different drugs were able to modify the Na^+–K^+-dependent ATPase in lower molar concentrations than those in the adenylate cyclase concentrations. These results a priori suggested the existence of a complex feedback system, which could be modified by mediators, hormones and drugs.

6.4.2. Regulatory mechanisms between the tissues levels of ATP, ADP, cAMP and AMP in the intact rat gastric mucosa (in vivo studies)

The tissue levels of ATP, ADP and AMP were enzymatically (Boehringer Ingelheim, Germany); while the cAMP by RIA (Beckton, Dikinson, Orengeburg, USA) was measured. The protein content was measured by the method of Lowry et al. (1951) in the tissue concentration of ATP, ADP and AMP (except for cAMP which was expressed as pmol/mg) in nmol/mg protein. The ratio of ATP/ADP and the values of adenylate pool (ATP+ADP+AMP) were calculated. From the ATP, ADP, AMP and adenylate pool, the values of "energy charge"[(ATP +0.5 ADP)/(ATP+ADP+AMP)] were calculated according to the method of Atkinson's formula (1968). This value is theoretically 1 when all adenosine compounds are in phosphorylated form, and its value is 0 when all adenosine nucleotides are in dephosphorylated form.

http://dx.doi.org/10.5772/60101

	ATP-ADP transformation		ATP-cAMP transformation	
Drugs	Effects	Doses (M)	Effects	Doses (M)
Acetylcholine	Stimulation	10^{-7} M →	Inhibition	10^{-4} M →
Parasympatholytics:				
Atropine	Inhibition	10^{-11} M →	Stimulation	10^{-8} M →
Isopropamide	Inhibition	10^{-8} M →	Stimulation	10^{-5} M →
Gastrixon	Inhibition	10^{-7} M →	Stimulation	10^{-4} M →
Epinephrine	Inhibition	10^{-9} M →	Stimulation	10^{-7} M →
β-blocker (Visken)	Stimulation	10^{-4} M →	Inhibition	10^{-5} M →
Histamine	Inhibition	10^{-11} M →	Stimulation	10^{-8} M →
Cimetidine	Stimulation(?)	10^{-4} M →	Inhibition	10^{-6} M →
Pentagastrin	Inhibition	10^{-11} M →	Stimulation	10^{-9} M →
PGE_1	Inhibition	10^{-11} M →	Stimulation	10^{-9} M →
PGE_2	Inhibition	10^{-11} M →	Stimulation	10^{-9} M →
Ouabain	Inhibition	10^{-8} M →	Stimulation	10^{-4} M →
cAMP	Inhibition	10^{-13} M →		
AMP	Inhibition	10^{-8} M →		

*Direct effects of the membrane-bound ATP-splitting enzyme activities.

Table 29. Pharmacological effects on the transformation of ATP into ADP by membrane ATPase and the ATP–cAMP transformation by adenylate cyclase from rat and human gastric, fundic, antral, duodenal and jejunal mucosa. [Mózsik and Jávor: Dig. Dis. Sci 33:92–105, 1988* (with kind permission).]

Some general aspects of the biochemical approach need to be emphasized for the establishment of the theoretical base of the feedback systems between the tissue levels of ATP, ADP, AMP and cAMP:

1. Simultaneous determinations of the tissue ATP, ADP, AMP and cAMP and lactate may be used for a correct evaluation of the role of membrane-bound ATP-dependent energy systems in both development and prevention of ulcer. No such conclusions can be derived from the determination of ATP or cAMP alone;

2. The tissue hypoxia produced by two characteristic biochemical properties: (a) a significant increase in the level of lactate in tissue and (b) failure of the ATP resynthesis due to impaired oxidative phosphorylation by tissue hypoxia. A significant decrease in tissue ATP level was observed in many experimental models, but without an increase in the lactate level (Mózsik et al., 1976 a, b, c, d; Mózsik and Vizi, 1976 a, b; Mózsik et al., 1979 a, b, c, d, e, f, g; Mózsik et al., 1981 a, b, c, d, e; Nagy et al., 1983). The simultaneous measurements of ATP–membrane, ATPase–ADP and ATP–adenylate cyclase–cAMP systems offer useful information on the energy turnover. If there was increased activity of ATP-splitting enzymes together with increased concentration of ADP and cAMP, it would be indicative of increased ATP breakdown in one or another direction, or in both pathways (Mózsik and Vizi, 1976 a, b; Mózsik et al., 1978c; Mózsik et al., a, b, c, d, e, f, g; Mózsik et

al., 1983 a, b, c). If the ATP level had been found at a significantly higher level, this would indicate an increased extent of oxidative phosphorylation. These findings however do not indicate the presence of tissue hypoxia in the gastrointestinal mucosa;

3. The balance between the membrane-bound ATP-dependent energy systems can be modified by hormones, mediators and drugs, under physiological and pathophysiological conditions (Mózsik et al., 1979 a, b, c, d, e, f, g; Mózsik et al., 1983 a, b, c). The major effects produced by these agents can be evaluated as steps in the injury to the gastrointestinal mucosa. It is important to note that the ATP–ADP and ATP–cAMP energy systems are affected by different dose–response curves of drugs. For example, the doses required to produce 50% inhibition of ATP–ADP and ATP–cAMP transformation from affinity curves (pD_2) and those required to express intrinsic activities (pA_2) using ouabain as having an activity ($\alpha = 1.00$) differ significantly in both systems (Tables 26, 29);

4. Data are scarce for the two ATP-dependent energy systems (Robinson et al., 1957; Schwartz et al., 1975; Sutherland and Rall, 1975, 1960; Butcher and Sutherland, 1971). Their correlations were evaluated by responses to various hormones, mediators and drugs by the gastric mucosa in rats and human subjects. These responses show that feedback mechanisms exist between the membrane-bound energy systems (Mózsik et al., 1979 a, b, d, e, f, g; Mózsik, 1969 a, b);

5. The system is characterized mainly by the following:

   a. ATP is a common substrate for both Na^+–K^+-dependent membrane ATPase and adenylate cyclase (Mózsik, 1969 a, b);

   b. the drugs which stimulate membrane ATPase activity, inhibit the transformation of ATP into cAMP by adenylate cyclase (Mózsik, 1969 a, b);

   c. drugs and hormones inhibiting the membrane ATPase activity stimulate the adenylate cyclase activity directly and vice versa (Mózsik et al., 1973 a, b; Mózsik et al., 1974 a, b, c; Mózsik et al., 1979 a, b, c, d, e, f ; Mózsik et al., 1981 a, b, c);

   d. the increased transformation of ATP into ADP indirectly inhibits the extent of ATP–cAMP transformation (Mózsik et al., 1983b; Morón et al., 1983; Mózsik et al., 1983 b, c);

   e. the decrease in transformation of ATP into ADP by various agents leads to the indirect stimulation of the transformation of ATP into cAMP (Mózsik et al., 1979 a);

   f. the increase in ATP transformation into cAMP leads to an indirect inhibition of ATP–ADP transformation (Mózsik et al., 1979 a, b, c, d, e, f, g, h);

   g. AMP and cAMP directly inhibit the transformation of ATP into AMP by direct inhibition of membrane ATPase activity (Mózsik, 1969a, 1970);

   h. the inhibition in the transformation of ATP into cAMP is the result of the indirect stimulation in the transformation of ATP into ADP (Mózsik et al., 1987 a, b);

http://dx.doi.org/10.5772/60101

i. the extent of cAMP transformation through regulation of phosphodiesterase by drugs may be regulated by both ATP–ADP and ATP–cAMP transformation.

6. The extent of phosphorylation and/or dephosphorylation can be estimated by the Atkinson's formula (1968).

The critical evaluation of the results of these observations offers a significant possibility for the biochemical background of gastrointestinal tract.

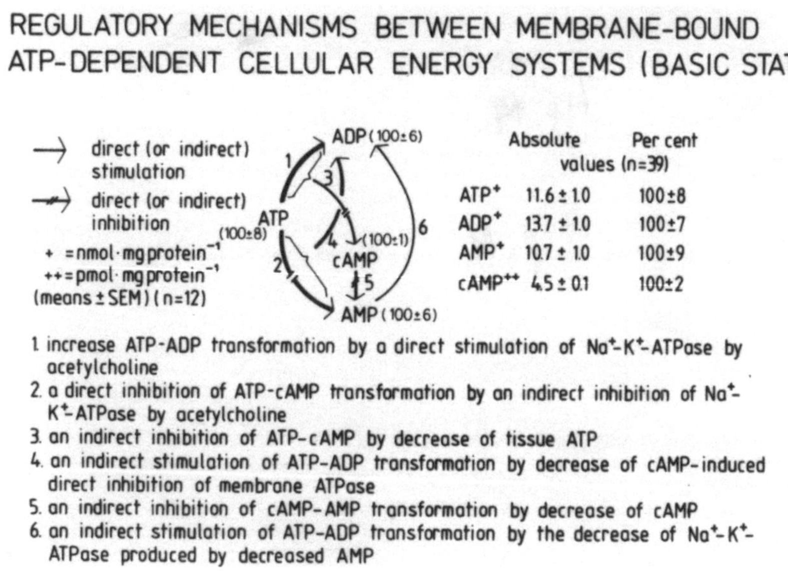

Figure 36. Main regulatory steps to membrane-bound ATP-dependent energy systems in rats under the physiological conditions. [Mózsik et al., Ann N Y Acac Sci. 597: 264–281, 1990a (with kind permission).]

6.4.3. Cholinergic and adrenergic influences on the regulatory mechanisms between the tissue levels of ATP, ADP, cAMP and AMP in the intact rat stomach

Under the physiological conditions, the ATP–ADP transformation is the first-line regulation in the active movements of cations (Na^+, K^+) across the cell membrane, and this ATP decrease in the membrane ATPase results in an indirect inhibition on the ATP–cAMP transformation. Furthermore, the acetylcholine (ACh) alone directly inhibits the adenylate cyclase activity (Mózsik, 1969 a, b). The decrease in cellular level of cAMP relatively enhances the extent of the ATP–ADP transformation, and in the meantime further decreases the extent of ATP–cAMP transformation (Figure 38).

Epinephrine directly enhances the adenylate cyclase activity and it directly inhibits the membrane ATPase activity in smaller doses (Mózsik, 1970). During the epinephrine effect, the extent of ATP–cAMP transformation will increase, and in the meanwhile the ATP–ADP transformation will decrease (Figures 16, 17).

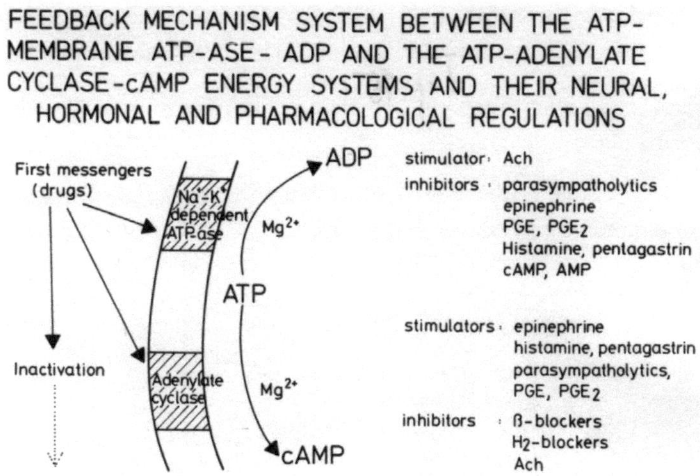

Figure 37. Pharmacological regulations (first messengers) of membrane-bound ATP-dependent energy systems (second messengers) in the rat and human gastric mucosa under the physiological conditions. [Mózsik et al., Acta Medica Acad Sci Hung 36, 1–29, 1979 (with kind permission).]

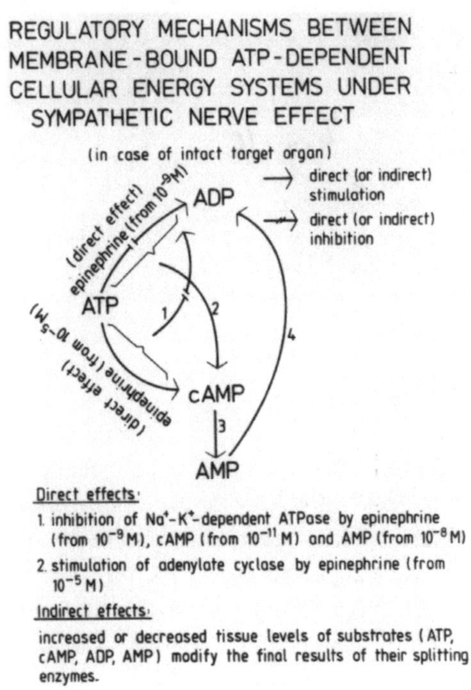

Figure 38. Epinephrine-induced direct and indirect regulatory mechanisms on the transformation of ATP–ADP by membrane ATPase and of ATP–cAMP by adenylate cyclase and of ADP–AMP and cAMP–AMP transformation in the gastric mucosa in intact rats. [Mózsik et al., Ann N Y Acad Sci 579, 264–281, 1990a (with kind permission).]

http://dx.doi.org/10.5772/60101

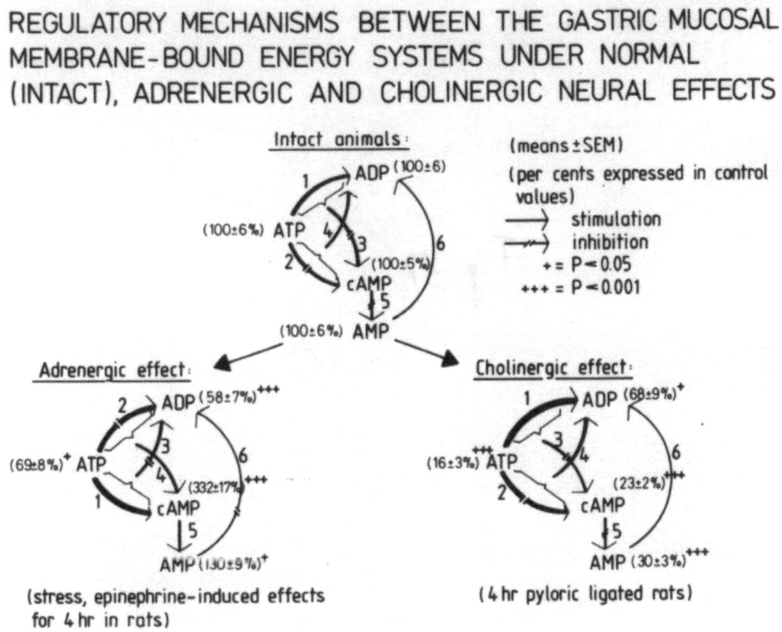

Figure 39. Regulatory mechanisms between the cellular ATP, ADP, cAMP and AMP in the rat gastric mucosa under normal (intact), adrenergic and cholinergic neural effects.

6.4.4. The effects of "surgical" and "chemical" vagotomy on the energy metabolism of gastric mucosa in intact rats

The aims of these studies were as follows:

a. To evaluate the effects of acute "chemical" and "surgical" vagotomy on the gastric mucosal biochemistry in rats;

b. To find correlations between these tissue biochemical parameters after "surgical" and "chemical" vagotomy (without the application of any damaging agents) in intact rats.

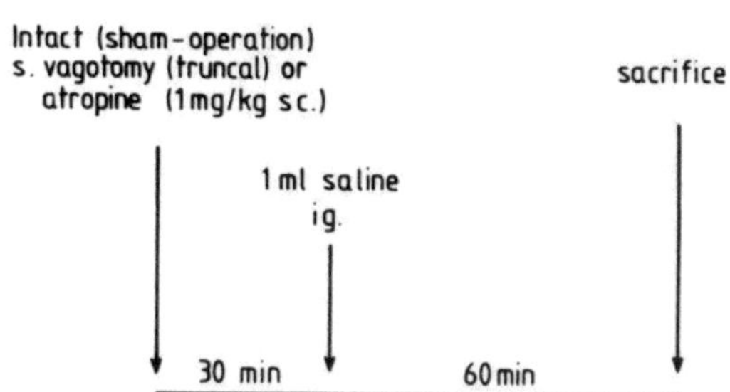

Figure 40. Experimental design of these experiments. [Mózsik, Sütő, Vincze: J. Clin. Gastroenterol S135–S139, 1992b (with kind permission).]

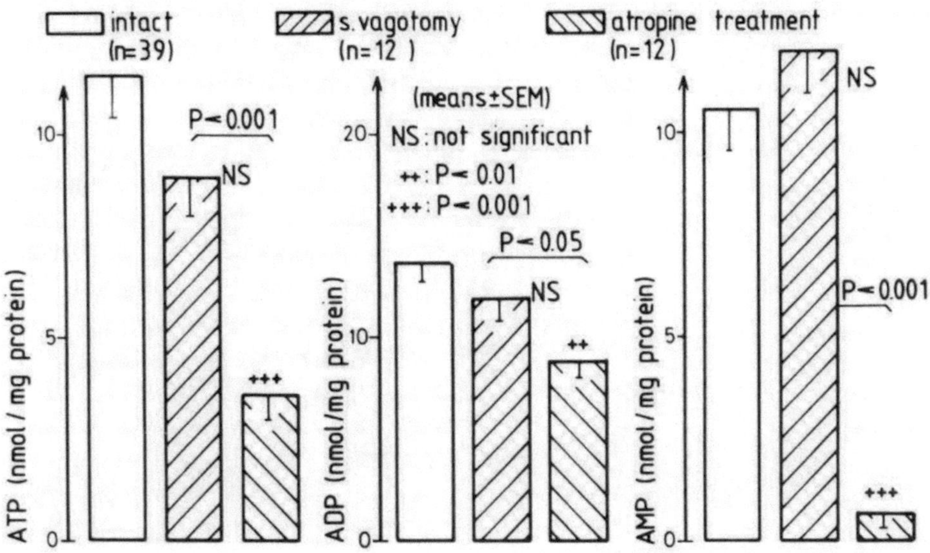

Figure 41. Surgical and chemical vagotomy-induced changes in the gastric mucosal levels of adenosine triphosphate (ATP), adenosine diphosphate (ADP) and adenosine monophosphate (AMP) in rats (without giving any necrotizing agents). *P* values are between the intact (sham-operated) versus surgical and chemical vagotomized rats. [Mózsik, Sütő, Vincze: J. Clin. Gastroenterol 14(Suppl.2):S135–S139, 1992b (with kind permission).]

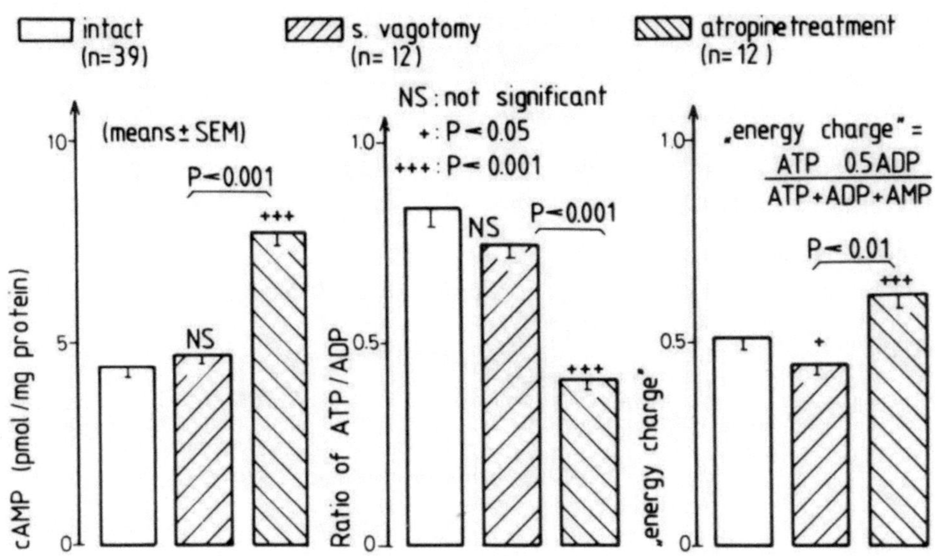

Figure 42. "Surgical" and "chemical" vagotomy-induced changes in the tissue levels of cyclic adenosine monophosphate (cAMP), ratio of ATP/ADP and "energy charge" in the gastric fundic mucosa of rats (without application of any necrotizing agents). For further explanations, see Figure 41. [Mózsik, Sütő, Vincze: J. Clin. Gastroenterol 14(Suppl.2): S135–S139, 1992b (with kind permission).]

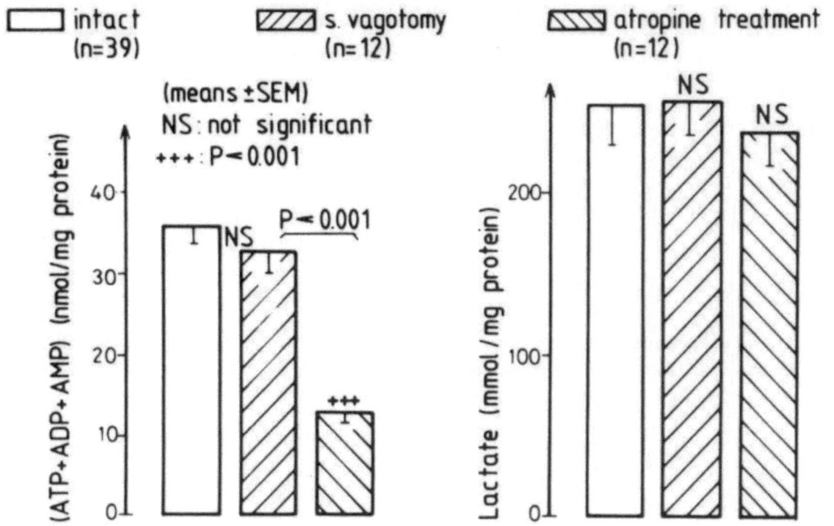

Figure 43. "Surgical" and "chemical" vagotomy-induced changes in the gastric mucosal levels of the adenylate pool (ATP+ADP+AMP) and lactate. For further explanation, see Figure 41. [Mózsik, Sütő, Vincze: J. Clin. Gastroenterol 14(Suppl.2): S135–S139, 1992b (with kind permission).]

	Transformations of ATP - ADP	ATP - cAMP	cAMP - AMP
Intact vagus	↑↑↑	↓↓↓	↓↓↓
Surgical vagotomy	0	0	0
	P<0.05	P<0.001	P<0.001
Pharmacological vagotomy	↓↓	↑↑↑	↓↓↓

Figure 44. Surgical" and "chemical" vagotomy-induced changes in the gastric mucosal membrane-bound ATP-dependent energy systems of rats (without application of any necrotizing agents). *P* values are presented between intact (sham-operated) versus "surgical" and "chemical" vagotomized groups: ↑ , increase; ↓ , decrease. Abbreviations: 0, not significant; ↓ ↓, $P < 0.01$; ↑ ↑ ↑ (↓ ↓ ↓) : $P < 0.001$. (Mózsik, Sütő, Vincze: J. Clin. Gastroenterol 14(Suppl.2): S135-S139, 1992b) (with kind permission).

The results in this chapter clearly indicate that the acute "surgical" and "chemical" (acute administration of atropine) vagotomy produce significantly different changes in the gastric mucosal energy systems (similar conclusions were obtained from our biochemical observations carried out earlier).

Membrane-bound ATP-dependent (ATP-splitting) systems			
Mg^{2+}-Na^+-K^+-dependent ATPase			
Compounds	Mg^{2+}-dependent	Na^+-K^+-dependent	Adenylate cyclase
Acetylcholine	No effect	Stimulation	Inhibition
Atropine	No effect	Inhibition	Stimulation
cAMP	No effect	Inhibtion	No effect
AMP	Stimulation	Inhibition	No effect

Table 30. Effect of compounds on membrane- bound ATP-dependent systems. [Mózsik, Jávor: Dig. Dis. Sci. 33:92–105, 1988; Mózsik, Nagy, Tárnok, Vizi: Acta Med. Acad. Sci. Hung. 36: 1–29, 1979) (with kind permission).]

Author details

Gyula Mozsik[1*] and Imre Szabó[2]

*Address all correspondence to: gyula.mozsik@aok.pte.hu

1 First Department of Medicine, Medical and Health Centre, University of Pécs, Hungary

2 Associate Professor at the First Department of Medicine, University of Pécs, Hungary

Chapter 7

Biochemical Examination of the Human Gastrointestinal Tract

Gyula Mozsik and Imre Szabó

Additional information is available at the end of the chapter

http://dx.doi.org/10.5772/60102

The forthcoming biochemical observations were from the resecates of the patients who underwent surgical intervention because of peptic ulcer disease. These observations were done during 1969–1976, when only the parasympatholytics were used in the medical treatment of patients with peptic ulcer.

The resecates of the gastrointestinal tract were divided into two parts: one was used for classical histopathological examinations (with the permission from Professor György Romhányi, Head of the Department of Pathology and of Professor Tihamer Gy. Karlinger, Head of First Department of Surgery, Pécs University, Hungary),, awhile the other part was used for biochemical examinations. Different parts from the mucosa and musculature were separated from each other immediately after the surgical resection of the GI tract, and these parts were put immediately into liquid nitrogen.

All biochemical parameters of the GI tissue samples (normal and ulcerated antral, duodenal and jejunal mucosa and three gastric fundic mucosa and musculature, if we received fundic tissues) were maintained in the same time in all the received tissue samples.

It is very important to emphasize that, on the one hand, all biochemical parameters maintained from the same tissue samples, and on the other hand, all tissue samples were biochemically examined. It is also important to note that the weight of these tissue samples was about 0.25–0.5 g wet tissue (these examinations cannot be carried out from biopsy materials).

The methodologies were detailed in the original published papers.

These patients had typical ulcer histories and endoscopic pictures. These patients received medical treatment (by dominant internists) for about 4 weeks before surgery. The patients who were suspected to have malignant ulcers did not receive any tissue samples from the resecates (because of necessary histopathological examinations).

7.1. Correlation between the gastric fundic mucosal Na^+-K^+-dependent ATPase activity versus gastric basal acid output (BAO) in humans

In the gastric basal acid output (BAO) and maximal acid output (MAO), there are different associations with cations and protein secretion from the serosa to the mucosa: the H^+, chloride, K^+, Mg^{2+}, Ca^{2+} and albumin increase significantly, while the Na indicates a decrease (Myren, 1968; Semb and Myren, 1968; Wright and Hirschowitz, 1976). These called for attention to study the correlations between the classical membrane-bound ATP-dependent energy systems and gastric BAO and MAO.

There was no doubt that after the administration of pentagastrin or histamine (given in doses) to produce gastric MAO values, the changes in the contents of the gastric juice cations became much higher than those in gastric BAO. These data also suggested that there is some correlation between the membrane-bound ATP-dependent energy systems and the gastric BAO and MAO values.

In 45 patients with peptic ulcer (20 patients with gastric and 25 patients with duodenal ulcer), the gastric H^+ was measured without the administration of any drug (basal acid output, BAO), and its value was expressed in mEq/L. These patients underwent resection of the stomach for peptic ulcer. During the surgery, a piece was cut from the fundic part of the stomach. The gastric mucosa and the muscular layer were separated from each other, and the membrane ATPase was prepared from fundic gastric mucosa with differential centrifugation (20.000 × g and 40.000 × g) and treatment with 2.0 M NaI solution as per our method (Mózsik and Øye, 1969). The membrane ATPase activity was measured in an incubation system at 37 °C by the liberation of inorganic phosphorus (Mózsik, 1969b). The Na^+–K^+-dependent ATPase activity was calculated as the difference between the total (obtained in the presence of Mg^{2+}, Na^+ and K^+) and Mg^{2+}-dependent system (obtained in the presence of Mg^{2+}) (Figure 45).

The Na^+–K^+-dependent ATPase differs from the H^+–K^+-dependent ATPase, independently from the similarities of protein structures (see Sections 5.1, 5.2), and the mitochondrial ATP is a common substrate for both these enzymes. Our enzyme was prepared from the whole gastric fundic mucosa; H^+–K^+–ATPase is located only in the parietal cells, which are highly specialized epithelial cells in the inner cell lining of the stomach. H^+–K^+–ATPase can be separated from the Na^+–K^+-pump enzyme based on specific immunological studies (Saccomani et al., 1979b; Yao and Forte, 2004; Dunbar and Caplan, 2001; Sachs et al., 1995; https.//www.nlm.nil.gov/cgi/mesh/2011/MB_cgi?&term=Potassium+Hydrogen+ATPase).

There is no doubt that both the active transport of Na^+ and K^+ (Na pump) and the gastric acid secretion are energy-dependent processes (obtained from the ATP transformation into ADP); however, the sodium pump is a general function of all cells, while the H^+–K^+–ATPase is responsible only for gastric acid secretion.

We never participated in the study of H^+–K^+–ATPase; however, it is true that the presence of Na^+–K^+–ATPase was proved earlier in the rat and human gastrointestinal (gastric) mucosa (Mózsik and Øye, 1969).

http://dx.doi.org/10.5772/60102

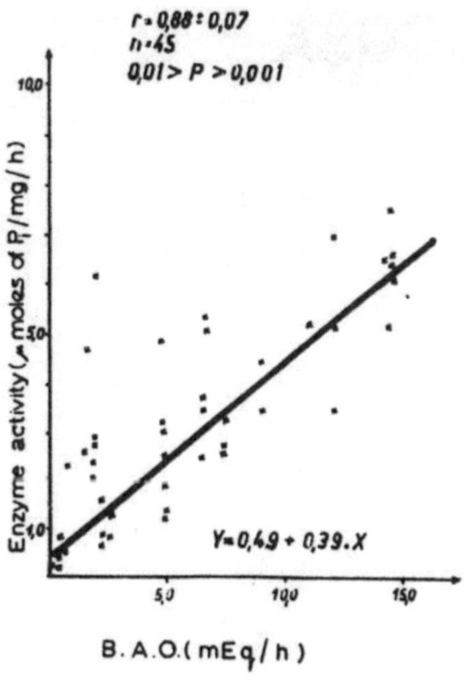

Figure 45. Correlation between the Na^+–K^+-dependent ATPase activity from human fundic mucosa (ordinate) and basal acid output (BAO) (abscissa) in 45 patients with peptic ulcer. The enzyme activities are expressed as P_i (μMol/mg protein/hour). [Mózsik, Nagy, Tárnok, Vizi F, Kutas J: Experientia (Basel) 30: 1024–1025, 1974 (with kind permission).]

We used the Na^+–K^+-dependent ATPase system as a key enzyme participating in the regulation of cell functions, of course, in the gastric mucosal cells. The function of Na^+–K^+–ATPase represents only one side of the ATP splitting process (as energy source), while the actual level of tissue ATP indicates the other side of energy source system (namely, the ATP resynthesis). These processes occur together in all cells and tissues. Both Na^+ and K^+ are involved in both the classical sodium pump and the gastric acid secretion.

Our results presented here are related dominantly to the function of the classical sodium pump in the human gastric mucosa. It is interesting and important to note that the activity of Na^+–K^+-dependent ATPase is closely associated with the gastric acid secretion.

7.2. Interaction of cholinergic function with Mg^{2+}-Na^+-K^+-dependent ATPase system of cells in the human fundic gastric mucosa

This section deals with the effects of some cholinergic and anticholinergic drugs on the membrane-bound ATPase enzyme (Mózsik et al., 1974c).

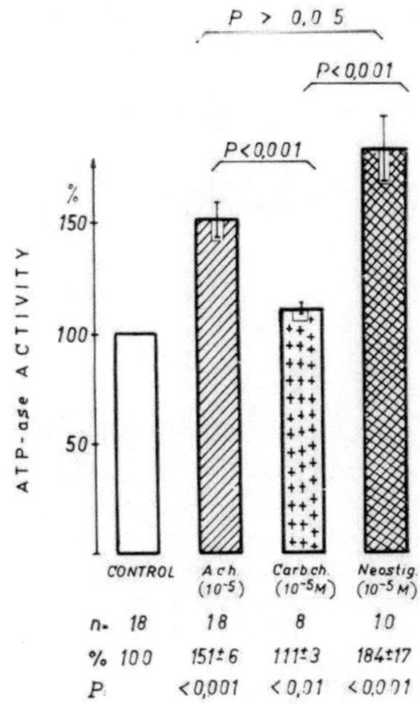

Figure 46. Effects of acetylcholine (Ach), carbamylcholine (Carb.ch.) and neostigmine (Neostig.) on the total ATPase activity in the human gastric fundic mucosa. The enzyme activity is expressed in percentage of total ATPase activity (=100%) without any drug [Mózsik, Nagy, Kutas, Tárnok: Scand. J. Gastroenterol. 9: 741–745, 1974 (with kind permission).]

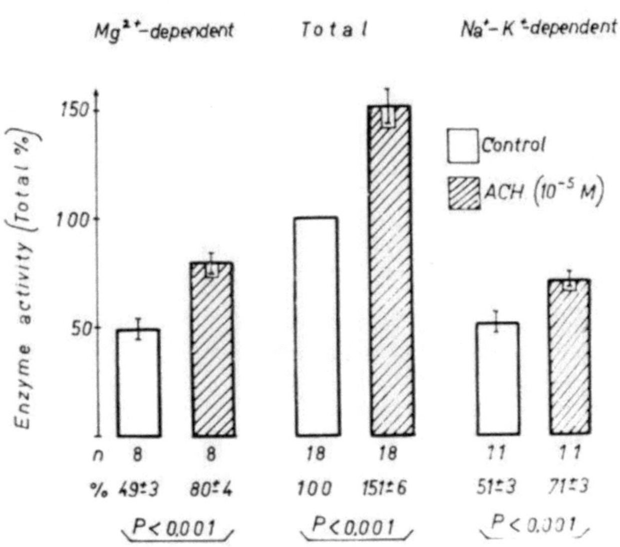

Figure 47. Effects of acetylcholine on Mg^{2+}-dependent, total and Na^{+}–K^{+}-dependent ATPase prepared from the human gastric fundic mucosa. The results are presented in percentage of total ATPase (=100%) activity without the administration of any drugs. [Mózsik, Nagy, Kutas, Tárnok: Scand. J. Gastroenterol. 9: 741–745, 1974 (with kind permission).]

http://dx.doi.org/10.5772/60102

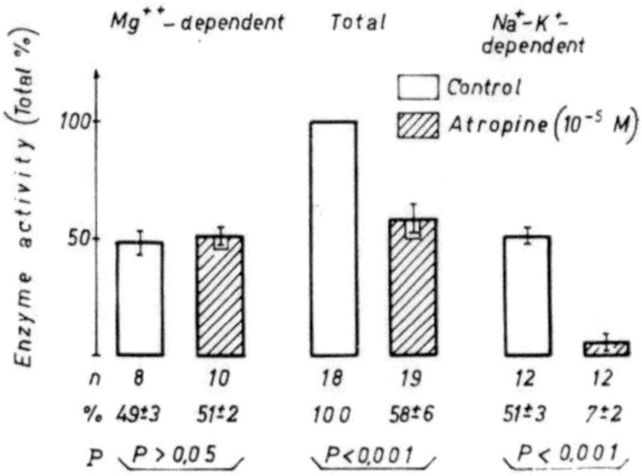

Figure 48. Effects of atropine on Mg^{2+}-dependent, total and Na^+–K^+-dependent ATPase prepared from the human gastric fundic mucosa. The results are presented in percentage of total ATPase (=100%) activity without the administration of any drugs. [Mózsik, Nagy, Kutas, Tárnok: Scand. J. Gastroenterol. 9: 741–745, 1974 (with kind permission).]

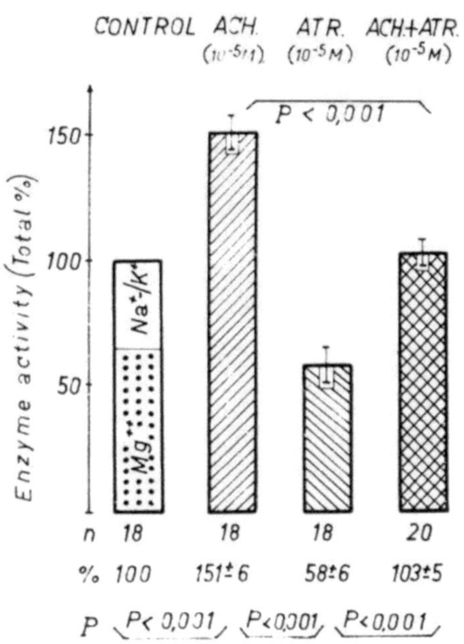

Figure 49. Comparative inhibitory effect of different parasympatholytics on the total membrane ATPase prepared from the human gastric fundic mucosa. The results are presented in percentage of total ATPase (=100%) activity without the administration of any drugs. [Mózsik, Nagy, Kutas, Tárnok: Scand. J. Gastroenterol. 9: 741–745, 1974 (with kind permission).]

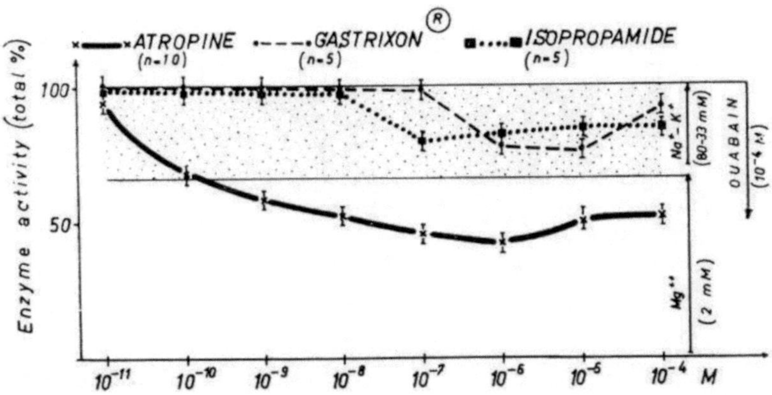

Figure 50. Comparative inhibitory effect of different parasympatholytics on the total membrane ATPase activity prepared from the human gastric fundic mucosa. The results are presented in per cent of total ATPase (= 100 per cent) activity without application of any drugs. (Mózsik, Nagy, Kutas, Tárnok: Scand. J. Gastroenterol. 9: 741-745, 1974) (with kind permission).

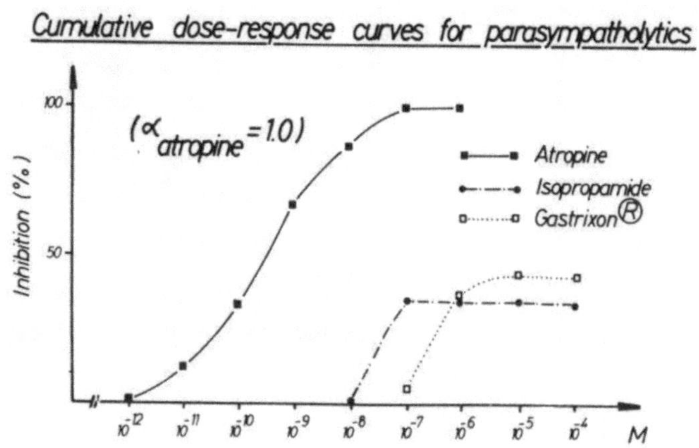

Figure 51. Cumulative dose–response curves for parasympatholytics inhibiting the Na^+–K^+-dependent ATPase prepared from the human gastric fundic mucosa. The intrinsic activity (α) of atropine was found to be equal to 1.0 on Na^+–K^+-dependent ATPase activity. Each point represents the average of 10 measurements (chemical structures: isopropamide, 2,2-diphenyl-4-diiso-propylamino-methyliodide; Gastrixon^R, methyl-tropinium-bromide-xanthene-9-carboxylate). [Mózsik, Kutas, Nagy, Tárnok, Vizi: Acta Physiol. Sand. Special Suppl. 199–208, 1978 (with kind permission).]

http://dx.doi.org/10.5772/60102

Parasympatholytics	Affinity (pD_2)	Intrinsic activity (α)
Atropine	9.50	1.00
Isopropamide	7.50	0.36
Gastrixon^R	6.40	0.43

Table 31. Values of affinity (pD_2) and intrinsic activities (α) for parasympatholytics inhibiting the Na^+–K^+-dependent ATPase prepared from the human gastric fundic mucosa. The intrinsic activity of atropine was found to be equal to 1.0.

The results presented above indicate clearly the following:

1. During the cholinergic activation, the enzyme system of sodium pump (the transformation of ATP into ADP by membrane ATPase) is in working state (acetylcholine, carbamylcholine, neostigmine);

2. The parasympatholytics inhibit the function of membrane ATPase prepared from the human gastric fundic mucosa;

3. The different parasympatholytics produced different extents on the inhibition of membrane ATPase activity.

7.3. Inhibitory effects of histamine, pentagastrin, PGE_1 and PGE_2 on Na^+-K^+-dependent ATPase prepared from human gastric mucosa

The gastric acid secretory responses are characterized by the so-called basal acid secretory responses (e.g., without the administration of any drug to stimulate the gastric acid secretion) (basal acid output, BAO) and maximal gastric acid secretory responses (maximal acid output, MAO). The MAO can be produced by the administration of histamine (0.04 mg/kg body weight, given subcutaneously) (Kay's test) or pentagastrin (6 μg/kg given subcutaneously).

The effect of histamine was studied on the typical membrane ATPase prepared from the gastric fundic mucosa of patients with gastric (8 patients) and duodenal (6 patients) ulcer, before resection of their stomach: BAO value = 3.86 ± 1.14 mEg/h and MAO = 16.30 ± 2.25 mEg/h.

Histamine was used in 10^{-7} M concentration to test its effect only on Mg^{2+}-dependent part and Na^+–K^+-dependent part (Figure 52).

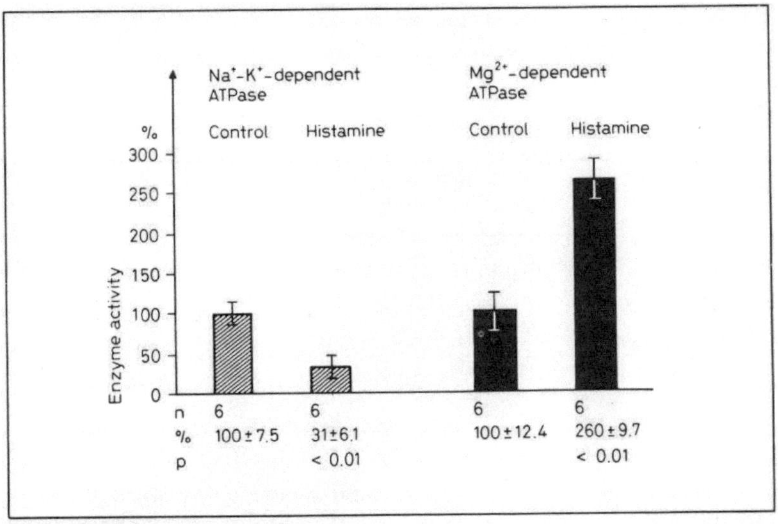

Figure 52. Histamine (10^{-7} M) effects on only Mg^{2+}-dependent ATPase and on Na^+-K^+-dependent ATPase activity. The results (means±SEM) are presented as per cent of control values. (Mózsik, Nagy, Tárnok, Jávor, Kutas: Pharmacology 12: 193-200, 1974) (with kind permission).

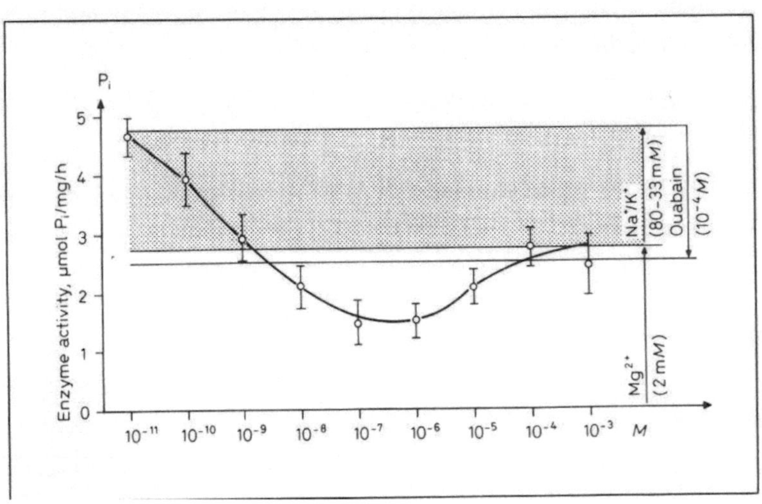

Figure 53. Inhibition of total ATPase from the human gastric fundic mucosa by histamine. The results of 14 patients are expressed in means ± SEM. The left ordinate shows the enzyme activity (µmol P_i /mg membrane protein/h, while the abscissa indicates the histamine concentration (M). The right side of the figure demonstrates the "chemical marker behavior" of this membrane fraction taken from 14 patients' gastric fundic mucosa. [Mózsik, Nagy, Tárnok, Jávor, Kutas: Pharmacology 12: 193–200, 1974 (with kind permission).]

http://dx.doi.org/10.5772/60102

The inhibition of total membrane ATPase activity was caused by histamine in a concentration of 10^{-7} to 10^{-3} M.

Similar observations were noted in pentagastrin, and the same type of inhibition of membrane ATPase was obtained as that of histamine.

The effects of prostaglandin E_1 and E_2 were studied on the Mg^{2+}- dependent and Na^+–K^+-dependent ATPase prepared from the human gastric fundic mucosa (Figures 54, 55), and significant inhibitory actions were produced by PGE_1 and PGE_2 in concentrations of 10^{-10} to 10^{-6} M.

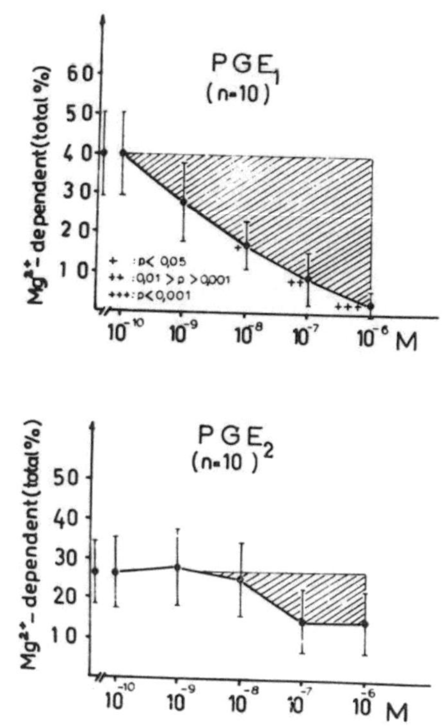

Figure 54. Inhibitory effects of prostaglandin E_1 (top) and E_2 (bottom) on Mg^{2+}-dependent ATPase prepared from the human gastric fundic mucosa. The results are expressed as percentage value of total ATPase activity (=100%). The abscissa indicates the concentrations of prostaglandins (M). Each point represents the means ± SEM of 10 observations. [Mózsik, Kutas, Nagy, Németh: Eur. J. Pharmacol. 29: 133–137, 1974 (with kind permission).]

7.4. Correlations between the magnitudes of drug actions versus magnitudes of Na^+-K^+-dependent ATPase prepared from the human gastric fundic mucosa and from the small intestinal mucosa

It was clear to conclude that the magnitudes of drugs actions depend on the membrane enzyme activity. Because the membrane ATPase activity significantly changes on the activity of target organ, the drug actions depend on the activity of the target organ (Nagy et al., 1976, 1981 a, b).

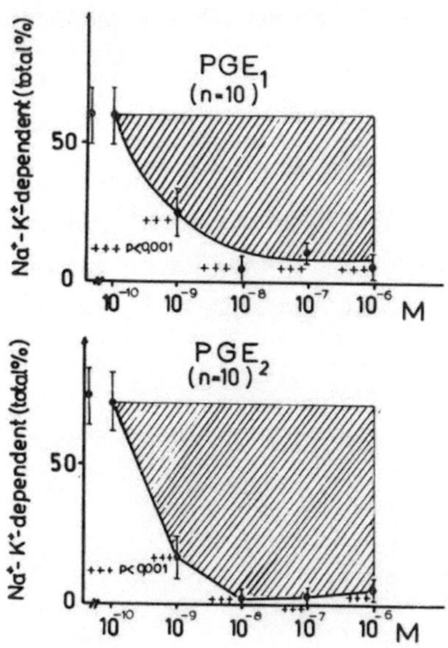

Figure 55. Inhibitory effects of prostaglandin E_1 (top) and E_2 (bottom) on Na^+–K^+-dependent ATPase prepared from the human gastric fundic mucosa. The results are expressed as percentage value of total ATPase activity (=100%). The abscissa indicates the concentrations of prostaglandins (M). Each point represents the means ± SEM of 10 observations. [Mózsik, Kutas, Nagy, Németh: Eur. J. Pharmacol. 29: 133–137, 1974 (with kind permission).]

Drug:	Drug effect:	Tested dose:	r:	Regression line:	p value:	n:
AcH	stimulation	10^{-4} M	0.98	Y=0.5X−0.8	<0.001	7
Atropine	inhibition	10^{-7} M	0.97	Y=1.35X+0.49	<0.001	19
cAMP	inhibition	10^{-9} M	0.78	Y=1.34X−1.63	<0.05	8
Epinephrine	inhibition	10^{-7} M	0.68	Y=1.10X+0.12	<0.05	10
Histamine	inhibition	10^{-7} M	0.87	Y=0.96X+0.88	<0.01	9
Ouabain	inhibition	10^{-7} M	0.93	Y=1.03X+0.20	<0.001	45
	inhibition	10^{-4} M	0.93	Y=1.20X+1.03	<0.001	45
Pentagastrin	inhibition	10^{-7} M	0.94	Y=0.85X+0.11	<0.02	10

Affinity (pD_2) values: Ach=5.50 ; Atr. =9.50; cAMP=11.30 ; Epinephr. =8.60 ; Hist.=9.70 ; Pentagast.=10.55 ; Ouabain=7.50 (9.20−6.50)

Table 32. Correlations between the magnitudes of drug actions and the magnitudes of Na^+–K^+–ATPase prepared from the human gastric fundic mucosa.

7.5. Correlations between the magnitudes Na^+-K^+-dependent ATPase, tissue levels of ATP, ADP in the human gastric fundic mucosa versus values of gastric basal acid ouput (BAO) in humans

We prepared the membrane ATPase from the human gastric fundic mucosa and, simultaneously, directly measured the tissue level of ATP, ADP, lipid phosphates, ribonucleic acid and deoxyribonucleic acid. The tissue levels of ATP, ADP, lipid phosphates and ribonucleic acid

http://dx.doi.org/10.5772/60102

were expressed in accordance to 1.0 mg deoxyribonucleic acid (DNA). The membrane ATPase activity was assayed (Mózsik and Øye, 1969) by *in vitro* method (Figures 56, 58). The different correlations were expressed in consequence of mathematical analyses: BAO versus Na^+–K^+-dependent ATPase ($r = 0.88$, $n = 45$; $P<0.001$); BAO versus tissue level of ATP ($r = 0.53$, $n = 28$, $P<0.01$); ATP versus Na^+–K^+–ATPase ($r = 0.55$, $n = 32$, $P<0.001$); ATP versus ADP ($r = 0.99$, $n = 32$, $P <0.001$); BAO versus ADP ($r = 0.59$, $n = 28$, $P<0.001$) (Mózsik et al., 1979 a, b, 1981d, 1978b) (Figure 56).

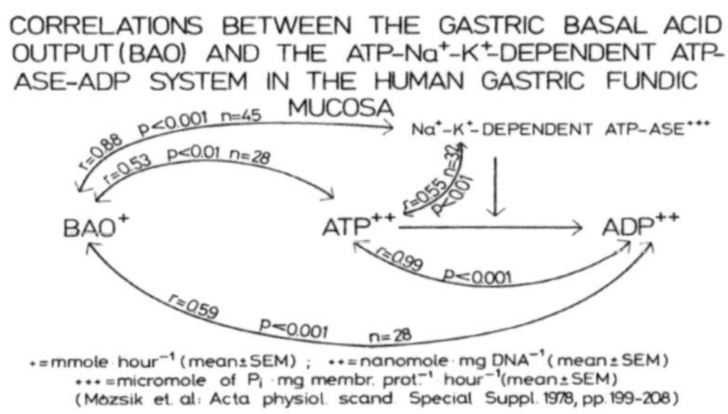

Figure 56. Biochemical regulatory pathways between Na^+–K^+-dependent ATPase, tissue levels of ATP, ADP in the human gastric fundic mucosa dependent on the gastric BAO values (means ± SEM). [Mózsik, Tárnok, Kutas (1981) in Gáti, Szollár, Ungváry (eds.) Advances in Physiological Sciences Vol. 12. Nutrition, Digestion, Metabolism. pp. 117–128. 1981 (with kind permission).]

7.6. Correlation between gastric basal acid output (BAO) versus gastric maximal acid ouput (MAO) in humans

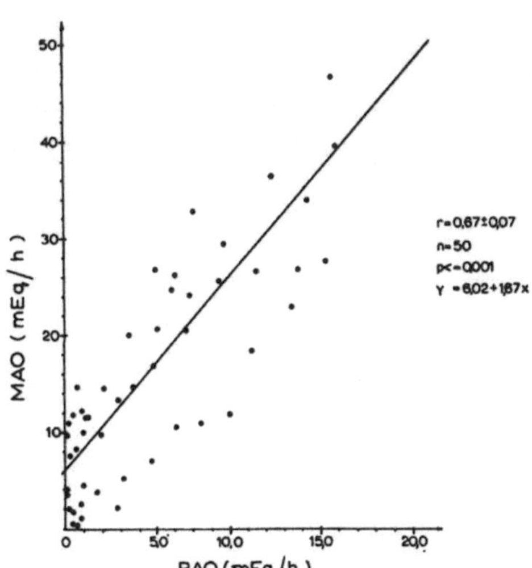

Figure 57. Correlation between the gastric basal acid output (BAO) versus gastric maximal acid output (MAO) in patients examined biochemically. [Mózsik, Vizi, Nagy, Bero, Tárnok, Kutas (1976): Na^+–K^+-dependent ATPase system and the H^+ secretion by the human gastric mucosa. In: Mozsik Gy., Javor T. (eds). Progress in Peptic Ulcer. Budapest, Akadémiai Kiadó, pp. 37–72 (with kind permission).]

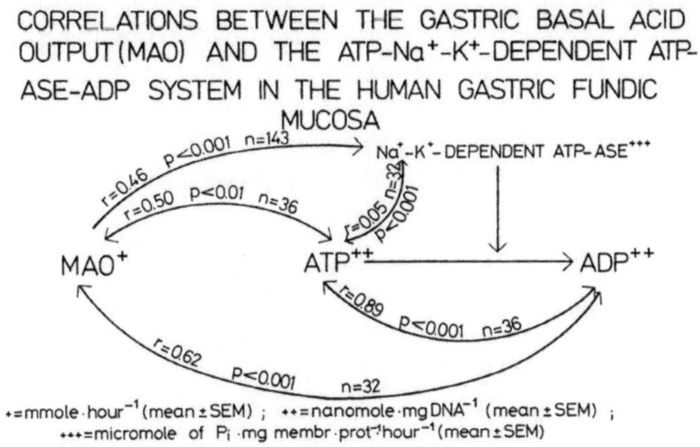

Figure 58. Biochemical regulatory pathways between Na^+–K^+-dependent ATPase, tissue levels of ATP, ADP in the human gastric fundic mucosa dependent on the gastric maximal acid output (MAO) values. For further explanation, see Figure 56 (with kind permission).

7.7. Correlations between Na^+-K^+-dependent ATPase activity, tissue level of ATP, ADP in the human gastric fundic mucosa versus gastric maximal acid output (MAO) in humans

Figure 58 indicates the results of different correlation calculations versus MAO values.

We found positive and significant correlations between the following parameters:

a. MAO versus Na^+–K^+-dependent ATPase;

b. MAO versus tissue level of ATP;

c. Na^+–K^+-dependent ATPase versus ATP;

d. ATP versus ADP;

e. MAO versus ADP. (Andrási, 1997; Bódis et al., 1977 a, b; Levine, 1971; Mózsik et al., 1978b).

7.8. Affinity and intrinsic activity curves of acetylcholine, histamine and pentagastrin on the Na^+-K^+-dependent ATPase prepared and on the adenylate cyclase prepared from human gastric mucosa

The contradictory effects of drugs on Na^+–K^+-dependent ATPase and adenylate cyclase were demonstrated earlier (Mózsik, 1969 a, b, 1970, 1974 a, b, 1979 b, c, e).

Table 33 indicates affinity (pD_2) and intrinsic activity (pA_2) curves for the actions of acetylcholine, histamine and pentagastrin. The table also indicates the contradictory actions of these agents on Na^+–K^+-dependent and adenyl cyclase systems.

We hypothesized a feedback system between the membrane ATPase and adenylate cyclase in the development of gastric BAO and MAO (Figure 59).

http://dx.doi.org/10.5772/60102

Mediators	Actions	Affinity values (pD_2)	Intrinsic activities (α)	(pA_2)
ATP – membrane ATP-ase – ADP				
Ach	Stimulation	5.50	1.00_{Ach}	5.50
Histamine	Inhibibion	9.70	$1.00_{Ouabain}$	9.70
Pentagastrin	Inhibition	10.55	$0.87_{Ouabain}$	10.55
ATP – adenylate cyclase – cAMP				
Ach	Inhibition	5.30	$-0.70_{Pentagastrin}$	5.30
Histamine	Stimulation	9.30	$1.00_{Pentagastrin}$	9.30
Pentagastrin	Stimulation	9.40	1.00	9.40

Table 33. Actions of acetylcholine, histamine and pentagastrin in human beings.

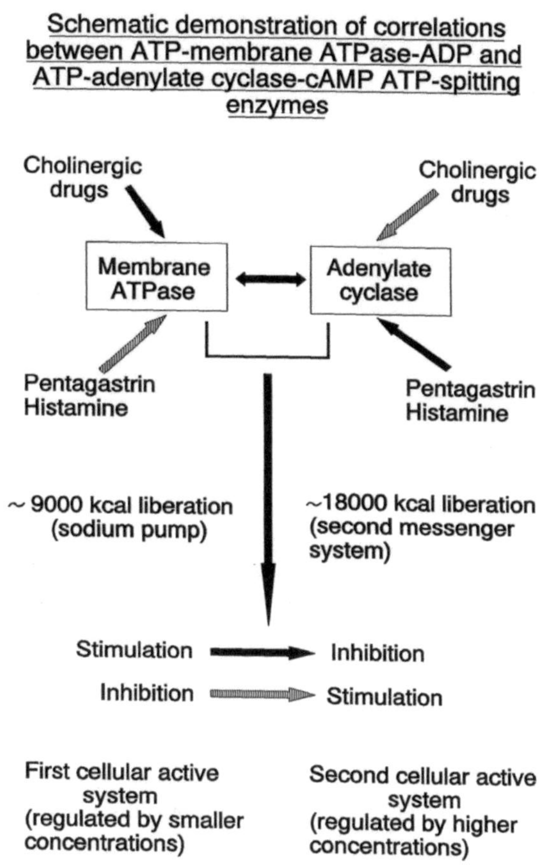

Figure 59. Our suggestion to demonstrate the correlations between the ATP-dependent membrane-bound energy systems and the gastric BAO and MAO values regulated by acetylcholine, pentagastrin and histamine. [Mózsik, Debreceni, Juricskay, Karádi, Nagy (1997) In: Gaginella T.S., MózsikGy., Rainsford K.D. (eds) Biochemical Pharmacology as an Approach to Gastrointestinal Disorders, Kluwer Academic Publishers, Dordrecht, Boston, London. pp. 199–222 (with kind permission).]

7.9. Energetical and biochemical gradients between the gastric fundic, antral and duodenal mucosa in dependence of gastric BAO values in peptic ulcer patients

7.9.1. Energetical and biochemical gradients in the gastric fundic mucosa and musculature in peptic ulcer patients in dependence of gastric basal secretory responses

The biochemical examinations were carried out in resecates of stomach (fundus, antrum) and small intestine (duodenum, jejunum) in patients with chronic peptic ulcer, who underwent surgical intervention.

The gastric BAO and MAO (subcutaneously given 6 μg/kg body weight of pentagastrin) were measured before the surgical intervention.

The examined patients were divided into three groups, according to the BAO values (Table 34). These patients underwent resection of stomach (and some part from duodenum; in patients with jejunal ulcer, who underwent surgery previously, Billroth II-type gastric resection was carried out, and jejunal ulcer appeared later). Immediately after resection, different tissue samples were separated from the obtained tissues, and they were put into liquid nitrogen.

Groups of patients	Basal acid outputs (BAO)	Maximal acid outputs (MAO)
BAO < 2.0 mEq/ h	0.27 ± 0.0.1 (n = 12)	7.95 ± 1.38 (n = 12)
BAO 2.00 to 4.0 mEq/h	2.81 ± 0.10 (n = 9)	15.69 ± 0.76 (n=9)
BAO > 4.0 mEq/h	5.33 ± 0.24 (n = 11)	18.76 ± 2.15 (n=11)

Table 34. Gastric secretory responses in patients in whom the biochemical examinations were carried out. The gastric acid secretory responses are presented in mEq/h (means ± SEM), *n* indicates the number of patients. [Mózsik, Vizi, Kutas: Scand. J. Gastroenterol. 11: 205–211, 1976 (with kind permission).]

The following biochemical examinations were carried out from different tissue samples:

1. Determination of membrane (Mg^{2+}–Na^{+}–K^{+}-dependent) ATPase;
2. Separation and determination of adenine–adenosine, adenosine triphosphate (ATP), adenosine diphosphate (ADP) and adenosine monophosphate (AMP);
3. Separation and determination of lipid phosphates;
4. Separation and determination of nucleic acids.

The details of these methodological problems are presented in a paper (Mózsik et al., 1976b).

It is important to note and emphasize the following:

http://dx.doi.org/10.5772/60102

1. The number of biochemically evaluated tissue samples in different figures is different (e.g., in case of gastric fundic mucosa vs. musculature), which is dependent on the *in situ* situation at the time of surgical intervention;

2. We had no possibility for direct measurement of cyclic AMP from these tissue samples in these series of observations;

3. All biochemical examinations (including the preparative works) were carried out in all tissue samples obtained in one patient.

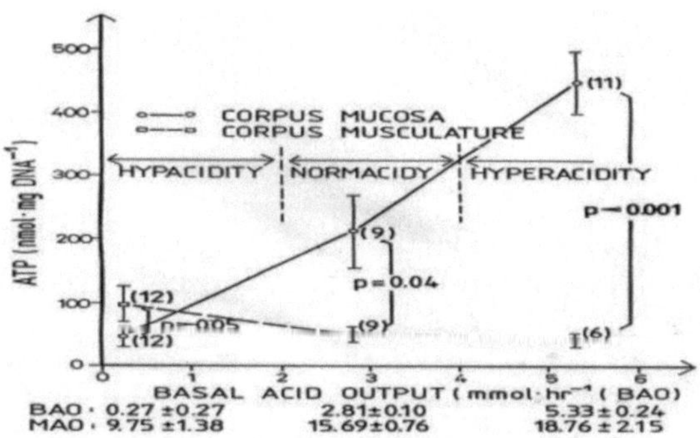

Figure 60. Tissue levels of adenosine triphosphate (ATP) in the gastric fundic mucosa and musculature prepared from patients with peptic ulcer depending on the gastric acid secretory responses. The results are presented in nmol/mg DNA (means ± SEM). The results are based on the results published in a paper (Mózsik, Vizi, Kutas: Scand. J. Gastroenterol. 11: 205–211, 1976) (with some modification).

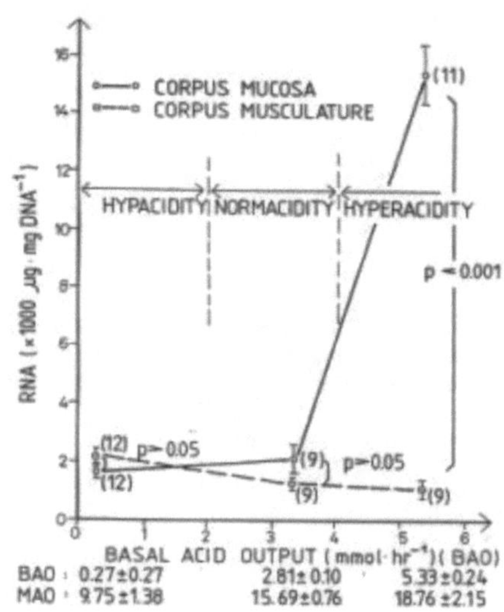

Figure 61. Tissue levels of ribonucleic acid (RNA) in the gastric fundic mucosa and musculature prepared from patients with peptic ulcer depending on the gastric acid secretory responses. The results are presented in mg RNA/mg DNA (means ± SEM).The results are based on the results published in a paper (Mózsik, Vizi, Kutas: Scand. J. Gastroenterol. 11: 205–211, 1976) (with some modification). The numbers in parenthesis indicate the number of patients.

ATP-MEMBRANE ATP-ASE-ADP SYSTEM IN THE HUMAN GASTRIC CORPUS MUCOSA AND MUSCULATURE ON DEPENDENCE OF GASTRIC SECRETORY RESPONSES

	BAO<2.0		2–4		BAO>4	
CORPUS MUCOSA						
ATP+	48±17	(12)	213±69	(9)	447±46	(11)
ATP-ASES: Mg2+-dependent++	0.95±0.14	(62)	2.56±0.43	(28)	3.90±0.56	(59)
ATP-ASES: Mg2+Na+-K+-dependent++	2.19±0.27	(62)	4.54±0.60	(28)	9.14±1.19	(59)
ATP-ASES: Na+-K+-dependent++	1.24±0.19	(62)	2.04±0.34	(28)	5.24±0.72	(59)
ADP+	65±23	(12)	211±40	(9)	446±60	(11)
CORPUS MUSCULATURE						
ATP+	99±37	(12)	49±11	(9)	39±10	(6)
ATP-ASES: Mg2+-dependent++	1.17±0.30	(33)	0.77±0.29	(6)	1.10±0.20	(11)
ATP-ASES: Mg2+Na+-K+-dependent++	2.03±0.39	(33)	1.47±0.51	(6)	1.83±0.20	(11)
ATP-ASES: Na+-K+-dependent++	0.86±0.21	(33)	0.70±0.26	(6)	0.73±0.26	(11)
ADP+	123±38	(12)	74±14	(9)	33±7	(6)

BAO (mmol·hr^{-1}): BAO<2.0; 2–4; BAO>4

+ = nmol·mgDNA^{-1} (means ±SEM); ++ = μmol of P_i · mg membr. prot.$^{-1}$ · hr^{-1} (means±SEM)

Figure 62. ATP–membrane ATPase–ADP system in the human gastric fundic mucosa and musculature prepared in the stomach resecates obtained from patients with peptic ulcer. The results are based on the results published in a paper (Mózsik, Vizi, Kutas: Scand. J. Gastroenterol. 11: 205–211, 1976 and Mózsik, Vizi, Kutas: Scand. J. Gastroenterol. 12: 461–464, 1977) (with some modification). The numbers in parenthesis indicate the number of patients.

ATP MEMBRANE ATP-ASE-ADP SYSTEM IN THE HUMAN ANTRAL MUCOSA AND MUSCULATURE ON DEPENDENCE OF GASTRIC SECRETORY RESPONSES

	BAO<2.0		2–4		BAO>4	
ANTRUM MUCOSA						
ATP+	46±24	(12)	32±5	(9)	16±2	(11)
Mg2+-dependent++	2.00±0.35	(51)	1.60±0.20	(6)	1.56±0.42	(6)
Mg2+Na+-K+-dependent++	2.65±0.40	(51)	2.40±0.30	(6)	2.52±0.69	(6)
Na+-K+-dependent++	0.65±0.10	(51)	0.86±0.30	(6)	0.96±0.22	(6)
ADP+	64±25	(12)	25±2	(9)	31±8	(11)
ANTRUM MUSCULATURE						
ATP+	107±41	(6)	88±28	(9)	37±3	(6)
Mg2+-dependent++	1.54±0.30	(21)	1.33±0.20	(6)	1.01±0.33	(5)
Mg2+Na+-K+-dependent++	3.36±0.31	(21)	3.10±0.30	(6)	2.02±0.50	(5)
Na+-K+-dependent++	1.82±0.12	(21)	1.73±0.29	(6)	1.01±0.30	(5)
ADP+	129±56	(6)	138±38	(9)	23±2	(6)

BAO (mmol·hr^{-1}): BAO<2.0; 2–4; BAO>4

+ = nmol · mg DNA^{-1} (means ±SEM); ++ = μmol of P_i · mg membr. prot.$^{-1}$ · hr^{-1} (means±SEM)

Figure 63. Correlations between the membrane ATPase activity, tissue levels of ATP and ADP in the human gastric fundic mucosa and musculature in patients with different gastric (hypacid, normacid and hyperacid) secretory responses depending on the gastric basal acid output (BAO) (means ± SEM). The results are based on the results published in a paper (Mózsik, Vizi, Kutas: Scand. J. Gastroenterol. 11: 205–211, 1976 and Mózsik, Vizi, Kutas: Scand. J. Gastroenterol. 12: 461–464, 1977) (with some modification).

http://dx.doi.org/10.5772/60102

MAIN CHANGES IN METABOLISM OF GASTRIC MUCOSA (A) AND MUSCULATURE (B) IN PATIENTS WITH DIFFERENT GASTRIC SECRETORY RESPONSES (BAO)
(means±SEM)

BAO (mmol·hr⁻¹)	<2 (n=12) A	<2 (n=12) B	2-4 (n=9) A	2-4 (n=9) B	>4 (n=11) A	>4 (n=11) B
CORPUS						
[a] ATP·ADP⁻¹	0.74±0.05	0.80±0.06	1.01±0.07	0.66±0.05	1.00±0.02	1.18±0.07
[b] Lipid-P·DNA⁻¹	0.36±0.04	0.43±0.04	404±0.10	0.33±0.04	13 58±0.70	1.40±0.30
[b] RNA·DNA⁻¹	1.74±0.08	2.03±0.15	2.00±0.24	1.24±0.06	15.28±1.00	714±0.84
[a] „energy charge"	0.43±0.04	0.46±0.03	0.33±0.04	0.42±0.03	0.03±0.01	0.14±0.02
ANTRUM						
[a] ATP·ADP⁻¹	0.72±0.06	0.83±0.06	1.29±0.08	0.64±0.05	0.52±0.04	1.60±0.10
[b] Lipid-P·DNA⁻¹	0.16±0.05	0.85±0.08	0.26±0.06	0.31±0.04	0.43±0.03	0.34±0.04
[b] RNA·DNA⁻¹	1.39±0.10	1.75±0.11	1.05±0.05	296±0.02	2.03±0.15	1.24±0.06
[a] „energy charge"	0.45±0.04	0.51±0.04	0.39±0.03	0.46±0.07	0.07±0.01	0.27±0.03

a=values are in nmoles·mg DNA⁻¹ ; b=values are in mg·mg DNA⁻¹
„energy charge"=(ATP+0.5 ADP)·(ATP+ADP+AMP)⁻¹

Figure 64. The changes in the biochemistry of gastric fundic mucosa and musculature in patients with different gastric BAO values. The results are expressed as means ± SEM/1.0 mg deoxyribonucleic acid (DNA) (means ± SEM). The results are based on the results published in a paper (Mózsik, Vizi, Kutas: Scand. J. Gastroenterol. 11: 205–211, 1976 and Mózsik, Vizi, Kutas: Scand. J. Gastroenterol. 12: 461–464, 1977) (with some modification). The numbers in parenthesis indicate the number of patients.

7.9.2. Energetical and biochemical gradients in the gastric antral and duodenal mucosa and musculature in patients with peptic ulcer in dependence of gastric basal acid secretory responses

There was an energy gradient in the corpus, antrum and duodenum mucosa depending on the gastric basal and maximal acid secretory activities (Mózsik et al., 1976 a, b, c, 1979 b, 1981a) (Figures 65–66; Tables 35–37).

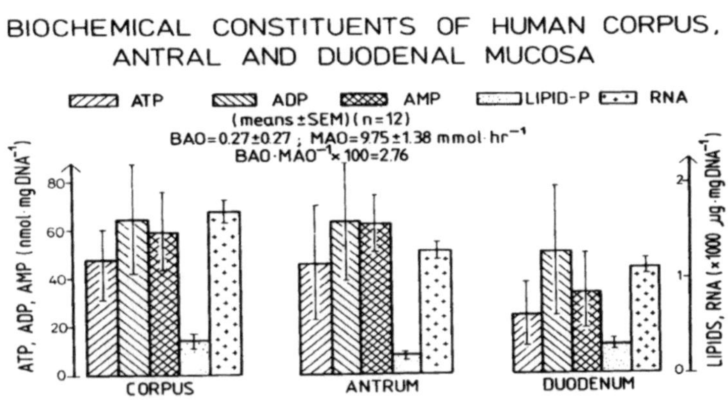

Figure 65. Biochemical parameters in the corpus, antrum and duodenum in patients with gastric hypacidity (BAO, MAO) (means ± SEM) (Mózsik, Vizi, Kutas: Scand. J. Gastroenterol. 12: 461–464, 1976) (with some modification).

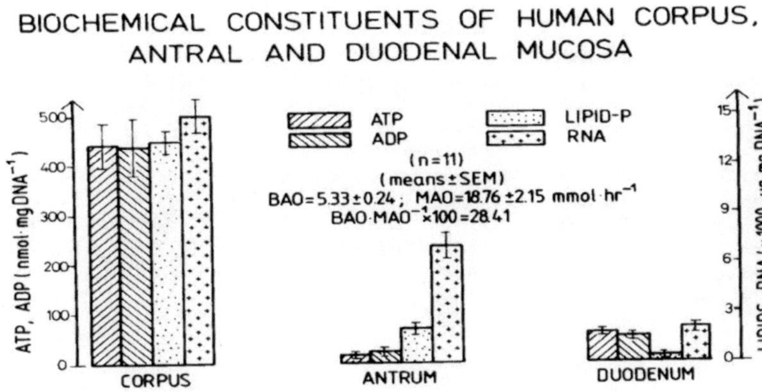

Figure 66. Biochemical gradients in the gastric fundic, antral and duodenal mucosa in patients with hyperacidity (means ± SEM). (Mózsik, Vizi, Kutas: Scand. J. Gastroenterol. 12: 461–464, 1976) (with some modification).

	Corpus (12)[b]	Antrum (12)[b]	Duodenum (12)[b]	p^1 [c]	p^2 [c]	p^3 [c]
ATP[d]	48±17	46±24	24±14	NS[e]	NS	NS
ADP[d]	65±23	64±25	51±28	NS	NS	NS
ATP/ADP	0.74±0.05	0.72±0.06	0.47±0.06	NS	<0.01	<0.01
AMP[d]	60±17	63±12	34±16	NS	NS	NS
ATP+ADP+AMP[d]	173±25	173±18	109±12	NS	<0.01	<0.02
Energy charge[f]	0.43±0.04	0.45±0.04	0.45±0.08	NS	NS	NS
Adenine-adenosine[d]	718±179	549±229	435±207	NS	NS	NS
Lipid-P[g]	358±46	163±50	306±43	<0.02	NS	NS
RNA[g]	1741±81	1397±107	1133±41	=0.02	=0.04	<0.001

[a] ATP,adenosine triphosphate; ADP,adenosine diphosphate; AMP,adenosine monophosphate; lipid-P, lipid phosphates; RNA,ribonucleic acid.
[b] Numbers in parentheses indicate numbers of patients.
[c] p^1,corpus versus antrum; p^2,antrum versus duodenum; p^3,corpus versus duodenum.
[d] Values=nanomoles of substrates per 1.0 mg deoxyribonucleic acid (means±S.E.M.).
[e] Not significant.
[f] Adenylate pool energy charge (ATP+0.5 ADP/ATP+ADP+AMP).
[g] Values=micrograms of substrates per 1.0 mg deoxyribonucleic acid (means±S.E.M.).

Table 35. Substrate levels in the gastric mucosa of the corpus, antrum and duodenum of patients with BAO values <2.0 mEq/h (BAO = 0.27 ± 0.27; MAO = 9.75 ± 1.38)[a]. [Mózsik, Vizi, Kutas: Scand. J. Gastroenterol. 12: 461–464, 1977 (with kind permission).]

http://dx.doi.org/10.5772/60102

	Corpus (9)[b]	Antrum (9)[b]	Duodenum (9)[b]	p^{1} [c]	p^{2} [c]	p^{3} [c]
ATP[d]	213±69	32±5	25±3	=0.02	NS[e]	=0.02
ADP[d]	211±40	25±2	29±6	<0.001	NS	<0.001
ATP/ADP	1.01±0.07	1.29±0.08	0.86±0.07	NS	<0.001	NS
AMP[d]	545±75	57±15	60±7	<0.001	NS	<0.001
ATP+ADP+AMP[d]	969±100	114±18	114±11	<0.001	NS	<0.001
Energy charge[f]	0.33±0.04	0.39±0.03	0.43±0.11	NS	NS	NS
Adenine-adenosine[d]	4327±1908	353±39	326±48	<0.001	NS	<0.001
Lipid-P[g]	4047±108	269±60	261±50	<0.001	NS	<0.001
RNA[g]	2008±543	1050±53	933±32	NS	NS	=0.06

[a] ATP,adenosine triphosphate; ADP,adenosine diphosphate; AMP,adenosine monophosphate; lipid-P, lipid phosphates; RNA, ribonucleic acid.
[b] Numbers in parentheses indicate numbers of patients.
[c] p^1,corpus versus antrum; p^2,antrum versus duodenum; p^3,corpus versus duodenum.
[d] Values=nanomoles of substrates per 1.0 mg deoxyribonucleic acid (means±S.E.M.).
[e] Not significant.
[f] Adenylate pool energy charge (ATP+0.5 ADP/ATP+ADP+AMP).
[g] Values=micrograms of substrates per 1.0 mg deoxyribonucleic acid (means±S.E.M.).

Table 36. Substrate levels in the gastric mucosa of the corpus, antrum and duodenum of patients with 2.0<BAO<4.0 mEq/h (BAO = 2.81 ± 0.10; MAO = 15.69 ± 0.76)[a]. [Mózsik, Vizi, Kutas: Scand. J. Gastroenterol. 12: 461–464, 1977 (with kind permission).]

	Corpus (11)[b]	Antrum (11)[b]	Duodenum (11)[b]	p^{1} [c]	p^{2} [c]	p^{3} [c]
ATP[d]	447±46	16±4	60±2	<0.001	<0.001	<0.001
ADP[d]	446±60	31±8	63±6	<0.001	<0.001	<0.001
ATP/ADP	1.00±0.02	0.52±0.04	0.95±0.10	<0.001	<0.001	NS[e]
AMP[d]	19606±720	381±70	38±6	<0.001	<0.001	<0.001
ATP+ADP+AMP[d]	20449±200	428±38	224±21	<0.001	<0.001	<0.001
Energy charge[f]	0.03±0.01	0.07±0.01	0.40±0.07	NS	<0.001	<0.001
Adenine-adenosine[d]	13394±569	3212±1311	370±27	<0.001	=0.05	<0.001
Lipid-P[g]	13588±708	1406±300	91±18	<0.001	<0.001	<0.001
RNA[g]	15289±1000	7141±847	1961±21	<0.001	<0.001	<0.001

[a] ATP,adenosine triphosphate; ADP,adenosine diphosphate; AMP,adenosine monophosphate; lipid-P, lipid phosphates; RNA,ribonucleic acid.
[b] Numbers in parentheses indicate numbers of patients.
[c] p^1,corpus versus antrum; p^2,antrum versus duodenum; p^3,corpus versus duodenum.
[d] Values=nanomoles of substrates per 1.0 mg deoxyribonucleic acid (means±S.E.M.).
[e] Not significant.
[f] Adenylate pool energy charge (ATP+0.5 ADP/ATP+ADP+AMP)).
[g] Values=micrograms of substrates per 1.0 mg deoxyribonucleic acid (means±S.E.M.)

Table 37. Substrate levels in the gastric mucosa of the corpus, antrum and duodenum of patients with BAO values >4.0 mEq/h (BAO = 5.33 ± 0.24; MAO = 18.76 ± 2.15)[a]. [(Mózsik, Vizi, Kutas: Scand. J. Gastroenterol. 12: 461–464, 1977 (with kind permission).]

7.10. Comparative biochemistry of ulcerated and non-ulcerated mucosal tissues in peptic (antral, duodenal, jejunal) ulcer patients

The membrane ATPase activity and tissue levels of ATP and ADP were measured around the gastric antral, duodenal and jejunal ulcer patients (after partial gastrectomy).

The ATPase activity and tissue levels of ATP and ADP were significantly higher around the gastric antral, duodenal and jejunal mucosa than those obtained in the non-ulcerated (control) mucosa (Mózsik et al., 1976 d, f, 1981 a, c, 1987 a, b, 2000) (Figures 65, 66; Tables 35–37).

7.10.1. Mucosal biochemistry of chronic ulcerated and non-ulcerated antral mucosa in patients with chronic antral ulcer

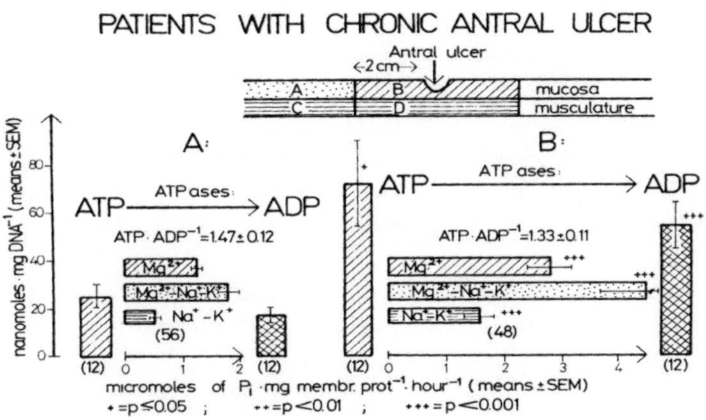

Figure 67. Changes in the extents of ATP–ADP transformation in the antral mucosa of patients with chronic antral ulcer in the ulcerated and non-ulcerated (control) mucosa (means ± SEM). [Mózsik, Kutas, Nagy, Tárnok, 1979; Mózsik, Kutas, Nagy, Tárnok, Acta Medica Acad. Sci. Hung. 36: 1–29, 1979 and Acta Medica Acad. Sci. Hung. 38: 129–134, 1984 (with kind permission).]

7.10.2. Mucosal biochemistry of ulcerated and non-ulcerated duodenal mucosa in patients with chronic duodenal ulcer

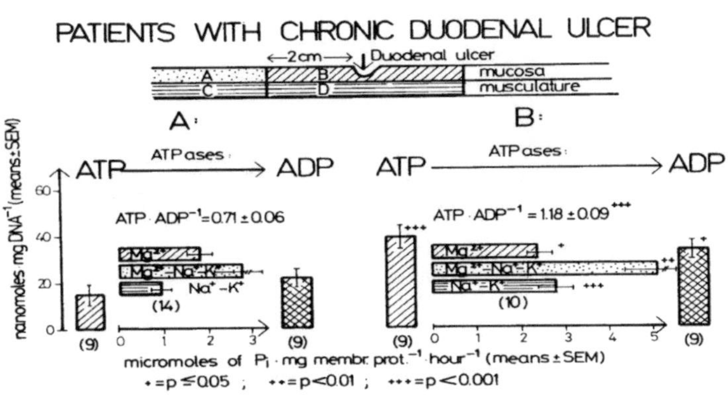

Figure 68. Changes in the extent of ATP–ADP transformation in the duodenal mucosa of patients with chronic duodenal ulcer, in the ulcerated and non-ulcerated duodenal mucosa (means ± SEM). [Mózsik, Kutas, Nagy, Tárnok: Acta Medica Acad. Sci. Hung. 37: 39–49, 1979 (with kind permission).]

http://dx.doi.org/10.5772/60102

7.10.3. Mucosal biochemistry of ulcerated and non-ulcerated jejunal mucosa in patients with chronic jejunal ulcer

It was clear to conclude that the magnitudes of drugs actions depend on the membrane enzyme activity. Because the membrane ATPase activity significantly changes on the activity of target organ, the drug actions depend on the activity of the target organ (Nagy et al.,1976, 1981 a, b).

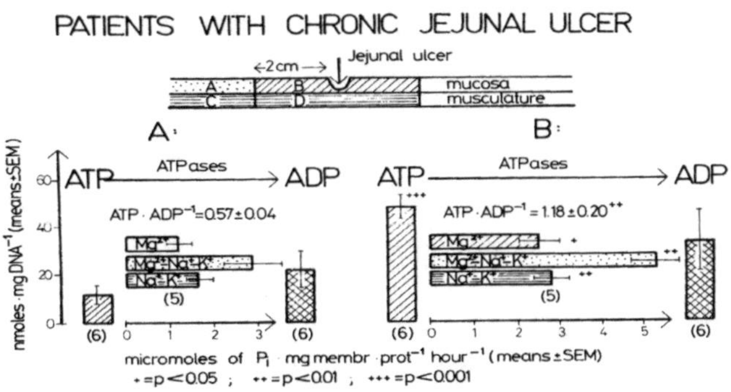

Figure 69. Changes in the extent of ATP–ADP transformation in the jejunal mucosa of patients who underwent partial gastrectomy (according to the method of Billroth II) around the jejunal ulcerated mucosa and non-ulcerated jejunal mucosa (means ± SEM). [Mózsik, Nagy, Tárnok, Kutas: Acta Medica Acad. Sci. Hung. 38, 129–134, 1981 (with kind permission).]

7.10.4. Exclusion of tissue hypoxia in the tissues around the chronic gastric, duodenal and jejunal mucosa in patients

Figures 70 and 71 clearly indicate that the tissue levels of mucosal levels of ATP and ADP are significantly higher in the ulcerated antral, duodenal and jejunal mucosa than those obtained in the control (non-ulcerated) mucosa specimen (the measurements were done simultaneously in patients).

As we indicated earlier, the membrane ATPase activity was also significantly higher in these ulcerated mucosa specimens than that in the control (non-ulcerated) mucosa. Against these biochemical changes, the values of "energy charge" remained the same (Figure 72).

These results demonstrated earlier in Figures 70–72 clearly indicate the following:

1. The extent of ATP–ADP breakdown is significantly higher in the ulcerated antral, duodenal and jejunal mucosa specimens than that in the control (non-ulcerated) mucosa specimens. This fact can be proven by the increased membrane ATPase activity and by increased level of ADP;

2. No impaired phosphorylation can be found in the ulcerated mucosa specimens, which can be proven by increased tissue levels of ATP in time when the ATP–ADP breakdown was significantly increased (significantly higher membrane ATPase activity and increased level of ADP);

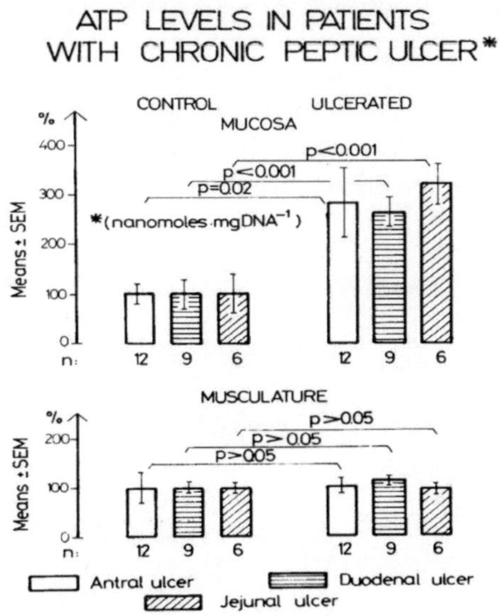

Figure 70. Comparative demonstration in the changes of the tissue levels of ATP in the ulcerated versus non-ulcerated antral, duodenal and jejunal mucosa (the musculature is located under the examined mucosa tissues) (means ± SEM). [Mózsik el al., in Mózsik, Hänninen, Jávor (eds.) Advances in Physiological Sciences. Vol. 29. Gastrointestinal Defence Mechanism, Pergamon Press, Oxford-Akadémiai Kiadó, Budapest. pp. 213–288, 1981 (with kind permission).]

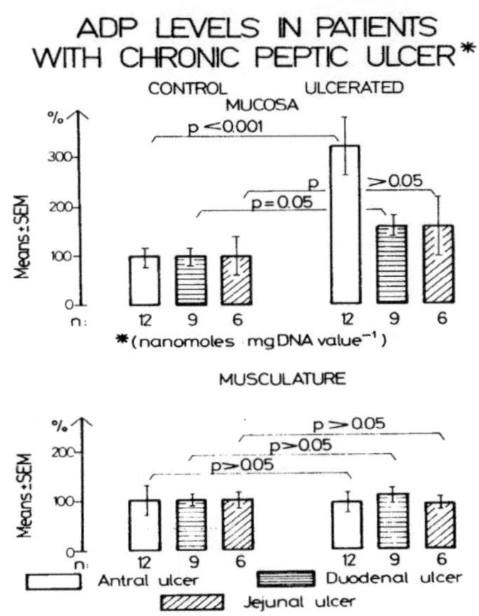

Figure 71. Comparative demonstration in the changes of tissue levels of ADP in the ulcerated and non-ulcerated antral, duodenal and jejunal mucosa (the musculature is located under the examined mucosa tissues). (Mózsik et al., In: Mózsik, Hänninen, Jávor (eds.) Advances in Physiological Sciences. Vol. 29. Gastrointestinal Defence Mechanism, Pergamon Press, Oxford- Akadémiai Kiadó, Budapest. pp. 213–288, 1981). For further explanation, see Figure 70.

http://dx.doi.org/10.5772/60102

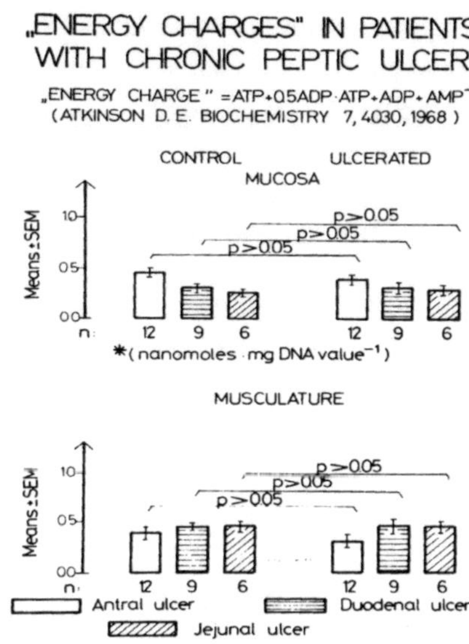

Figure 72. Critical evaluation of the "energy charge" in the mucosa around the chronic antral, duodenal and jejunal mucosa versus Non-ulcerated mucosa (the musculature located under the studies mucosa tissues). [Mózsik el al., in Mózsik, Hänninen, Jávor (eds.) Advances in Physiological Sciences. Vol.29. Gastrointestinal Defence Mechanism, Pergamon Press, Oxford- Akadémiai Kiadó, Budapest. pp. 213–288, 1981 (with kind permission).] For further explanation, see Figure 70.

3. The extent of ATP–cAMP transformation was significantly higher in the ulcerated antral, duodenal and jejunal mucosa around the chronic ulcer;

4. The tissue levels of ATP were significantly higher in the mucosa – around the chronic antral, duodenal and jejunal ulcer – that those in the control (non-ulcerated) mucosa, while the extents of both ATP–ADP and ATP–cAMP transformations were increased in the ulcerated antral mucosa specimens;

5. The higher ATP tissue levels (in time when the ATP breakdown was increased in both directions) can be obtained by the intact oxidative phosphorylation pathway;

6. The biochemical components of gastric mucosal tissue were expressed in accordance to 1.0 mg DNA, which represents the same number of cells (Figure 297). The values of adenine–adenosine, ATP, ADP and AMP were increased in the gastric fundic mucosa in patients with increased gastric secretory responses (BAO, MAO) and in the mucosa around chronic antral, duodenal and jejunal ulcers.

No physiological data are available in the literature to prove the presence of decreased GMBF in the gastric fundic mucosa in patients with gastric hyperacidity, and nobody found an increased tissue level of lactate. All experts accept the increased energy turnover (increased extents of ATP–ADP and ATP–cAMP transformation) in these gastric fundic mucosa specimens.

The results of animal experiments clearly indicated that the biochemical components differ significantly in the glandular stomach in comparison with the values in the forestomach. When we analyzed the time -sequence of biochemical changes, development of gastric hyperacidity and ulcer development, we first obtained the gastric hyperacidity and then the ulcer development. The same tendency was obtained in the changes of gastric mucosal biochemistry in both parts of the stomach, and these changes appeared before the development of gastric hyperacidity in 24-hour pylorus-ligated rats (Mózsik and Vizi, 1976 a, b).

A significant biochemical gradient was biochemically proved in the gastric fundic, antral, duodenal and jejunal mucosa depending on the gastric secretory responses (BAO, MAO).

Author details

Gyula Mozsik[1*] and Imre Szabó[2]

*Address all correspondence to: gyula.mozsik@aok.pte.hu

1 First Department of Medicine, Medical and Health Centre, University of Pécs, Hungary

2 Associate Professor at the First Department of Medicine, University of Pécs, Hungary

Chapter 8

Animal Models Used to Study the Different Mechanisms Involved in the Gastric Mucosal Damage and in the Protection

Gyula Mozsik and Imre Szabó

Additional information is available at the end of the chapter

http://dx.doi.org/10.5772/60505

8.1. 24-hour pylorus-ligated rats

8.1.1. 24-hour pylorus-ligated rats alone

The peak of the membrane ATPase appears earlier than the gastric hypersecretion (Figure 73). When we prepared the membrane ATPase from the forestomach (rumen), we also found its peak earlier than the ulcer development (Shay et al., 1945) (Figure 74).

It is interesting to note that the changes in the membrane ATPase reached its peak at the same time in both stomach parts after pylorus-ligation (4 hours after the pyloric ligation). When we compared the sequence of biochemistry, gastric hypersecretion and ulcer development, we found a similar sequence to that in patients with antral, duodenal and jejunal ulcers.

The membrane ATPase can be specifically inhibited by ouabain application. This principal argument offers an approach to the changes in the gastric acid output and concentration) and ulcer development (Figures 75, 76).

The tissue level of cAMP decreased significantly in both parts of the rat stomach (Mózsik et al., 1978 a, c; Mózsik et al., 1979 a, b, c, d, e, f).

8.1.2. 24-hour pylorus-ligated rats after bilateral surgical vagotomy

After a 24-hour bilateral surgical vagotomy, the gastric acid secretory responses and gastric ulcer significantly decreased (Table 38), meanwhile the ATP--ADP transformation significantly decreased in both glandular part and the forestomach (Figures 77, 78).

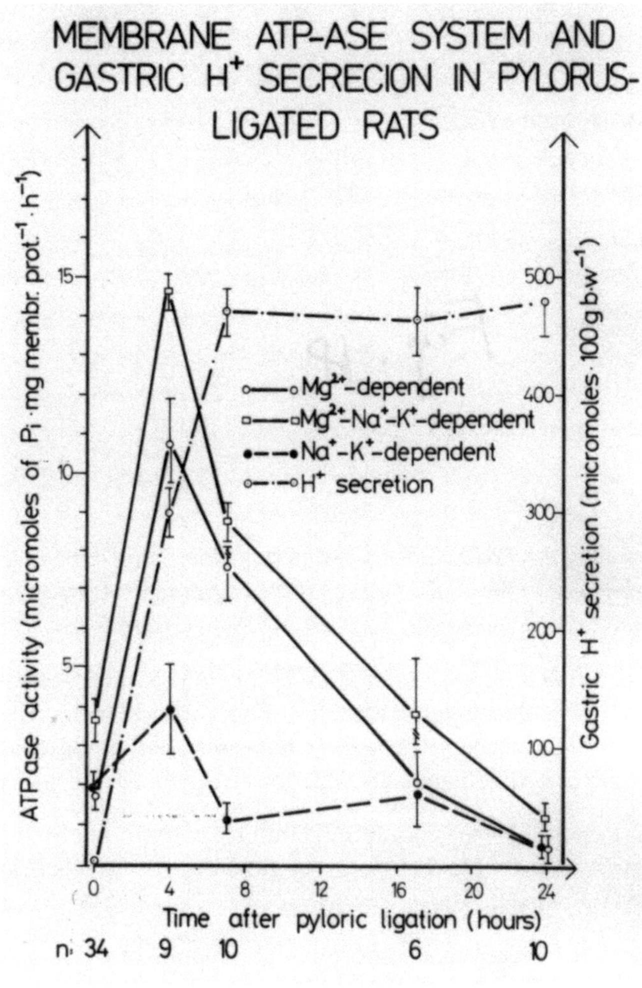

Figure 73. Correlations between the changes in membrane ATPase activity and H^+ output in 24-hour pylorus-ligated rats (means ± SEM) [Mózsik and Vizi: Amer. J. Dig. Dis. 21:449-454, 1976a) (with kind permission)].

http://dx.doi.org/10.5772/60505

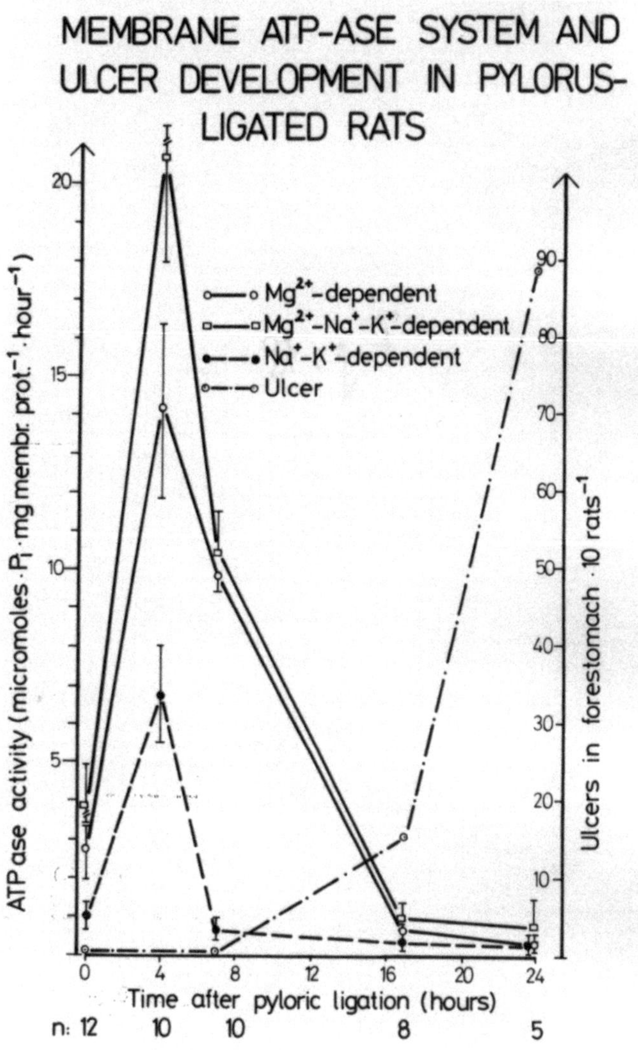

Figure 74. Correlation between the changes in membrane ATPase prepared from the forestomach and ulcer development in 24-hour pyloru-ligated rats (means ± SEM) [Mózsik Gy. and Vizi: Amer. J. Dig. Dis. 21:449-454, 1976a)(with kind permission)].

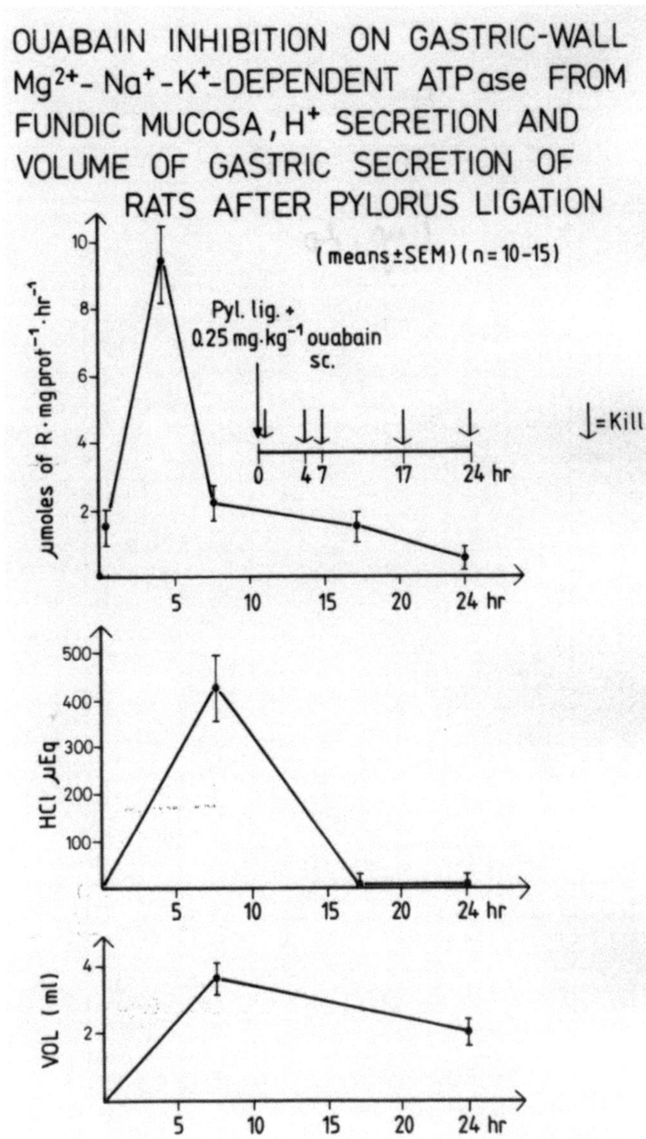

Figure 75. Ouabain-induced inhibition of the membrane ATPase prepared from gastric fundic mucosa, volume of gastric secretion and H^+ output in 24-hour pylorus-ligated rats dependent upon time after pyloric ligation (means ± SEM). [Mózsik and Vizi: Amer. J. Dig. Dis. 21:449–454, 1976a (with kind permission).]

http://dx.doi.org/10.5772/60505

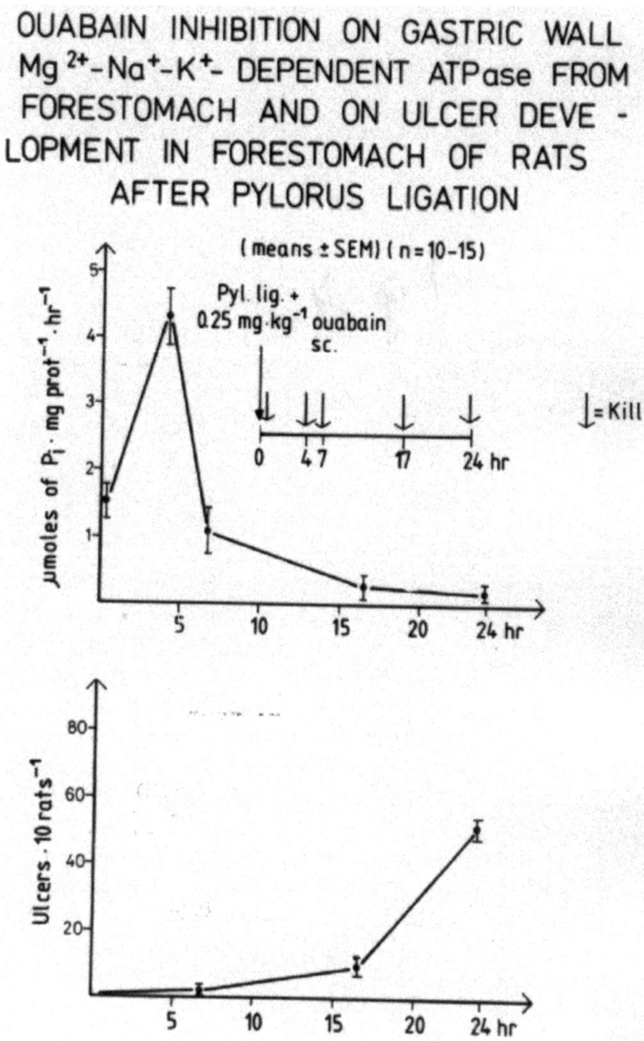

Figure 76. Ouabain-induced inhibition of the membrane ATPase prepared from the forestomach and ulcer development in 24-hour pylorus-ligated rats (means ± SEM) [Mózsik and Vizi: Amer. J. Dig. Dis. 21: 449–454, 1976a (with kind permission).]The tissue level of cAMP decreased significantly in both parts of the rat stomach (Mózsik et al., 1978 a, c; Mózsik et al., 1979 a, b, c, d, e, f).

Experimal parameters	Pylorus ligation alonc	Pylorus ligation + bilateral surgical vagotomy
Volume of gastric secretion (mL/24 h)	15.4 ± 2.1	2.0 ± 0.3*
H^+ output (μEq/ 24)	867 ± 50	130 ± 20*
H^+ concentration (mEq/L)	55.2 ± 2.6	65 ± 10
Total number of ulcer in the forestomach/ 10 rats	86	0

Table 38. Gastric secretory numbers (means ± SEM) and ulcer development (total ulcer/10 rats) in pylorus-ligated rats with and without bilateral surgical vagotomy. Abbreviation: * : $P < 0.001$. [Mózsik and Vizi: Dig. Dis. Sci. 22: 1072–1075, 1976b (with kind permission).]

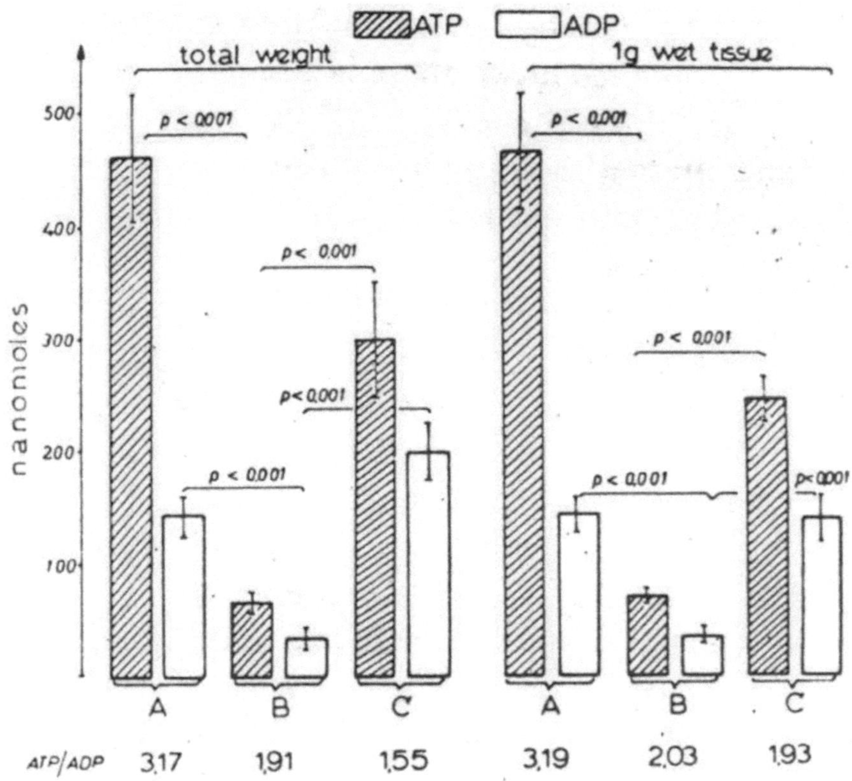

Figure 77. Changes in stomach wall ATP and ADP in the corpus of pylorus-ligated rats 24 hours after pylorus ligation, with and without bilateral surgical vagotomy. The results are expressed in nanomoles (means ± SEM of 10 rats). Abbreviations: A, sham-operated rats; B, pylorus-ligated rats; C, pylorus-ligated and surgically vagotomized rats. The ATP/ADP for A is significantly greater than that for B: $P < 0.001$. [Mózsik and Vizi: Dig. Dis. 22: 1072–1075, 1976b (with kind permission).]

http://dx.doi.org/10.5772/60505

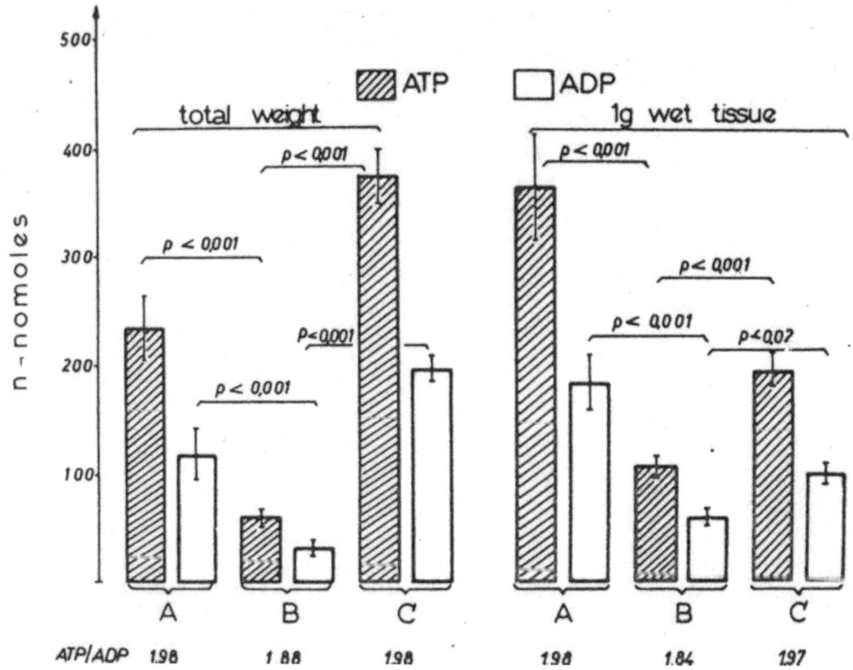

Figure 78. Changes in stomach wall ATP and ADP in the forestomach of rats 24 hours after pylorus ligation, with and without bilateral surgical vagotomy. The results are expressed in nanomoles (means ± SEM of 10 rats). Abbreviations: A, sham-operated rats; B, pylorus-ligated rats; C, pylorus-ligated and surgically vagotomized rats. The ATP/ADP for A is not significantly different from that for B. [Mózsik and Vizi: Dig. Dis. 22:1072–1075, 1976b (with kind permission).]

The stomach wall ATP and ADP have been studied in rats, with and without bilateral surgical vagotomy, 24 hours after pylorus ligation. It was observed that the amounts and concentrations significantly decreased in both parts (corpus + antrum and forestomach) in pylorus-ligated rats, whereas the amounts and concentrations remained significantly higher in pylorus-ligated + vagotomized rats. Changes in amounts and concentrations of ADP paralleled those of ATP. It has been concluded that a significant decrease of cellular ATP is necessary to produce gastric hypersecretion in ulceration in pylorus-ligated rats. This significant decrease of cellular ATP, in corpus + antrum and forestomach, can be prevented by bilateral surgical vagotomy (Mózsik and Vizi, 1976b).

8.2. Dynamic evaluation the changes of extra- and intracellular regulatory mechanisms of gastric cellular energy systems in pylorus-ligated rats without application of any drugs

As we mentioned earlier, the time period of 4 hours after pylorus ligation offers an ideal time to study the stimulatory or inhibitory actions of drugs, hormones and mediators given immediately after pylorus ligation (Figure 73). During this time period, gastric ulceration upon gastric hyperacidity never appears.

In the study, the fundus and forestomach in the rats were biochemically analyzed in depth to understand the drugs, hormones and mediators.

BIOCHEMICAL CONSTITUENTS IN THE GASTRIC FUNDIC MUCOSA OF UNTREATED RATS

BIOCHEMICAL CONSTITUENTS	MEANS ± SEM	N
ATP*	11.58 ± 1	39
ADP*	13.75 ± 1	39
$ATP \cdot ADP^{-1}$	0.84 ± 0.06	39
AMP*	10.73 ± 2	39
ATP+ADP+AMP*	36.06 ± 2	39
$\frac{ATP+0.5\,ADP}{ATP+ADP+AMP}$	0.51 ± 0.02	39
cAMP**	4.51 ± 0.10	39
LACTATE***	277 ±20	39

* nmoles · mg mucosal protein^{-1} (means ± SEM)
** pmoles · mg mucosal protein^{-1} (means ± SEM)
*** µmoles · mg mucosal protein^{-1} (means ± SEM)

Table 39. Biochemical constituents in the gastric fundic mucosa of intact rats.

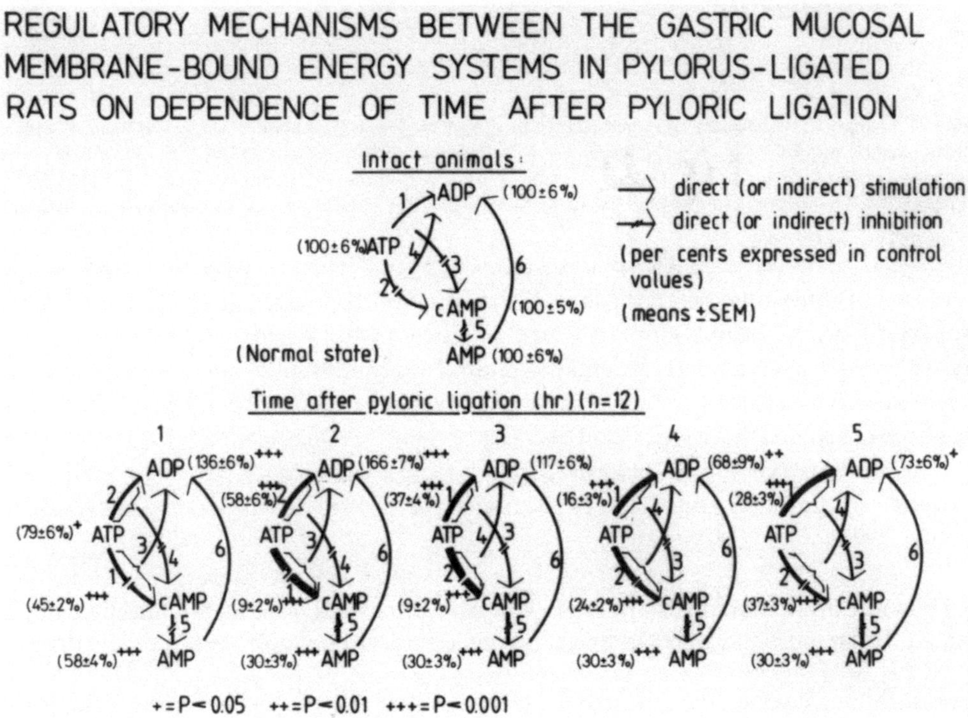

Figure 79. Changes in the cellular ATP, ADP, cAMP and AMP in the time period of first 5 hours dependent upon time after pyloric ligation. The observations were carried out on gastric fundic mucosa. The results obtained in sham-operated rats (normal state) were taken to be equal to 100% (means ± SEM). [Mozsik (2006) Molecular pharmacology and biochemistry of gastroduodenal mucosal damage and protection. In: Mózsik Gy. (Ed.) Discoveries in Gastroenterology (1960–2005). Akadémiai Kiadó, Budapest. pp. 139–224 (with kind permission).]

http://dx.doi.org/10.5772/60505

The tissue levels of ATP, ADP, cAMP and AMP and the regulatory mechanisms between them were measured at 1, 2, 3, 4 and 5 hours after pylorus ligation (Figure 79, Table 39).

8.2.1. Biochemical backgrounds of effect of atropine in 4 hours pylorus-ligated rats

The atropine dose-dependently decreases the gastric H⁺ output (Figure 80). In these observations, the ADP was decreased dose-dependently, whereas the cAMP and AMP were increased in the rat gastric fundic mucosa (Figure 81).

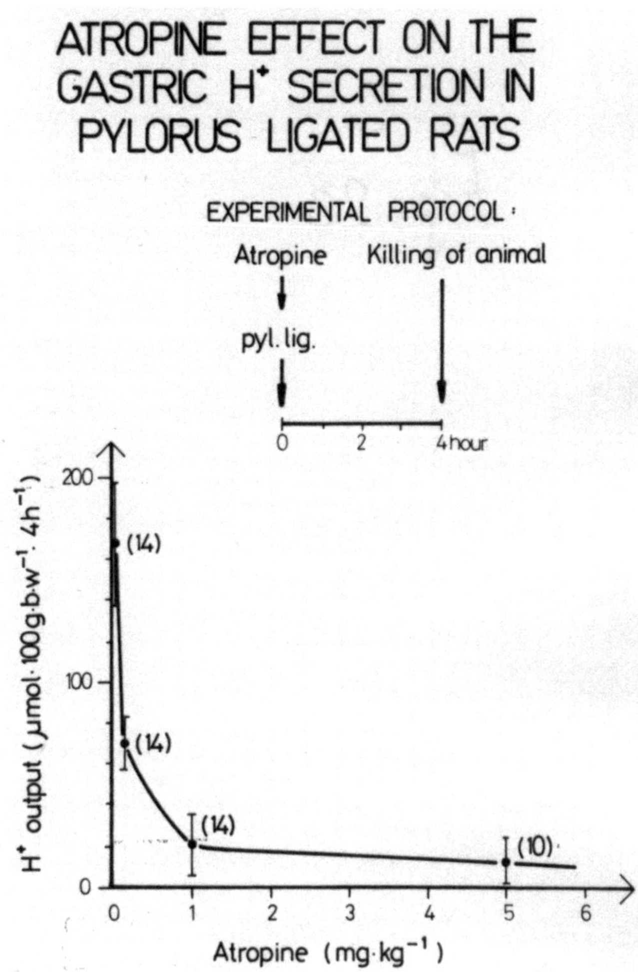

Figure 80. Dose-dependent inhibitory effect of atropine on the gastric acid secretion in 4-hour pylorus-ligated rats (means ± SEM). [Mózsik, Figler, Nagy, Patty, Tárnok (1981): Gastric and small intestinal energy metabolism in mucosal damage. In: Mózsik Gy., Hänninen O., Jávor T. (Eds.). Advances in Physiological Sciences. Vol. 29. Gastrointestinal Defence Mechanism. Pergamon Press, Oxford – Akadémiai Kiadó, Budapest. pp. 213–288 (with kind permission).]

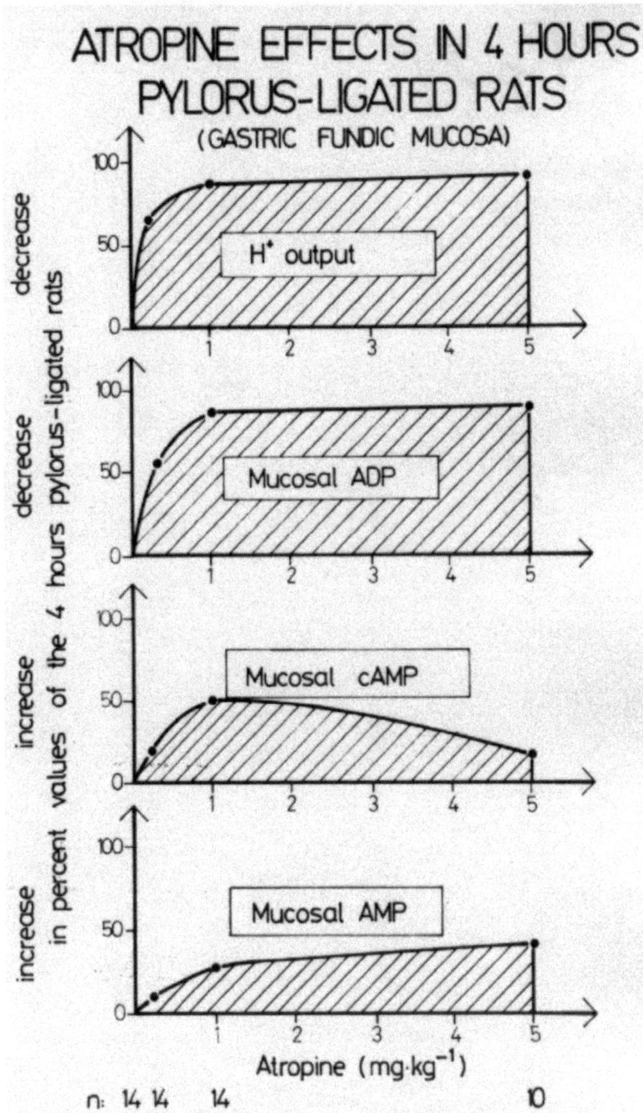

Figure 81. Atropine-induced changes in gastric H^+ output, gastric fundic mucosal levels of ATP, ADP and AMP in 4-hour pylorus-ligated rats. The results were expressed as percent values obtained immediately after pylorus ligation (=100%), except for gastric H^+ output, which was also expressed in percent values, but obtained at 4 hours after pylorus ligation (means ± SEM). [Mózsik, Figler, Nagy, Patty, Tárnok (1981): Gastric and small intestinal energy metabolism in mucosal damage. In: Mózsik Gy., Hänninen O., Jávor T. (Eds.). Advances in Physiological Sciences. Vol. 29. Gastrointestinal Defence Mechanism. Pergamon Press, Oxford – Akadémiai Kiadó, Budapest. pp. 213–288 (with kind permission).]

Similar changes were found in the forestomach during atropine treatment.

Schematic summary of atropine treatment-induced (given in different doses) gastric fundic mucosal damage in 4-hour pylorus-ligated rats (Figure 82).

http://dx.doi.org/10.5772/60505

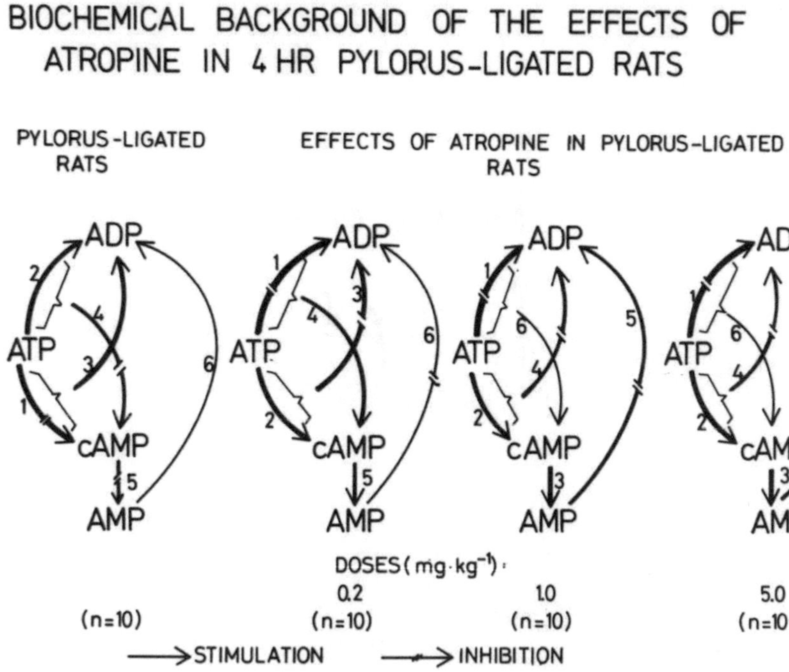

Figure 82. Biochemical changes in the regulatory steps of cellular energy systems in the gastric fundic mucosa produced by different (cytoprotective and antisecretory) doses of atropine in 4-hour pylorus-ligated rats.

8.2.2. Biochemical backgrounds of epinephrine in hours pylorus-ligated rats

Epinephrine dose-dependently decreased the gastric H^+ output and gastric fundic mucosal level of ADP, whereas the cAMP level was increased (Shay et al., 1945) (Figures 83–85).

Similar changes were found in the forestomach after epinephrine administration to those in the rat gastric fundic mucosa.

Figure 85 indicates the main steps of epinephrine-induced regulatory pathways in the tissue levels of ATP, ADP, cAMP and AMP in the gastric fundic mucosa of 4-hour pylorus-ligated rats.

8.3. Biochemistry of aspirin-induced mucosal damage and its prevention by different compounds

8.3.1. Biochemistry of aspirin-induced mucosal damage in 4 hours pylorus-ligated rats

Aspirin is a specific inhibitor of cyclooxygenase (COX-1; Mózsik et al., 2003).

Earlier, Davernport and coworkers proved that aspirin breaks the gastric mucosal barrier, which increases the H^+ backdiffusion.

We observed later (during the 1980s) that the transformation of ATP into ADP could be inhibited by aspirin administration (Figler et al., 1985, 1986, 1999).

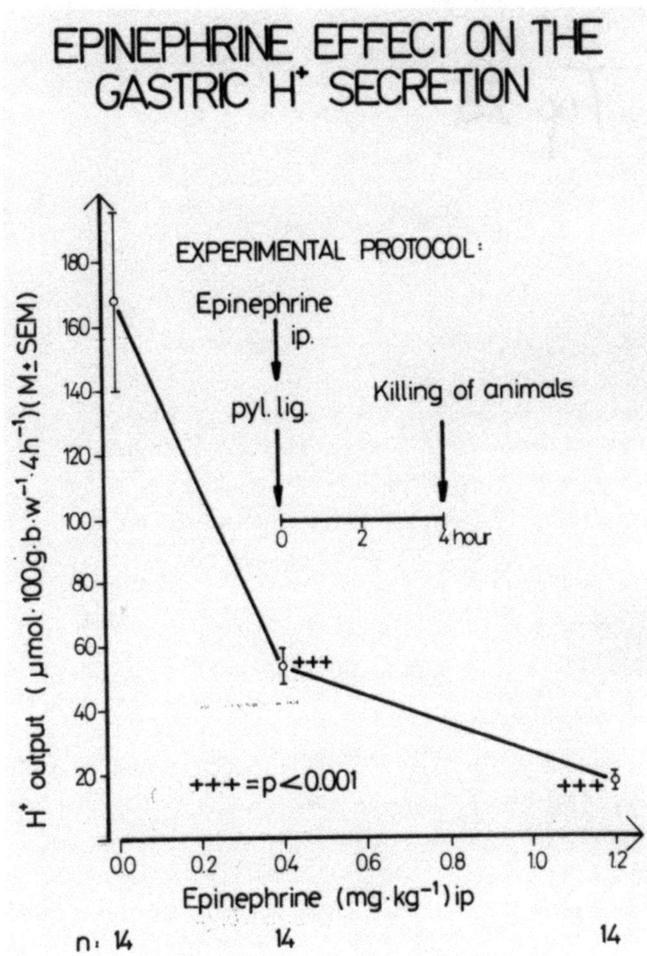

Figure 83. Dose-dependent inhibitory effect of epinephrine on the gastric acid secretion in 4-hour pylorus-ligated rats (means ± SEM). [Mózsik, Figler, Nagy, Patty, Tárnok (1981): Gastric and small intestinal energy metabolism in mucosal damage. In: Mózsik Gy., Hänninen O., Jávor T. (Eds.). Advances in Physiological Sciences. Vol. 29. Gastrointestinal Defence Mechanism. Pergamon Press, Oxford – Akadémiai Kiadó, Budapest. pp. 213–288 (with kind permission).]

http://dx.doi.org/10.5772/60505

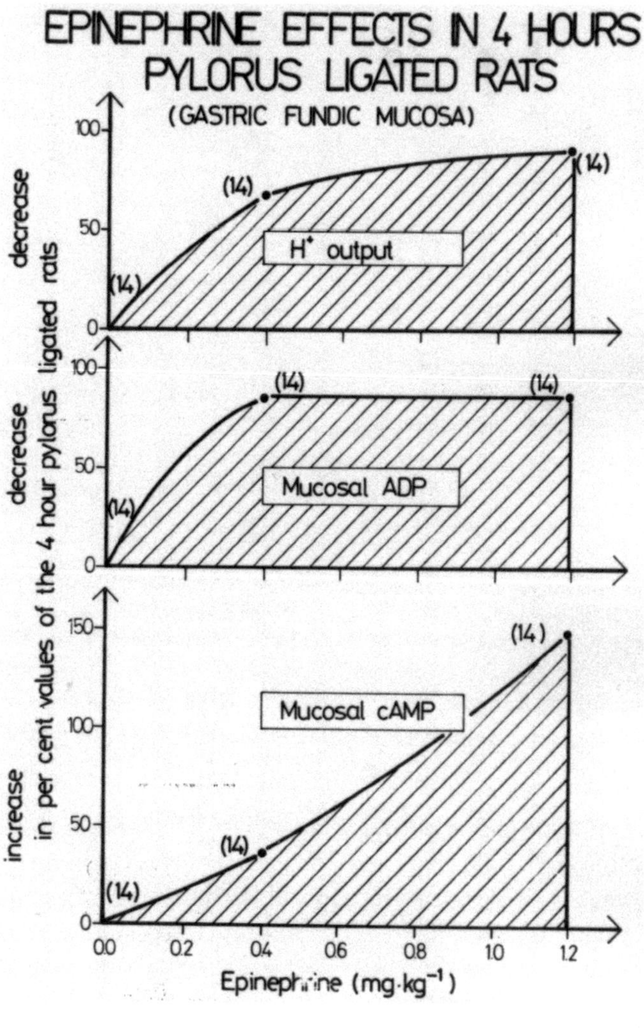

Figure 84. Epinephrine-induced changes in the fundic gastric mucosal levels of ADP and cAMP in comparison with the inhibition of gastric acid secretion (means ± SEM). [Mózsik, Figler, Nagy, Patty, Tárnok (1981): Gastric and small intestinal energy metabolism in mucosal damage. In: Mózsik Gy., Hänninen O., Jávor T. (Eds.). Advances in Physiological Sciences. Vol. 29. Gastrointestinal Defence Mechanism. Pergamon Press, Oxford – Akadémiai Kiadó, Budapest. pp. 213–288 (with kind permission).] For further explanation, see Figure 83.

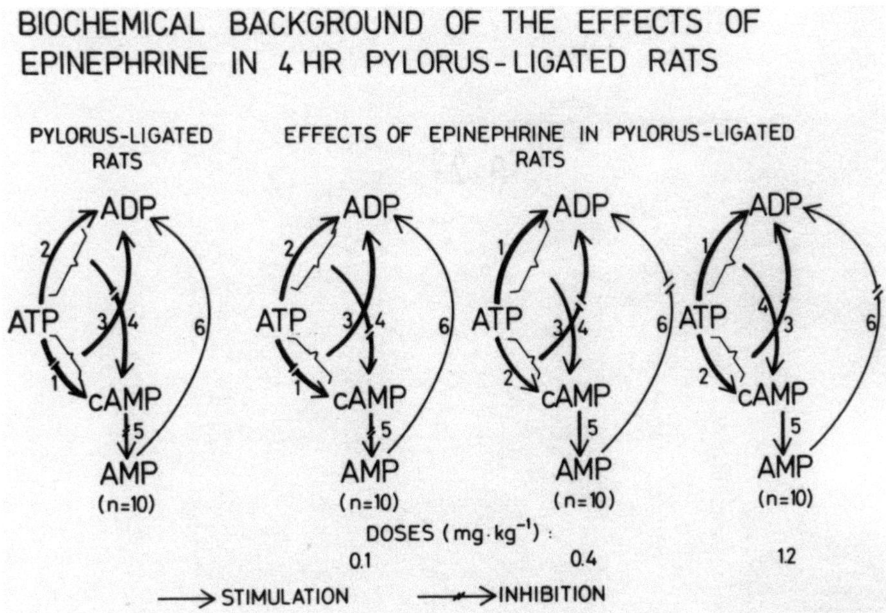

Figure 85. Epinephrine-induced changes in the regulatory mechanisms between the cellular ATP, ADP and AMP by different doses of epinephrine in 4-hour pylorus-ligated rats. The different doses of epinephrine were subcutaneously applied immediately after pyloric ligation (means ± SEM). For further explanation, see Figure 83.

In these studies, we analyzed the changes in the gastric H^+ output and changes in the rat gastric fundic mucosa after aspirin administration (200 mg/kg dissolved in 2 mL of 150 mmoles of H $^+$) given immediately after pylorus ligation.

Figure 83 demonstrates the effects of aspirin on 4-hour pylorus-ligated rats. The gastric H^+ output, obtained at 0, 1 and 3 hours, was less than the quantity given immediately after pyloric ligation. The difference between the given acid and the measured acid output was taken as a marker of gastric H^+ backdiffusion (Figure 86). This figure clearly indicates that the active gastric H^+ secretion starts only from the second hour (Figler et al., 1985, 1986, 1999) (Figures 87, 88).

The results presented in Figure 84 demonstrate the absolute values of volume (mL/100 g body weight/4 hours), H^+ output (μEq/100 b.w./4 hours) and glandular ulcer in 4-hour pylorus-ligated (A) and 4-hour pylorus-ligated plus aspirin (B) rats. The values of groups A and B are presented in Figure 87. The forthcoming figure (Figure 30) demonstrates the main changes in the rat gastric fundic mucosal biochemistry without (group A) and with (group B) aspirin administration (Figure 88).

Figure 89 demonstrates the correlations between the changes in the rat gastric fundic mucosal biochemistry without (group A) and with (group B) aspirin treatment. The values expressed

http://dx.doi.org/10.5772/60505

the differences between the pylorus-ligated versus pylorus-ligated plus aspirin-treated rats (Figures 88, 89).

We tried to summarize the changes in the regulatory pathways between the tissue levels of ATP, ADP, cAMP and AMP in intact (untreated), 4-hour pylorus-ligated and 4-hour pylorus-ligated plus aspirin-treated rats (Figure 90).

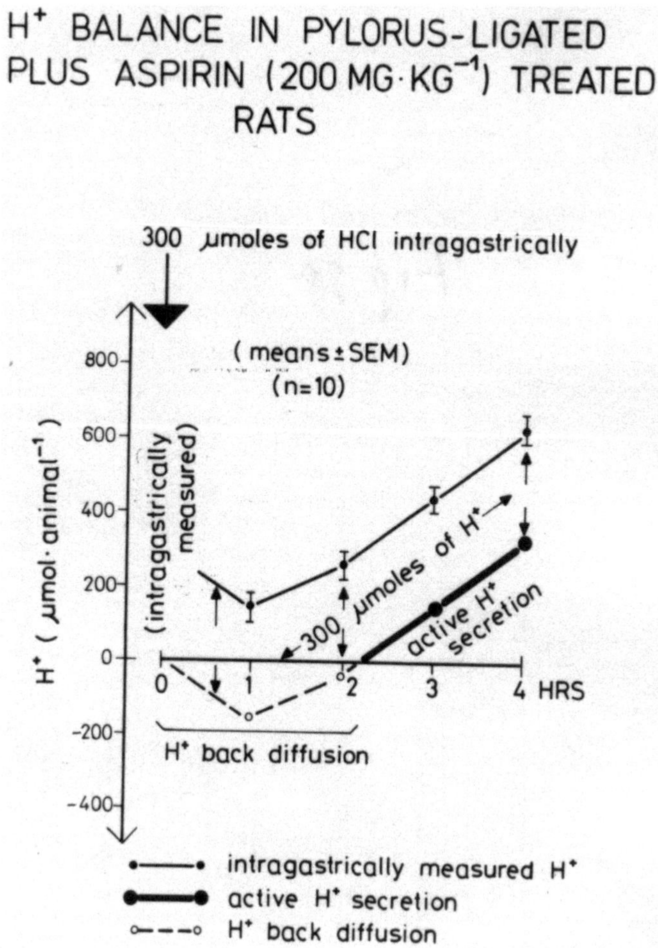

Figure 86. The balance between the aspirin-induced gastric H^+ backdiffusion and active H^+ secretion in 4-hour pylorus-ligated plus aspirin (200 mg/kg ig. in 2 mL = 300 µmoles of H^+)-treated animals (means ± SEM). [Figler, Jávor, Nagy, Patty, Mózsik 1986. Int. J. Tiss. React. 8: 15–22 (with kind permission).]

CHANGES IN GASTRIC SECRETORY RESPONSES AND DEVELOPMENT OF GASTRIC MUCOSAL LESIONS IN 4 HR PYLORUS-LIGATED (B) AND PYLORUS-LIGATED PLUS ASPIRIN-TREATED (B) RATS

	A (n=11)	B (n=10)	Δ(A-B)
Volume ($ml \cdot 100g^{-1} \cdot 4hr^{-1}$)	1.9 ± 0.1	$3.0 \pm 0.17^{++}$	+ 1.1 ± 0.1
H^+ output	150 ± 10	$110 \pm 10^{+}$	- 40 ± 10
($\mu Eq \cdot 100g^{-1} \cdot 4hr^{-1}$)	0 ± 0	$14.1 \pm 2.1^{+++}$	+ 14.1 ± 2.1
ULCER NUMBER	0 ± 0	$27.2 \pm 2.1^{+++}$	+ 27.2 ± 2.1

Figure 87. Changes in the volume (mL/100 g b.w./4 hours), acid output (μEq/100 g b.w./4 hours) in the 4-hour pylorus-ligated (A) versus. 4-hour pylorus-ligated plus aspirin-treated (B) rats. The Δ values expressed as difference between the groups of B versus A (means ± SEM). [(Figler, Jávor, Nagy, Patty, Mózsik 1986. Int. J. Tiss. React. 8: 15–22 (with kind permission).]

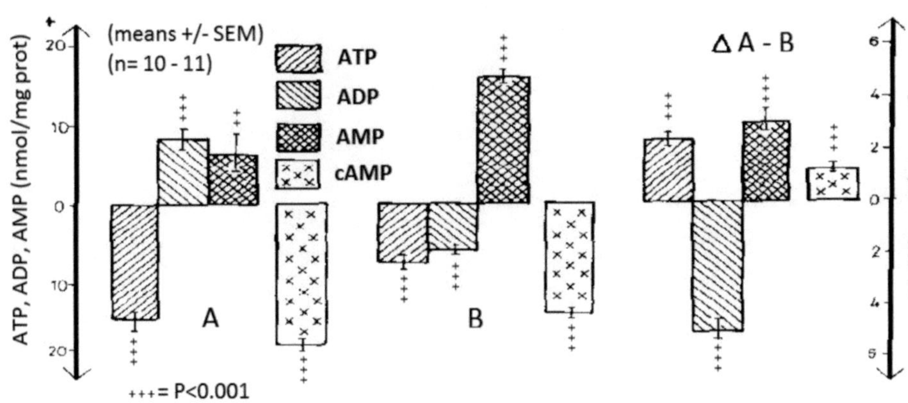

Figure 88. The changes in the gastric fundic mucosal levels of ATP, ADP, AMP and cAMP in 4-hour pylorus-ligated (A) and 4-hour pylorus-ligated plus aspirin-treated (B) rats expressed as absolute values. The values of groups A versus B were given as Δ values (means ± SEM). [Figler, Jávor, Nagy, Patty, Mózsik 1986. Int. J. Tiss. React. 8: 15–22 (with kind permission).]

http://dx.doi.org/10.5772/60505

CORRELATIONS BETWEEN CHANGES IN BIOCHEMISM OF GASTRIC MUCOSA IN 4 HR PYLORUS-LIGATED (A) AND PYLORUS-LIGATED PLUS ASPIRIN TREATED (B) RATS

	A	B	Δ A-B
ULCER NUMBER	-	↑↑↑	↓↓↓
ULCER SEVERITY	-	↑↑↑	↓↓↓
SECRETORY VOLUME	↑↑↑	↑↑↑	↓↓
H^+ output	↑↑↑	↑↑↑	↓
ATP	↓↓↓	↓↓↓	↑↑↑
ADP	↑↑↑	↓↓↓	↓↓
$ATP \cdot ADP^{-1}$	↓↓↓	NS	↑↑↑
AMP	↑↑	↑↑↑	↑↑↑
ADENYLATE POOL	NS	NS	NS
cAMP	↓↓↓	↓↓↓	↑↑↑
„ENERGY CHARGE" LACTATE	↓↓	↓↓	NS

NS = NOT SIGNIFICANT

↓ = 0.05 > P > 0.01 ↓↓ = 0.01 > P > 0.001 ↓↓↓ = P < 0.001

↑ = INCREASE ↓ = DECREASE

Figure 89. The summary of the changes in the rat gastric fundic mucosa and ulcer development in 4-hour pylorus-ligated and 4-hour pylorus-ligated plus aspirin-treated animals.

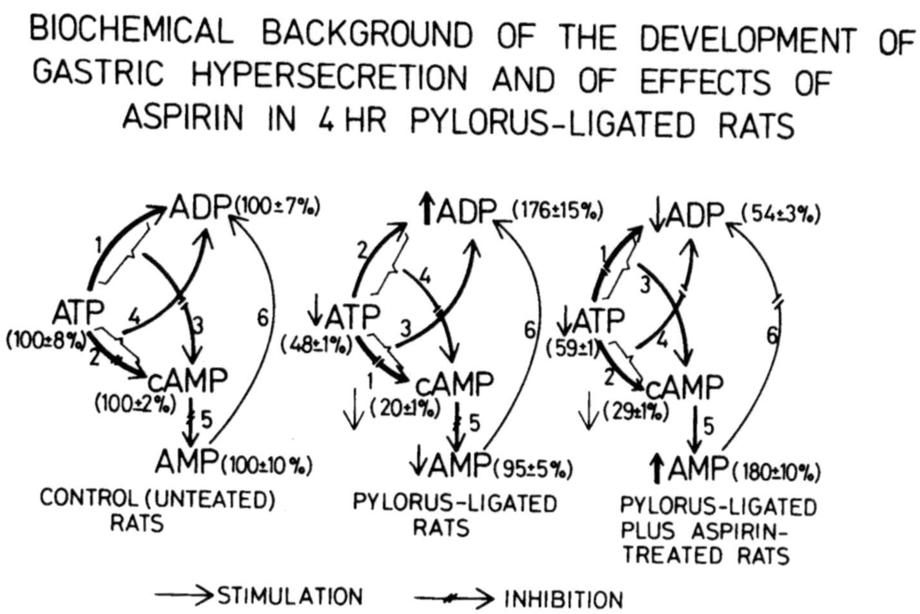

Figure 90. The details of the regulatory pathways in intact (left figure), in 4-hour pylorus-ligated (middle figure) and in 4-hour pylorus-ligated plus aspirin-treated rats (right figure) (means ± SEM).

8.3.2. Gastric mucosal-protective effect of atropine and its changes in biochemistry of gastric mucosa in 4-hour pylorus-ligated plus aspirin-treated rats

Following the observations presented before (as a section of 5.5.), the mucosal-protective effect of atropine was studied under the same experimental conditions. The gastric mucosal damage was produced after intragastric administration of 200 mg/kg aspirin (dissolved in 2 mL of 150 mmol HCl) immediately after pyloric ligation. The different doses of atropine (0.1, 0.5 and 1.0 mg/kg s.c.) given at the same time as that of aspirin in 4-hour pylorus-ligated rats (Figure 91).

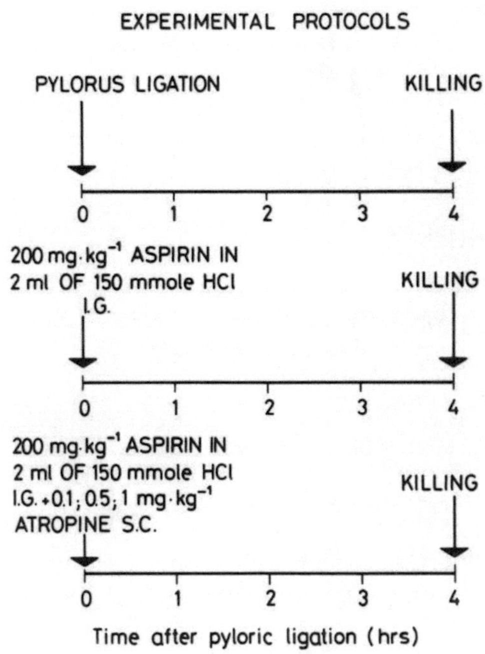

Figure 91. Experimental protocol for studies examined the mucosal-protective effect of atropine (given in doses of 0.1, 0.5 and 1.0 mg/kg subcutaneously immediately after pyloric ligation plus aspirin administration). [Figler et al., 1985, Digestion 31, 145–146 (with kind permission).]

The volume, concentration of H^+, gastric acid output (Figure 92) and the number and sum of ulcers (Figure 93) could be decreased dose-dependently by the application of atropine (Figure 93).

The results of biochemical measurements [tissue levels of ATP, ADP and AMP (Figure 94)], adenylate pool, "energy charge", ratio of ATP/ADP (Figure 95), tissue level of cAMP (Figure 96) and lactate (Figure 97) are provided.

The results clearly indicate that the ATP transformation is inhibited by atropine; however, its value decreases by the increase of atropine doses. In the background, the ATP transformation pathway will lead to an increase in ATP–cAMP transformation, whereas the ratio of ATP/ADP and "energy charge" increases; however, the adenylate pool and tissue level of lactate remained unchanged (Figure 98).

http://dx.doi.org/10.5772/60505

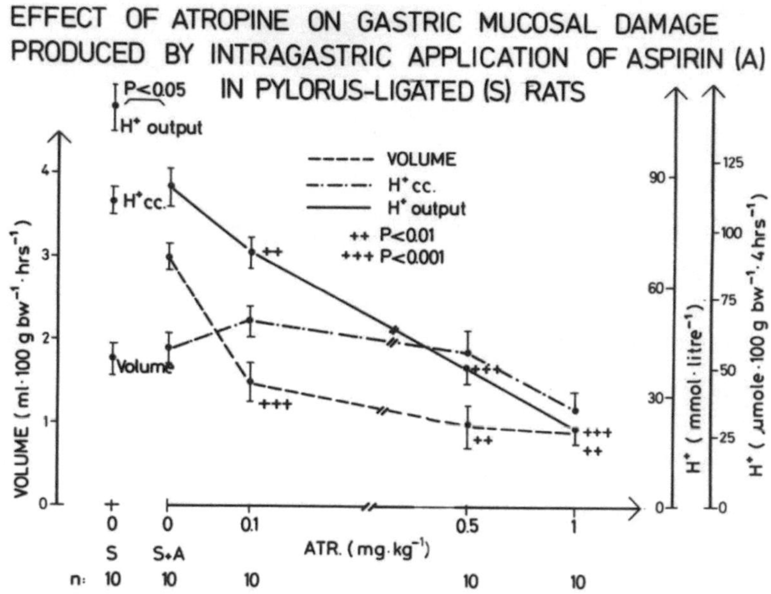

Figure 92. Changes in gastric secretory responses in 4-hour pylorus-ligated plus aspirin-treated rats after application of different doses of atropine. The results are expressed as means ± SEM. Abbreviations: S, surgical interventions; S + A, surgical intervention plus aspirin treatment, *n*, indicates the number of animals. [Figler et al., 1985, Digestion 31, 145–146 (with kind permission).]

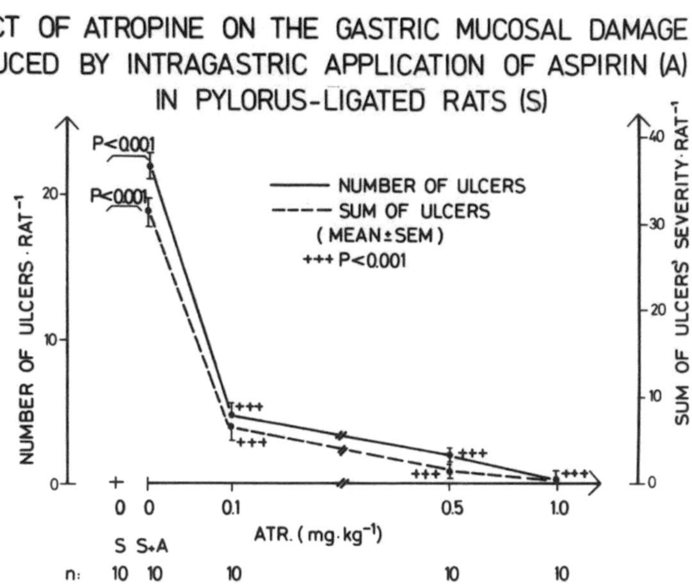

Figure 93. Dose-dependent gastric mucosal-preventive effects of different doses of atropine in 4-hour pylorus-ligated plus aspirin-treated rats. The results are presented as means ± SEM. Abbreviations: S, surgical intervention; S + A, surgical intervention plus aspirin treatment; *n*, indicates the number of animals. [Figler et al., 1985, Digestion 31, 145–146 (with kind permission).]

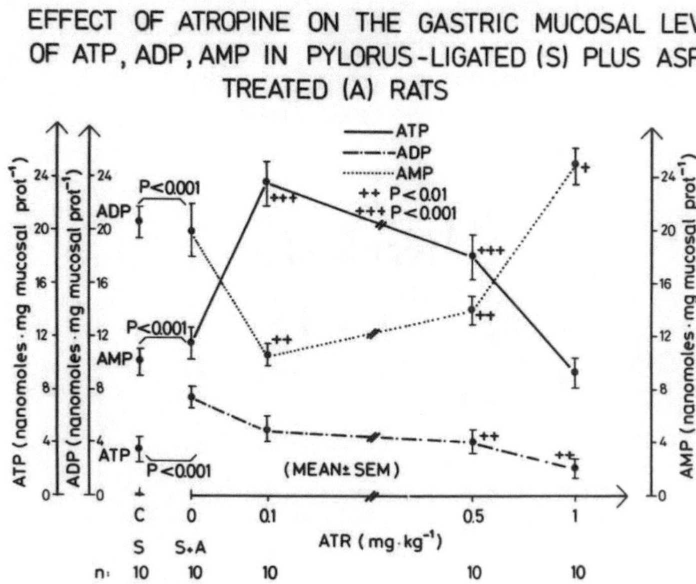

Figure 94. Atropine treatment-induced changes in adenylate pool, ratio of ATP/ADP and "energy charge" in the gastric mucosal tissues in 4-hour pylorus-ligated plus aspirin-treated rats. The results are expressed as means ± SEM. Abbreviations: S, surgical intervention; S + A, surgical intervention plus aspirin treatment; *n*, indicates the number of animals. [Figler et al., 1985, Digestion 31, 145–146 (with kind permission).]

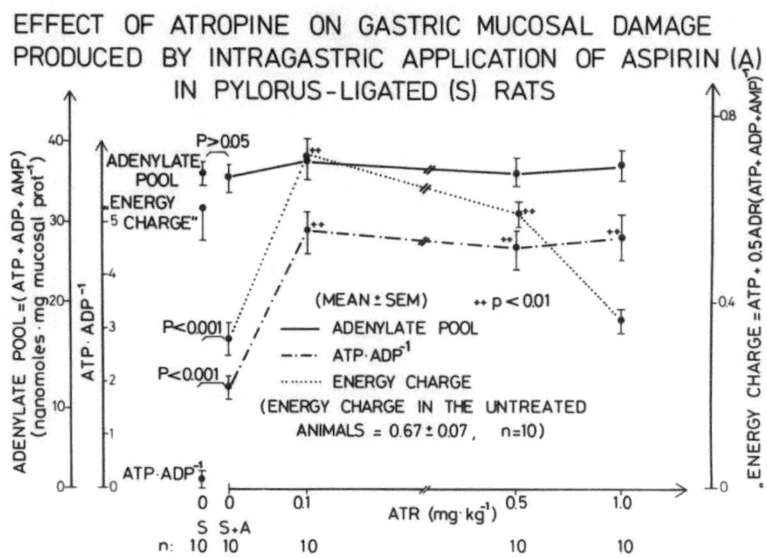

Figure 95. Atropine treatment-induced changes in adenylate pool, ratio of ATP/ADP and "energy charge" in the gastric mucosal tissues in 4-hour pylorus-ligated plus aspirin-treated rats. The results are expressed as means ± SEM. Abbreviations: S, surgical intervention; S + A, surgical intervention plus aspirin treatment; *n*, indicates the number of animals. [Figler et al., 1985, Digestion 31, 145–146 (with kind permission).]

http://dx.doi.org/10.5772/60505

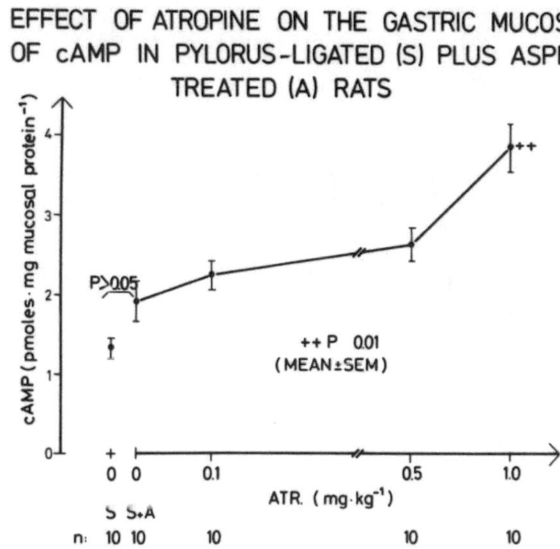

Figure 96. Atropine-induced changes in tissue level of cAMP in the gastric mucosa in 4-hour pylorus-ligated plus aspirin-treated rats. The results are expressed as means ± SEM. Abbreviations: S, surgical intervention; S + A, surgical intervention plus aspirin treatment; *n*, indicates the number of animals. [Figler et al., 1985, Digestion 31, 145–146 (with kind permission).]

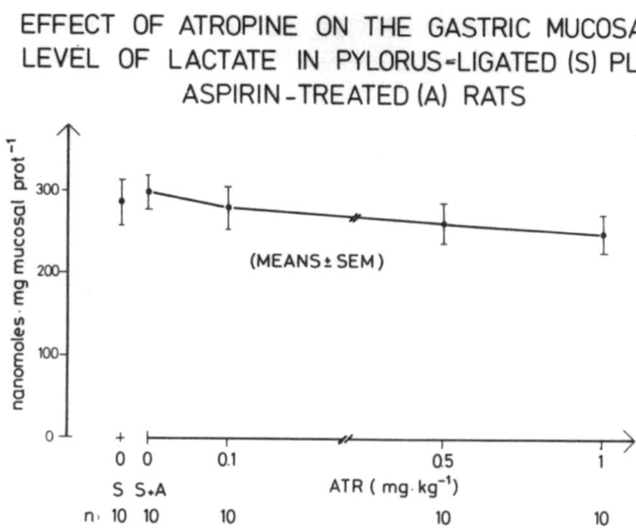

Figure 97. Effect of atropine treatment on the tissue level of lactate in the gastric mucosa of 4-hour pylorus-ligated plus aspirin-treated rats. The results are expressed as means ± SEM. Abbreviations: S, surgical intervention; S + A, surgical intervention plus atropine treatment; *n*, indicates the number of animals. [Figler et al., 1985, Digestion 31, 145–146 (with kind permission).]

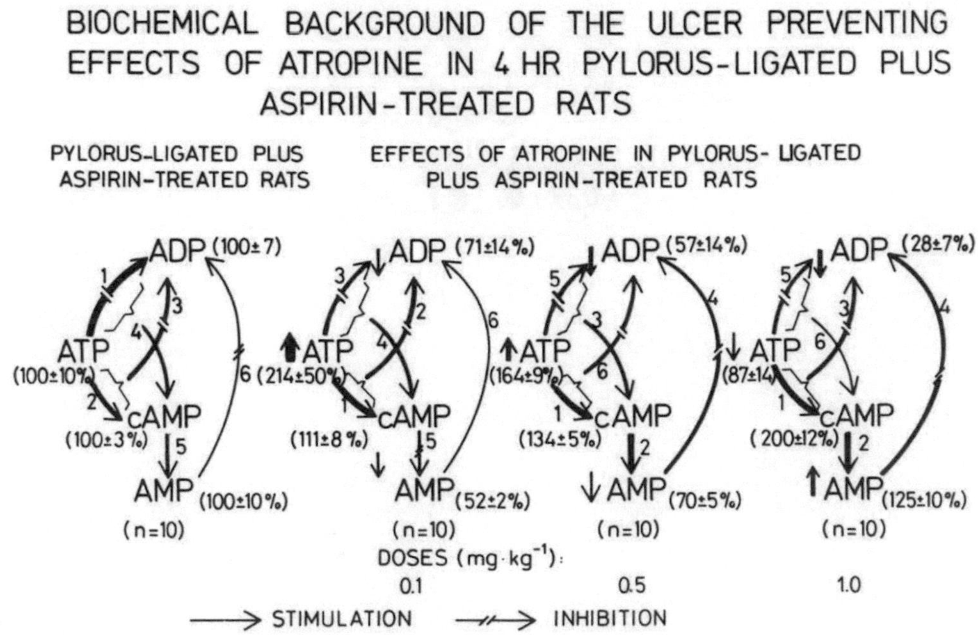

Figure 98. Schematic representation of changes in the extra- and intercellular feedback mechanisms, which exist after application of different doses of atropine. The different steps in the regulatory mechanisms were expressed by the results based on the changes in perpetual values of tissue levels of ATP, ADP, AMP and cAMP of the pathological (pylorus-ligated plus aspirin-treated) values (and these were taken as 100%).

Consequently, the intracellular regulatory mechanism between the energy systems also significantly changes in the gastric mucosa during the development of gastric mucosal protection by atropine.

8.3.3. Gastric mucosal-protective effects of vitamin A and β-carotene and their biochemical backgrounds in 4-hour pylorus-ligated plus aspirin-treated rats

In the previous sections (5.5. and 5.5.1.), the biochemical changes in the gastric mucosa and gastric secretory responses were studied in the 4-hour pylorus-ligated plus aspirin-treated rats during the time of development of gastric mucosal damage (5.5.) and prevention by atropine (5.5.1).

In this chapter, the 4-hour pylorus-ligated plus aspirin-treated ulcer model was further used; however, the actions of mechanisms of two scavengers (namely vitamin A and β-carotene) were studied. As indicated earlier, these compounds have no gastric secretory inhibitory actions neither in animals (Jávor et al., 1983) nor in human beings (Mózsik et al., 1986). Consequently, the scavenger action versus cytoprotection phenomenon were together studied in the aspirin animal model.

The experimental protocol and different measurements (gastric secretory responses, gastric mucosal lesions and biochemical measurements) are presented in Figure 99.

http://dx.doi.org/10.5772/60505

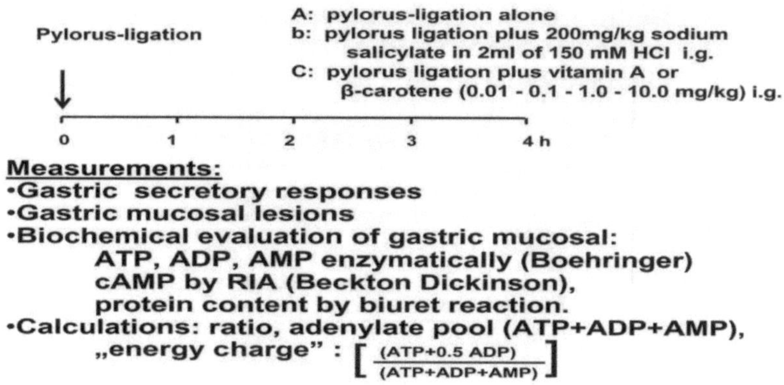

Figure 99. Experimental protocol (design) for the studies of actions of mechanisms of gastric mucosal protection of orally administered vitamin A and β-carotene (vitamin A and β-carotene were dissolved in oleum helianthi and given intragastrically in doses of 0.01, 0.1, 1.0 and 10.0 mg/kg by a flexible nasogastric tube). [Mozsik et al. Inflammopharmacology 11:560–562, 2003 (with kind permission).]

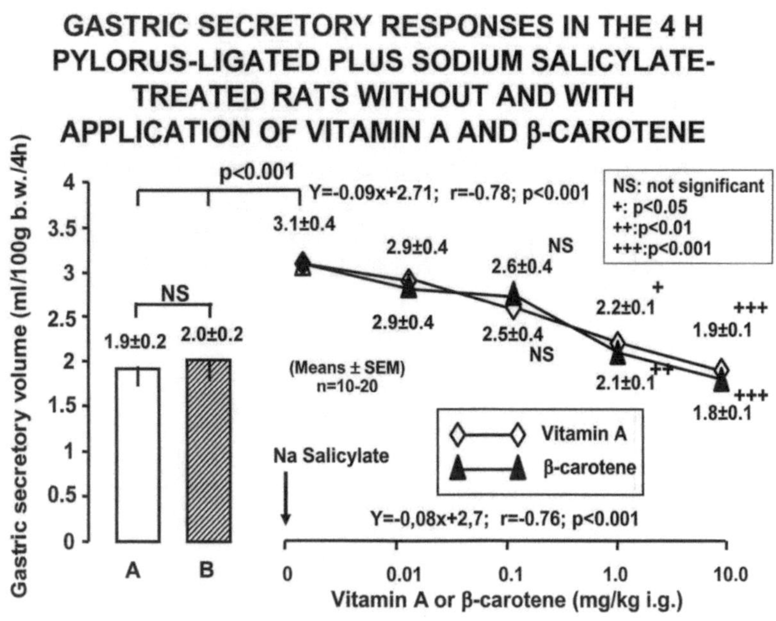

Figure 100. Changes in the volume of gastric secretion in 4-hour pylorus-ligated (A) and aspirin-treated (B) rats with and without vitamin A and β-carotene treatment (right side of the figure). The detailed results are presented in the figure. [Mozsik et al. Inflammopharmacology 11:560–562, 2003 (with kind permission).]

The volume of gastric secretion and acid output did not change in 4-hour pylorus-ligated plus aspirin-treated rats (B) versus pylorus-ligated rats alone (A), the volume decreased after the application of higher doses (1.0 and 10.0 mg/kg) (Figure 100); however, no changes were found in the gastric acid secretion (Figure 101).

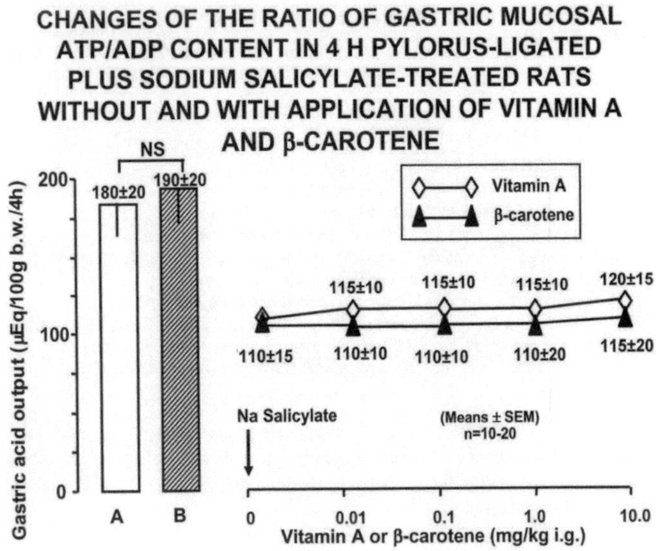

Figure 101. No change in the gastric acid secretion in 4-hour pylorus-ligated ligated plus aspirin-treated rats after intragastrically given vitamin A and β-carotene. [Mozsik et al. Inflammopharmacology 11:560–562, 2003 (with kind permission).]

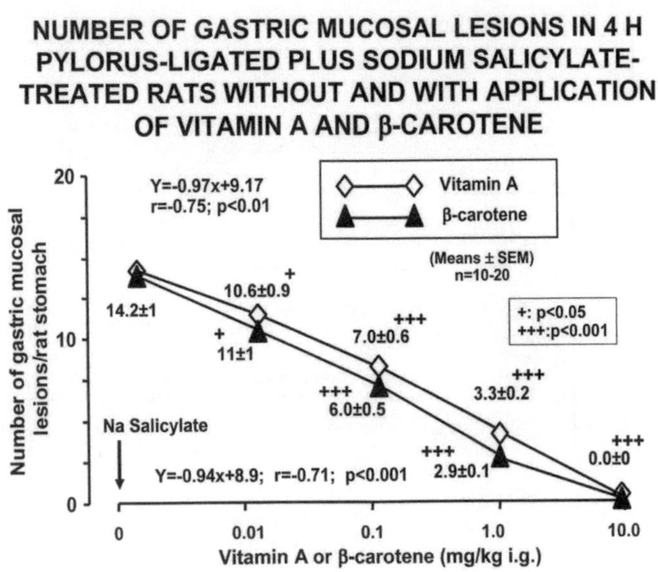

Figure 102. Gastric mucosal-preventive effect (on number of lesions) of vitamin A and β- carotene on 4-hour pylorus-ligated plus aspirin-treated rats. [Mozsik et al. Inflammopharmacology 11:560–562, 2003 (with kind permission).]

Both vitamin A and β-carotene dose-dependently prevented the number (Figure 102) and severity (Figure 103), which differ from the decrease of gastric acid secretion (Figure 101).

http://dx.doi.org/10.5772/60505

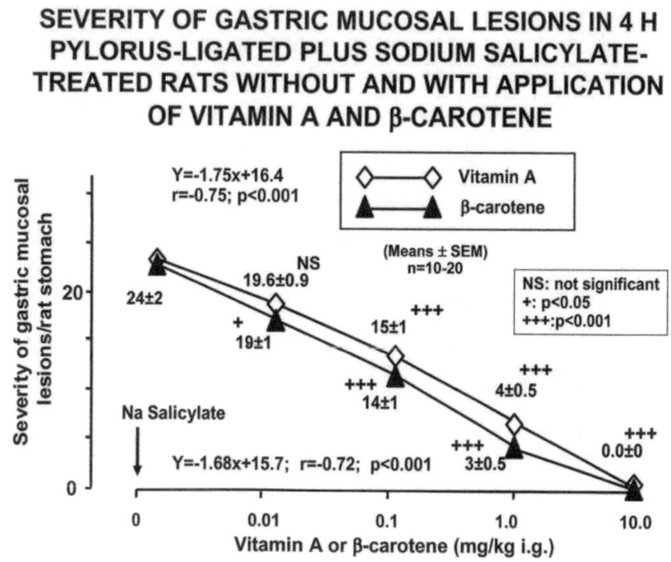

Figure 103. Gastric mucosal (severity)-preventive effects of vitamin A and β-carotene on 4-hour pylorus-ligated plus aspirin-treated rats. [Mozsik et al. Inflammopharmacology 11:560–562, 2003 (with kind permission).]

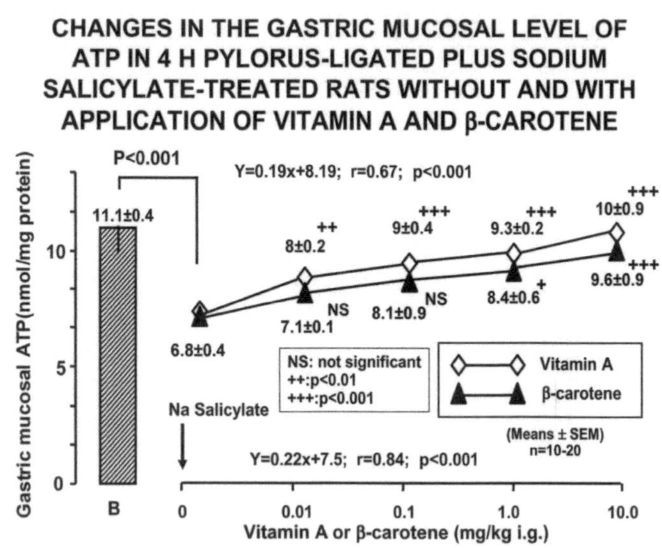

Figure 104. Changes in the gastric mucosal ATP in 4-hour pylorus-ligated and aspirin-treated rats after intragastric administration of vitamin A and β-carotene (given intragastrically in different doses). [Mozsik et al. Inflammopharmacology 11:560–562, 2003 (with kind permission).]

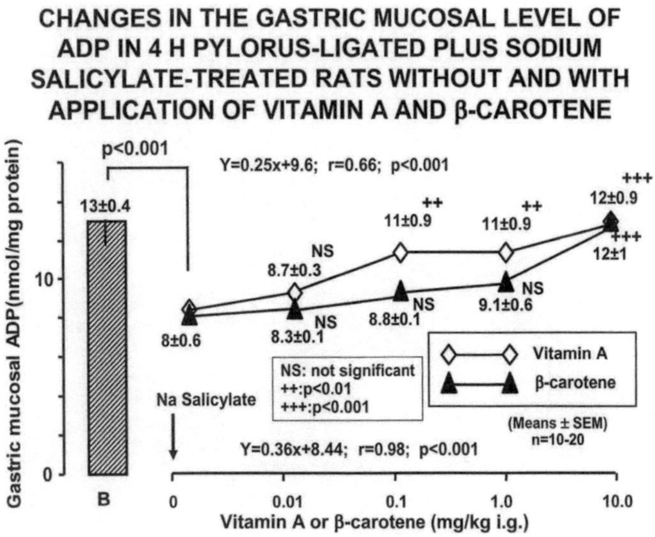

Figure 105. Changes in the gastric mucosal ADP in 4-hour pylorus-ligated plus aspirin-treated rats after administration of vitamin A and β-carotene (given intragastrically in different doses). [Mozsik et al. Inflammopharmacology 11:560–562, 2003 (with kind permission).]

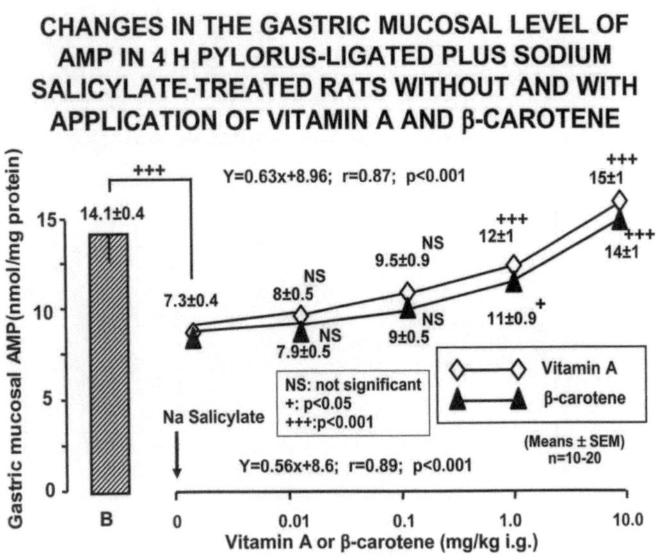

Figure 106. Changes in the gastric mucosal AMP in 4-hour pylorus-ligated plus aspirin-treated rats after administration of vitamin A and β-carotene (given intragastrically in different doses). [Mozsik et al. Inflammopharmacology 11:560–562, 2003 (with kind permission).]

http://dx.doi.org/10.5772/60505

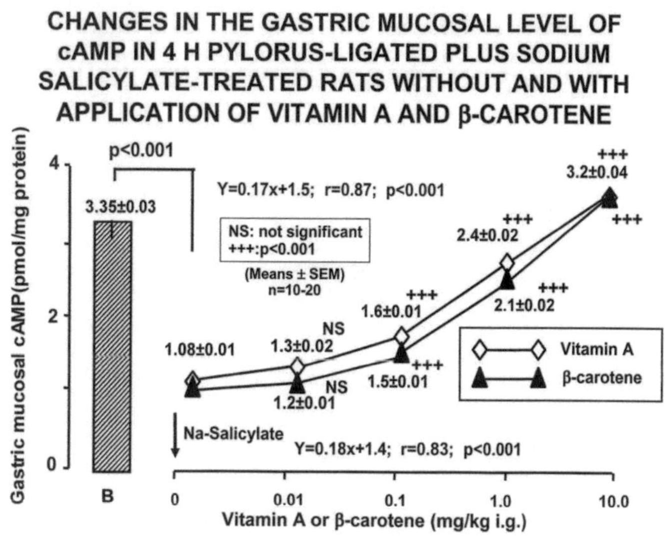

Figure 107. Changes in the gastric mucosal cAMP in 4-hour pylorus-ligated plus aspirin-treated rats after administration of vitamin A and β-carotene (given intragastrically in different doses). [Mozsik et al. Inflammopharmacology 11:560-562, 2003 (with kind permission).]

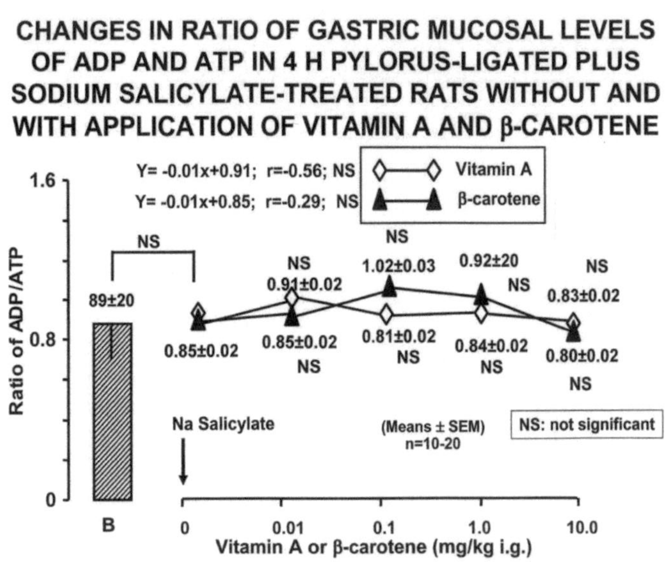

Figure 108. ATP/ADP ratio in the gastric mucosa in 4-hour pylorus-ligated plus aspirin-treated rats after administration of vitamin A and β-carotene (given intragastrically in different doses). [Mozsik et al. Inflammopharmacology 11:560–562, 2003 (with kind permission).]

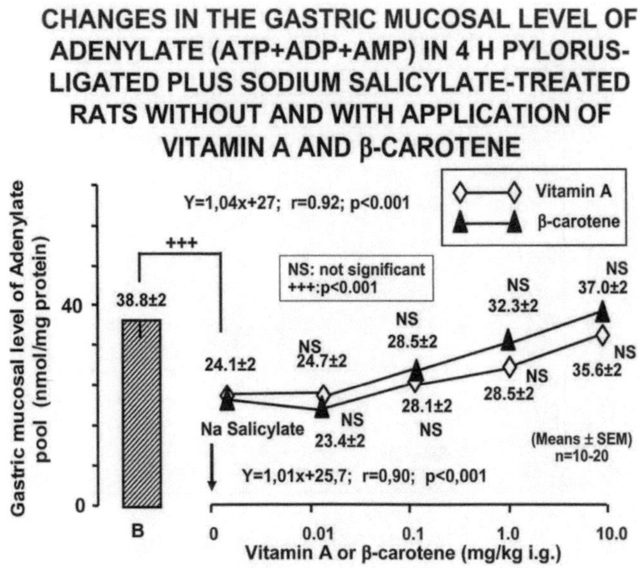

Figure 109. Changes in the gastric mucosal levels of adenylate pool (ATP + ADP + AMP) in 4-hour pylorus-ligated plus aspirin-treated rats after administration of vitamin A and β-carotene (given intragastrically in different doses). [Mozsik et al. Inflammopharmacology 11:560–562, 2003 (with kind permission)].

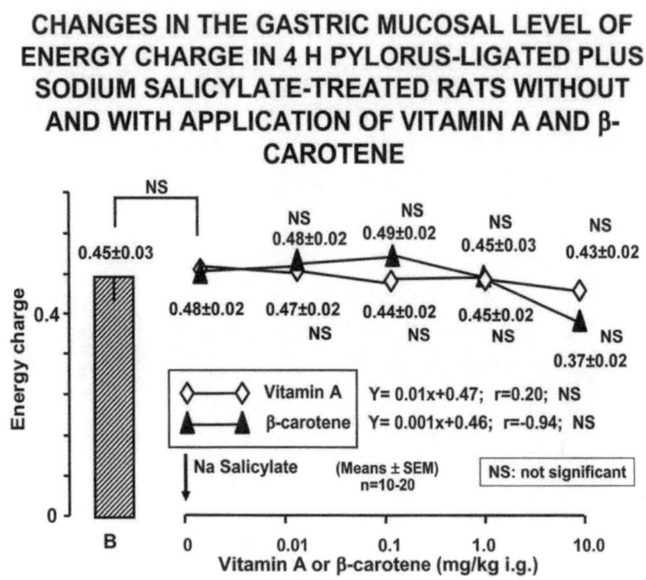

Figure 110. Changes in the gastric mucosal level of "energy charge" in 4-hour pylorus-ligated plus aspirin-treated rats after administration of vitamin A and β-carotene (given intragastrically in different doses). [Mozsik et al. Inflammo-pharmacology 11:560–562, 2003 (with kind permission).]

http://dx.doi.org/10.5772/60505

The tissue level of ATP (Figure 104), ADP (Figure 105), AMP (Figure 106) and cAMP (Figure 107) dose-dependently increased by intragastric administration of vitamin A and β-carotene in the animal model, whereas the ratio of ATP/ADP (Figure 108), adenylate pool (ATP+ADP +AMP) (Figure 109) and "energy charge" (Figure 110) did not change.

The actions of vitamin A and β-carotene on the gastric secretory responses, mucosal damage and biochemical parameters of gastric mucosal tissues produced by intragastric administration (in doses of 0.01, 0.1, 1.0 and 10.0 mg/kg) are summarized in Table 40.

Parameters	Vitamin (A)			β-carotene (B)		
	Regressio	R	P value	Regressio	R	P value
Gastric secretory volume	Y=-0.09x+2.71	-0.78	P<0.001	Y=-0,08x+2,7	-0.76	P<0.001
Gastric acid secretion	No significant action			No significant action		
Number of gastric ulcers	Y=-0.97x+9.17	-0.75	P<0.001	Y=-0.9x+8.9	-0.71	P<0.001
Severity of gastric ulcer	Y=-1.75x+16.4	-0.75	P<0.001	Y=-1.68x+15.7	-0.72	P<0.001
ATP	Y=0.19x+8.19	0.76	P<0.001	Y=0.22x+7.5	0.84	P<0.001
ADP	Y=-0.25x+9.6	0.66	P<0.001	Y=0.36x+8.44	0.98	P<0.001
ATP/ADP	Y=-0.01x+0.913	0,56	P<0.01	Y=0,1x+0.84	0.46	P<0.001
AMP	Y=0.63x+8.96	0.87	P<0.001	Y=0.56x+8.6	0.89	P<0.001
Adenylate pool	No significant action			No significant action		
cAMP	Y=1.17x+1.5	0.87	P<0.001	Y=0.18x+1.4	0.83	P<0.001
Energy charge	No significant action			No significant action		

Table 40. Correlation between gastric mucosal-preventive effects of vitamin A and β-carotene (given in doses of 0.01, 0.1, 1.0 and 10.0 mg/kg i.g.) versus the changes in gastric secretory responses and biochemical parameters in the gastric mucosa of rats treated with sodium salicylate (200 mg/kg dissolved in 2 mL of 150 mmol/L i.g.) in 4-h pylorus-ligated rats). [Mozsik et al. Inflammopharmacology 11:560–562, 2003 (with kind permission).]

8.4. Effect of indomethacin (IND) in 4-hour rats

8.4.1. Biochemical mechanisms of indomethacin-induced gastric mucosal damage in rats (4 hours)

The value of ED_{50} was identified for indomethacin (Djahanguiri, 1969; Karádi and Mózsik, 2000) and their value was obtained in 20 mg/kg. When IND (20 mg/kg s.c.) was given immediately after pylorus ligation, no significant decrease was obtained neither in gastric volume nor in gastric H^+ output. The tissue levels of ATP, AMP and cAMP decreased significantly (Király et al., 1992 a, b; Morón et al., 1982, 1983, 1984 a, b, c; Mózsik et al., 1992 b, f; Rumi et al., 2001 a, b) (Figures 111–114).

The number of ulcers in the glandular stomach was 15 ± 2, and the severity was 16 ± 2 in the indomethacin-treated animals.

The following changes in the cellular ATP-dependent energy systems were obtained in the gastric fundic mucosa of 4-hour indomethacin-treated rats: significant decrease of ATP ($P < 0.001$) and AMP ($P < 0.05$) and cAMP ($P < 0.001$), ratio of ATP/ADP ($P < 0.001$), adenylate pool ($P < 0.05$), ADP increased ($P < 0.0.5$) and changes were found in "energy charge" and tissue level of lactate. The correlation between the decrease of cAMP and indomethacin-induced gastric mucosal damage will be detailed in Section 8.4.4.

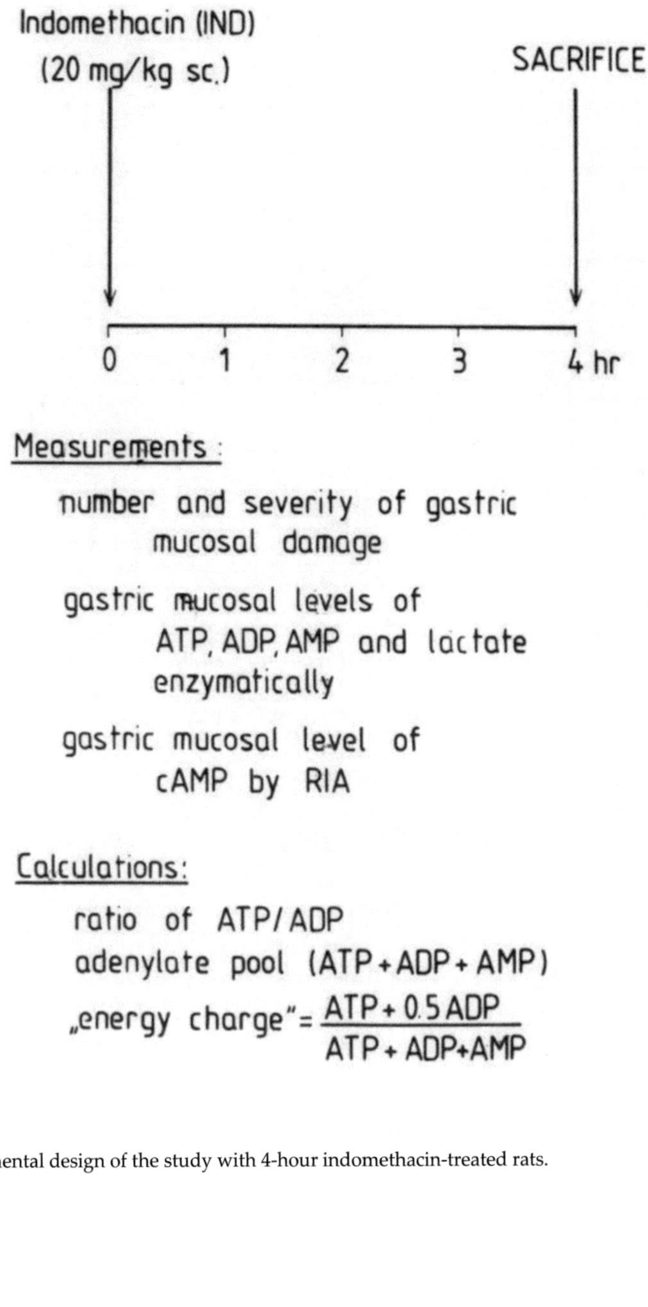

Figure 111. Experimental design of the study with 4-hour indomethacin-treated rats.

http://dx.doi.org/10.5772/60505

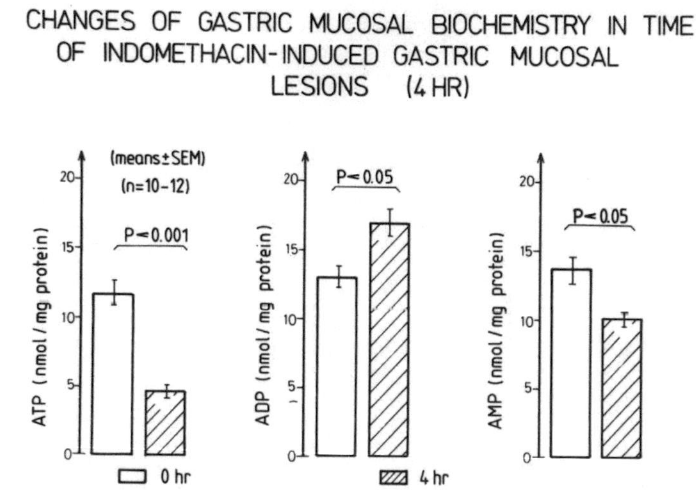

Figure 112. Changes in tissue levels of gastric mucosal ATP, ADP and AMP in 4-hour indomethacin-treated rats.

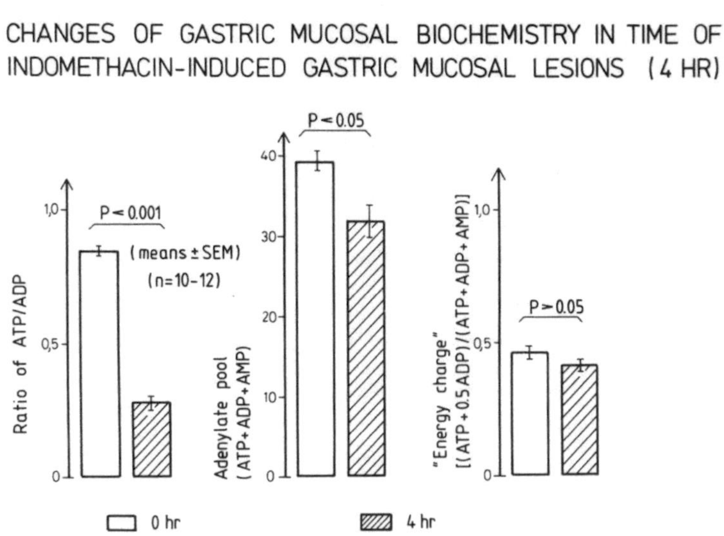

Figure 113. Changes in ratio of ATP/ADP, adenylate pool (ATP + ADP + AMP) and "energy charge" [(ATP + 0.5 ADP)/(ATP + ADP + AMP)] in gastric fundic mucosa of 4-hour indomethacin-treated rats.

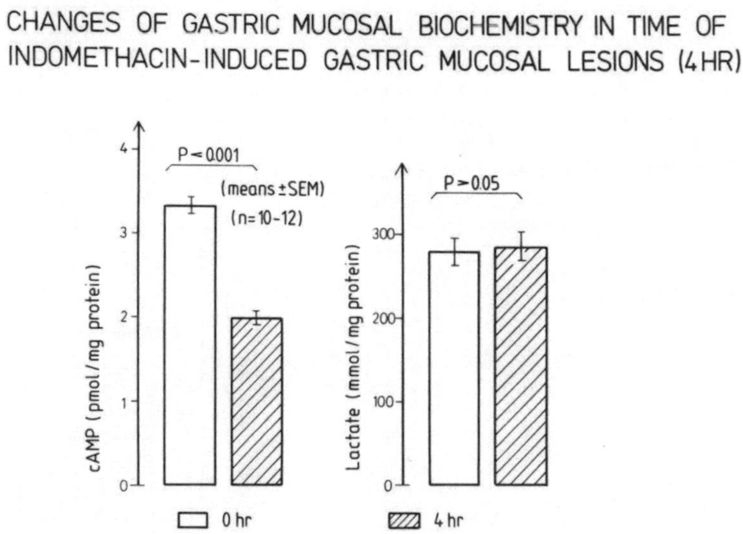

Figure 114. Changes in tissue levels of cAMP and lactate in the gastric fundic mucosa of 4-hour indomethacin-treated rats.

8.4.2. Comparative biochemical studies between the gastric-protective effects and biochemical mechanisms (tissue levels of ATP, ADP, cAMP and AMP) of atropine and cimetidine in the gastric mucosa of rats treated with indomethacin

Both atropine and cimetidine decreased dose-dependently and significantly the number (Figure 115) and severity (Figure 116).

It was interesting to note that atropine dose-dependently increased, whereas cimetidine decreased the tissue level of ATP (Figure 117), and the tissue levels of ADP could be decreased by atropine and increased by cimetidine (Figure 118). Consequently, these atropine- and cimetidine-induced changes in the tissue levels of ATP and ADP significantly modified the ratio of ATP/ADP (Figure 119), the AMP increased dose-dependently by atropine, whereas its value dose-dependently decreased (Mózsik et al., 1992f) (Figure 120).

The values of adenylate pool (ATP + ADP + AMP) were unchanged (Figure 121). The "energy charge" also did not change because of treatment with atropine or cimetidine (Figure 122). The tissue level of cAMP dose-dependently increased by atropine, whereas its value decreased by cimetidine (Figure 123).

When we measured the tissue level of lactate, we found no significant changes in case of atropine or in cimetidine (Figure 124). In the gastric juice, we could not demonstrate the presence of parenterally applied Evans blue (Figure 125).

Figures 126 (a, b) demonstrate the difference in actions of atropine and cimetidine in 4-hours rats. Although both drugs inhibit the IND-induced gastric mucosal damage, however, their biochemical effects completely differed from each other's.

http://dx.doi.org/10.5772/60505

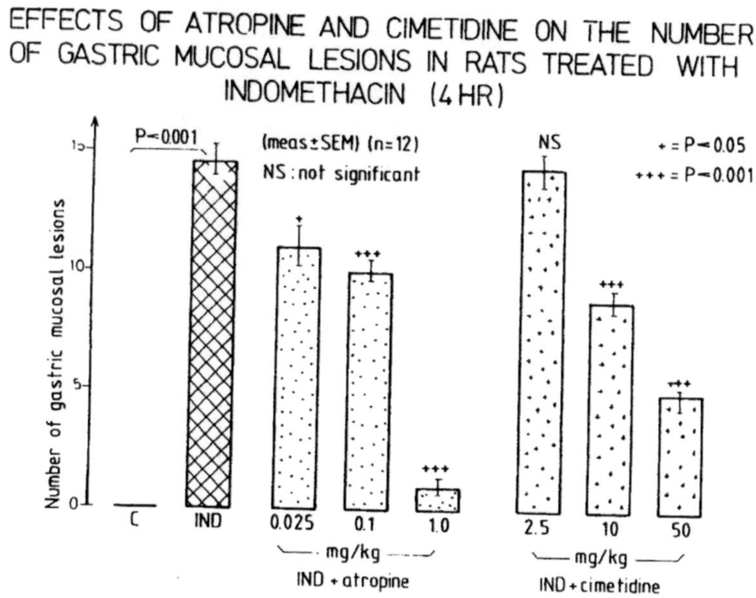

Figure 115. Effects of atropine and cimetidine on the number of gastric mucosal lesions in 4-hour indomethacin (IND)-treated rats. The small doses of atropine (0.025 mg/kg) and cimetidine (2.5 mg/kg) represent the cytoprotective dose of both drugs. C: indicates the results obtained from the saline-treated rats, IND: indicates the groups of animals treated with IND (20 mg/kg s.c.) alone or with atropine and cimetidine. *P* values are between the IND-treated versus IND plus atropine or IND-treated plus cimetidine-treated groups (means ± SEM). [Mózsik et al.: Exp. Clin. Gastroenterol. 3, 205–215, 1992a (with kind permission).]

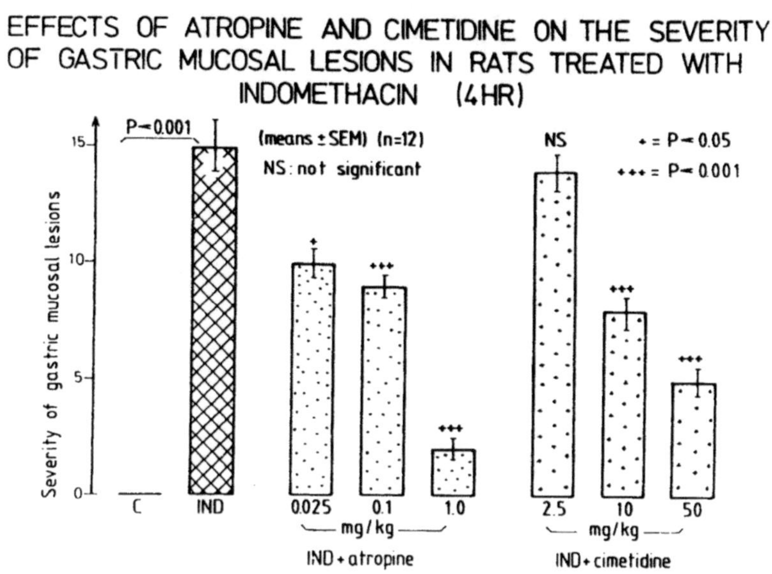

Figure 116. Effects of atropine or cimetidine on the severity of gastric mucosal damage produced by IND (means ± SEM). [Mózsik et al.: Exp. Clin. Gastroenterol. 3, 205–215, 1992a (with kind permission).]

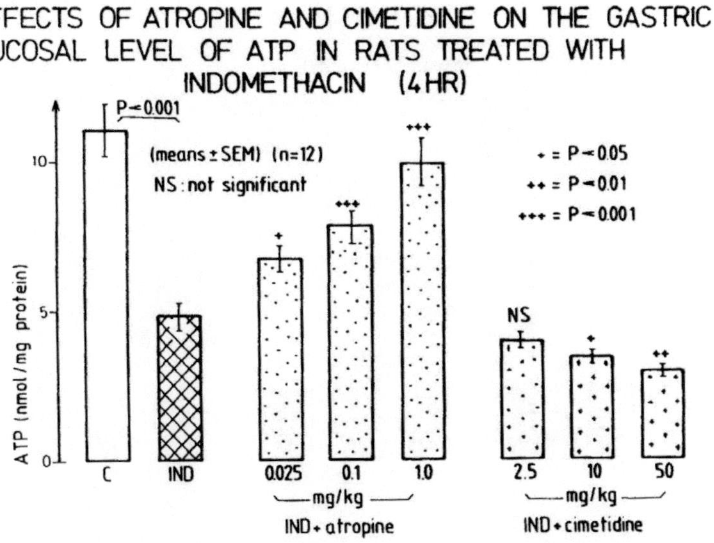

Figure 117. Changes in the gastric mucosal level of ATP produced by atropine and cimetidine in 4-hour IND-treated rats (means ± SEM). [Mózsik et al.: Exp. Clin. Gastroenterol. 3, 205–215, 1992a (with kind permission).] For further explanation, see Figure 115.

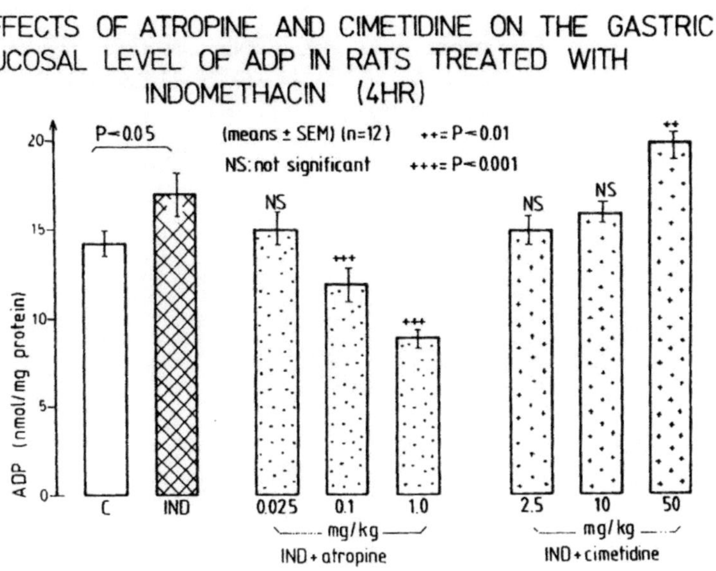

Figure 118. Changes in the gastric mucosal levels of ADP produced by atropine or cimetidine in 4-hour IND-treated rats (means ± SEM). [Mózsik et al.: Exp. Clin. Gastroenterol. 3, 205–215, 1992a (with kind permission).] For further explanation, see Figure 115.

http://dx.doi.org/10.5772/60505

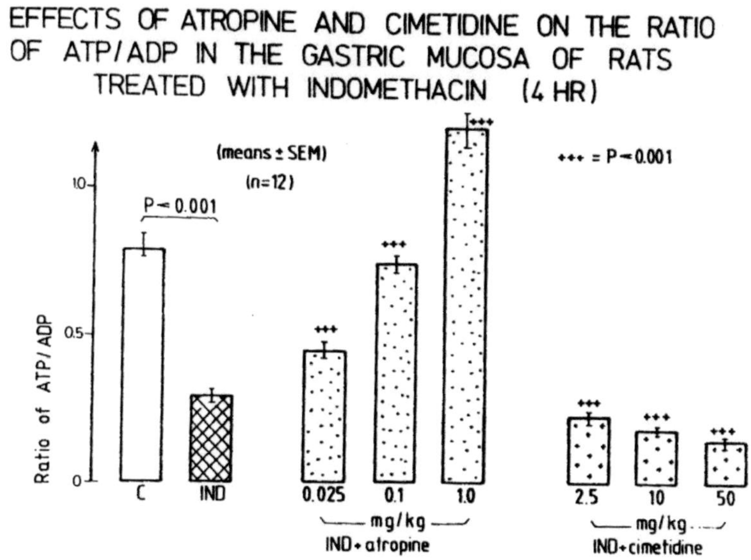

Figure 119. Changes in the ratio of ATP/ADP of gastric mucosa in 4-hour IND-treated rats produced by atropine or cimetidine (means ± SEM). [Mózsik et al.: Exp. Clin. Gastroenterol. 3, 205–215, 1992a (with kind permission).] For further explanation, see Figure 115.

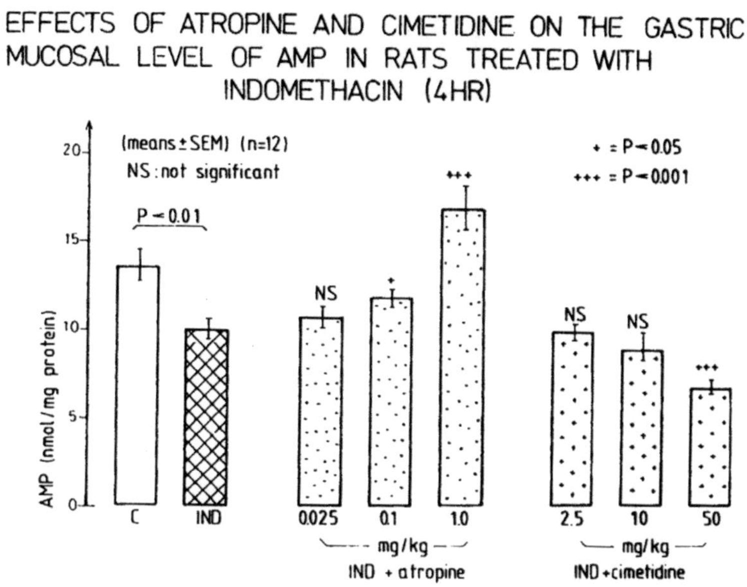

Figure 120. Changes in the gastric mucosal level of AMP produced by atropine or cimetidine in 4-hour IND-treated rats (means ± SEM). [Mózsik et al.: Exp. Clin. Gastroenterol. 3, 205–215, 1992a (with kind permission).] For further explanation, see Figure 115.

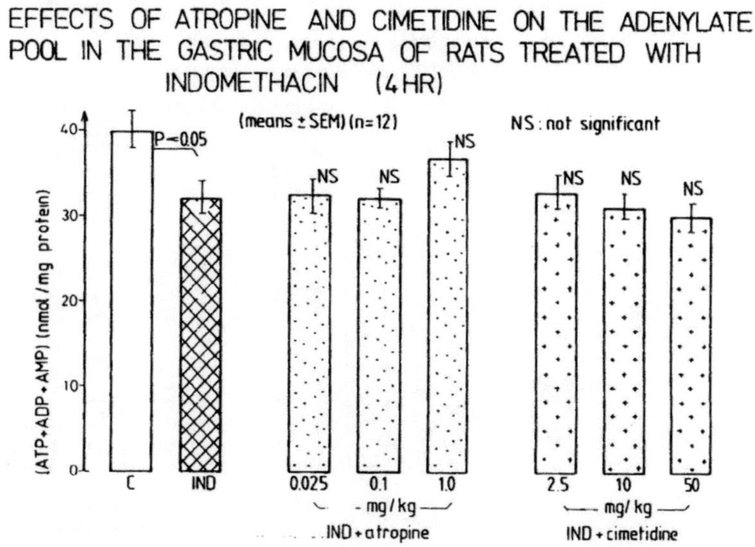

Figure 121. Changes in the gastric mucosal level of adenylate pool (ATP + ADP + AMP) produced by atropine or cimetidine in 4-hour IND-treated rats (means ± SEM). [Mózsik et al.: Exp. Clin. Gastroenterol. 3, 205–215, 1992a (with kind permission).] For further explanation, see Figure 115.

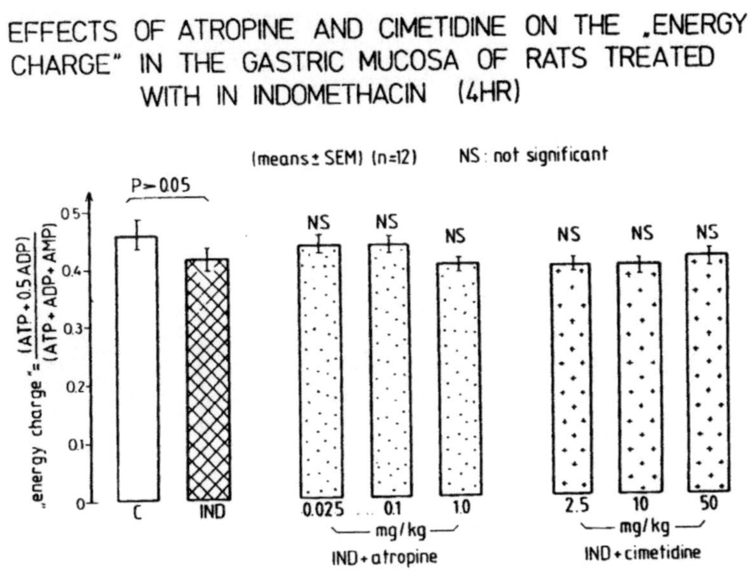

Figure 122. Changes in the values of "energy charge" produced by atropine or cimetidine in 4-hour IND-treated rats (means ± SEM). [Mózsik et al.: Exp. Clin. Gastroenterol. 3, 205–215, 1992a (with kind permission).] For further explanation, see Figure 115.

http://dx.doi.org/10.5772/60505

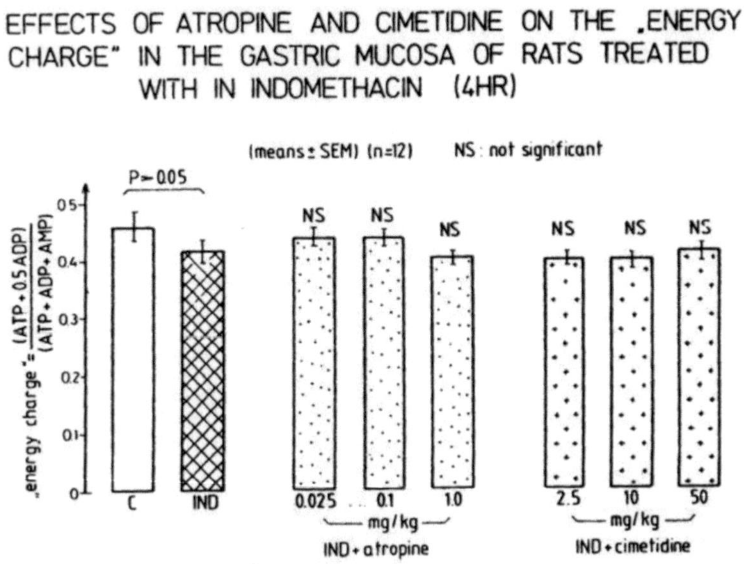

Figure 123. Changes in the gastric mucosal level of cAMP produced by atropine or cimetidine in 4-hour IND-treated rats (means ± SEM). [Mózsik et al.: Exp. Clin. Gastroenterol. 3, 205–215, 1992a (with kind permission).] For further explanation, see Figure 126 a, b.

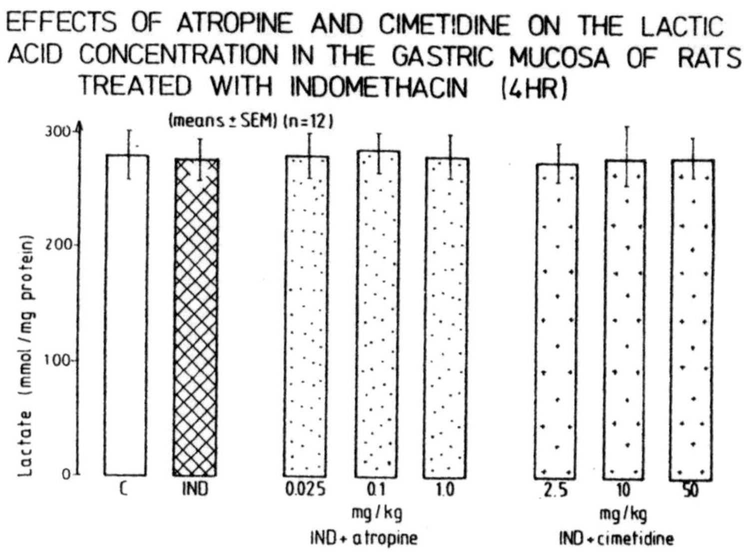

Figure 124. Changes in the gastric mucosal levels of lactate produced by atropine or cimetidine in 4-hour IND-treated rats (means ± SEM). [Mózsik et al.: Exp. Clin. Gastroenterol. 3, 205–215, 1992a (with kind permission).]

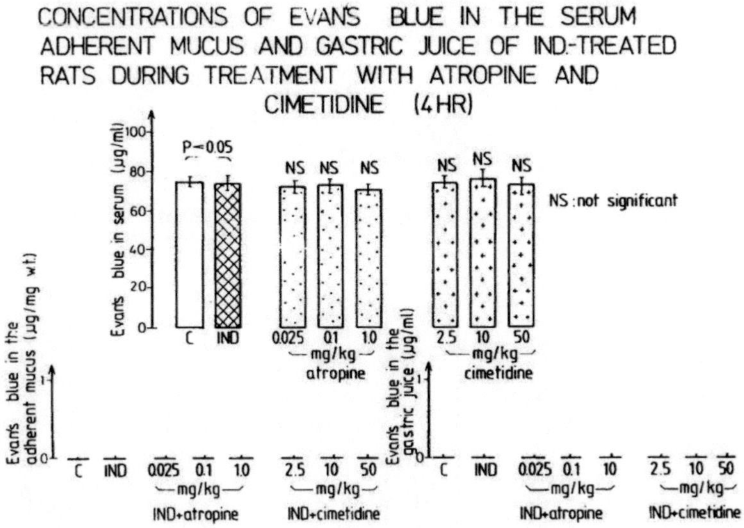

Figure 125. Concentration of Evan's blue in the serum, adherent gastric mucus and gastric juice produced by atropine or cimetidine in 4-hour IND-treated rats (means ± SEM). [Mózsik et al.: Exp. Clin. Gastroenterol. 3, 205–215, 1992a (with kind permission).] For further explanation, see Figure 115.

P values untreated vs. IND. and IND vs. IND plus atropine or cimetidine

	IND	IND + atropine			IND + cimetidine		
		0.025	0.1	1.0	2.5	10	50
		mg/kg					
ulcer number	↑↑↑	↓	↓↓↓	↓↓↓	NS	↓↓↓	↓↓↓
ulcer severity	↑↑↑	↓	↓↓↓	↓↓↓	NS	↓↓↓	↓↓↓
ATP	↓↓↓	↑	↑↑↑	↑↑↑	NS	↓	↓↓
ADP	↑	NS	↓↓↓	↓↓↓	NS	NS	↑↑
ATP/ADP	↓↓↓	↑↑↑	↑↑↑	↑↑↑	↓↓↓	↓↓↓	↓↓↓
AMP	↓↓	NS	↑	↑↑↑	NS	NS	↓↓↓
ATP+ADP+AMP	↓	NS	NS	NS	NS	NS	NS
„energy charge"	NS	NS	NS	NS	NS	NS	NS
cAMP	↓↓↓	NS	↑↑↑	↑↑↑	↓↓↓	↓↓↓	↓↓↓
Lactate	NS	NS	NS	NS	NS	NS	NS

NS: not significant ↑: increase ↓: decrease
↑(↓): $P < 0.05$ ↑↑(↓↓): $P < 0.01$ ↑↑↑(↓↓↓): $P < 0.001$

Figure 126. (a) Summary of the biochemical results obtained in the gastric fundic mucosa produced by atropine or cimetidine in 4-hour IND-treated rats (means ± SEM). [Mózsik et al.: Exp. Clin. Gastroenterol. 3, 205–215, 1992a (with kind permission).] For further explanation, see Figure 115. (b) Feedback mechanism between the membrane-bound ATP-dependent energy systems produced by cytoprotective and antisecretory doses of atropine or cimetidine in 4-hour IND-treated rats (means ± SEM). [Mózsik et al.: Exp. Clin. Gastroenterol. 3, 205–215, 1992a (with kind permission).]

These results clearly proved that the changes in the biochemical parameters in gastric fundic mucosa are significantly opposite in case of administration of atropine and cimetidine in 4-hour indomethacin-treated rats.

http://dx.doi.org/10.5772/60505

8.4.3. Biochemical backgrounds of gastric mucosal-protective effect of vitamin A in 4-hour indomethacin-treated rats

Vitamin A, β-carotene and other retinoids are not able to decrease the gastric acid outputs neither in pylorus-ligated rats nor in healthy human subjects. It was interesting to study the effects of vitamin A in 4-hour pylorus-ligated plus indomethacin-treated rats. In these studies, the tissue levels of ATP, ADP, cAMP and AMP were measured besides the inhibitory effects on the number and severity of IND-induced gastric mucosal damage (Figures 127,128).

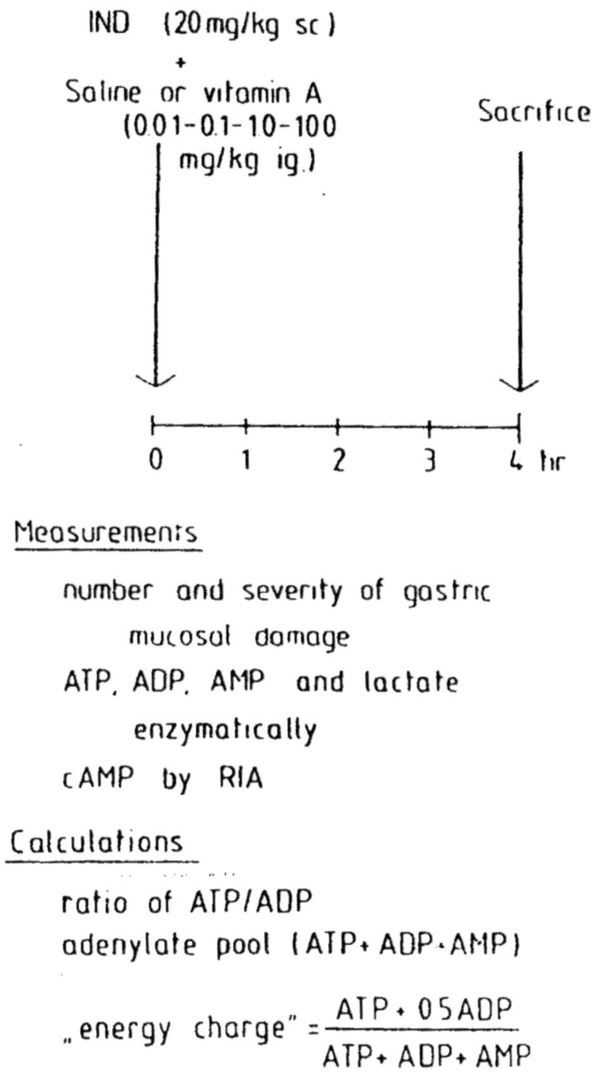

Figure 127. Experimental protocol for the study of gastroprotective and metabolic effects of vitamin A on 4-hour IND-treated rats. [Mózsik et al.: Int. J. Tiss. Reac. 11, 65–71, 1989c (with kind permission).]

Vitamin A dose-dependently decreased in both the number and severity of IND-induced gastric mucosal damage (Figure 128). During the development of gastric mucosal effect, the tissue levels of ATP significantly decreased in association with the significant increase of tissue ADP (Mózsik and Jávor, 1991; Mózsik et al., 1989c, 1996a) (Figure 129).

No change was obtained in the adenylate pool (Figure 130). It was interesting to note that the dose-dependent increase of cAMP (Figure 131) also increased slightly the "energy charge" and the ratio of ATP/ADP (Figure 132).

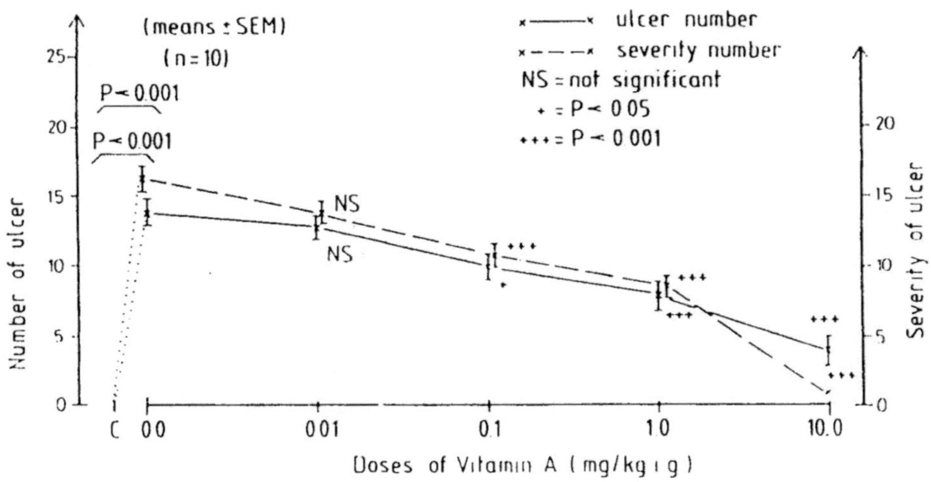

Figure 128. Changes in the number and severity of gastric mucosal lesions prevented by the application of different doses of vitamin A in 4-hour IND-treated rats (means ± SEM). [Mózsik et al.: Int. J. Tiss. Reac. 11, 65–71, 1989c (with kind permission).]

When the changes in tissue levels of ATP, ADP, AMP and cAMP and the number of gastric mucosal damage were simultaneously compared, similar changes were obtained as those by atropine (Figure 133).

8.4.4. Gastroprotective effect of β-carotene differs from the prostaglandin system in 4-hour indomethacin-treated rats

The details of the gastric mucosal-protective effect of vitamin A were studied – in a dose-dependent manner – in the previous Section (8.4.3). In this section, the correlations between the gastric mucosal-protective effect of β-carotene (as a provitamin for vitamin A), gastric mucosal levels of PGE_2 and cAMP were analyzed depending on the application of different doses of β-carotene and on time (the examinations were carried out at the 1, 2, 3 and 4 hours after indomethacin application) in indomethacin-treated rats. Earlier, it was proved that the carotenoids (including the β-carotene) prevent the chemically induced gastric mucosal damage (Jávor et al., 1983) by cytoprotection (without decreasing the gastric acid secretion).

http://dx.doi.org/10.5772/60505

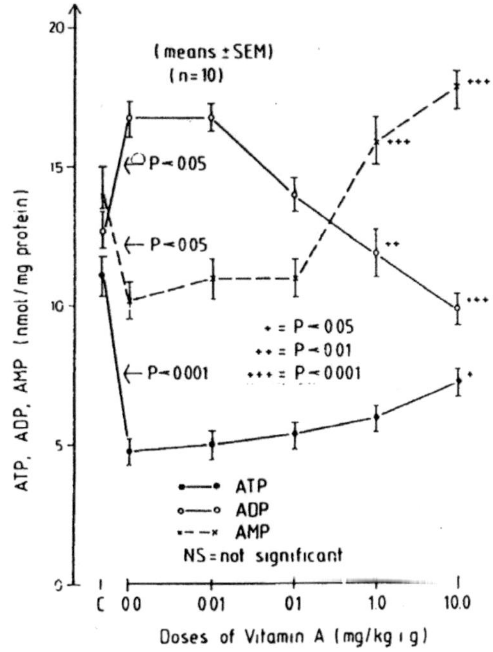

Figure 129. Changes in the gastric mucosal levels of ATP, ADP, AMP produced by vitamin A in 4-hour IND-treated rats (means ± SEM). [Mózsik et al.: Int. J. Tiss. Reac. 11, 65–71, 1989c (with kind permission).]

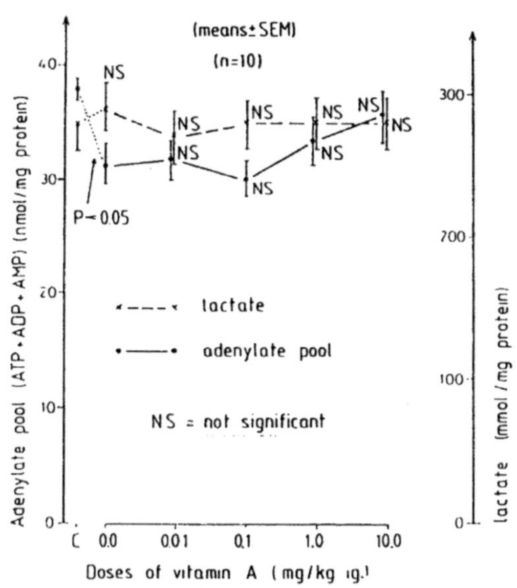

Figure 130. Changes in the gastric mucosal levels of adenylate pool and lactate produced by vitamin A in 4-hour IND-treated rats (means ± SEM). [Mózsik et al.: Int. J. Tiss. Reac. 11, 65–71, 1989c (with kind permission).]

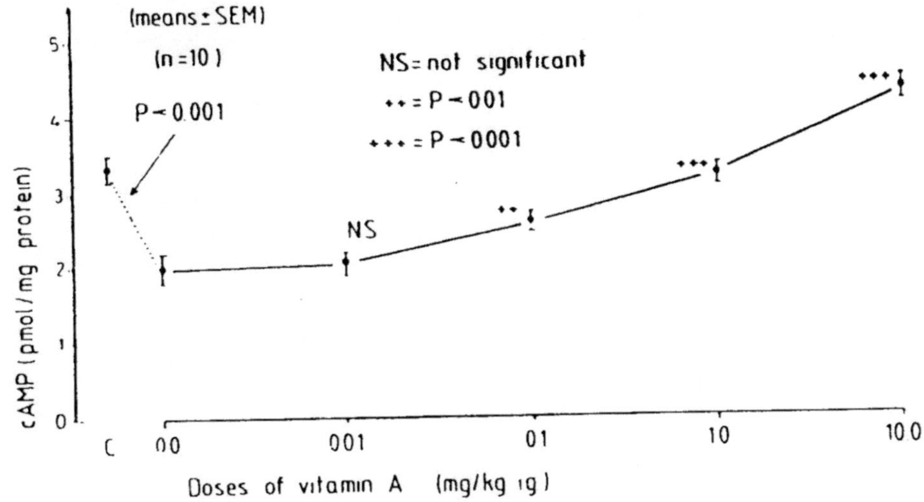

Figure 131. Changes in the gastric mucosal level of cAMP produced by vitamin A in 4-hour IND-treated rats (means ± SEM). [Mózsik et al.: Int. J. Tiss. Reac. 11, 65–71, 1989c (with kind permission).]

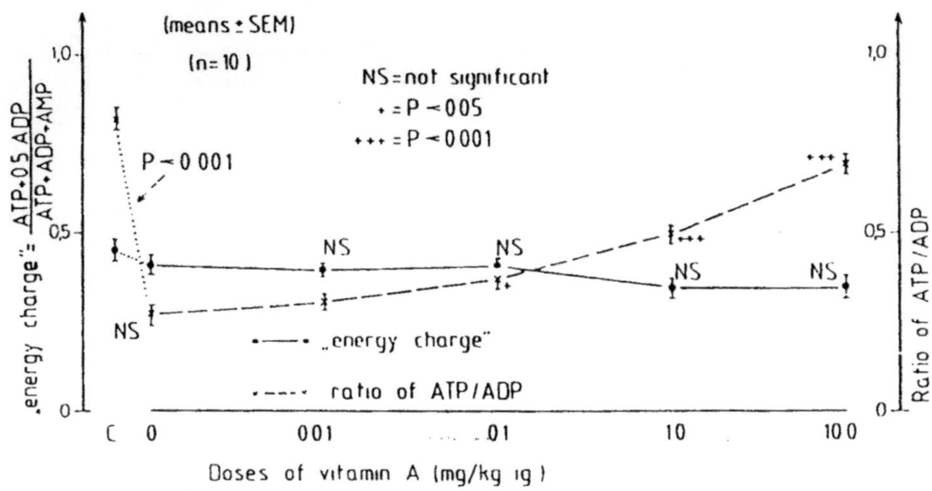

Figure 132. Changes in the gastric mucosal "energy charge" and ratio of ATP/ADP produced by vitamin A in 4-hour IND-treated rats (means ± SEM). [Mózsik et al. Int. J. Tiss. Reac. 11, 65–71, 1989c (with kind permission).]

The aims of these observations were as follows:

1. To evaluate the details of β-carotene-induced gastric mucosal prevention in rat model experiment;
2. Indomethacin produces inhibitory effect of the prostaglandin synthesis (and we proved this in rats in Section 8.4.3.) in 4-hour indomethacin-treated rats;

http://dx.doi.org/10.5772/60505

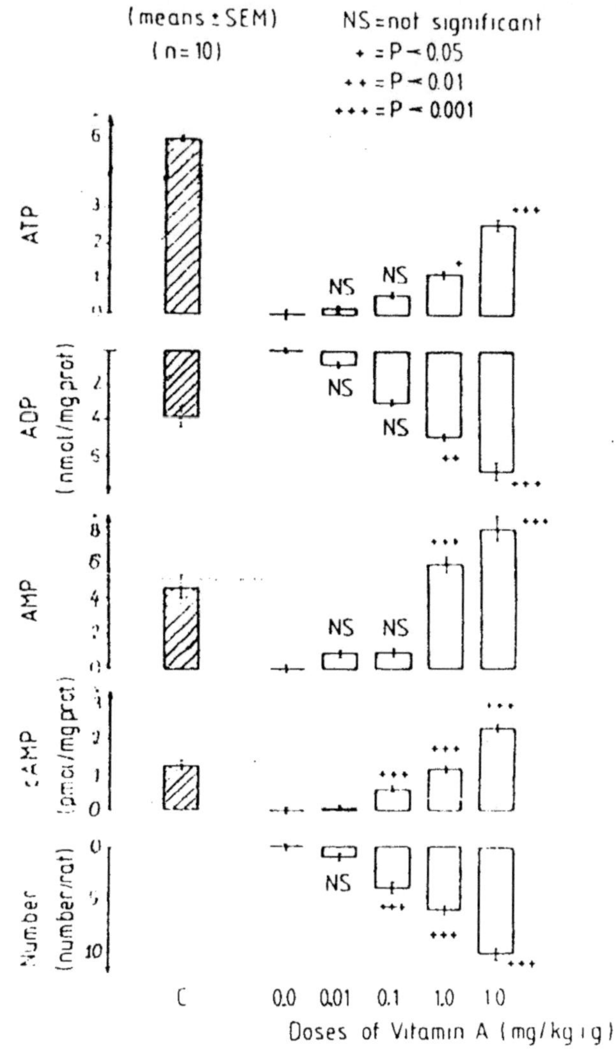

Figure 133. Regulatory pathways between the IND-induced gastric mucosal damage and vitamin A-induced changes in the 4-hour indomethacin-treated rat gastric fundic mucosa (means ± SEM). [Mózsik et al.: Int. J. Tiss. Reac. 11, 65–71, 1989c (with kind permission).]

3. To evaluate the possible correlations between the changes (decrease vs. development of indomethacin ulcer and increase vs. mucosal protection) of tissue levels of PGE_2 in indomethacin-treated rats;

4. To find (and to prove) the existence of β-carotene-induced mucosal protection versus changes (increase) in the gastric mucosal level of PGE_2 system; and

5. Is it really a well-established scientific fact that β-carotene produces only the scavenger pathway?

The experimental protocols (Figure 134) and the main results are presented in Figure 135.

Figure 136 indicated that a close correlation exists between the gastric fundic mucosal level of cAMP at 4 hours of experiments. We also indicated in many experiments that the responsible biochemical changes appeared earlier than the macroscopic appearance of gastric mucosal damage. So it was suggested that a similar correlation exists between the cAMP level in the gastric fundic mucosa versus clinical appearance of gastric mucosal damage, therefore the correlation between the tissue level of cAMP in the gastric fundic mucosa at 1 hour versus macroscopic images (number and severity) at 4 hours after indomethacin administration. Figures 137 and 138 clearly proved these correlations were clearly positive between these parameters.

When β-carotene (given intragastrically at doses of 0.1, 1.0 and 10 mg/kg dissolved in oleum helianthi) was given, then both the number (Figure 139) and severity (Figure 140) decreased dose-dependently. Interestingly, β-carotene produced a dose-dependent increase in the gastric fundic mucosal level of cAMP at 1 hour and at 4 hours after indomethacin administration (Figure 141).

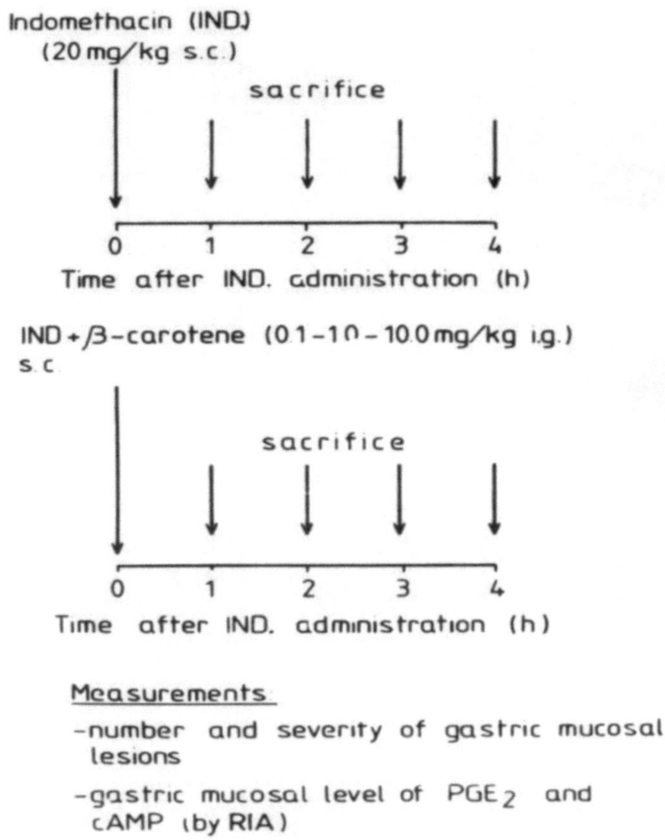

Figure 134. Design of the animal experiments in rats. [Mózsik, Bódis, Karádi, Király, Nagy, Rumi, Sütő, Szabó (1998). Inflammopharmacology 6: 27–40 (with kind permission).]

http://dx.doi.org/10.5772/60505

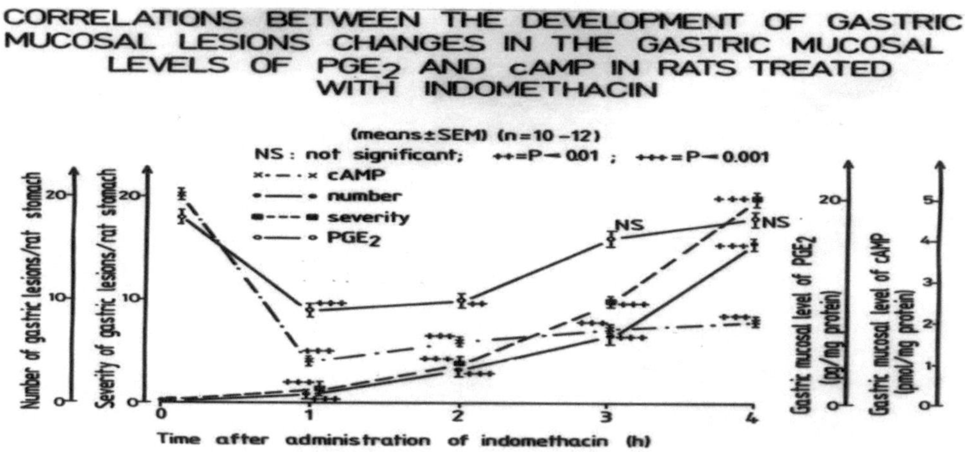

Figure 135. Correlations between the development of gastric mucosal damage (number and severity), changes in the tissue levels of PGE_2 and cAMP in the gastric fundic mucosa of 4-hour indomethacin-treated rats (at 0, 1, 2, 3 and 4 hours after administration of indomethacin). [Mózsik, Bódis, Karádi, Király, Nagy, Rumi, Sütő, Szabó (1998). Inflammopharmacology 6: 27–40 (with kind permission).]

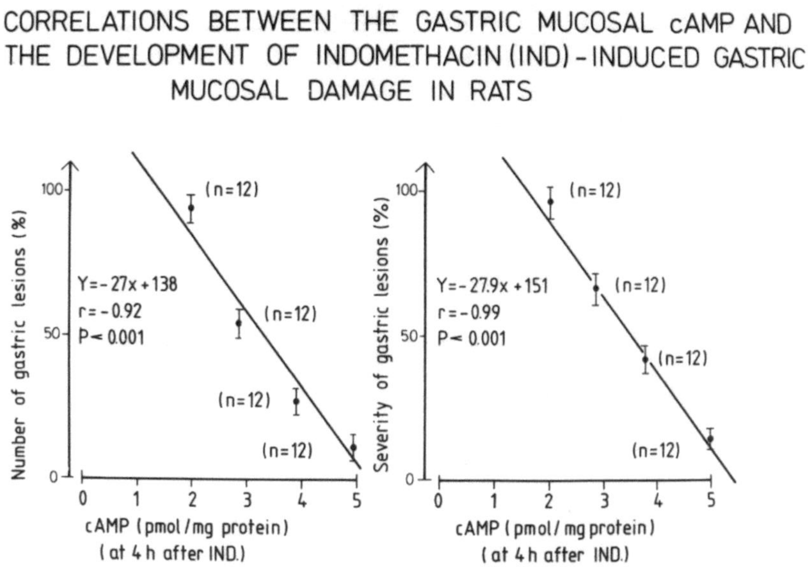

Figure 136. Correlation between the decrease of gastric mucosal level of cAMP (at 4 hours) versus number (and severity) (at 4 hours) in the gastric fundic mucosal damage in 4-hour indomethacin-treated rats. [Mózsik, Bódis, Karádi, Király, Nagy, Rumi, Sütő, Szabó (1998). Inflammopharmacology 6: 27–40 (with kind permission).]

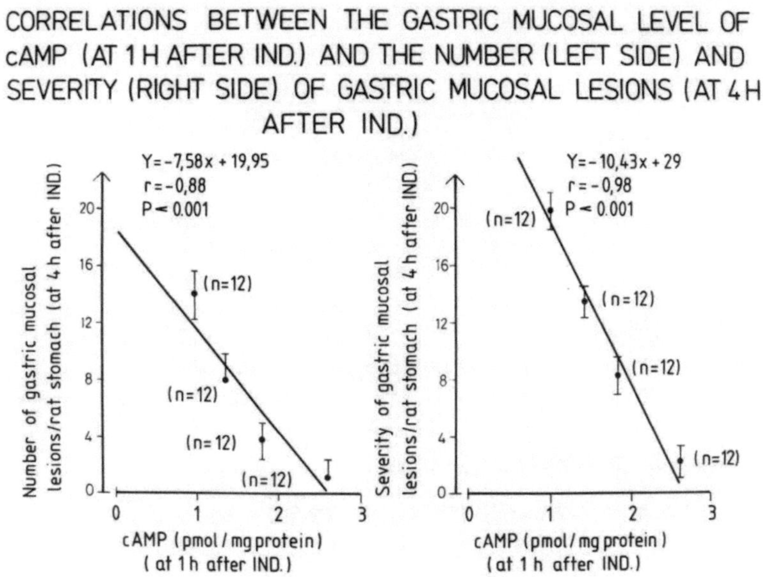

Figure 137. Correlations between the decrease of gastric fundic mucosal level of cAMP at 1 hour versus gastric mucosal damage (number and severity) at 4 hours in 4-hour indomethacin-treated rats. [Mózsik, Bódis, Karádi, Király, Nagy, Rumi, Sütő, Szabó (1998). Inflammopharmacology 6: 27–40 (with kind permission).]

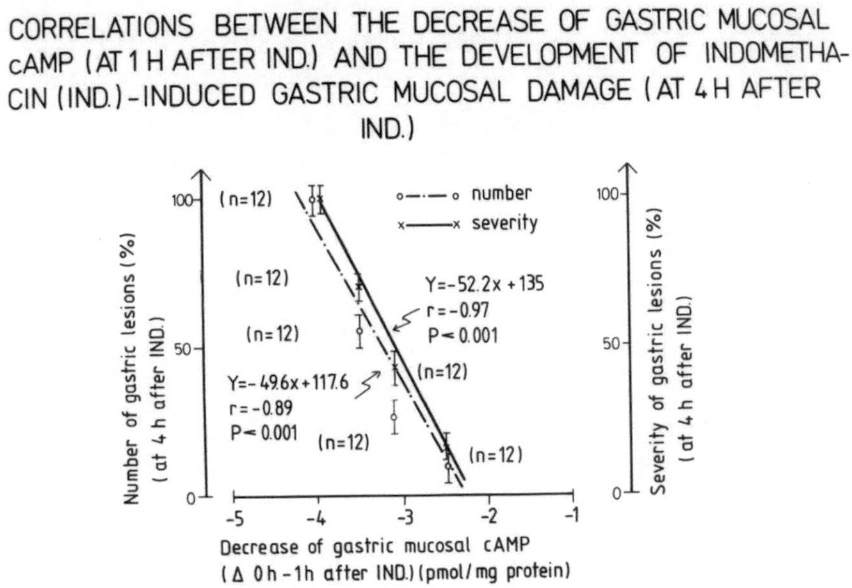

Figure 138. Similar results were obtained between the Δ values of decrease in gastric fundic mucosal level of cAMP (Δ 0–1 hour after IND) versus number and severity (expressed in percent values) (at 4 hours after IND) in 4-hour indomethacin-treated rats. This figure indicates that the existence of this correlation is practically the same in cases of both development of number and severity of gastric mucosal damage in 4-hour indomethacin-treated rats. [Mózsik, Bódis, Karádi, Király, Nagy, Rumi, Sütő, Szabó (1998). Inflammopharmacology 6: 27–40 (with kind permission).]

http://dx.doi.org/10.5772/60505

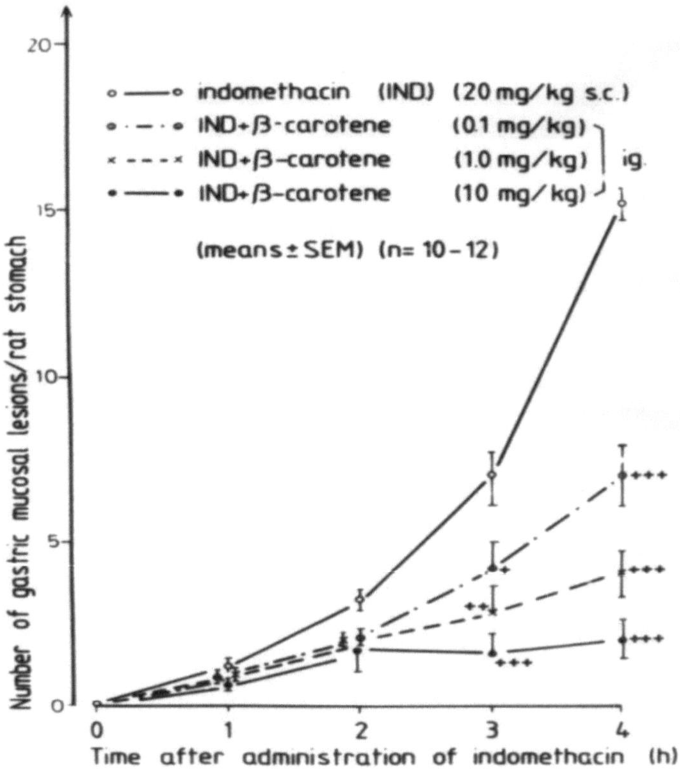

Figure 139. β-carotene-induced gastric fundic mucosal protection in 4-hour indomethacin-treated rats. The ordinate indicates the number of lesions, while the abscissa shows the time (in hours) after indomethacin administration. [Mózsik, Bódis, Karádi, Király, Nagy, Rumi, Sütő, Szabó (1998). Inflammopharmacology 6: 27–40 (with kind permission).]

No similar correlations were obtained between the changes in the gastric fundic mucosal PGE_2 level versus development of the gastric mucosal damage (and/or protection). The conclusions are as follows:

1. The decrease of cAMP in the gastric fundic mucosa appears at 1 hour after administration of indomethacin, and its level shows a moderate increase in the time period from 1 to 4 hours in 4-hour indomethacin-treated rats;

2. The extent of decrease of tissue levels of PGE_2 and cAMP differ significantly (including the different time periods) in 4-hour indomethacin-treated rats;

3. β-carotene, in a dose-dependent manner, prevents the indomethacin-induced gastric mucosal damage in association with dose- and time-dependent increase of gastric fundic mucosal cAMP level; however, no increase in gastric fundic mucosal PGE_2 was obtained during β-carotene-induced gastric mucosal damage;

4. β-carotene-induced gastric mucosal protection (in indomethacin model) differs from the gastric mucosal level of PGE_2;

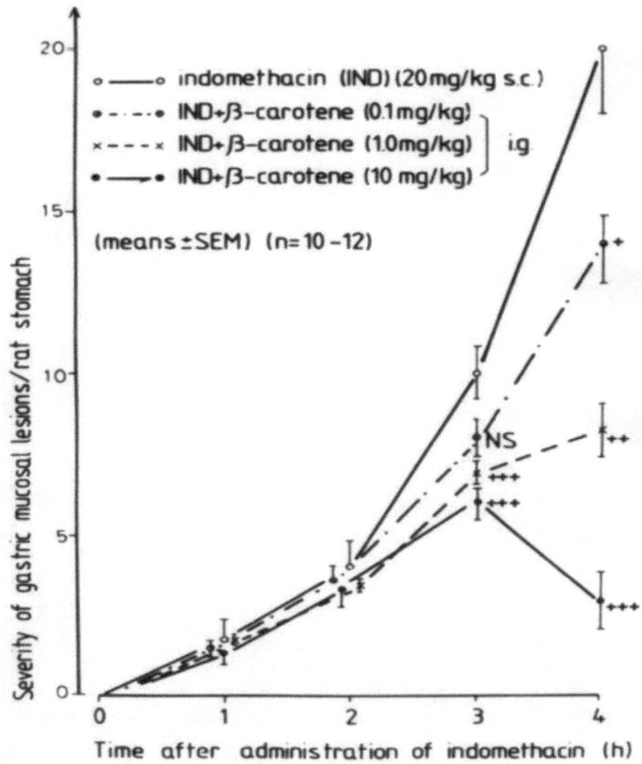

Figure 140. β-carotene-induced gastric fundic mucosal protection in 4-hour indomethacin-treated rats. The ordinate indicates the severity of lesions, while the abscissa shows the time (in hours) after indomethacin administration. [Mózsik, Bódis, Karádi, Király, Nagy, Rumi, Sütő, Szabó (1998). Inflammopharmacology 6: 27–40 (with kind permission).]

5. The decrease in gastric fundic mucosal cAMP is a responsible intracellular signal for the development of indomethacin-induced gastric mucosal damage, and the increase of cAMP by β-carotene is responsible for the development of β-carotene-induced gastric mucosal protection;

6. The treatment with vitamin A and β-carotene produces gastric mucosal protection against indomethacin-induced mucosal damage by a very complex extra- and intracellularly existing regulatory systems of the membrane-bound ATP-dependent energy systems in the rat gastric mucosa (Mózsik et al., 1990 a, b, c).

8.5. Changes in the gastric mucosal energy systems during 5-hour stress in rats

The aims of this study were as follows:

1. To evaluate the changes in the membrane-bound ATP-dependent energy systems during the development of stress-induced gastric mucosal damage;

2. To prove (or to exclude) the presence of tissue hypoxia in the rat gastric mucosa during development of gastric mucosal damage;

http://dx.doi.org/10.5772/60505

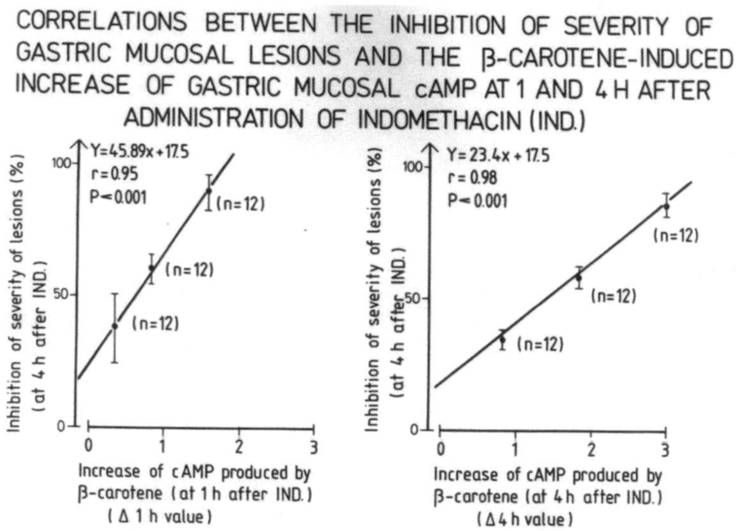

Figure 141. Correlations between the Δ values of gastric fundic mucosal level of cAMP at 1 hour (left figure) and at 4 hours (right figure) versus mucosal-protective effect of β-carotene on the severity of gastric mucosal damage (expressed in percent values) in 4-hour indomethacin-treated rats. [Mózsik, Bódis, Karádi, Király, Nagy, Rumi, Sütő, Szabó (1998). Inflammopharmacology 6: 27–40 (with kind permission).]

3. To present further evidence of a feedback mechanism existing between ATP-ADP and ATP-cAMP transformations;

4. To analyze the different biochemical changes in the gastric mucosa before and after macroscopic appearance of gastric mucosal damage; and

5. To study the direct effect of epinephrine, cAMP and AMP on Na^+-K^+-dependent ATPase prepared from the rat gastric fundic mucosa.

The animals were forced to swim in water below the body temperature (24 °C) for maximally 5 hours. They were sacrificed at 0, 1, 2, 3, 4 and 5 hours after the introduction of stress. The stress produced gastric mucosal lesions in the glandular portion of the stomach (its incidence is 100%). After sacrificing the animals (at the different times after the introduction of stress) (Figure 142), the number (and severity) of gastric mucosal lesions was registered and different biochemical examinations were carried out from the rat gastric fundic mucosa as the following:

1. The measurements of tissue levels of ATP, ADP, AMP, lactate and cAMP (and different calculations of the obtained results were performed between the results obtained in the measurements);

2. The preparation of membrane (Mg^{2+}-dependent and Na^+–K^+-dependent) ATPase was prepared and its activity was measured;

3. The effects of epinephrine, cAMP and AMP were measured on the Na^+–K^+-dependent ATPase activity prepared from the rat gastric fundic mucosa (for details, see Mózsik et al., 1990a).

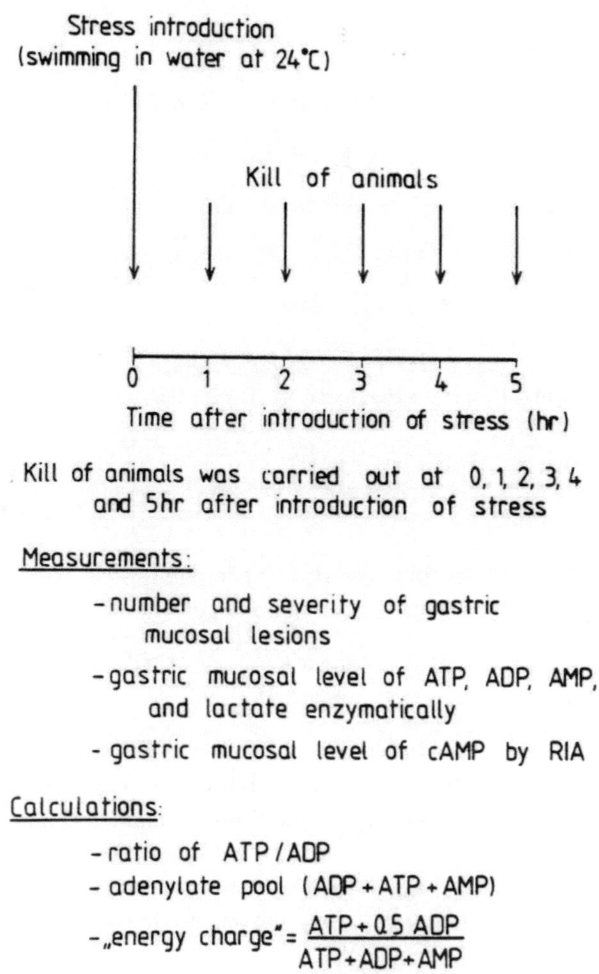

Figure 142. Experimental protocol of study of stress-induced gastric ulcer in rats [Mózsik et al., Ann N Y Acad Sci 597: 264–281, 1990a (with kind permission).]

The macroscopic appearance of gastric fundic mucosal lesions could be detected at the 2nd hour after the introduction of stress (Nagy et al., 1982, 1983; Mózsik et al., 1990a) (Figure 143). The results of biochemical examinations are presented in Figures 114–156 and Table 41.

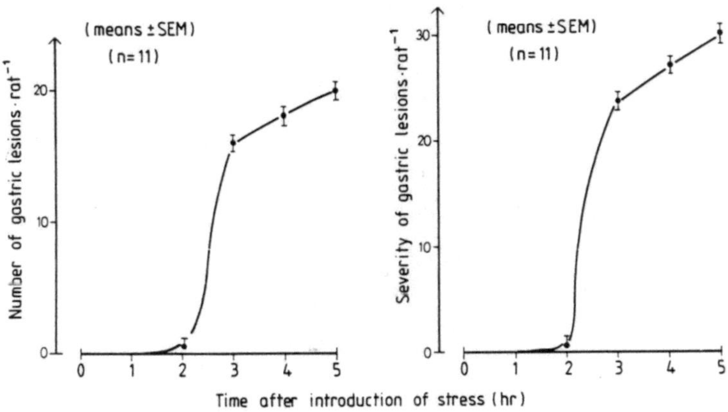

Figure 143. Macroscopic appearance of gastric mucosal lesions (number and severity) after the introduction of stress (means ± SEM) [Mózsik et al., Ann N Y Acad Sci 597: 264–281, 1990a (with kind permission).]

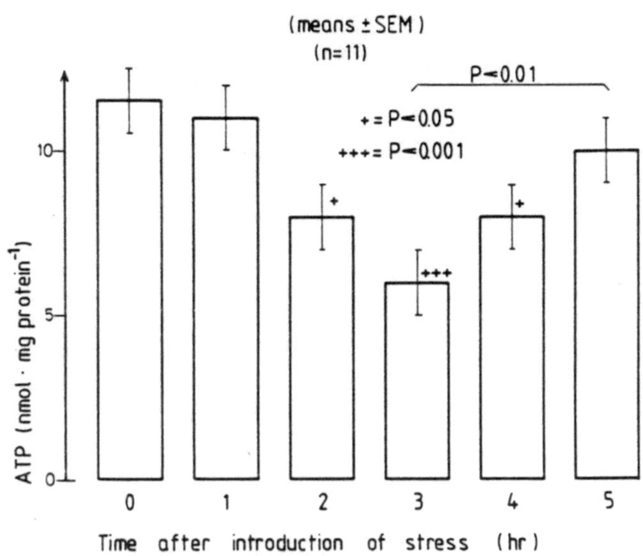

Figure 144. Changes in gastric mucosal level of adenosine triphosphate (ATP) during the development of stress-induced gastric mucosal lesions in rats. [Mózsik et al., Ann N Y Acad Sci 597: 264–281, 1990a (with kind permission).]

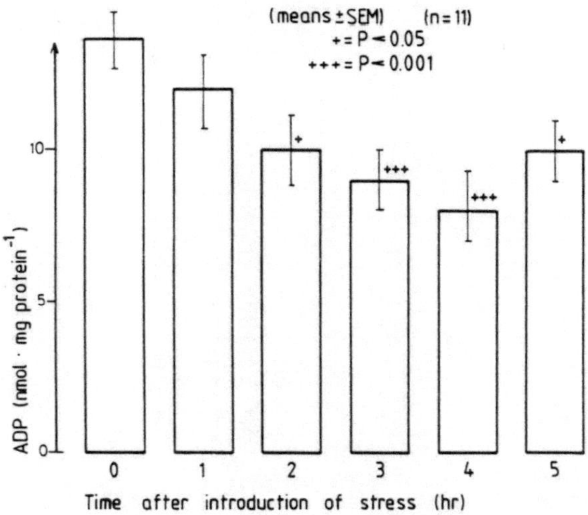

Figure 145. Changes in gastric mucosal level of adenosine diphosphate (ADP) during the development of stress-induced gastric mucosal lesions in rats. [Mózsik et al., Ann N Y Acad Sci 597: 264–281, 1990a (with kind permission).]

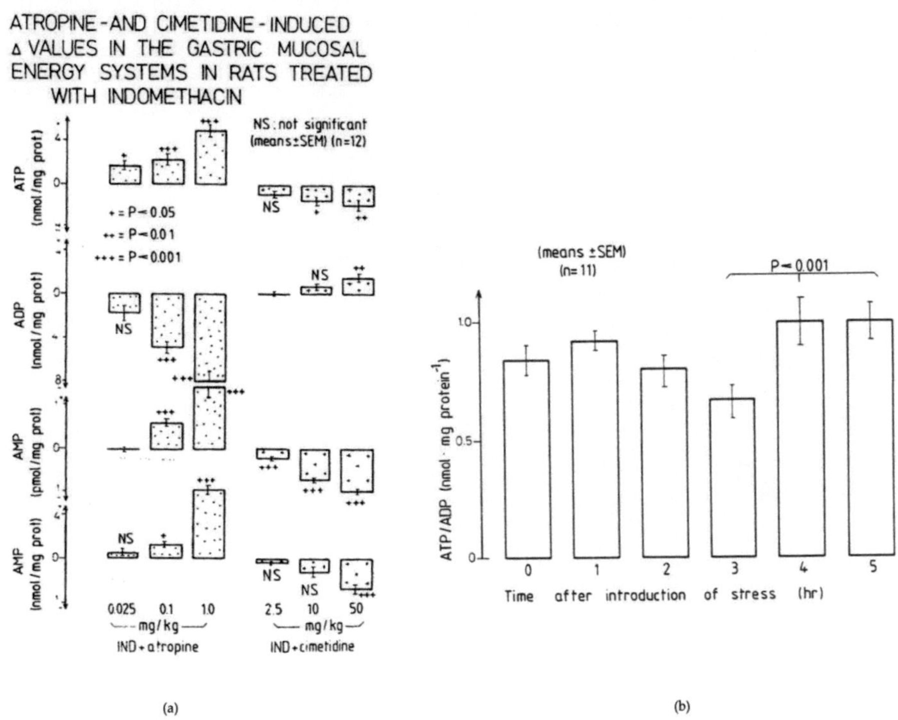

Figure 146. Stress-induced changes in the ratio of ATP–ADP (ATP/ADP) in the gastric mucosa of rats. [Mózsik et al., Ann N Y Acad Sci 597: 264–281, 1990a (with kind permission).]

http://dx.doi.org/10.5772/60505

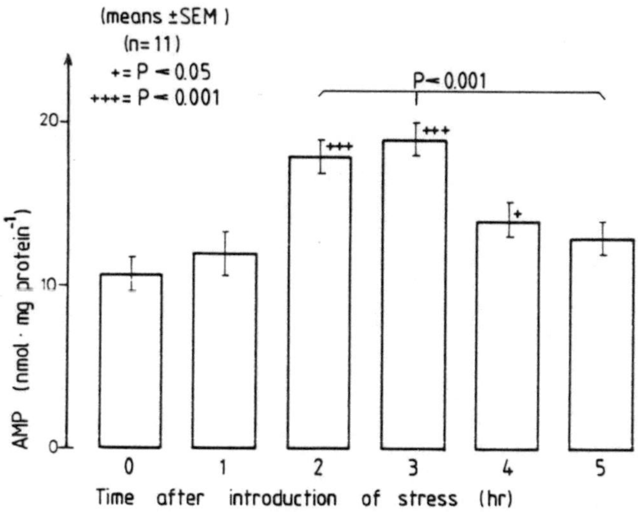

Figure 147. Changes in gastric mucosal level of adenosine monophosphate (AMP) during the development of stress-induced gastric mucosal lesions in rats. (Mózsik et al., Ann N Y Acad Sci 597: 264–281, 1990a (with kind permission).]

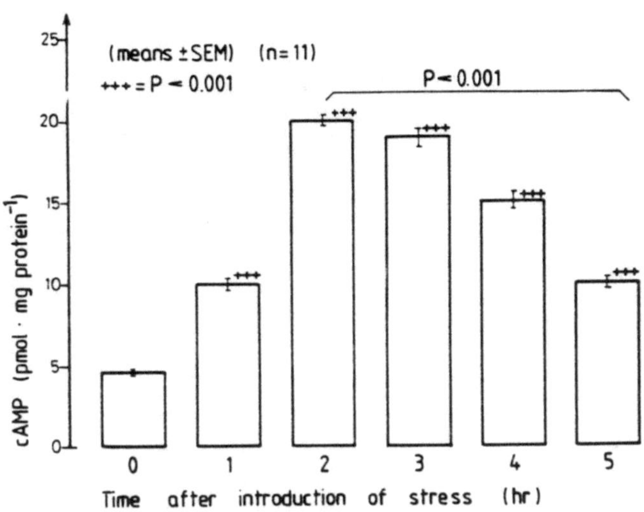

Figure 148. Changes in gastric mucosal level of cyclic adenosine monophosphate (cAMP) during the development of stress-induced gastric mucosal lesions in rats. [Mózsik et al., Ann N Y Acad Sci 597: 264–281, 1990a (with kind permission).]

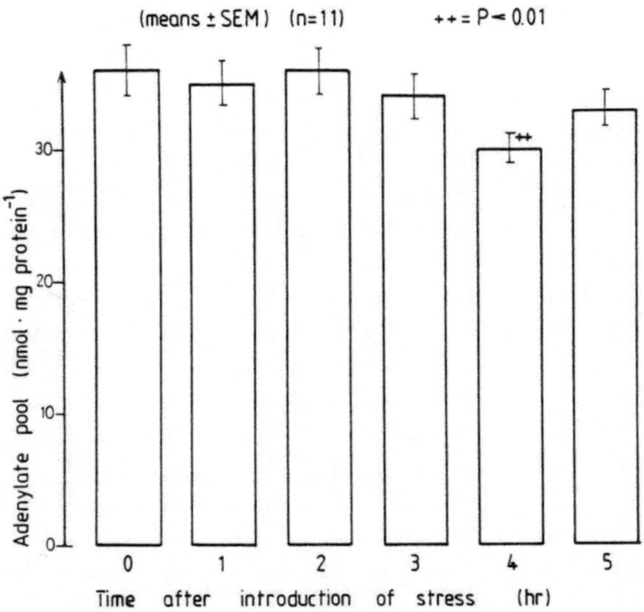

Figure 149. Tissue levels of adenylate pool (ATP + ADP + AMP) in the gastric mucosa during the development of stress-induced gastric mucosal lesions in rats. [Mózsik et al., Ann N Y Acad Sci 597: 264–281, 1990a (with kind permission).]

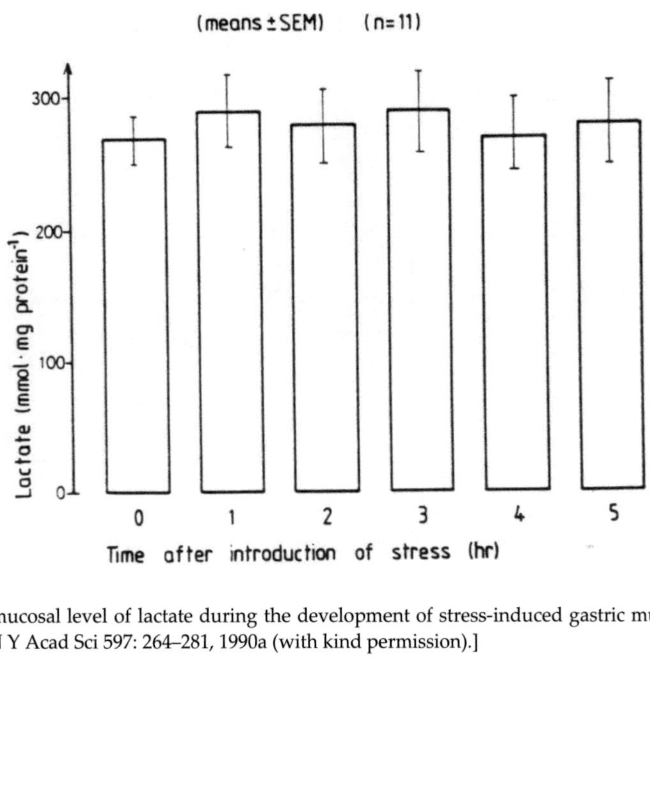

Figure 150. Gastric mucosal level of lactate during the development of stress-induced gastric mucosal lesions in rats. [Mózsik et al., Ann N Y Acad Sci 597: 264–281, 1990a (with kind permission).]

http://dx.doi.org/10.5772/60505

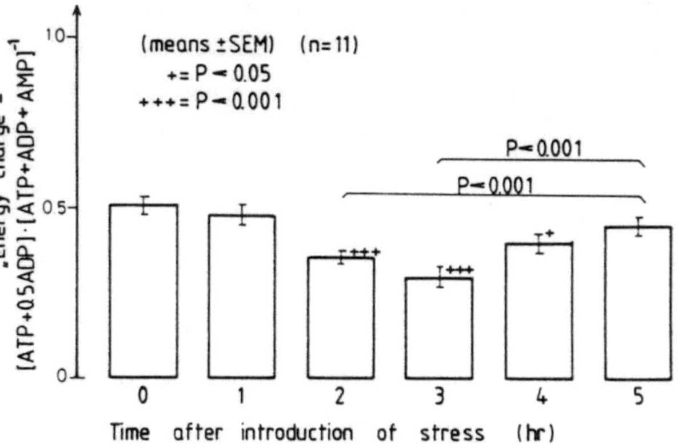

Figure 151. Changes in the gastric mucosal level of "energy charge" [(ATP + 0.5 ADP)/(ATP + ADP + AMP)] during the development of stress-induced gastric mucosal lesions in rats. [Mózsik et al., Ann N Y Acad Sci 597: 264–281, 1990a (with kind permission).]

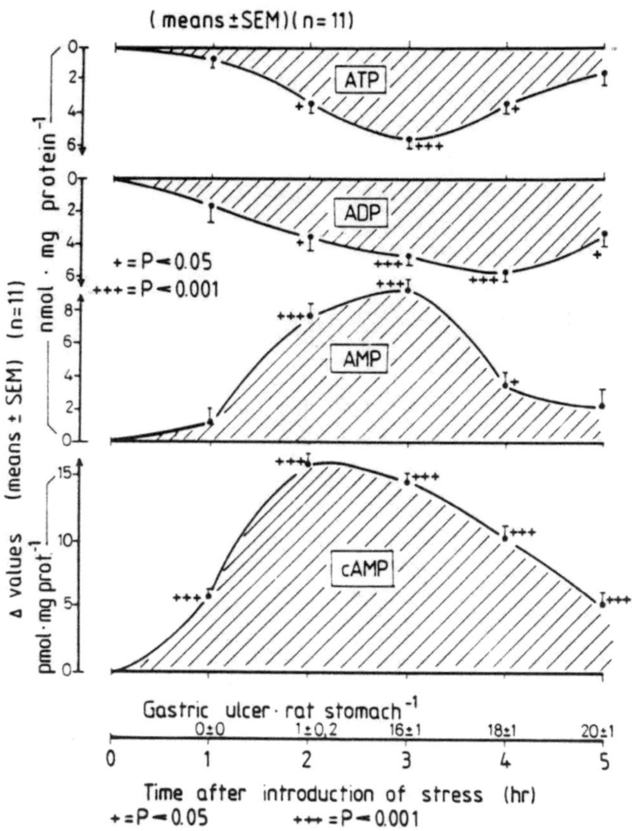

Figure 152. Correlations between changes in energy systems and development of gastric mucosal lesions in rats. Changes in the gastric mucosal levels of ATP, ADP, AMP and cAMP are expressed as Δ values. [Mózsik et al., Ann N Y Acad Sci 597: 264–281, 1990a (with kind permission).]

It was interesting to note that cAMP decreased significantly in 24 and 4 hours, with the increased level of cAMP being associated with gastric mucosal prevention in many models (pylorus-ligated plus IND-treated animals and the effects of atropine and vitamin A) (Mózsik et al., 1978c; 1979 a, b; 1988a, b; 1992 a, b, c, d, e; 1996 a, b; 1997 b, c; 1998).

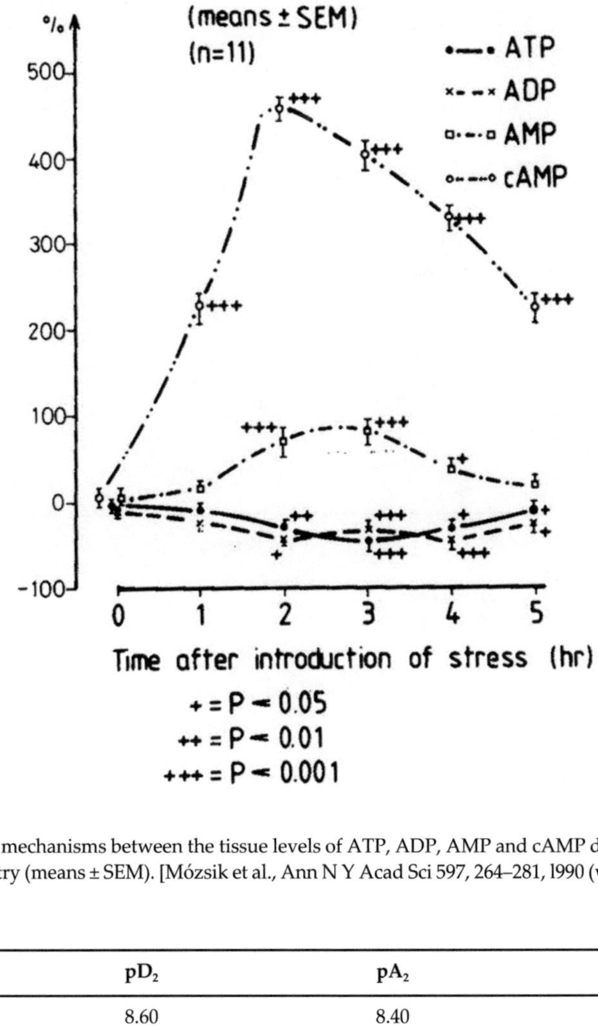

Figure 153. Regulatory mechanisms between the tissue levels of ATP, ADP, AMP and cAMP during stress-induced gastric mucosal biochemistry (means ± SEM). [Mózsik et al., Ann N Y Acad Sci 597, 264–281, 1990 (with kind permission).]

Drugs	pD_2	pA_2	α
Epinephrine	8.60	8.40	0.41
cAMP	11.80	10.00	0.48
AMP	8.80	8.70	0.90
Oabain	5.90	5.80	1.00

Table 41. Values of affinities (pD_2) and intrinsic activities (pA_2) ($\alpha_{atropine} = 1.00$) for epinephrine, cAMP, AMP and ouabain on Na^+–K^+-dependent ATPase activity prepared from the rat gastric fundic mucosa. The necessary dose to produce 50% action of affinity (pD_2) and intrinsic activity (pA_2) is expressed in [–] molar values. [Mózsik et al., Ann N Y Acad Sci 59, 264–281, 1990a (with kind permission).]

http://dx.doi.org/10.5772/60505

We followed the changes in the ratio of ATP/ADP and "energy charge" (Figure 154). No significant change in ATP/ADP was found.

MEAN STEPS OF THE BIOCHEMICAL BACKGROUNDS OF THE DEVELOPMENT OF STRESS-INDUCED GASTRIC MUCOSAL DAMAGE IN RATS

(UNTREATED RATS)

$ATP \cdot ADP^{-1}$: 0.84 ± 0.06

„Energy charge"=0.51±0.02

(n=11)

	Time after introduction of stess (hr)				
	1	2	3	4	5
$ATP \cdot ADP^{-1}$	0.92±0.09	0.80±0.08	0.67±0.08	1.00±0.10	1.00±0.08
„energy charge"	0.48±0.03	0.36±0.01^{+++}	0.30±0.02^{+++}	0.40±0.02^{+}	0.45±0.02
	(n=11)	(n=11)	(n=11)	(n=11)	(n=11)

+ = P < 0.05

+++ = P < 0.001

Figure 154. Changes in the ratio of ATP/ADP and in "energy charge" dependent upon time after the introduction of stress (means ± SEM). [Mózsik et al., Ann N Y Acad Sci 59, 264–281, 1990a (with kind permission).]

CHANGES IN THE RAT GASTRIC MUCOSAL BIOCHEMISTRY DURING DEVELOPMENT OF STRESS ULCER PRODUCED BY SWIMMING IN THE WATER

	Time after introduction of streess (hr)					
	0	1	2	3	4	5
Ulcer number				↑↑↑	↑↑↑	↑↑↑
Ulcer severity				↑↑↑	↑↑↑	↑↑↑
ATP			↓	↓↓↓	↓	
ADP			↓	↓↓↓	↓↓↓	↓
$ATP \cdot ADP^{-1}$						
AMP			↑↑↑	↑↑↑	↑	
ATP+ADP+AMP					↓	
„energy charge"			↓↓↓	↓↓↓	↓	
cAMP		↑↑↑	↑↑↑	↑↑↑	↑↑↑	↑↑↑
Lactate						

↑ = increase ↓ = decrease

↑(↓)= P < 0.05 ↑↑ ↑(↓↓ ↓)= P < 0.001

Figure 155. Time-sequence changes between the macroscopic development of gastric mucosal damage and biochemical parameters in the gastric fundic mucosa dependent upon time after the introduction of stress (means ± SEM). [Mózsik et al., Ann N Y Acad Sci 59, 264–281, 1990a (with kind permission).]

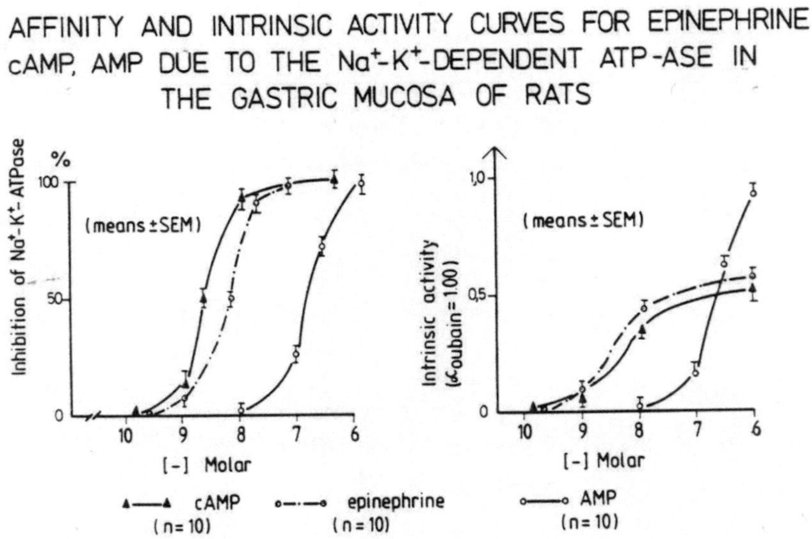

Figure 156. Affinity and intrinsic activity curves for inhibition by epinephrine, cAMP, AMP and ouabain of Na^+–K^+-dependent ATPase prepared from the rat gastric fundic mucosa. [Mózsik et al., Ann N Y Acad Sci 59, 264–281, 1990a (with kind permission).]

The results presented in this chapter are as follows:

1. Gastric mucosal lesions appeared and increased gradually 3 hours after the introduction of stress;
2. The extent of ATP–cAMP and cAMP–AMP transformations was increased considerably during the development of stress ulcer;
3. The extent of ATP–ADP transformation was completely inhibited;
4. The activity of Na^+–K^+-dependent ATPase from the rat gastric fundic mucosa could be inhibited by epinephrine, cAMP and AMP;
5. The ratio of ATP/ADP was unchanged during the first time period (from 0 to 3 hours), after its value increased;
6. The value of "energy charge" (e.g., the extent of phosphorylation and/or dephosphorylation) of cells was decreased at 2 and 3 hours, after which its value returned to a normal level;
7. There was no increase in the tissue level of lactate;
8. Several biochemical changes (decrease of ATP, ADP and "energy charge", increase of cAMP and AMP) preceded the macroscopic appearance of stress ulcer.

http://dx.doi.org/10.5772/60505

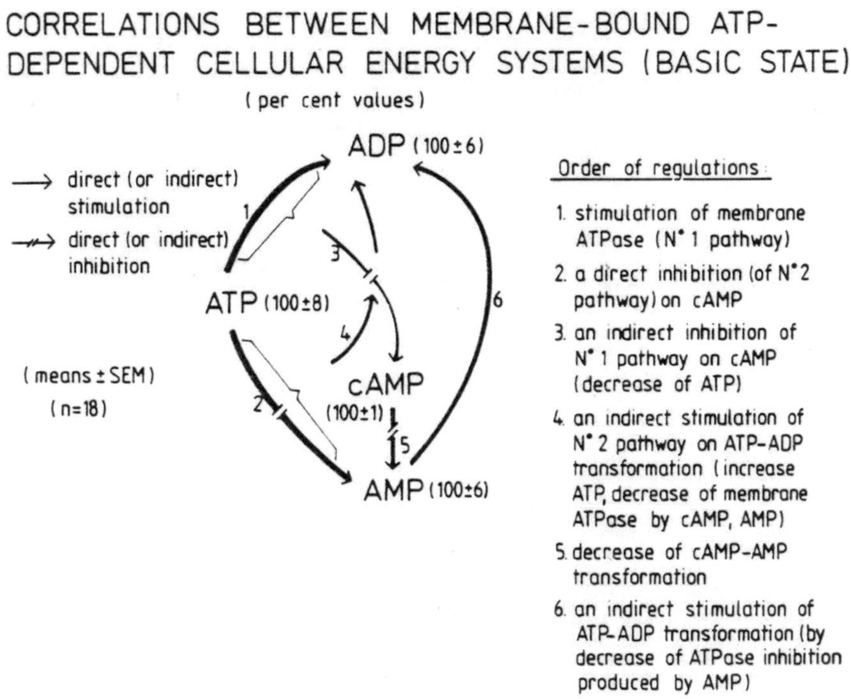

Figure 157. Suggested extra- and intracellular regulatory steps existing between the Na^+–K^+-dependent ATPase (transformation of ATP into ADP) and adenylate cyclase (transformation of ATP into cAMP) under physiological (basic) state of the target organ. It is important to emphasize that the different drugs, hormones and mediators ("first messengers") are able to modify the in smaller concentrations the Na^+–K^+-dependent ATPase system, and only in higher doses the adenylate cyclase, and the ATP as a common substrate cellular components for the function of both enzymes in presence of Mg^{2+}. [Mózsik et al., Ann N Y Acad Sci 59, 264–281, 1990a (with kind permission).]

For a better understanding, the existence of feedback extra- and intracellular regulatory mechanism system between the different membrane-bound ATP-dependent energy systems (under physiological and pathological conditions existing in the gastric fundic tissues) and the different (suggested) regulatory steps are demonstrated in Figures 157–160.

8.6. Reserpine ulcer and gastric mucosal biochemistry in rats

Reserpine liberates epinephrine and norepinephrine in the rats. If the animals receive reserpine (5 mg/kg) after 6 hours, visible ulceration will appear in the glandular stomach (Mózsik et al., 1983c) (Figure 161).

It was interesting to note that significant changes could be detected before the ulcer development; the peaks of the biochemical measurements were obtained at 6–12 hours after reserpine administration (Figures 162–164), whereas the peak of ulceration was obtained at 24 hours after reserpine administration.

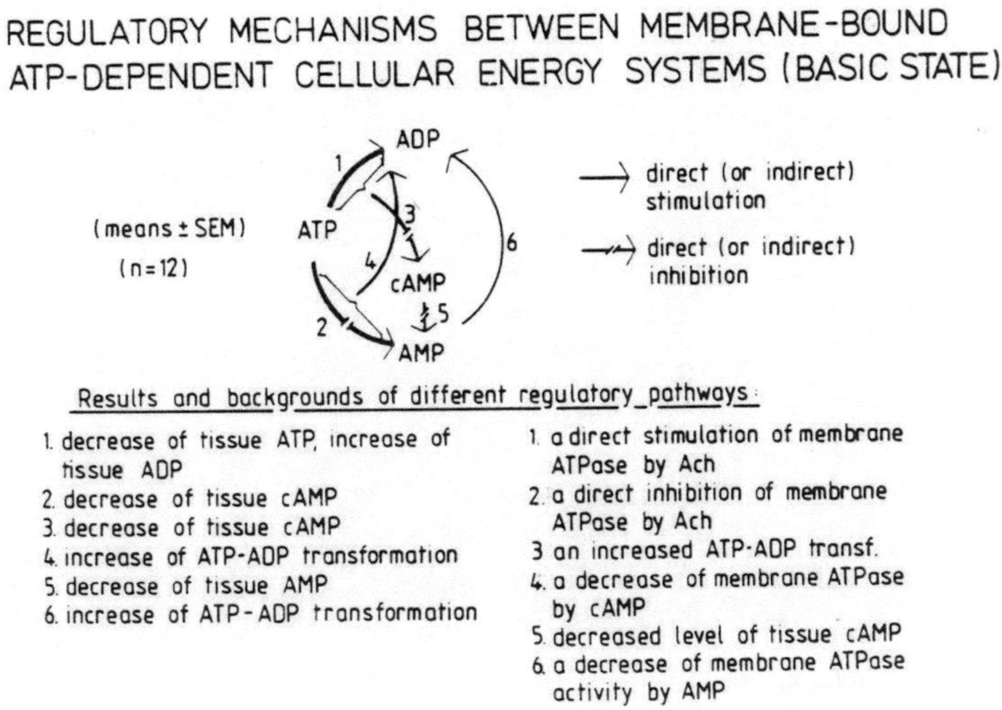

Figure 158. A detailed summary of the existence of the extra- and intracellular regulatory steps between the Na^+–K^+-dependent ATPase (ATP transformation of ATP into ADP) and adenylate cyclase (ATP transformation into cAMP) enzymes in the gastric fundic mucosa under physiological (basic) state. [Mózsik et al., Ann N Y Acad Sci 59, 264–281, 1990a (with kind permission).]

8.7. NaOH-, NaCl-, HCl- and ethanol-induced gastric mucosal damage in rats (1 hour): different chemically induced gastric mucosal damage versus same changes in the gastric mucosal biochemical backgrounds

The gastric fundic mucosal damage was first produced by Chaudhury and Jacobson (1978) and Robert and coworkers (1979), when they clearly indicated that the gastric mucosal damage was prevented by small doses of prostaglandins (PGs) without the presence of any inhibitory effect on the gastric acid secretion in rats. This event was the first evidence for that the gastric mucosal prevention can be separated from the importance of gastric acid secretion (that was the old dogma in the treatment of PUD). This step in the gastroenterological research offered a better understanding of patients' problems to the existing principal basic (experimental) research. Furthermore, these types of experimental approaches provide new results, which were responsible, and simple methods (Morón et al., 1983, 1984c; Mózsik et al, 1980; 1981a; 1983b; 1984 a, b, c, d; 1989 a, b, c, d, e; 1990b).

http://dx.doi.org/10.5772/60505

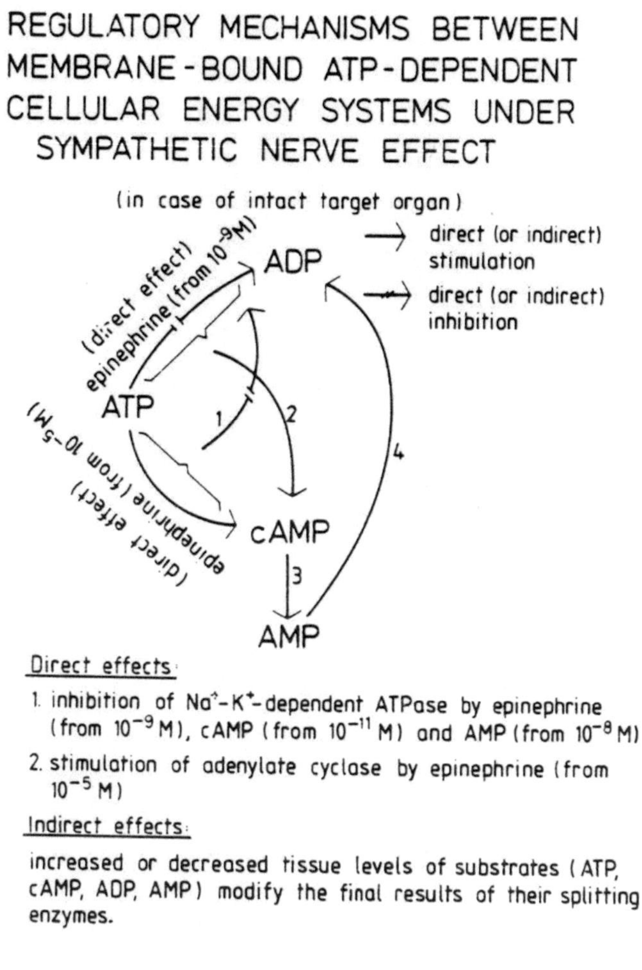

Figure 159. The epinephrine-induced changes in Na^+–K^+-dependent ATPase, adenylate cyclase prepared from the rat gastric fundic mucosa and in the tissue levels of ATP, ADP, AMP and cAMP in the rat gastric fundic mucosa. [Mózsik et al., Ann N Y Acad Sci 59, 264–281, 1990a (with kind permission).]

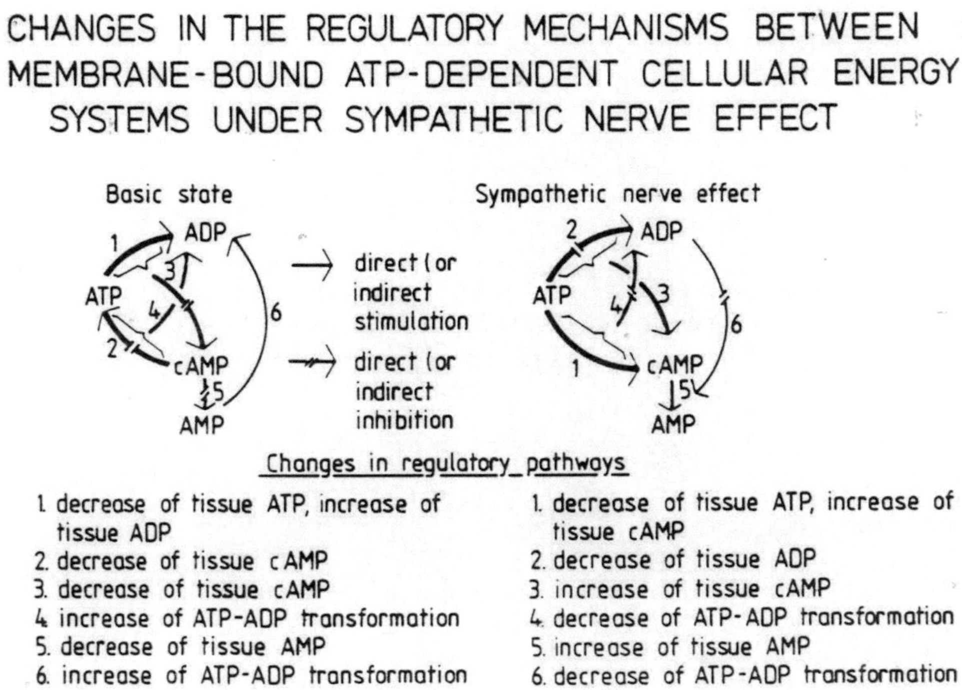

Figure 160. Summary of the changes in the feedback mechanism system during stress-induced gastric ulcer in rats (in comparison with each step to the existing physiological state). [Mózsik et al., Ann N Y Acad Sci 59, 264–281, 1990a (with kind permission).]

8.7.1. A model study of ethanol-induced injury to gastric mucosa in rats

Rats were given 96% ethanol intragastrically, and they were sacrificed at 0, 1, 5, 15, 30 and 60 minutes later. At each time period, the number and severity of mucosal lesions were recorded. At the same time intervals, the tissue levels of ATP, ADP, AMP and lactate were determined in homogenates of gastric mucosa by enzymatic methods. Tissue content of cAMP was determined by RIA (Becton Dickinson, Orangeburg, USA). The protein content was measured by the method of Lowry et al. (1951). The tissue levels of ATP, ADP, AMP and lactate are expressed as nmoles/mg protein, except for cAMP, which is expressed as pmoles mucosal protein. The ratio of ATP/ADP, values of adenylate pool (ATP + ADP + ANP) and "energy charge" [(ATP + 0.5 ADP)/(ATP + ADP + AMP)] were calculated from the individual values (Figures 165–173, Table 42).

http://dx.doi.org/10.5772/60505

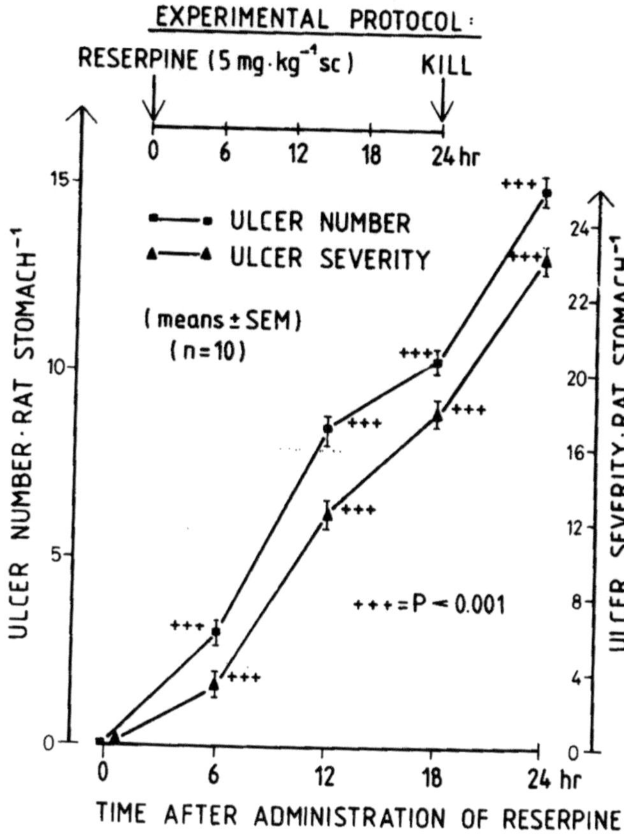

Figure 161. Ulcer (number and severity) development in reserpine (5 mg/kg s.c.)-induced gastric fundic mucosal lesions dependent upon time after reserpine administration (means ± SEM). [Mózsik et al., Acta Physiol Hung 62, 107–112, 1983c (with kind permission).]

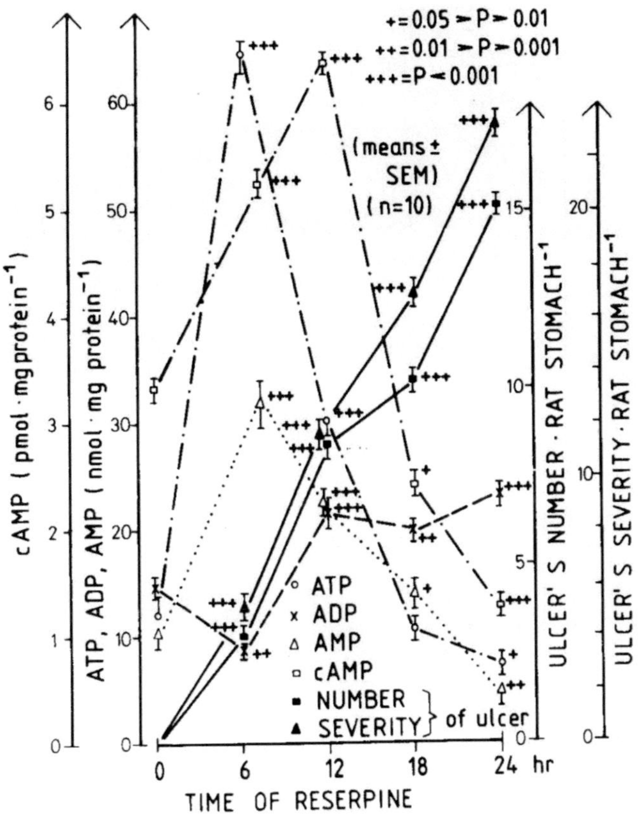

Figure 162. The time sequence between the biochemical changes (tissue levels of ATP, ADP, AMP and cAMP) versus gastric fundic mucosal damage ulcer (number and severity) in reserpine-treated rats (means ± SEM). [Mózsik et al., Acta Physiol Hung 62, 107–112, 1983c (with kind permission).]

http://dx.doi.org/10.5772/60505

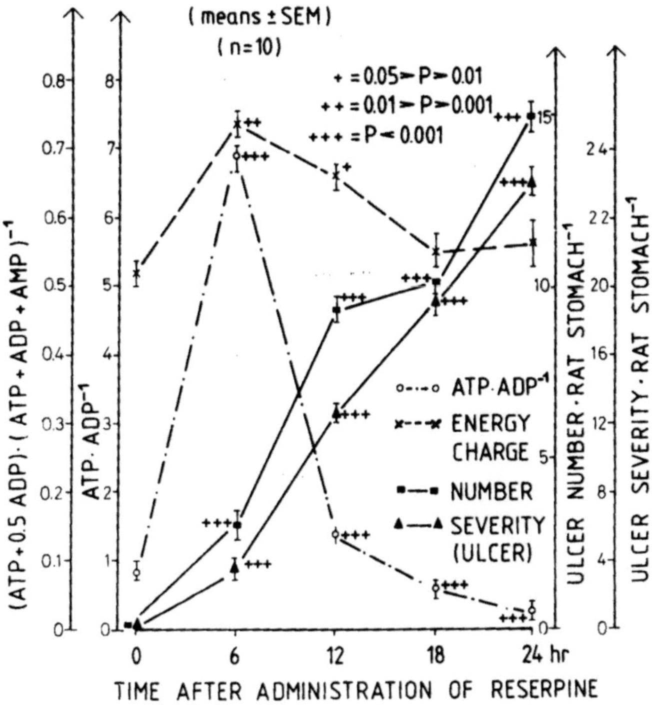

Figure 163. Correlations between the changes in "energy charge" and ratio of ATP/ADP versus gastric fundic mucosal damage (number and severity) produced by reserpine administration dependent on time after reserpine administration (means ± SEM). [Mózsik et al., Acta Physiol Hung 62, 107–112, 1983a (with kind permission).]

	Time periods after ethanol administration (min)			
	0 to 5	5 to 15 (Δ 10 min)	15 to 30 (Δ 15 min)	30 to 60 (Δ 30 min)
Number of gastric mucosal lesions	5.85 ± 0.60 (5.85)*	3.67 ± 1.00 (1.82)*	1.30 ± 0.40 (0.32)*	3.00 ± 0.80 (0.50)*
Severity of gastric mucosal esions	28 ± 2 (28)*	9 ± 1 (4.5)*	13 ± 1 (4.3)*	12 ± 2 (2)*

Table 42. Changes in macroscopically appearing gastric mucosal damage produced by intragastric administration of ethanol and time dependence after administration (means ± SEM) (n=12).* = average value per 5 minutes corresponding to different time periods after ethanol administration. [Mózsik and Javor: Dig. Dis. Sci. 33:92–105, 1988 (with kind permission).]

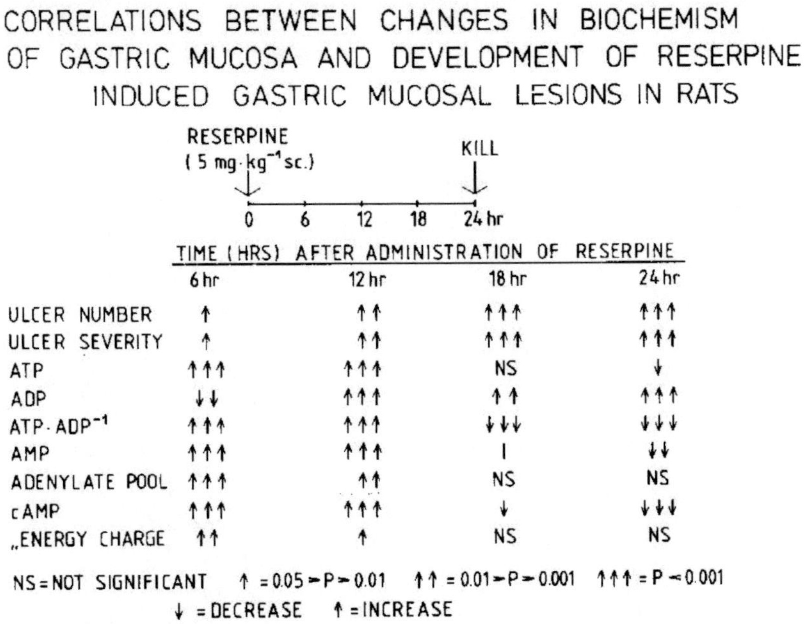
CORRELATIONS BETWEEN CHANGES IN BIOCHEMISM OF GASTRIC MUCOSA AND DEVELOPMENT OF RESERPINE INDUCED GASTRIC MUCOSAL LESIONS IN RATS

TIME (HRS) AFTER ADMINISTRATION OF RESERPINE	6 hr	12 hr	18 hr	24 hr
ULCER NUMBER	↑	↑↑	↑↑↑	↑↑↑
ULCER SEVERITY	↑	↑↑	↑↑↑	↑↑↑
ATP	↑↑↑	↑↑↑	NS	↓
ADP	↓↓	↑↑↑	↑↑	↑↑↑
$ATP \cdot ADP^{-1}$	↑↑↑	↑↑↑	↓↓↓	↓↓↓
AMP	↑↑↑	↑↑↑	I	↓↓
ADENYLATE POOL	↑↑↑	↑↑	NS	NS
cAMP	↑↑↑	↑↑↑	↓	↓↓↓
„ENERGY CHARGE	↑↑	↑	NS	NS

NS = NOT SIGNIFICANT ↑ = 0.05 > P > 0.01 ↑↑ = 0.01 > P > 0.001 ↑↑↑ = P < 0.001
↓ = DECREASE ↑ = INCREASE

Figure 164. The correlations between the changes in the tissue levels of ATP, ADP, AMP, adenylate pool, ratio of ATP/ADP, cAMP versus ulcer (number and severity) development dependent on time after reserpine administration (means ± SEM). [Mózsik et al., Acta Physiol Hung 62, 107–112, 1983a (with kind permission).]

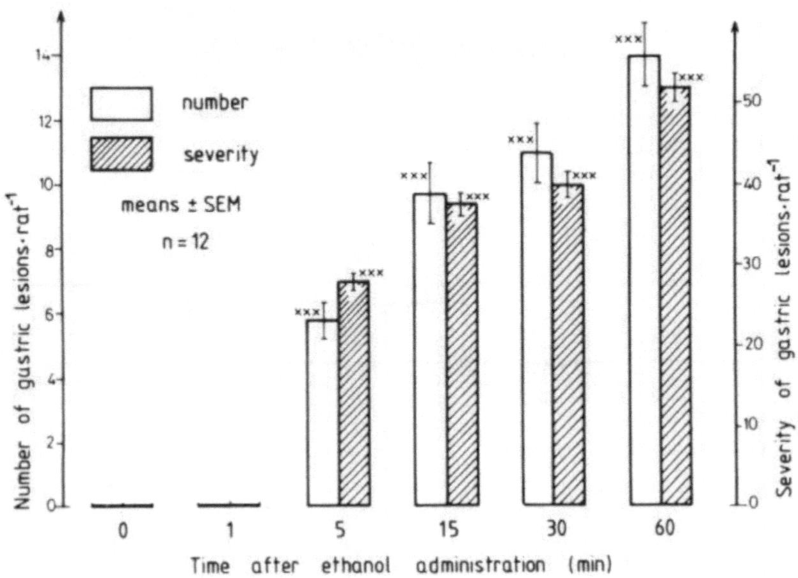

Figure 165. Macroscopic appearance of gastric mucosal damage in rats produced by intragastric administration of 96% ethanol. Time dependence after administration of ethanol. [Mózsik and Javor: Dig. Dis. Sci. 33:92–105, 1988 (with kind permission).]

http://dx.doi.org/10.5772/60505

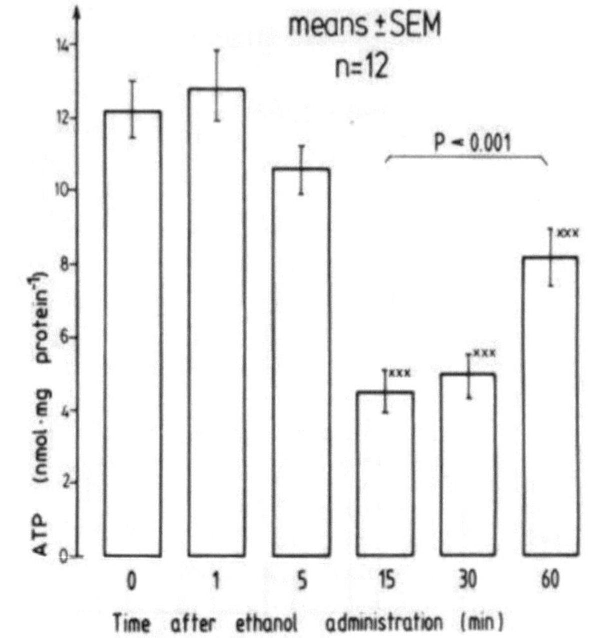

Figure 166. Changes in gastric mucosal level of ATP in rats after intragastric administration of 96% ethanol (1 mL). [Mózsik and Javor: Dig. Dis. Sci. 33: 92–105, 1988 (with kind permission).]

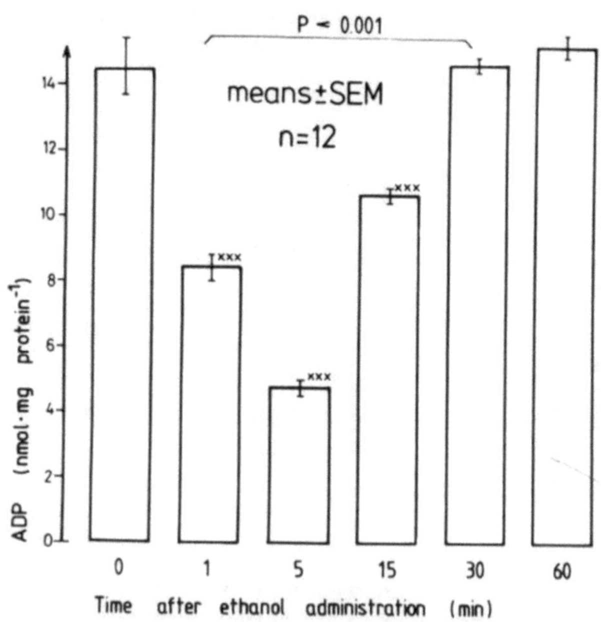

Figure 167. Changes in gastric mucosal level of ADP in rats after intragastric administration of 96% ethanol (1 mL). [Mózsik and Javor: Dig. Dis. Sci. 33: 92–105, 1988 (with kind permission).]

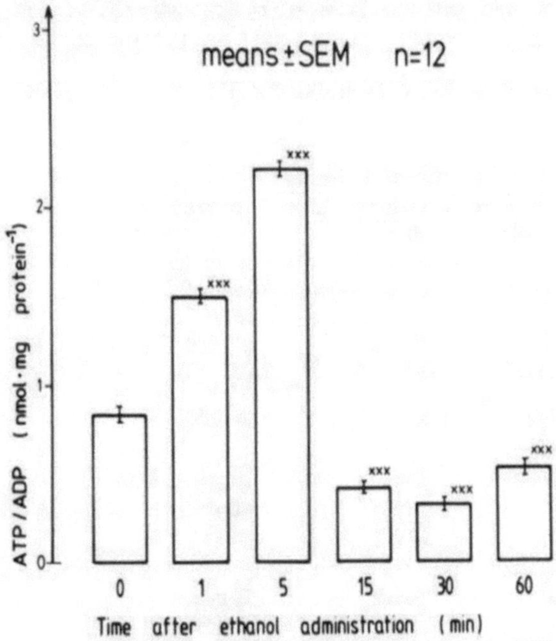

Figure 168. Changes in ratio of ATP/ADP in the gastric mucosa of rats after administration of 96% ethanol (1 mL). [Mózsik and Javor: Dig. Dis. Sci. 33: 92–105, 1988 (with kind permission).]

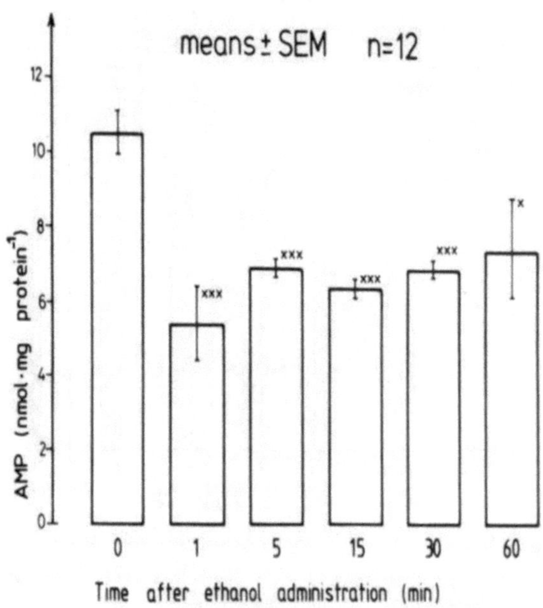

Figure 169. Changes in gastric mucosal level of AMP in rats after intragastric administration of 96% ethanol (1 mL). [Mózsik and Javor: Dig. Dis. Sci. 33: 92–105, 1988 (with kind permission).]

http://dx.doi.org/10.5772/60505

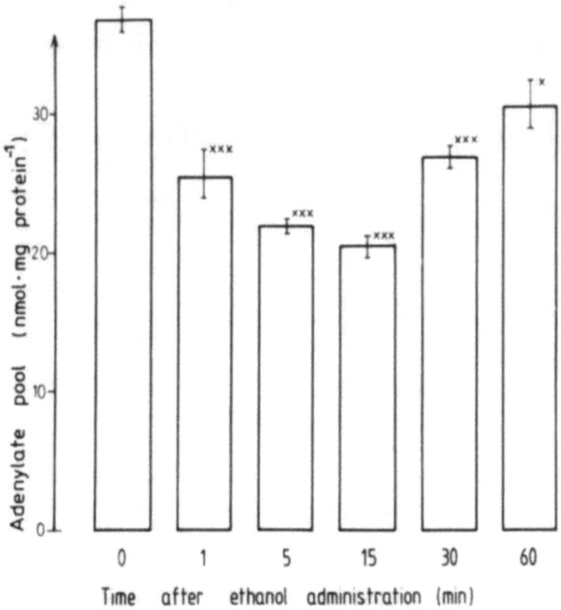

Figure 170. Changes in gastric mucosal level of adenylate pool of rats after intragastric administration of 96% ethanol (1 mL). [Mózsik and Javor: Dig. Dis. Sci. 33: 92–105, 1988 (with kind permission).]

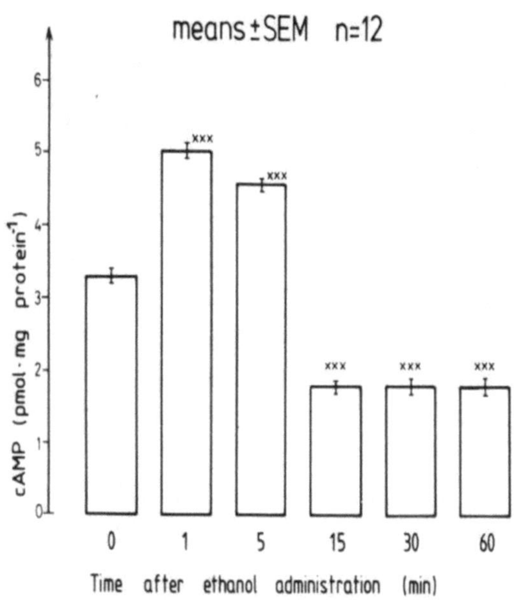

Figure 171. Changes in gastric mucosal level of cAMP of rats after intragastric administration of 96% ethanol (1 mL). [Mózsik and Javor: Dig. Dis. Sci. 33: 92–105, 1988 (with kind permission).]

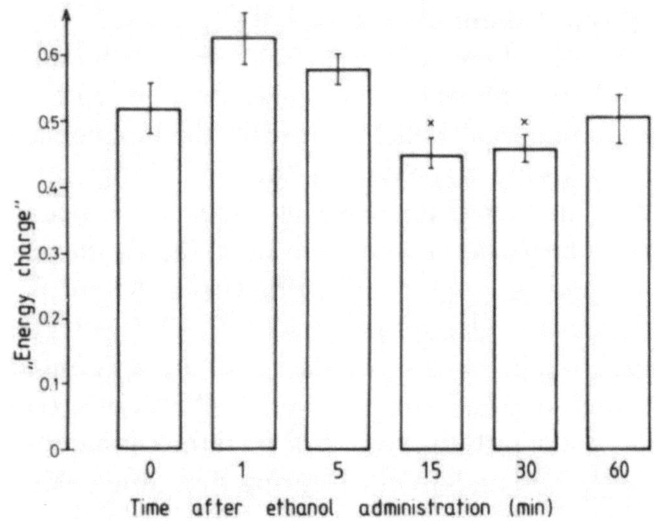

Figure 172. Changes in "energy charge" [(ATP + 0.5 ADP)/(ATP + ADP + AMP)] in the gastric mucosa after intragastric administration of 96% ethanol (1 mL). [Mózsik and Javor: Dig. Dis. Sci. 33: 92–105, 1988 (with kind permission).]

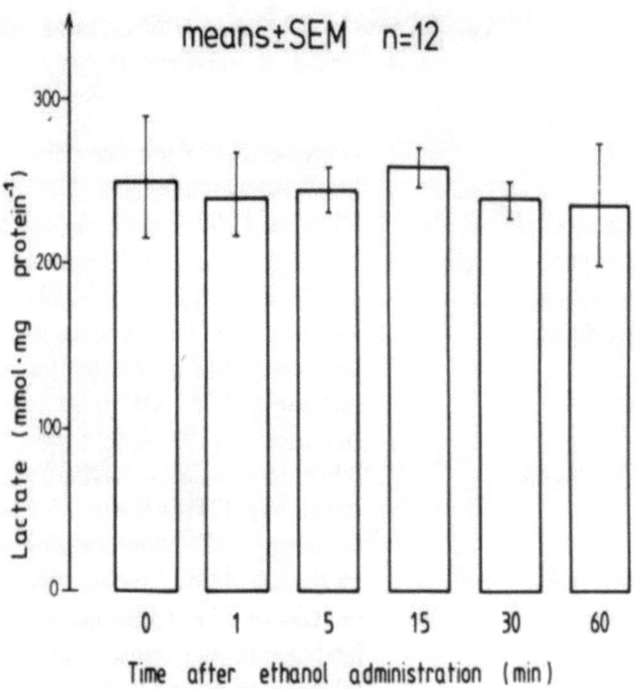

Figure 173. Gastric mucosal level of lactate in rats after intragastric administration of 96% ethanol (1 mL). [Mózsik and Javor: Dig. Dis. Sci. 33: 92–105, 1988 (with kind permission).]

http://dx.doi.org/10.5772/60505

The tissue level of ATP did not change during the first 5 min. It decreased from 15 to 60 minutes after ethanol administration, but then increased again at 60 minutes compared with levels at 15 and 30 minutes after ethanol administration. The tissue level of ADP decreased during the first 15 minutes and then returned to pretreatment values at 30 and 60 minutes after ethanol administration. The ratio of ATP/ADP increased over the first 5 minutes and then decreased. The tissue level of AMP was decreased during the first hour. The value of adenylate pool was decreased at all time intervals. The tissue level of cAMP increased at 1 and 5 minutes after ethanol administration and decreased thereafter. The extent of phosphorylation and/or dephosphorylation as estimated by Atkinson's formula was decreased at 15 and 30 minutes after ethanol administration. Surprisingly, there was no change in the tissue level of lactate independently of the presence of macroscopic mucosal injury.

Gastric mucosal damage appeared macroscopically after 5 min. It occurred to half the extent of that present after 1 hour following the exposure to ethanol. The tissue level of ATP did not decrease, whereas the ratio of ATP/ADP and tissue level of cAMP increased. There was no increase in the levels of ADP, AMP or lactate during the first 5 minutes after ethanol administration. It can be concluded that the presence of mucosal hypoxia before and at the time of appearance of macroscopic mucosal damage after ethanol administration can be excluded.

8.7.2. Extra- and intracellular regulatory mechanism system in the gastric mucosa during the development of ethanol-induced gastric mucosal damage in rats

If the changes in tissue levels of ATP, ADP, AMP and cAMP are expressed in percent values at 0 minute (intact animals) dependent upon time after the administration of ethanol, then two different characteristic changes can be found in the gastric mucosa: the cAMP level significantly increased together with of the inhibition of ATP transformation into ADP at 5 minutes; thereafter (from 5 to 60 minutes), the tissue level of cAMP decreased in association with increase in tissue level of ADP and gradually increasing tissue level of ATP by intact oxidative phosphorylation. The critical evaluation of these changes in the membrane-bound ATP-dependent energy systems offers us to demonstrate the existence of feedback systems between the ATP–ADP and ATP–cAMP transformations in the gastric mucosa during the development of ethanol-induced macroscopic damage (*in vivo* examinations) (Figure 174).

8.7.3. Comparison of development of gastric mucosal damage and gastric mucosal biochemistry in acid-dependent (HCl) and nonacid-dependent (ETOH) experimental models in rats

The time dependence of gastric fundic mucosal damage (number and severity) appeared in time order after the application of HCl or ethanol (ETOH). The extent of gastric fundic mucosal damage reaches its value in about 50% at 5 minutes after the administration of necrotizing agents (Figures 175, 176).

The extent of ATP–ADP transformation significantly increased at 0–5 minutes after the administration of necrotizing agents (Figures 177, 178), whereas the ATP–cAMP transformation decreased significantly (Figures 179). During this time period, no elevation was obtained in the tissue level of lactate (Figure 180). The different necrotizing agents were applied (presently HCl and ETOH); however, the biochemical changes in the rat gastric mucosa were found to be the same (Figure 181).

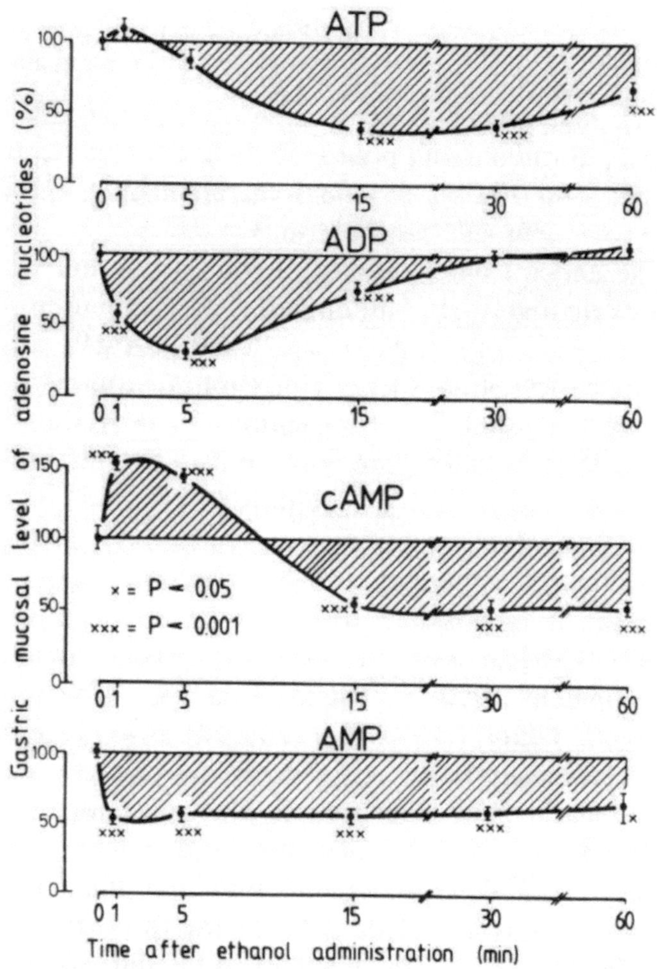

Figure 174. Feedback mechanisms between ATP–ADP, ATP–cAMP systems in the rat gastric mucosa after intragastric administration of 96% (1 mL) ethanol. [Mózsik and Javor: Dig. Dis. Sci. 33: 92–105, 1988 (with kind permission).]

http://dx.doi.org/10.5772/60505

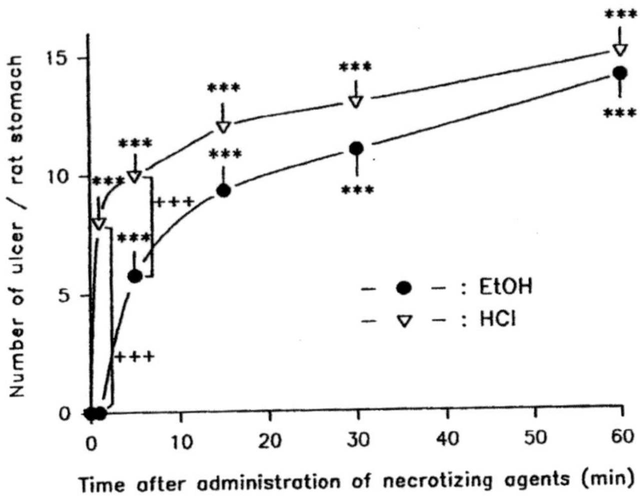

Figure 175. Macroscopic appearance of the number of gastric mucosal damage in rats treated with ethanol (ETOH) (1 mL of 96 v/v and HCl (1 mL, 0.6 M HCl i.g.) dependent on time after administration of necrotizing agents. The results were expressed as means ± SEM of 12 animals. *P* values were calculated as results between 0 versus different times (*) and results obtained at the same time in ETOH and HCl models (+) (means ± SEM; $P < 0.5$; $P < 0.001$; $P < 0.100$). [Gasztonyi et al., Inflammopharmacology 4, 351–360, 1996 (with kind permission).]

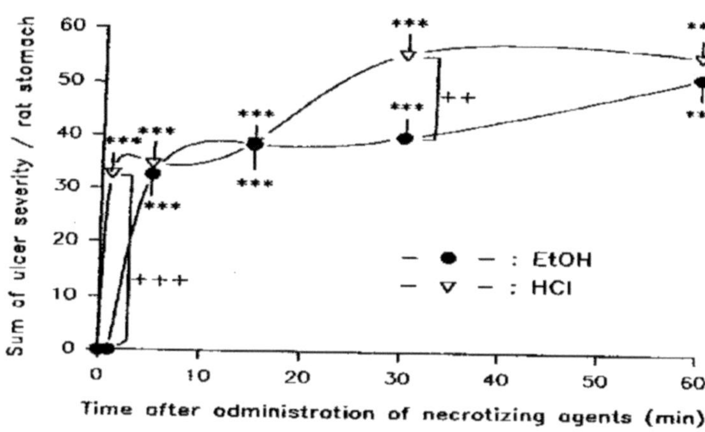

Figure 176. Macroscopic appearance of sum of gastric mucosal damage in rats with ETOH and HCl models (means ± SEM). [Gasztonyi et al., Inflammopharmacology 4, 351–360, 1996 (with kind permission).]

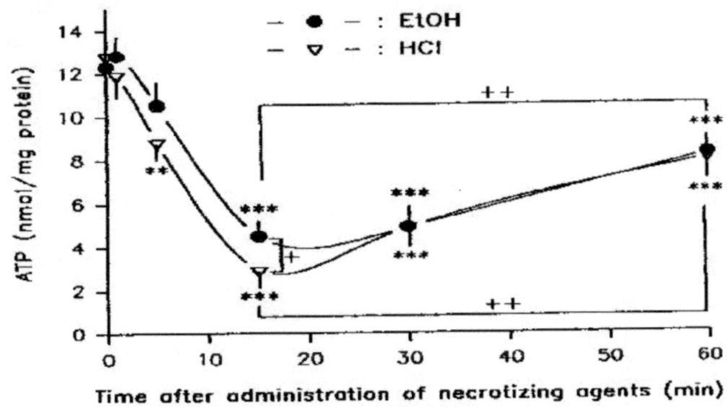

Figure 177. Changes in the gastric mucosal level of ATP in rats with ETOH- and HCl-treated rats after application of necrotizing agents (means ± SEM). [Gasztonyi et al., Inflammopharmacology 4, 351–360, 1996 (with kind permission).]

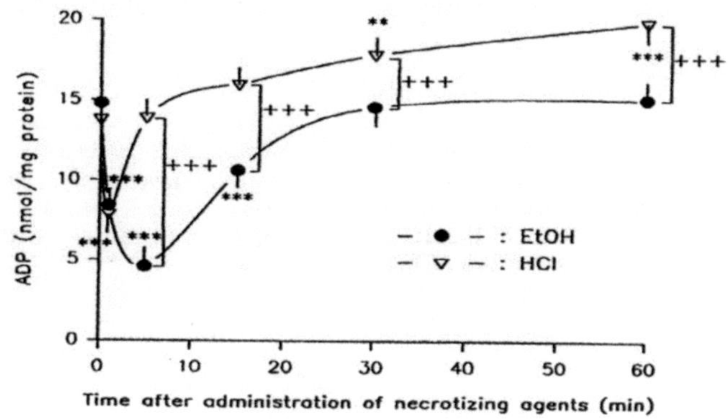

Figure 178. Changes in the gastric mucosal level of ADP in ETOH- and HCl-treated rats dependent upon time after application of necrotizing agents (means ± SEM). [Gasztonyi et al., Inflammopharmacology 4, 351–360, 1996 (with kind permission).]

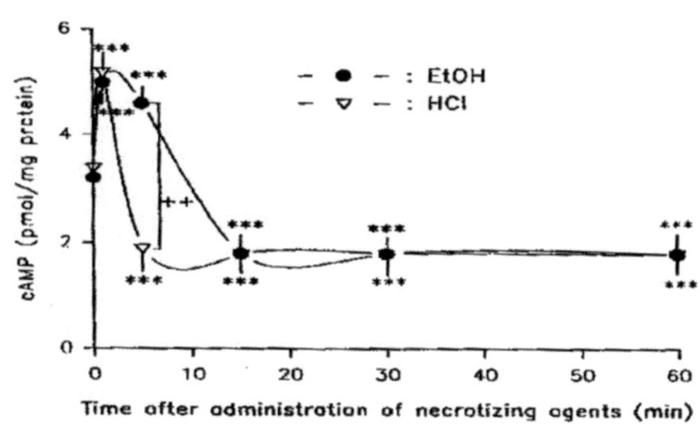

Figure 179. Changes in gastric mucosal cAMP of rats treated with ETOH or HCl dependent on time after administration of necrotizing agents (means ± SEM). [Gasztonyi et al., Inflammopharmacology 4, 351–360, 1996 (with kind permission).]

http://dx.doi.org/10.5772/60505

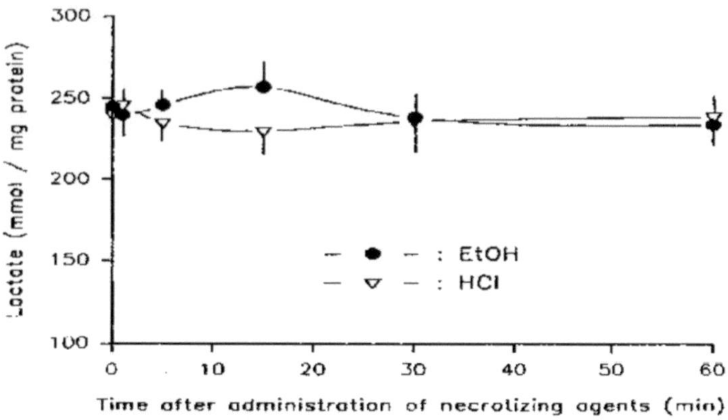

Figure 180. Gastric mucosal level of lactate in rats treated with ETOH and HCl dependent upon time after application of necrotizing agents (means ± SEM). For further explanation, see Figure 175. [Gasztonyi et al., Inflammopharmacology 4, 351–360, 1996 (with kind permission).]

The biochemical measurements were carried out in the HCl-, NaOH-, NaCl- and ethanol-induced models, and the summary of these results is given in Figure 182. Although the necrotizing agents differ significantly, the biochemical changes in the rat gastric mucosa are quite similar (Figure 182). Very similar changes were obtained in the ratio of ATP/ADP and "energy charge" (Figure 183).

Examined parameters	1		5		15		30		60	
	min after administration of HCl (A) and EtOH (B)									
	A	B	A	B	A	B	A	B	A	B
Number of ulcers	↑↑↑	NS	↑↑↑	↑↑↑	↑↑↑	↑↑↑	↑↑↑	↑↑↑	↑↑↑	↑↑↑
Severity of ulcers	↑↑↑	NS	↑↑↑	↑↑↑	↑↑↑	↑↑↑	↑↑↑	↑↑↑	↑↑↑	↑↑↑
ATP	NS	NS	↓↓	NS	↓↓↓	↓↓↓	↓↓↓	↓↓↓	↓↓↓	↓↓↓
ADP	↓↓↓	↓↓↓	NS	↓↓↓	NS	↓↓↓	↑↑	NS	↑↑	NS
cAMP	↑↑↑	↑↑↑	↑↑↑	↓↓↓	↓↓↓	↓↓↓	↓↓↓	↓↓↓	↓↓↓	↓↓↓
Lactate	NS	NS	NS	NS	NS	NS	NS	NS	NS	NS

NS: not significant ↑↑↑/↓↓↓ (increase/decrease): $p<0.001$
↑↑/↓↓: $p<0.01$

Figure 181. Changes in the gastric fundic mucosal levels of biochemistry, gastric mucosal damage (number and severity) in ETOH or HCl models (means ± SEM). [Gasztonyi et al., Inflammopharmacology 4, 351–360, 1996 (with kind permission).]

CORRELATIONS BETWEEN CHANGES IN BIOCHEMISM OF GASTRIC MUCOSA AND DEVELOPMENT OF NECROTIZING AGENTS-INDUCED GASTRIC MUCOSAL LESIONS IN RATS

	96 % ETHANOL-	0.6 M HCl-	0.2 M NaOH-	25 % NaCl-
	INDUCED	GASTRIC	MUCOSAL	LESIONS
ULCER NUMBER	↑↑↑	↑↑↑	↑↑↑	↑↑↑
ULCER SEVERITY	↑↑↑	↑↑↑	↑↑↑	↑↑↑
ATP	↓↓	↓↓	↓↓↓	↓↓↓
ADP	NS	↑	↑	↑
ATP · ADP^{-1}	↓↓↓	↓↓↓	↓↓↓	↓↓↓
cAMP	↓↓↓	↓↓↓	↓↓↓	↓↓↓
AMP	↓	↓↓↓	NS	↓↓
ADENYLATE POOL	NS	NS	NS	NS
„ENERGY CHARGE"	NS	NS	↓↓	NS
LACTATE	NS	NS	NS	NS

NS = NOT SIGNIFICANT ↓ = 0.05 > P > 0.01 ↓↓ = 0.01 > P > 0.001 ↓↓↓ = P < 0.001

↑ = INCREASE ↓ = DECREASE

Figure 182. The schematic representation of regulatory pathways between the tissue levels of ATP, ADP, AMP and cAMP, values of ATP/ADP, "adenylate pool" and "energy charge" as well as the development of gastric mucosal lesions in chemicals [(1 mL from 96 v/v, 1 mL from 0.2 M NaOH, 1 mL from 25 v/v NaCl and 1 mL 0.6 M HCl)]. [Mózsik (2006): Molecular pharmacology and biochemistry of gastroduodenal mucosal damage and protection. In: Mózsik Gy. (Ed.) Discoveries in Gastroenterology (1960–2005). Akadémiai Kiadó, Budapest. pp. 139–224 (with kind permission).]

SCHEMATIC PRESENTATION OF THE INTERRELATIONSHIPS BETWEEN THE CELLULAR ENERGY SYSTEMS DURING THE DEVELOPMENT OF GASTRIC MUCOSAL DAMAGE BY 0.2 M NaOH (I), 25 % NaCl (II), 0.6 M HCl (III.), AND 96 % ETHANOL (IV)

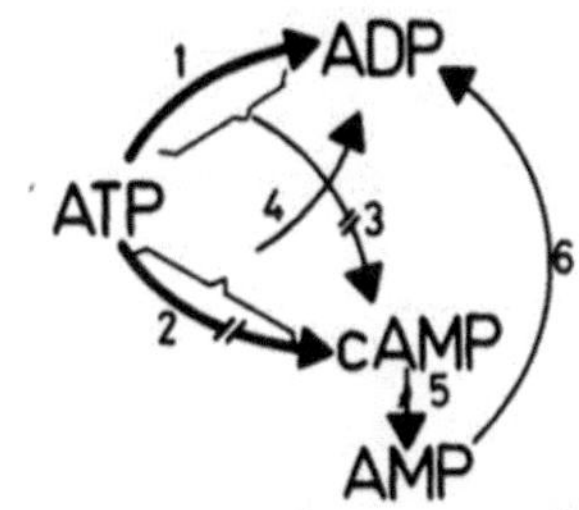

	C	I.	II.	III.	IV.
ATP · ADP^{-1}	0.84 ± 0.06	0.16 ± 0.01***	0.27 ± 0.02***	0.44 ± 0.03***	0.53 ± 0.04***
ENERGY CHARGE	0.52 ± 0.04	0.38 ± 0.03**	0.45 ± 0.02	0.53 ± 0.04	0.51 ± 0.04

→ STIMULATION —/→ INHIBITION

C = Control (untreated) ** = P<0.01 *** = P<0.001

Figure 183. The changes in the regulatory pathways between the tissue level of ATP, ADP, AMP and cAMP in the intact (untreated) and in HCl models. The same results were obtained in the HCl model, 25% NaCl and 96% ETOH (means ± SEM). [Mózsik (2006): Molecular pharmacology and biochemistry of gastroduodenal mucosal damage and protection. In: Mózsik Gy. (Ed.) Discoveries in Gastroenterology (1960–2005). Akadémiai Kiadó, Budapest. pp. 139–224 (with kind permission).]

8.7.4. Dynamism of extra- and intracellular regulatory mechanisms in the ethanol-induced gastric mucosal damage in 1-hour experiments dependent on time after intragastric application of ethanol

The changes in the regulatory pathways between the tissue levels of ATP, ADP, cAMP and AMP are indicated in Figure 184 dependent upon time after the administration of ethanol. This figure demonstrates well that the changes in the cellular energy systems significantly dynamically change from time to time in the rat gastric fundic mucosa; however, the ATP resynthesis worked well in this tissue.

The changes in the membrane-bound ATP-dependent energy systems in the gastric fundic mucosa were the same in the other models, independent from the kinds of intragastric application of 0.2 M NaOH, 25% NaCl, 0.6 M HCl and 96% ethanol.

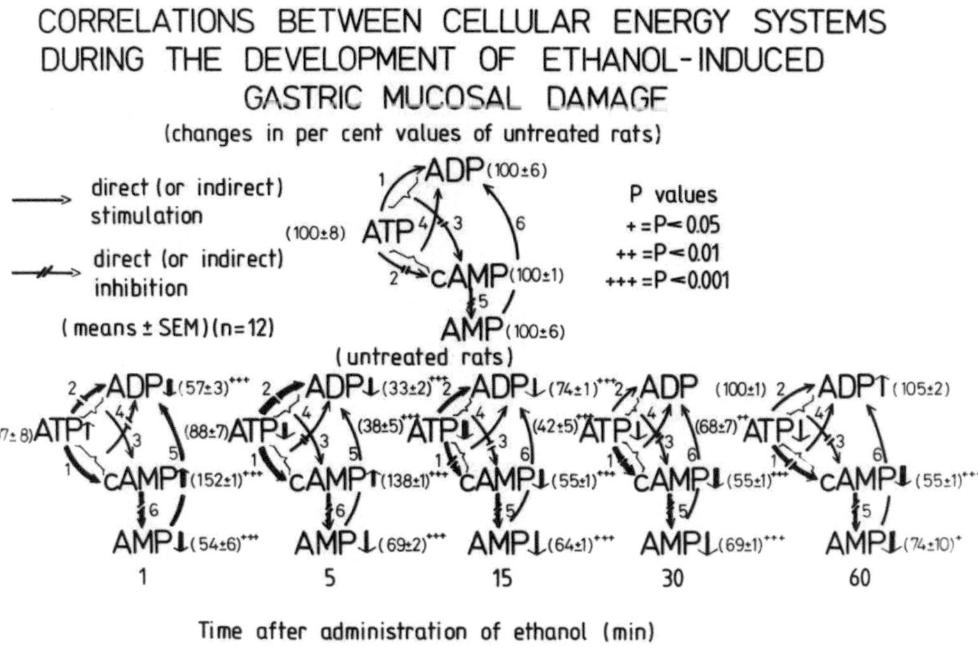

Figure 184. Changes in the cellular regulatory mechanisms of energy systems in ethanol (ETOH) induced in the rat gastric fundic mucosa dependent on time after intragastric administration of ETOH (1 mL from 96%). [Mózsik (2006): Molecular pharmacology and biochemistry of gastroduodenal mucosal damage and protection. In: Mózsik Gy. (Ed.) Discoveries in Gastroenterology (1960–2005). Akadémiai Kiadó, Budapest. pp. 139–224 (with kind permission).]

8.7.5. Biochemical backgrounds of gastric mucosal-protective effects of cytoprotective and antisecretory doses of atropine and cimetidine in acid-dependent model in rats (1-hour model)

After the classical cytoprotective agents (PGE_2 and PGI_2), the gastric mucosal-protective effect of different antisecretory drugs was studied (given in different doses) in animal experiments. It was suggested that all the drugs having antisecretory properties are able to produce gastric

mucosal protection without the presence of any antisecretory activities. We studied these problems in cases of atropine and cimetidine (Figure 185).

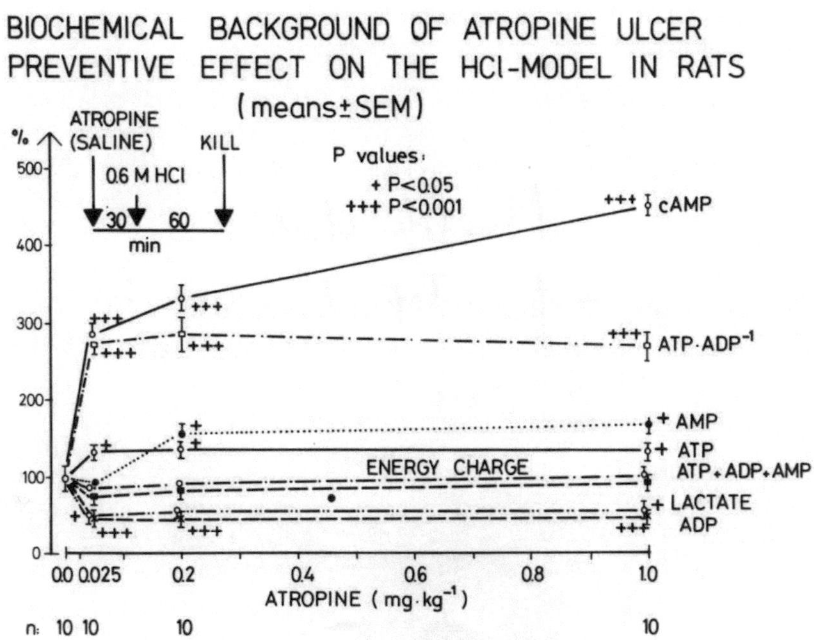

Figure 185. Changes in biochemical parameters of cellular energy systems and lactate in the gastric fundic mucosa in HCl model of rats. [Mózsik (2006): Molecular pharmacology and biochemistry of gastroduodenal mucosal damage and protection. In: Mózsik Gy. (Ed.) Discoveries in Gastroenterology (1960–2005). Akadémiai Kiadó, Budapest. pp. 139–224 (with kind permission).]

We studied the gastric mucosal-preventive effect of atropine (given in doses of 0.025, 0.2 and 1.0 mg/kg s.c.). The 0.025-mg/kg atropine indicated mucosal protection in the HCl model, together with significant changes in the gastric fundic mucosa, without the presence of inhibitory effect on gastric acid secretion. It was interesting to note that the gastric mucosal protection and the biochemical changes in the gastric fundic mucosa differ only in their extents.

The evaluation of quantitative changes produced by "cytoprotective" doses of atropine and cimetidine is presented in Figures 186 and 187.

These figures indicate that very complex intracellular mechanisms exist in the gastric fundic mucosa of rats produced by the gastric mucosal-protective effects of cytoprotective and antisecretory doses of atropine and cimetidine; however, it is clear that the original cellular regulatory mechanisms by PGI_2 (5 μg/kg), atropine (0.025 mg/kg) and cimetidine (2.5 mg/kg) also differ from each other (Figure 188).

http://dx.doi.org/10.5772/60505

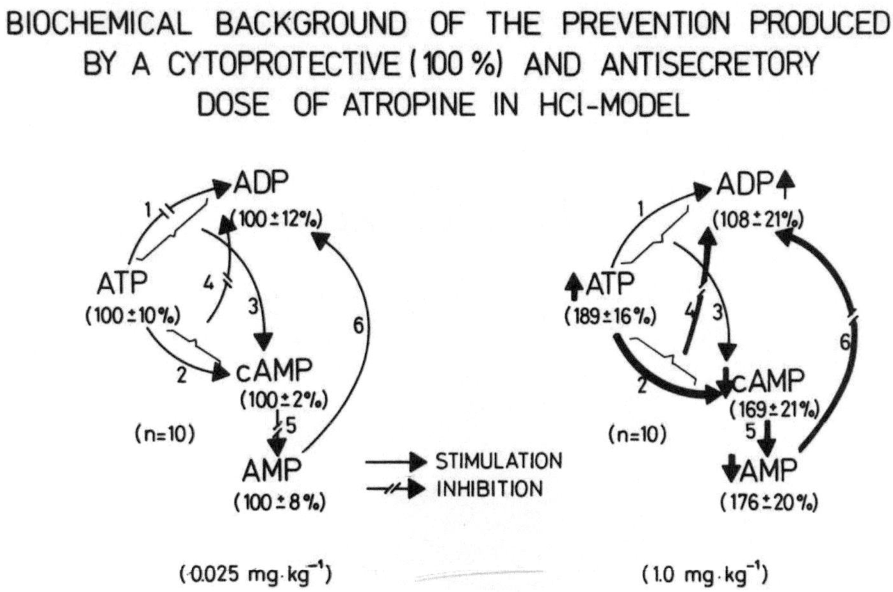

Figure 186. Comparison between changes in cellular energy systems of gastric fundic mucosa of rats produced by cytoprotective (0.025 mg/kg) and antisecretory (1.0 mg/kg) doses of atropine. The changes in the antisecretory dose of atropine are expressed in percent of cytoprotective dose (= 100%).

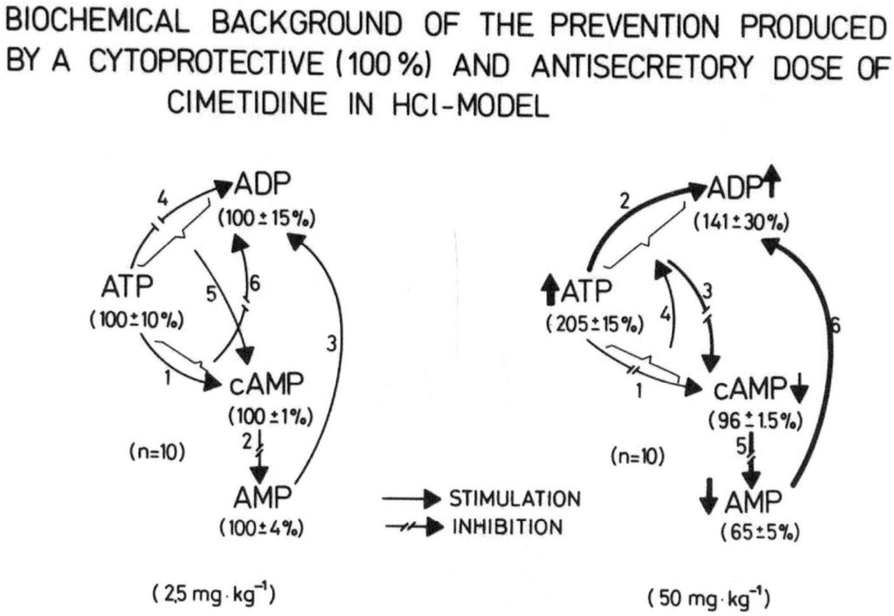

Figure 187. Comparison between changes in cellular energy systems of gastric fundic mucosa of rats produced by cytoprotective (2.5 mg/kg) and antisecretory (50 mg/kg) doses of cimetidine. The changes of antisecretory dose of atropine are expressed in percent of cytoprotective dose (= 100%).

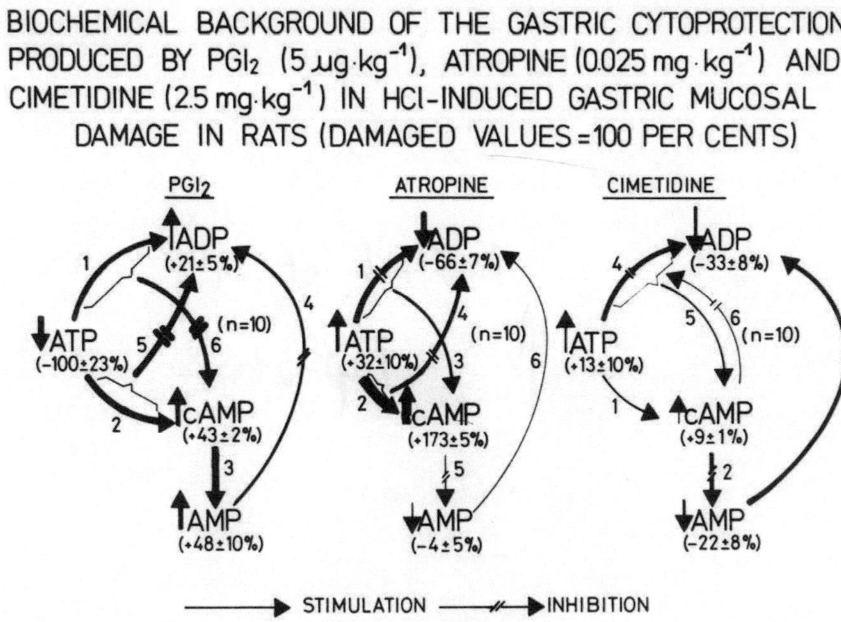

Figure 188. Comparison of the cellular regulatory mechanisms (steps) in the gastric fundic mucosa of rats produced by cytoprotective doses (5 µg/kg), atropine (0.025 mg/kg) and cimetidine (2.5 mg/kg). The changes in the different parameters of the cellular energy systems are presented in percent values of control (untreated) rats (100% values).

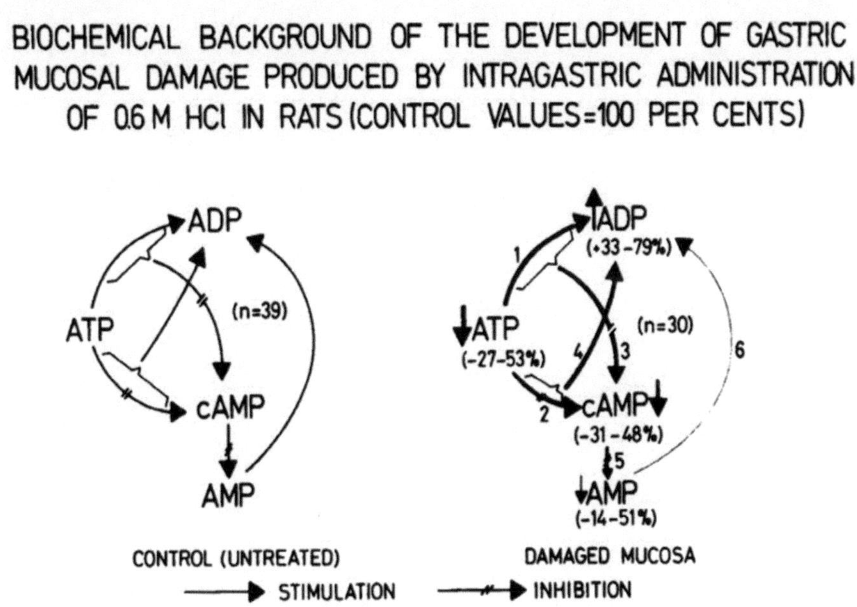

Figure 189. The extra- and intracellular regulatory mechanism system in intact (untreated) and in HCl-treated rats. The results obtained from the untreated rats were taken to be equal to 100%, and the changes in the HCl-treated rats expressed as changes in percent values in comparison with the normal (100) values.

http://dx.doi.org/10.5772/60505

Bilateral surgical vagotomy completely inhibited the volume and gastric H^+ output together with complete prevention of gastric ulcer (Mózsik and Vizi, 1976 a, b). It was surprising that the tissue level of ATP after surgical vagotomy remained (Mózsik and Vizi, 1976 a, b) neither in the glandular stomach nor in the forestomach. These results suggested that the tissue level of ATP must break down for the energy liberation and development of gastric secretory responses and ulcer development (Mózsik et al., 1993 a, b, 2001 a, b).

When the chemical vagotomy (i.g. atropine administration) was carried out, the tissue levels of ATP decreased significantly and the tissue levels of ADP and AMP were increased (Figures 80, 81). The tissue levels of cAMP were found to be significantly higher after chemical vagotomy than after bilateral surgical vagotomy (Karádi and Mózsik, 2000; Mózsik et al., 1981a, b; 1987a; 1996b; Vincze et al., 1992, 1993a) (Figures 81, 190).

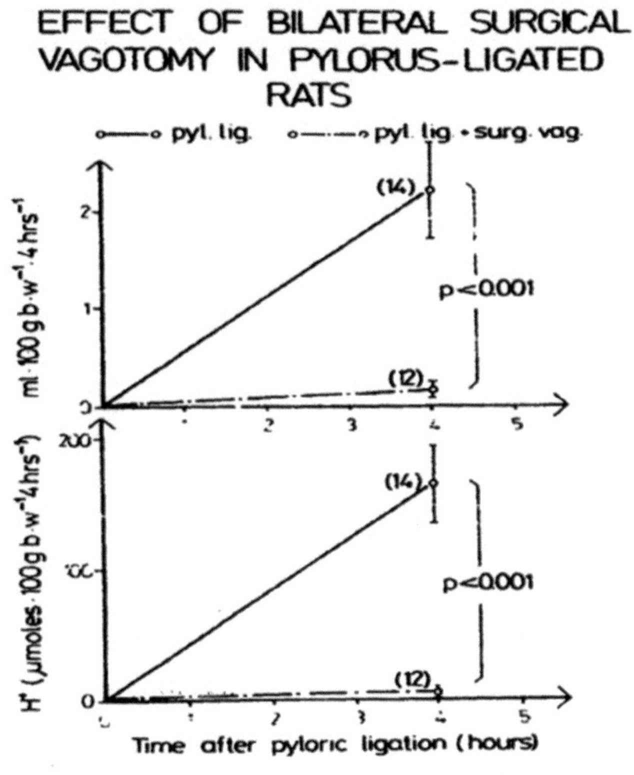

Figure 190. The effect of bilateral surgical vagotomy in the gastric secretory responses (volume and H^+ output) in 4-hour pylorus-ligated rats (means ± SEM). [Mózsik and Vizi, Am J Digest Dis 22, 1072–1075, 1976 (with kind permission).]

The best conclusions of these observations were as follows:

1. The ATP breakdown in the glandular stomach and forestomach is basically necessary to obtain gastric hypersecretion as well gastric ulceration;

2. Represents an intracellular regulatory mechanism to obtain a gastric hypersecretion;
3. In case of chemical vagotomy, the significant increase of mucosal cAMP probably represents an important regulatory step against the development of gastric hypersecretion (Karádi and Mózsik, 2000).

Previously, gastric ulceration was considered to appear as a result of extremely decreased tissue ATP produced by the impaired oxidative phosphorylation. However, we first demonstrated that the gastric ulceration in the forestomach appears as the consequence of active biochemical mechanisms of the gastric tissues (Mózsik et al., 1967 a, b; 1969 b, c).

These results also demonstrated that the intracellular mechanism systems differ significantly in the rat stomach after surgical and chemical vagotomy.

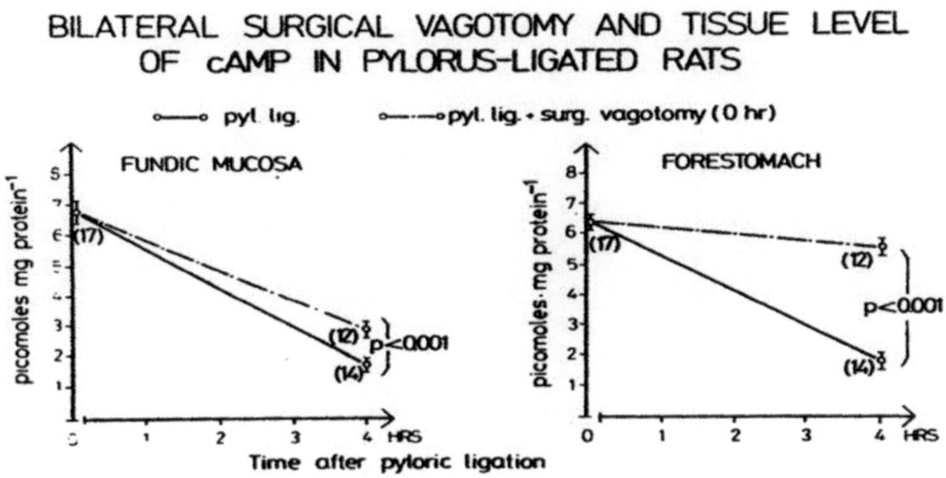

Figure 191. The effect of bilateral surgical vagotomy on the gastric tissue levels of cAMP in pylorus-ligated rats (means ± SEM). [Mózsik and Vizi, Amer J Digest Dis 22, 1072–1075, 1976 (with kind permission).]

8.8. "Surgical" and "chemical" vagotomy on the biochemistry of gastric mucosa in 1-hour rats

The results of these observations are presented in Section 4.3.2.

8.8.1. "Surgical" vagotomy inhibits the PGI_2 –induced gastric mucosal-protective effect in rats

The surgical vagotomy alone cannot produce any ulcer development in the rat stomach; however, Sikiric and coworkers found the appearance of ulcer in the rat stomach (Mózsik et al., 1981a; 1990 b, c; Karádi and Mózsik, 2000).

After bilateral surgical vagotomy, the extent of IND-induced gastric mucosal lesion was found to be increased, whereas the chemical vagotomy significantly decreased the gastric mucosal damage to chemicals.

http://dx.doi.org/10.5772/60505

The interpretation of these results led to the following conclusions:

a. The intact vagal nerve is basically necessary for the mechanisms involved in different chemically induced gastric mucosal damage;

b. The gastric mucosal-protective effects significantly differ from each other against chemically induced gastric mucosal damage.

These results were presented in a Satellite Symposium of the Congress of International Union of Physiological Sciences (IUPS) (Budapest, Hungary, 1980) [Mózsik, Hänninen and Jávor (1981) (eds.) Advances in the Physiological Sciences. Vol. 29, Gastrointestinal Mucosal Defence. Pergamon Press, Oxford – Akadémiai Kiadó, Budapest] (Figure 192).

These type of observations were published in the *Journal of Prostaglandins, Leucotrienes and Medicine* (Mózsik, Moron, Jávor, 9: 71–84, 1982), in which we also emphasized on the essential role of the intact vagal nerve for the development of gastric mucosal-preventive effect of prostacyclin against the chemically induced mucosal damage, e.g., this protective effect of prostacyclin was not present in these animal models. We concluded from the results of these observations that the intact vagal nerve is basically necessary for the gastric mucosal protection.

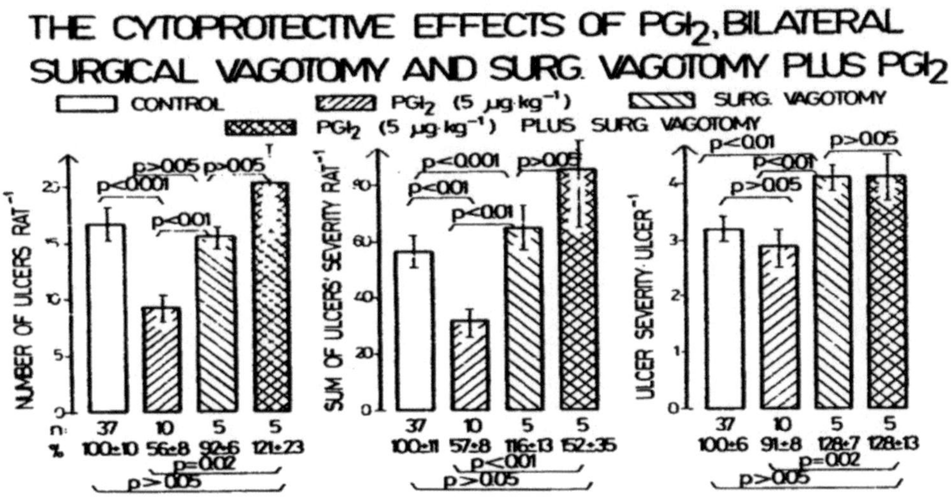

Figure 192. The presentation (first in the world) of PGI_2 gastric-protective effect disappears after bilateral surgical vagotomy in rats treated with ETOH (96 v/v) (means ± SEM). [Jávor et al., (1981) Gastric mucosal resistance to physical and chemical stress. In: Mózsik Gy., Hänninen O., Jávor T. (Eds.) Advances in the Physiological Sciences. Vol. 29. Gastrointestinal Mucosal Defence. Pergamon Press, Oxford – Akadémiai Kiadó, Budapest. pp. 141–159 (with kind permission).]

Similar observations were published by Miller (Amer J Physiol. 245: 601–623, 1983), and Henagen, Seidel and Miller cited our results in their forthcoming paper (Gastroenterology 84: 1186, 1983); however, from time to time, our priority has been the key role of the intact vagal

nerve in the gastric mucosal defense mechanisms (Karádi and Mózsik, 2001; Király et al., 1992b; Mózsik, 2006 a, b; Mózsik et al., 1990a, 1991a, 2001b; Vincze et al., 1992, 1993a, 1997).

However, it is important to emphasize that the "chemical vagotomy" (atropine treatment) does not clinically inhibit the appearance of prostaglandin- and prostacyclin-induced gastric mucosal protection against the chemically induced mucosal damage in animals.

We need to emphasize well that surgical vagotomy is widely used in the clinical practice of treatment of patients with peptic ulcer. We never accepted the application of surgical vagotomy in the medical practice and we emphasized the application of "chemical vagotomy" in the medical treatment of patients with peptic ulcer (see Chapter 2).

8.9. Biochemical backgrounds of the PGI_2–induced gastric mucosal protection against by different chemicals in rats

When small doses (5 and 50 μg/kg) of PG_2 were given, both the number (Figure 193) and severity (Figure 194) dose-dependently decreased and surprisingly the tissue level of ATP practically decreased to a value of zero (Figure 195). The tissue level of ADP (Figure 196), cAMP (Figure 197) and AMP (Figure 198) increased, and the values of ATP/ADP were practically zero (Mózsik et al., 1983b) (Figure 199).

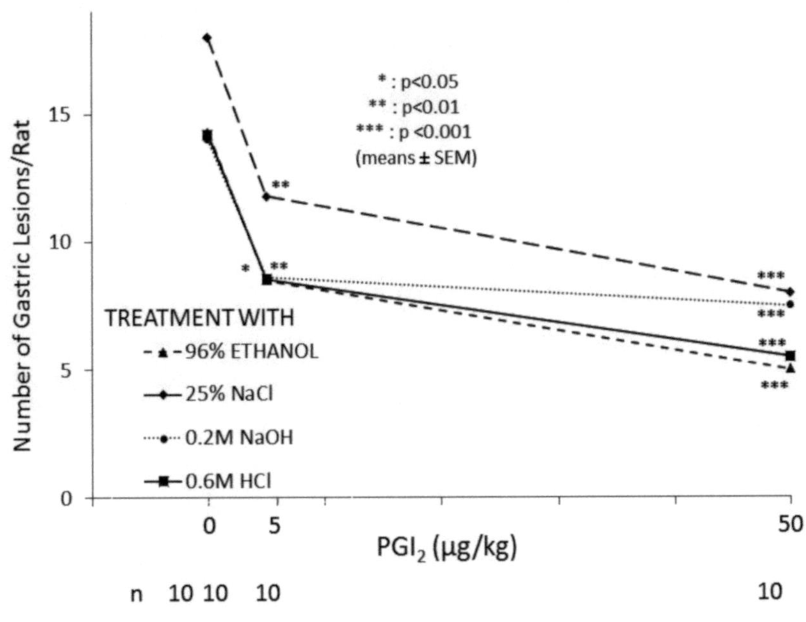

Figure 193. Preventive effects of PGI_2 on the number of gastric lesions produced by topical application of 0.2 M NaOH, 25%, 0.6 M HCl and 96% ethanol (means ± SEM). [Mózsik et al., Prostagland. Leucot. Med. 12, 423–436, 1983 (with kind permission).]

http://dx.doi.org/10.5772/60505

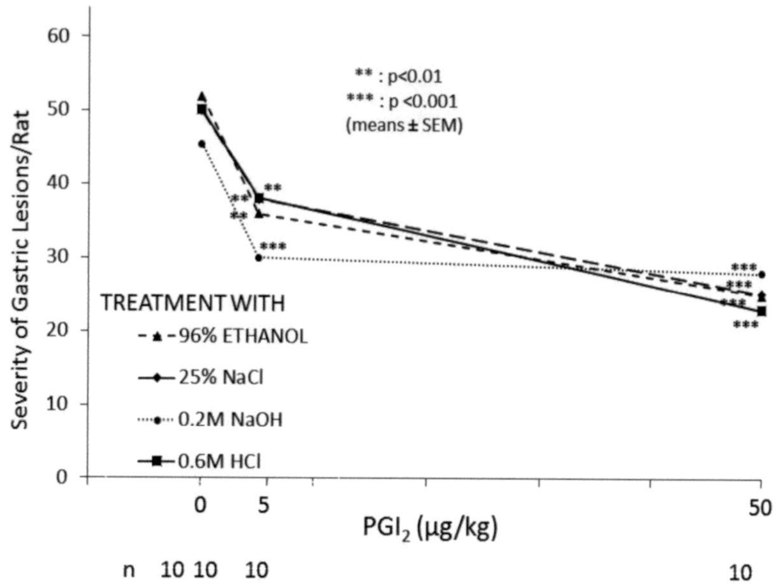

Figure 194. Gastric-preventive effects of PGI_2 on the severity in 0.2 M NaOH, 0.6 M HCl, 25% NaCl and 96% ethanol (means ± SEM). [Mózsik et al., Prostagland. Leucot. Med. 12, 423–436, 1983 (with kind permission).]

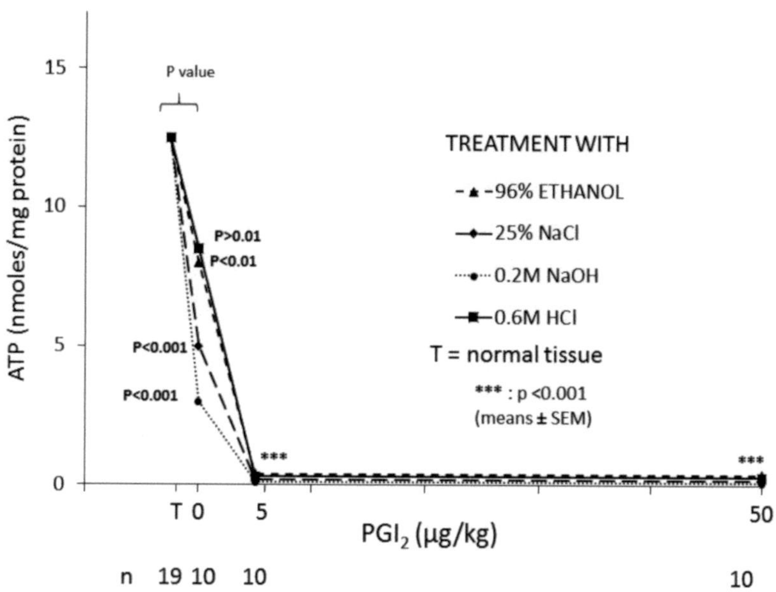

Figure 195. Changes in the gastric fundic mucosal level of ATP during development of gastric mucosal damage produced by different necrotizing agents (left side of the figure) and of different doses of PGI_2 (right side of figure). The differences in the results obtained in the normal pathological state (O) indicate the changes in the levels of ATP during the development of gastric mucosal damage (means ± SEM). [Mózsik et al., Prostagland. Leucot. Med. 12, 423–436, 1983 (with kind permission).]

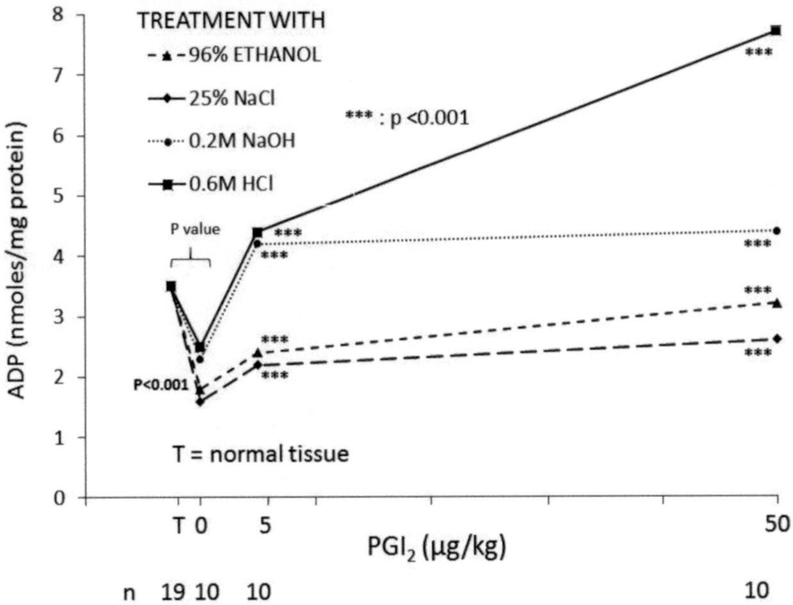

Figure 196. Changes in the gastric fundic mucosal level of ADP during mucosal damage produced by different necrotizing agents (left side) and of PGI_2-induced gastric mucosal protection (means ± SEM). [Mózsik et al., Prostagland. Leucot. Med. 12, 423–436, 1983 (with kind permission).]

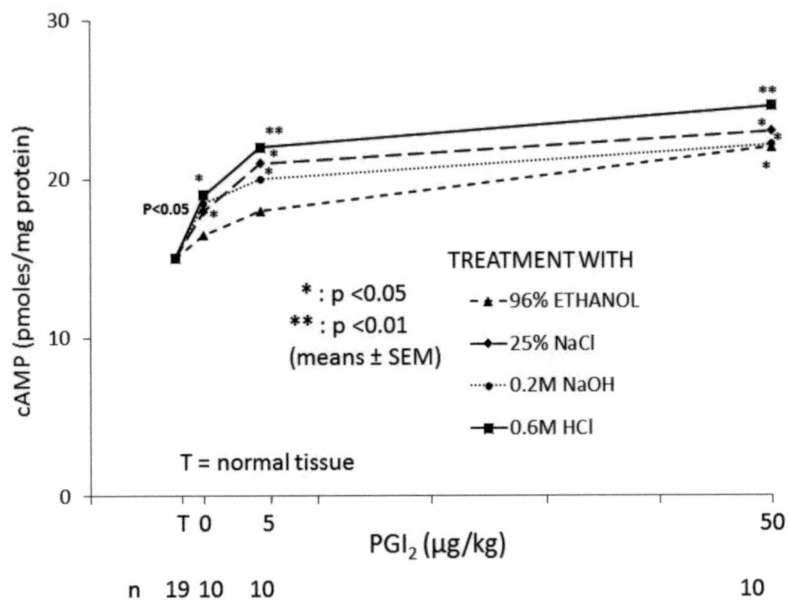

Figure 197. Changes in the gastric fundic mucosal level of cAMP during the development of gastric mucosal damage and of PGI_2-induced gastric cytoprotection (means ± SEM). [Mózsik et al., Prostagland. Leucot. Med. 12, 423–436, 1983 (with kind permission).]

http://dx.doi.org/10.5772/60505

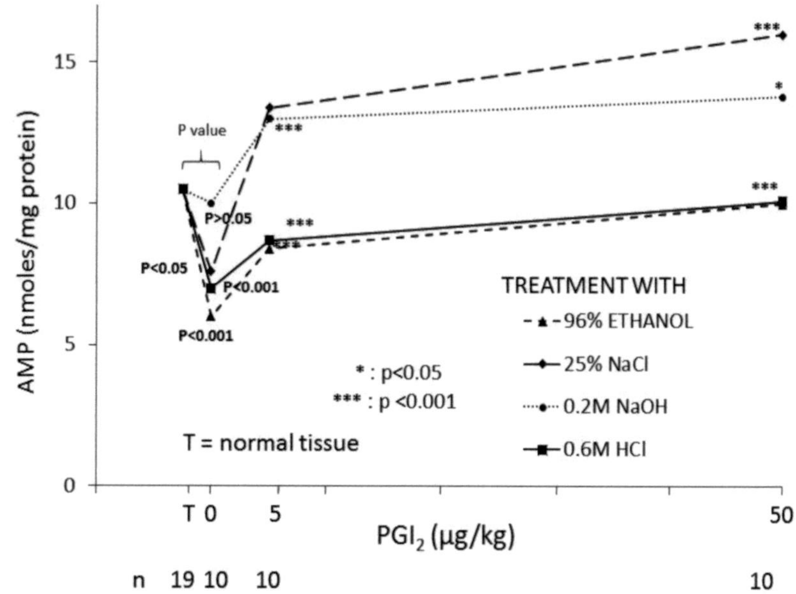

Figure 198. Changes in the gastric mucosal level of AMP during the development of gastric mucosal damage produced by different necrotizing agents and of PGI_2-induced gastric cytoprotection (means ± SEM). [Mózsik et al., Prostagland. Leucot. Med. 12, 423–436, 1983 (with kind permission).]

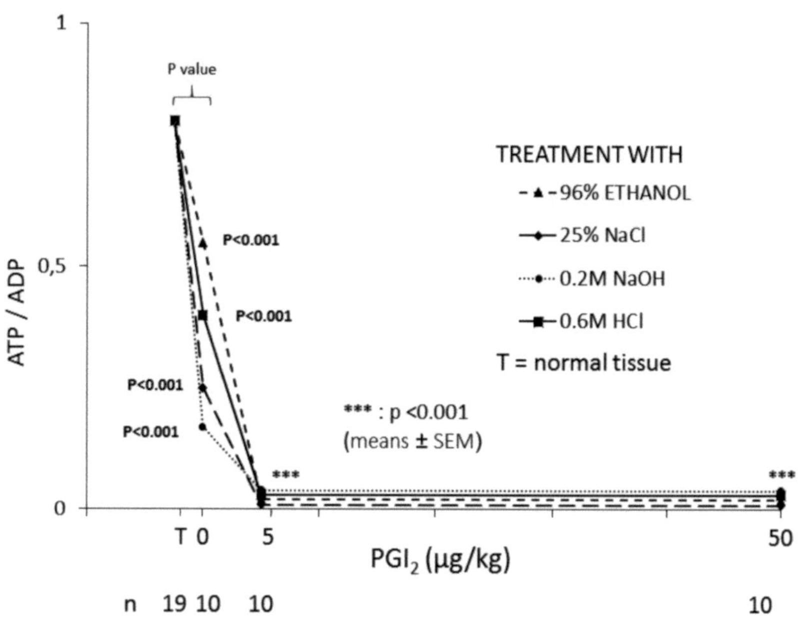

Figure 199. Changes in the ratio of ATP/ADP in the rat gastric fundic mucosa during the development of gastric mucosal damage produced by different necrotizing agents and of PGI_2-induced gastric cytoprotection (means ± SEM). [Mózsik et al., Prostagland. Leucot. Med 12, 423–436, 1983 (with kind permission).]

The results of these observations indicated the following:

1. The different chemically induced mucosal acute gastric mucosal damages are practically the same (during 1-hour time period) in relation to the time dependence of mucosal damage and its biochemical backgrounds (in membrane-bound ATP-dependent energy systems);
2. The prostacyclin-induced gastric mucosal-preventive effects are the same in different experimental models (produced by 0.6 M HCl, 0.2 M NaOH, 25% NaCl solution and 96% ethanol) in relation to time dependence of macroscopic detectable patterns of defensive actions and to changes in the membrane-bound ATP-dependent energy systems in the rat gastric mucosa;
3. It was very surprising to note that the tissue levels of ATP in the rat gastric mucosa practically reached the value of zero in the rat gastric mucosa, when the prostacyclin-induced mucosal-protective effects are present in the different animal models;
4. The prostacyclin (and other prostaglandins) inhibits the extent of ATP transformation into ADP (*in vitro* conditions) in smaller concentrations, whereas they stimulate the ATP transformation into cAMP. These steps of the regulatory steps of prostacyclin are present in different chemically induced experimental models (under *in vivo* conditions);
5. The results indicated similar changes in the regulatory feedback mechanisms of different chemical agents (drugs) to those we received in other experimental models.

8.10. Similarities and differences of PGI_2- and ß-carotene-induced gastric mucosal protections and their biochemical actions in an acid-dependent (HCl) and in a non-acid dependent (ETOH) experimental model in rats

8.10.1. Gastric mucosal protective effect of PGI_2 versus changes in the gastric mucosal energy systems in HCl model in rat

The experimental protocol and the obtained results are presented in Figure 200. The 5 µg/kg PGI_2 was found as ED_{50} value (Figure 201). The PGI_2 prevented the HCl-induced gastric mucosal damage (Figures 202, 203), and this inhibition appeared in the early period after the administration of HCl (Figures 203–211). In all biochemical parameters of the gastric mucosal biochemistry, the PGI_2 produced dose-dependent actions (Mózsik et al., 1983b; 1984a; 1989 a, b; 1990 b, c; 1998; Sütő et al., 1989; Vincze et al., 1993a, 1997; Garamszegi et al., 1989; Gasztonyi et al., 1996).

8.10.2. Gastric mucosal protective effect of PGI_2 versus changes in the gastric mucosal enery systems in ethanol (ETOH) model in rat

The dose of 5 µg/kg was also found as the value of ED5O in the ETOH model (Figure 213). The actions of PGI2 were found to be dose-dependent (Figures 214–222), except for the tissue level of lactate because its level was unchanged (Figure 222).

http://dx.doi.org/10.5772/60505

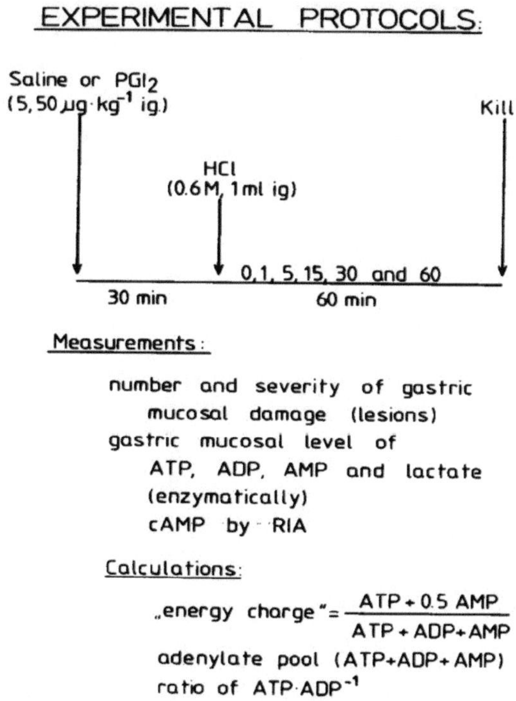

Figure 200. Experimental protocol for study of PGI_2-induced gastric mucosal-preventive effects and their biochemical changes in HCl model. [Mózsik Gy. (2006) Molecular pharmacology and biochemistry of gastroduodenal mucosal damage and protection. In: Mózsik Gy. (Ed.) Discoveries in Gastroenterology (1960–2005) Akadémiai Kiadó, Budapest. pp. 139–224 (with kind permission).]

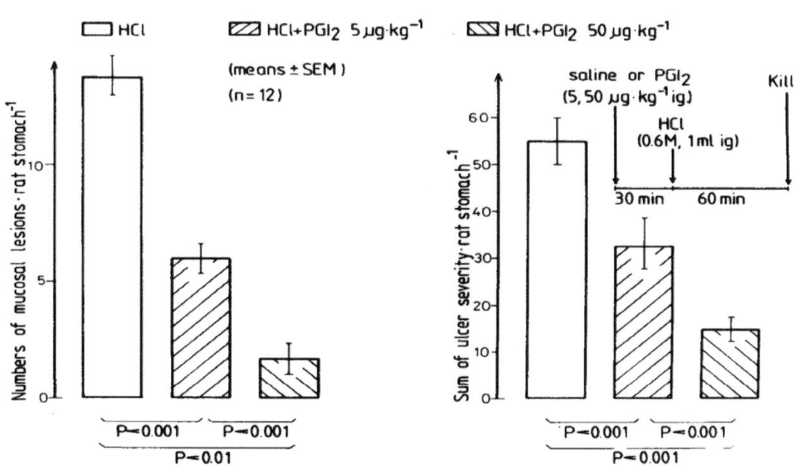

Figure 201. Determination of ED_{50} value for PGI_2 in HCl model (means ± SEM). [Mózsik Gy. (2006). Molecular pharmacology and biochemistry of gastroduodenal mucosal damage and protection. In: Mózsik Gy. (Ed.) Discoveries in Gastroenterology (1960–2005) Akadémiai Kiadó, Budapest. pp. 139–224 (with kind permission).]

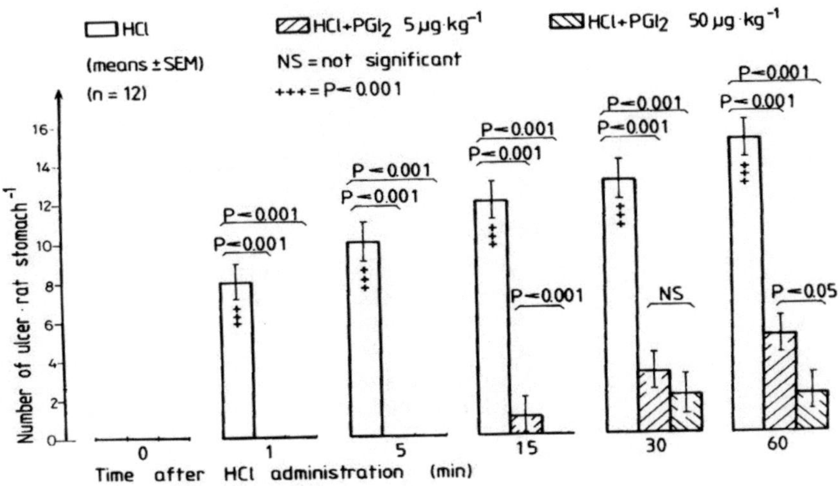

Figure 202. Inhibitory effect of PGI_2 on the number of gastric mucosal damage (means ± SEM) in the HCl model. [Mózsik Gy. (2006).Molecular pharmacology and biochemistry of gastroduodenal mucosal damage and protection. In: Mózsik Gy. (Ed.) Discoveries in Gastroenterology (1960–2005) Akadémiai Kiadó, Budapest. pp. 139–224 (with kind permission).]

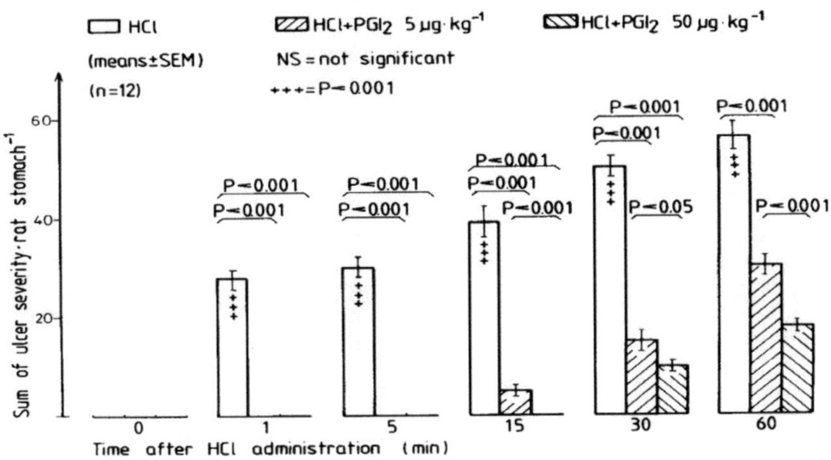

Figure 203. Inhibitory effect of PGI_2 on the sum of the ulcer severity in HCl model (means ± SEM). [Mózsik Gy. (2006). Molecular pharmacology and biochemistry of gastroduodenal mucosal damage and protection. In: Mózsik Gy. (Ed.) Discoveries in Gastroenterology (1960–2005) Akadémiai Kiadó, Budapest. pp. 139–224 (with kind permission).]

http://dx.doi.org/10.5772/60505

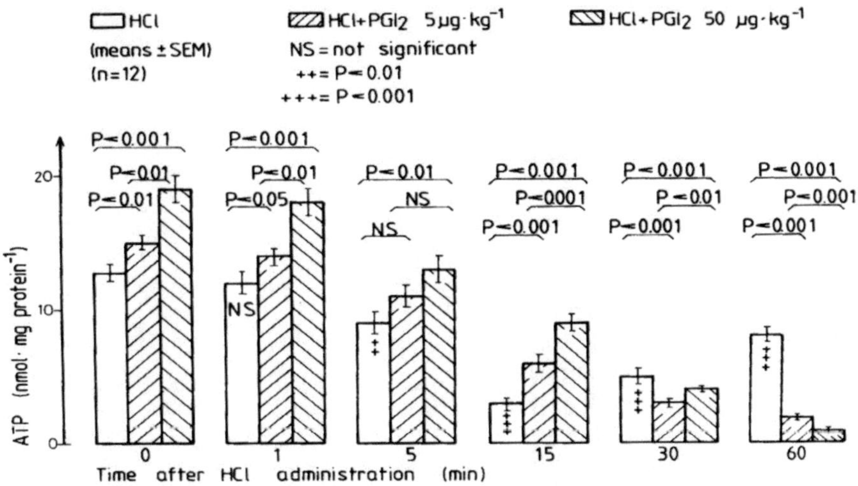

Figure 204. Dose–response changes produced by PGI_2 in the rat gastric fundic mucosal level of ATP (means ± SEM in HCl model). [Mózsik Gy. (2006). Molecular pharmacology and biochemistry of gastroduodenal mucosal damage and protection. In: Mózsik Gy. (Ed.) Discoveries in Gastroenterology (1960–2005) Akadémiai Kiadó, Budapest. pp. 139–224 (with kind permission).]

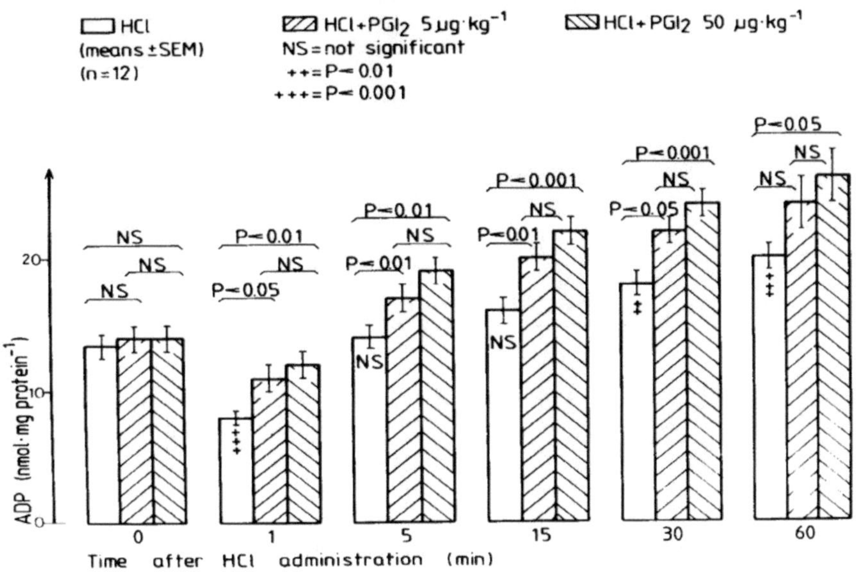

Figure 205. Dose–response changes produced by PGI_2 in the rat gastric fundic mucosal level of ADP in HCl model (means ± SEM). [Mózsik Gy. (2006). Molecular pharmacology and biochemistry of gastroduodenal mucosal damage and protection. In: Mózsik Gy. (Ed.) Discoveries in Gastroenterology (1960–2005) Akadémiai Kiadó, Budapest. pp. 139–224 (with kind permission).]

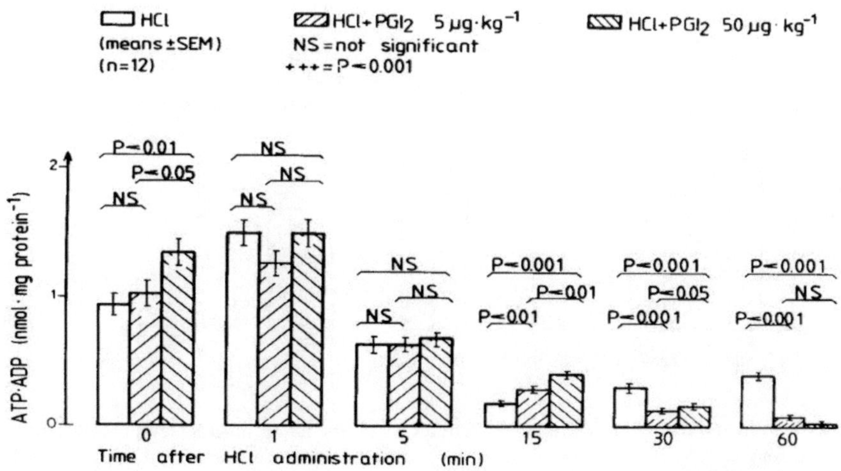

Figure 206. Changes in the values of ATP/ADP produced by PGI_2 in the rat gastric mucosa in HCl model (means ± SEM). [Mózsik Gy. (2006). Molecular pharmacology and biochemistry of gastroduodenal mucosal damage and protection. In: Mózsik Gy. (Ed.) Discoveries in Gastroenterology (1960–2005) Akadémiai Kiadó, Budapest. pp. 139–224 (with kind permission).]

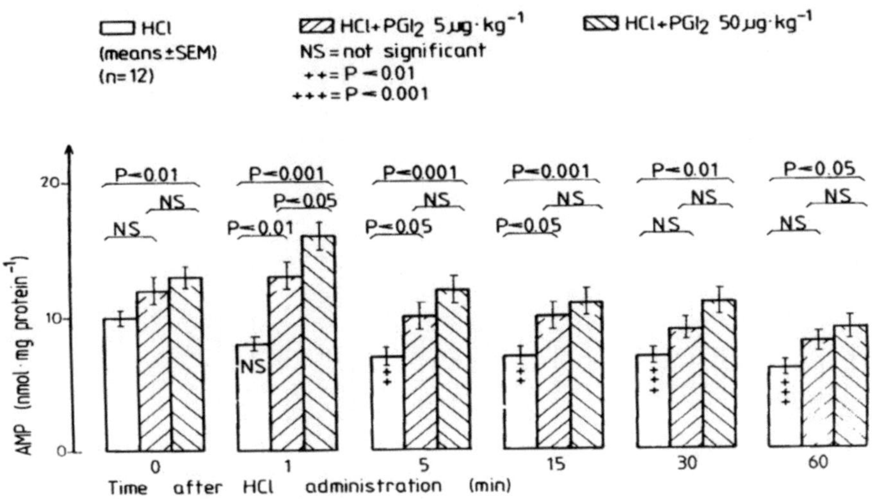

Figure 207. Dose–response changes in the rat gastric fundic mucosal level of AMP produced by PGI_2 in HCl model (means ± SEM). [Mózsik Gy. (2006). Molecular pharmacology and biochemistry of gastroduodenal mucosal damage and protection. In: Mózsik Gy. (Ed.) Discoveries in Gastroenterology (1960–2005) Akadémiai Kiadó, Budapest. pp. 139–224 (with kind permission).]

http://dx.doi.org/10.5772/60505

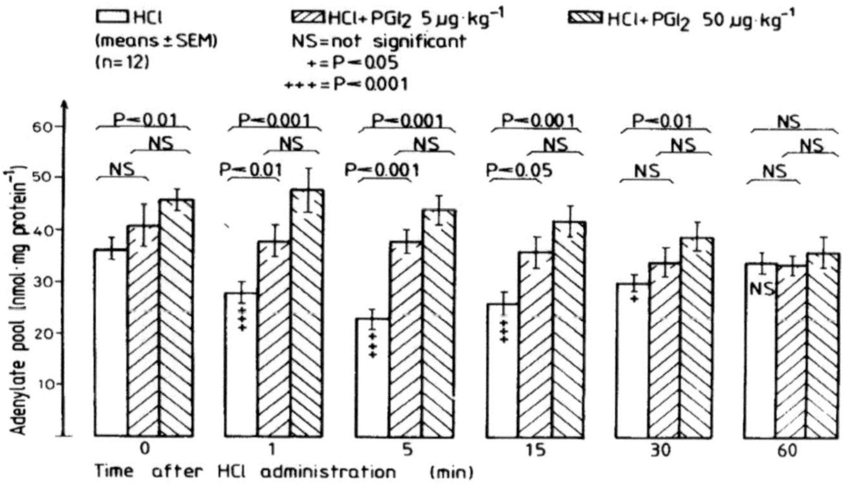

Figure 208. Dose–response changes in the rat gastric fundic mucosal levels of adenylate pool produced by PGI_2 in HCl model (means ± SEM). [Mózsik Gy. (2006). Molecular pharmacology and biochemistry of gastroduodenal mucosal damage and protection. In: Mózsik Gy. (Ed.) Discoveries in Gastroenterology (1960–2005). Akadémiai Kiadó, Budapest. pp. 139–224 (with kind permission).]

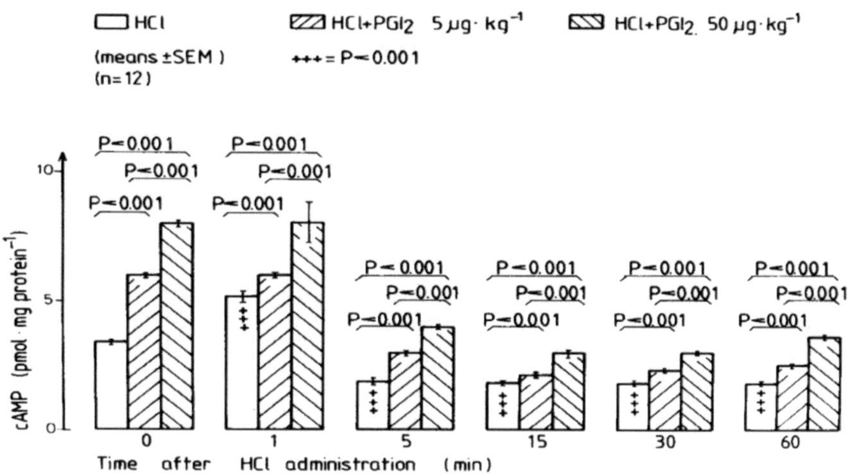

Figure 209. Dose–response changes in the rat gastric fundic mucosal levels of cAMP produced by PGI_2 in HCl model (means ± SEM). [Mózsik Gy. (2006). Molecular pharmacology and biochemistry of gastroduodenal mucosal damage and protection. In: Mózsik Gy. (Ed.) Discoveries in Gastroenterology (1960–2005). Akadémiai Kiadó, Budapest. pp. 139–224 (with kind permission).]

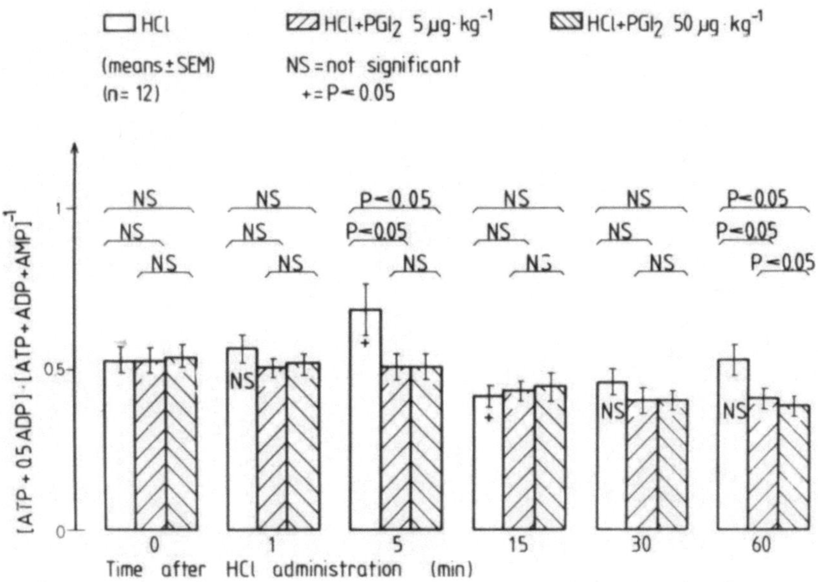

Figure 210. Changes in the rat gastric fundic mucosal level of "energy charge" produced by PGI_2 in HCl model (means ± SEM). [Mózsik Gy. (2006). Molecular pharmacology and biochemistry of gastroduodenal mucosal damage and protection. In: Mózsik Gy. (Ed.) Discoveries in Gastroenterology (1960–2005). Akadémiai Kiadó, Budapest. pp. 139–224 (with kind permission).]

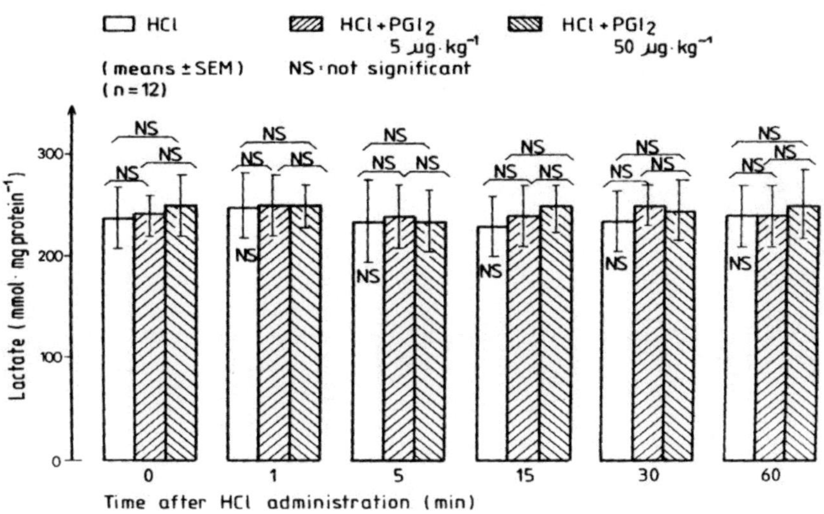

Figure 211. PGI_2-induced effects on the rat gastric fundic mucosal levels of lactate produced by PGI_2 in HCl model (means ± SEM). [Mózsik Gy. (2006). Molecular pharmacology and biochemistry of gastroduodenal mucosal damage and protection. In: Mózsik Gy. (Ed.) Discoveries in Gastroenterology (1960–2005). Akadémiai Kiadó, Budapest. pp. 139–224 (with kind permission).]

http://dx.doi.org/10.5772/60505

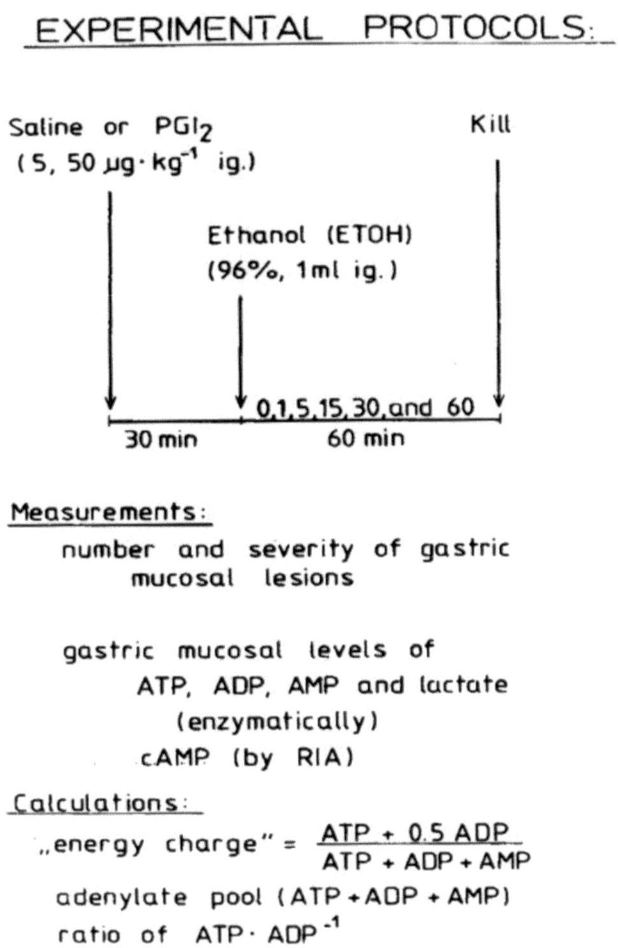

Figure 212. Experimental protocol for the study of gastric fundic mucosal-preventive effect of PGI_2 and its biochemical background in ethanol (ETOH) (nonacid-dependent) model. [Mózsik Gy. (2006). Molecular pharmacology and biochemistry of gastroduodenal mucosal damage and protection. In: Mózsik Gy. (Ed.) Discoveries in Gastroenterology (1960–2005). Akadémiai Kiadó, Budapest. pp. 139–224 (with kind permission).]

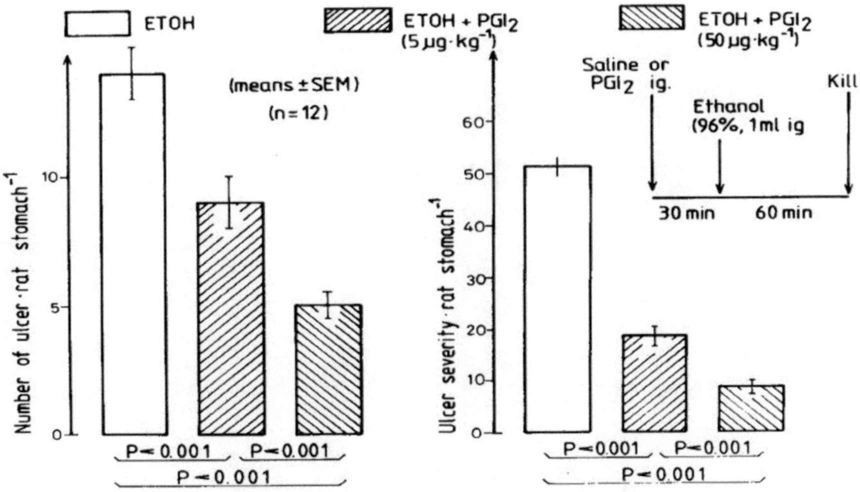

Figure 213. Determination of ED_{50} value for PGI_2 in ETOH model (means ± SEM). [Mózsik Gy. (2006). Molecular pharmacology and biochemistry of gastroduodenal mucosal damage and protection. In: Mózsik Gy. (Ed.) Discoveries in Gastroenterology (1960–2005). Akadémiai Kiadó, Budapest. pp. 139–224 (with kind permission).]

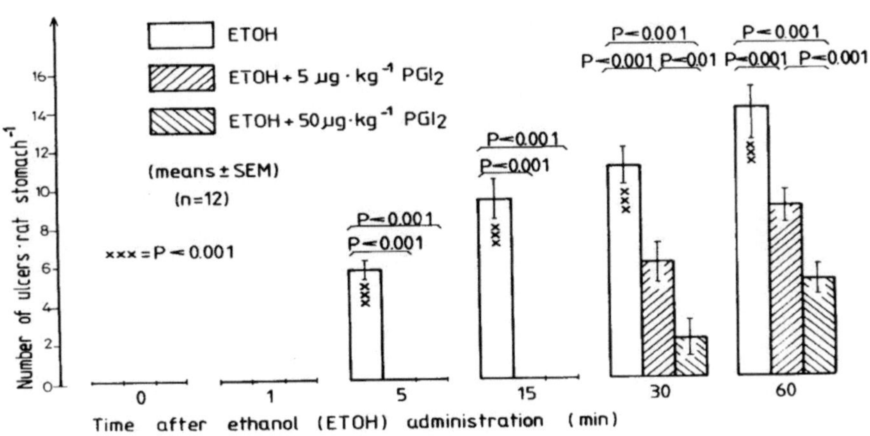

Figure 214. PGI_2-induced gastric mucosal-preventive effect (number) in ETOH model (means ± SEM). [Mózsik Gy. (2006). Molecular pharmacology and biochemistry of gastroduodenal mucosal damage and protection. In: Mózsik Gy. (Ed.) Discoveries in Gastroenterology (1960–2005). Akadémiai Kiadó, Budapest. pp. 139–224 (with kind permission).]

http://dx.doi.org/10.5772/60505

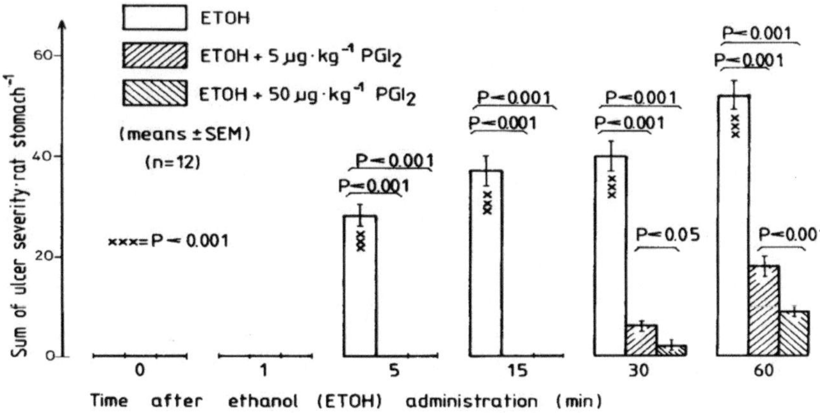

Figure 215. PGI_2-induced gastric mucosal-preventive effect on the severity in ETOH model (means ± SEM). [Mózsik Gy. (2006). Molecular pharmacology and biochemistry of gastroduodenal mucosal damage and protection. In: Mózsik Gy. (Ed.) Discoveries in Gastroenterology (1960–2005). Akadémiai Kiadó, Budapest. pp. 139–224 (with kind permission).]

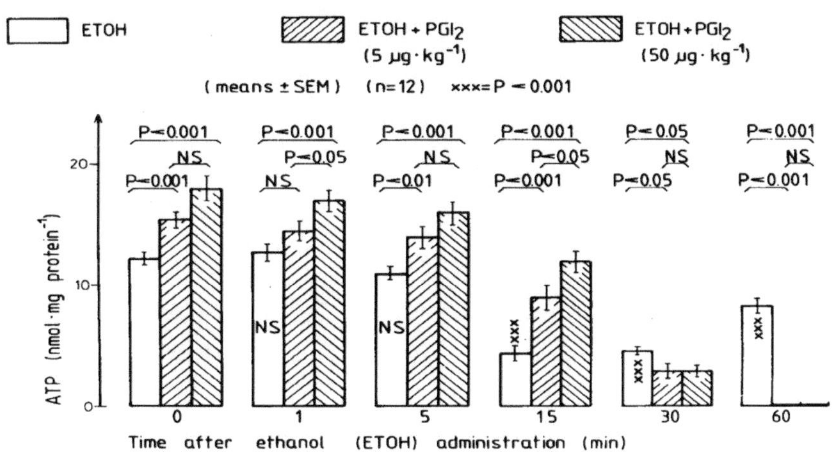

Figure 216. Dose-dependent changes produced by PGI_2 in the tissue levels of ATP of the rat gastric fundic mucosa in ETOH model (means ± SEM). [Mózsik Gy. (2006). Molecular pharmacology and biochemistry of gastroduodenal mucosal damage and protection. In: Mózsik Gy. (Ed.) Discoveries in Gastroenterology (1960–2005). Akadémiai Kiadó, Budapest. pp. 139–224 (with kind permission).]

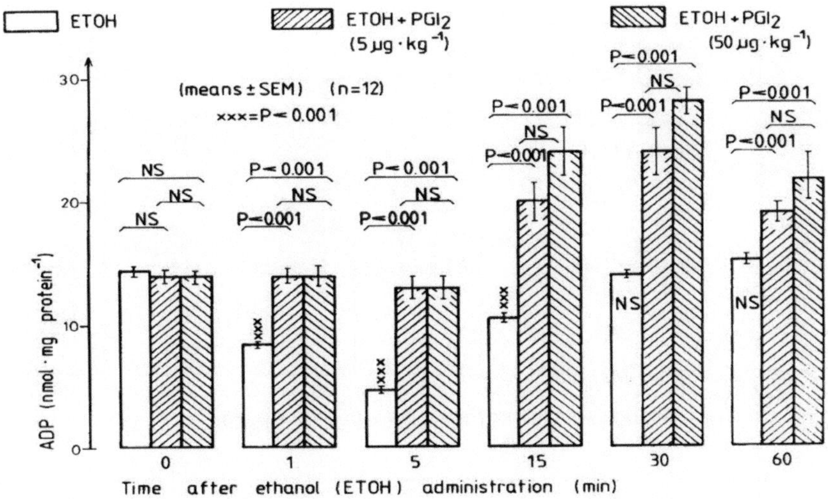

Figure 217. Dose-dependent changes produced by PGI_2 in the gastric fundic mucosal level of ADP in ETOH model (means ± SEM). [Mózsik Gy. (2006). Molecular pharmacology and biochemistry of gastroduodenal mucosal damage and protection. In: Mózsik Gy. (Ed.) Discoveries in Gastroenterology (1960–2005). Akadémiai Kiadó, Budapest. pp. 139–224 (with kind permission).]

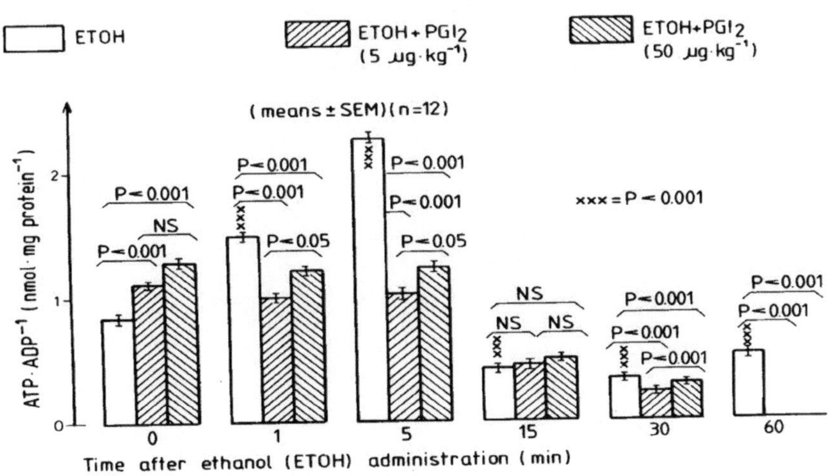

Figure 218. PGI_2-induced changes in the gastric fundic mucosal level of ATP/ADP in ETOH model (means ± SEM). [Mózsik Gy. (2006). Molecular pharmacology and biochemistry of gastroduodenal mucosal damage and protection. In: Mózsik Gy. (Ed.) Discoveries in Gastroenterology (1960–2005). Akadémiai Kiadó, Budapest. pp. 139–224 (with kind permission).]

http://dx.doi.org/10.5772/60505

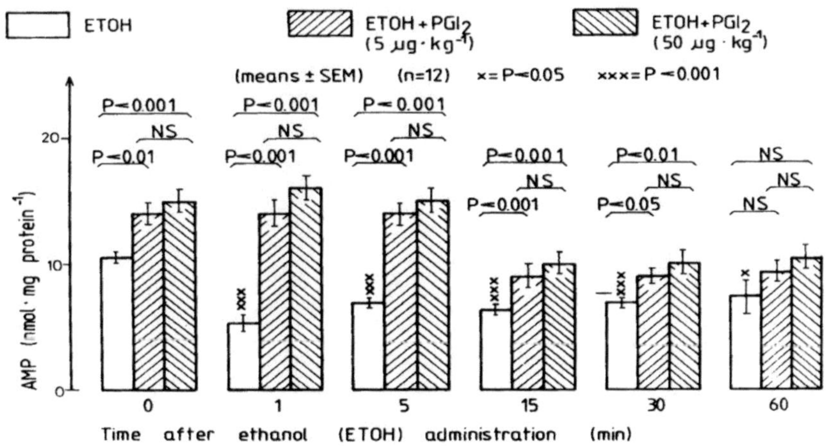

Figure 219. Dose-dependent changes in the rat gastric fundic mucosal level of AMP produced by PGI_2 in ETOH model (means ± SEM). [Mózsik Gy. (2006). Molecular pharmacology and biochemistry of gastroduodenal mucosal damage and protection. In: Mózsik Gy. (Ed.) Discoveries in Gastroenterology (1960–2005). Akadémiai Kiadó, Budapest. pp. 139–224 (with kind permission).]

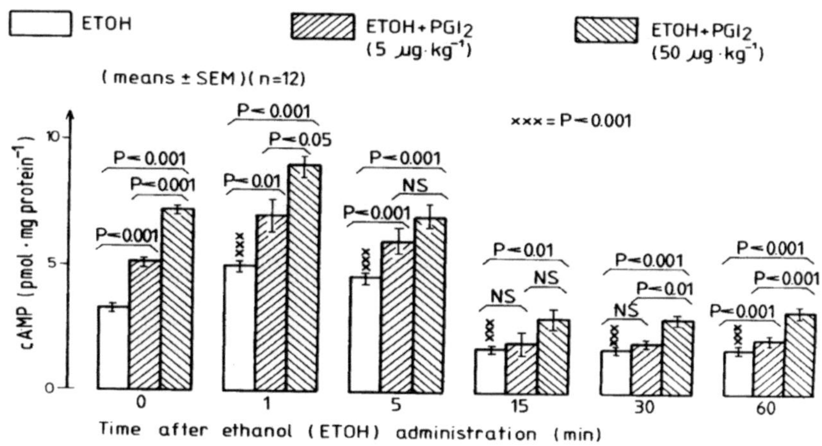

Figure 220. Dose-dependent changes in the rat gastric fundic mucosal level of cAMP produced by PGI_2 in ETOH model (means ± SEM). [Mózsik Gy. (2006). Molecular pharmacology and biochemistry of gastroduodenal mucosal damage and protection. In: Mózsik Gy. (Ed.) Discoveries in Gastroenterology (1960–2005). Akadémiai Kiadó, Budapest. pp. 139–224 (with kind permission).]

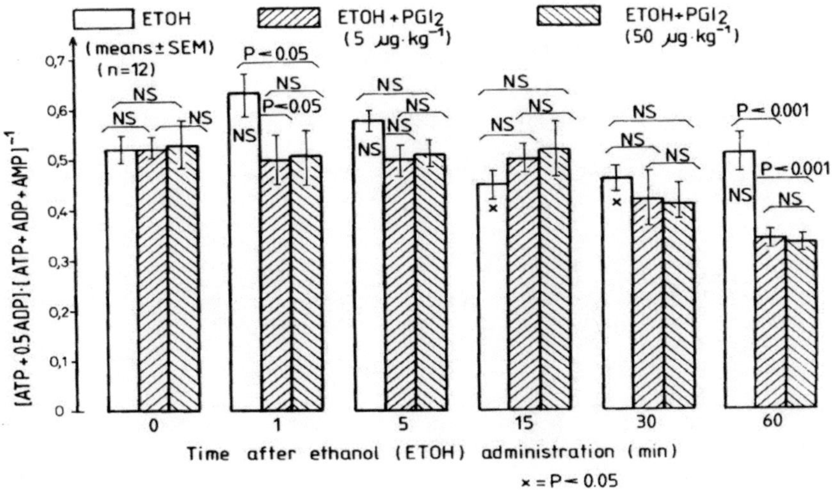

Figure 221. Changes in the rat gastric fundic mucosal level of "energy charge" produced by PGI_2 in ETOH model (means ± SEM). [Mózsik Gy. (2006). Molecular pharmacology and biochemistry of gastroduodenal mucosal damage and protection. In: Mózsik Gy. (Ed.) Discoveries in Gastroenterology (1960–2005). Akadémiai Kiadó, Budapest. pp. 139–224 (with kind permission).]

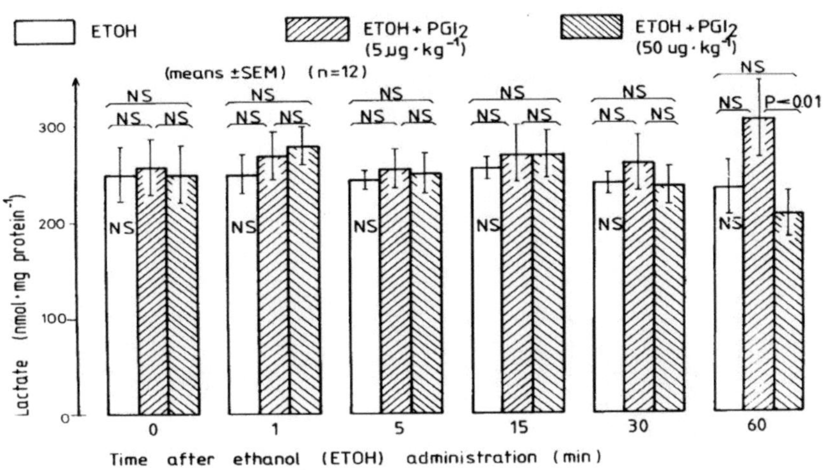

Figure 222. PGI_2-induced changes in the rat gastric fundic mucosal level of lactate in ETOH model (means ±SEM). [Mózsik Gy. (2006). Molecular pharmacology and biochemistry of gastroduodenal mucosal damage and protection. In: Mózsik Gy. (Ed.) Discoveries in Gastroenterology (1960–2005). Akadémiai Kiadó, Budapest. pp. 139–224 (with kind permission).]

It was interesting to note that the PGI_2-induced gastric mucosal-preventive effect appears in the first (0–15 min) time period as that obtained by PGI_2 in the HCl model.

http://dx.doi.org/10.5772/60505

The biochemically obtained results indicated dose-dependent actions on the tissue levels of ATP, ADP, AMP and cAMP and changes in the values of ratio of ATP/ADP, and the adenylate pool was found to be about the same.

8.10.3. Gastric mucosal-preventive effect of β-carotene versus changes in the gastric mucosal energy systems in HCl model in rats

β-carotene (given in 1 and 10 mg/kg doses i.g.) led to significant and dose-dependent prevention of the gastric mucosal damage (Figures 222, 223). The 1 mg/kg β-carotene produced the ED_{50} value in the HCl model (Figure 223). It was also interesting to note that β-carotene-induced gastric mucosal prevention appears later (from 15 to 60 min) (Figures 225, 226). The ATP–ADP transformation was decreased, whereas the ATP–cAMP transformation was increased (Figures 227–230). No significant changes were obtained in the adenylate pool (Figure 231) and the tissue level of lactate (Figure 232).

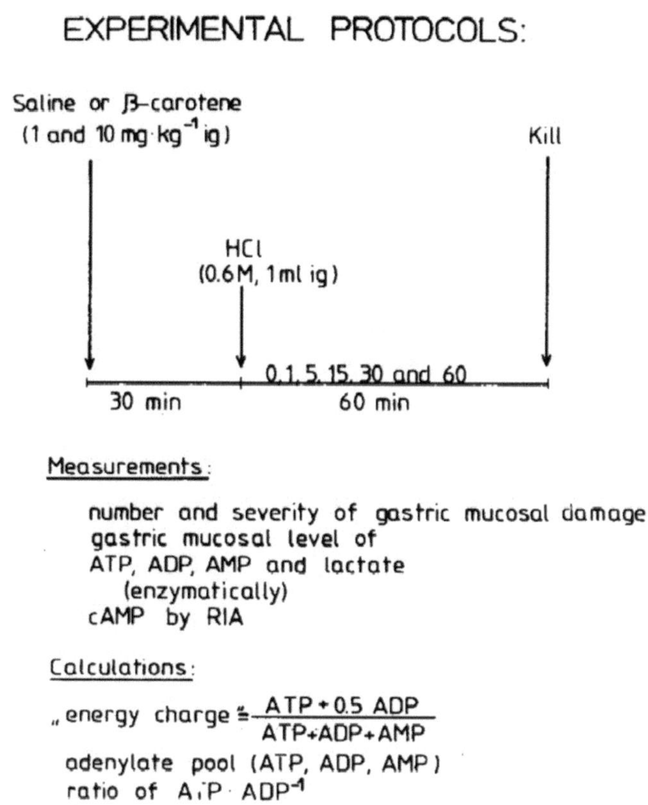

Figure 223. Experimental protocol for the study of gastric mucosal-preventive effects and their biochemistry produced by β-carotene in HCl model. [Mózsik Gy. (2006). Molecular pharmacology and biochemistry of gastroduodenal mucosal damage and protection. In: Mózsik Gy. (Ed.) Discoveries in Gastroenterology (1960–2005). Akadémiai Kiadó, Budapest. pp. 139–224 (with kind permission).]

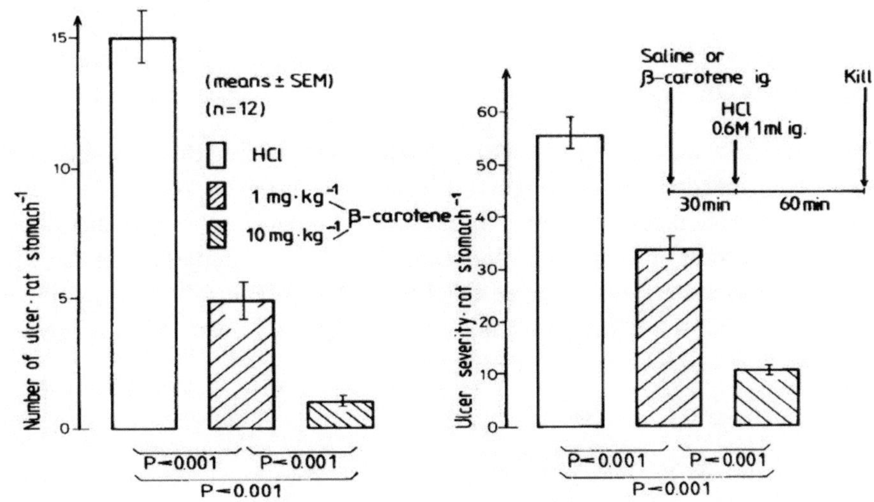

Figure 224. Determination of ED_{50} values for gastric fundic mucosal-preventive effects of β-carotene in HCl model (means ± SEM). [Mózsik Gy. (2006). Molecular pharmacology and biochemistry of gastroduodenal mucosal damage and protection. In: Mózsik Gy. (Ed.) Discoveries in Gastroenterology (1960–2005). Akadémiai Kiadó, Budapest. pp. 139–224 (with kind permission).]

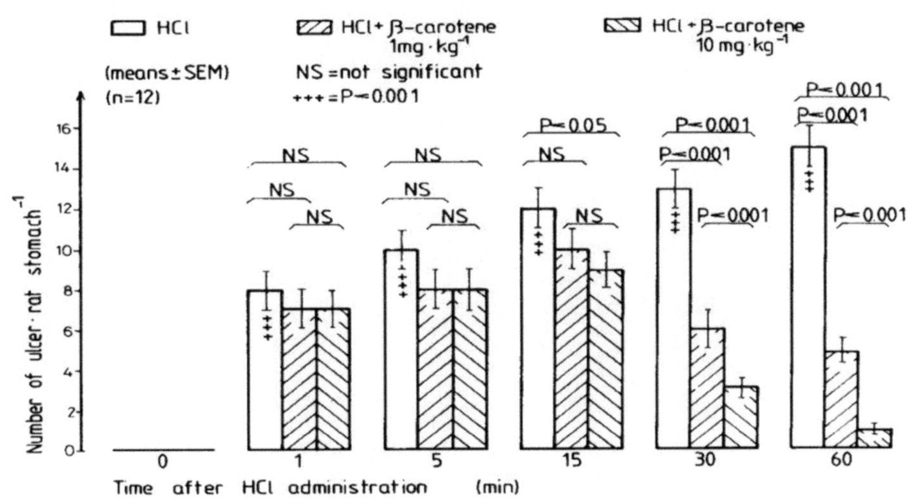

Dose-dependent gastric mucosal-preventive effect (number) of β-carotene in HCl model (means ± SEM). [Mózsik Gy. (2006). Molecular pharmacology and biochemistry of gastroduodenal mucosal damage and protection. In: Mózsik Gy. (Ed.) Discoveries in Gastroenterology (1960–2005). Akadémiai Kiadó, Budapest. pp. 139–224 (with kind permission).]

http://dx.doi.org/10.5772/60505

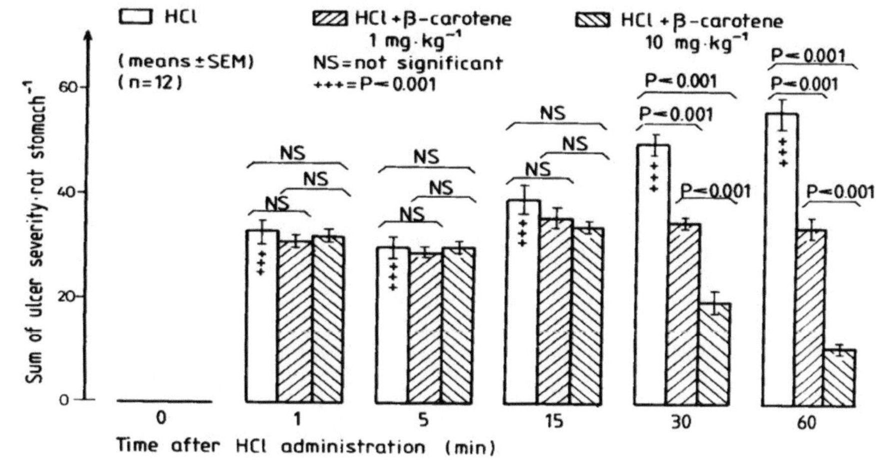

Figure 226. Dose-dependent gastric mucosal-protective effect (severity) of β-carotene in HCl model (means ± SEM). [Mózsik Gy. (2006). Molecular pharmacology and biochemistry of gastroduodenal mucosal damage and protection. In: Mózsik Gy. (Ed.) Discoveries in Gastroenterology (1960–2005). Akadémiai Kiadó, Budapest. pp. 139–224 (with kind permission).]

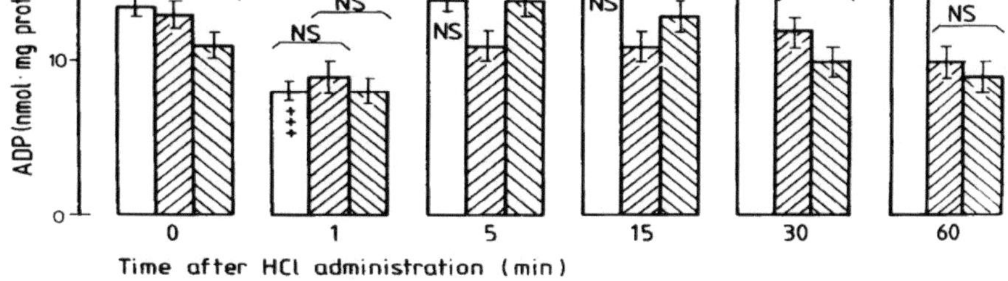

Figure 227. Dose-dependent changes in the rat gastric fundic mucosal level of ADP produced by β-carotene in HCl model (means ± SEM). [Mózsik Gy. (2006). Molecular pharmacology and biochemistry of gastroduodenal mucosal damage and protection. In: Mózsik Gy. (Ed.) Discoveries in Gastroenterology (1960–2005). Akadémiai Kiadó, Budapest. pp. 139–224 (with kind permission).]

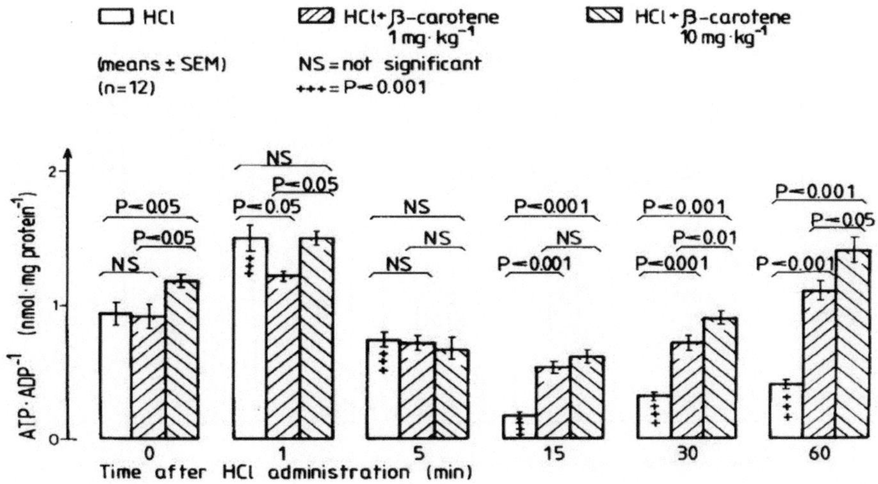

Figure 228. Changes in the gastric fundic mucosal level of ATP/ADP produced by β-carotene in HCl model (means ± SEM). [Mózsik Gy. (2006). Molecular pharmacology and biochemistry of gastroduodenal mucosal damage and protection. In: Mózsik Gy. (Ed.) Discoveries in Gastroenterology (1960–2005). Akadémiai Kiadó, Budapest. pp. 139–224 (with kind permission).]

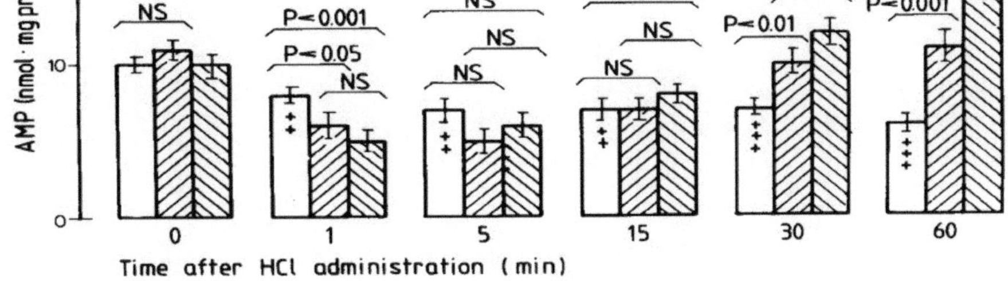

Figure 229. Changes in the rat gastric fundic mucosal level of AMP produced by β-carotene in HCl model (means ± SEM). [Mózsik Gy. (2006). Molecular pharmacology and biochemistry of gastroduodenal mucosal damage and protection. In: Mózsik Gy. (Ed.) Discoveries in Gastroenterology (1960–2005). Akadémiai Kiadó, Budapest. pp. 139–224 (with kind permission).]

http://dx.doi.org/10.5772/60505

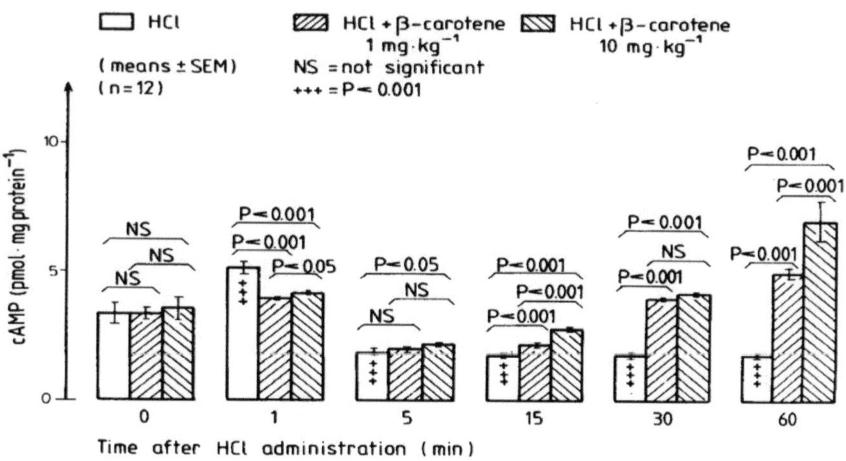

Figure 230. Changes in the rat gastric fundic mucosal level of cAMP produced by β-carotene in HCl model (means ± SEM). [Mózsik Gy. (2006). Molecular pharmacology and biochemistry of gastroduodenal mucosal damage and protection. In: Mózsik Gy. (Ed.) Discoveries in Gastroenterology (1960–2005). Akadémiai Kiadó, Budapest. pp. 139–224 (with kind permission).]

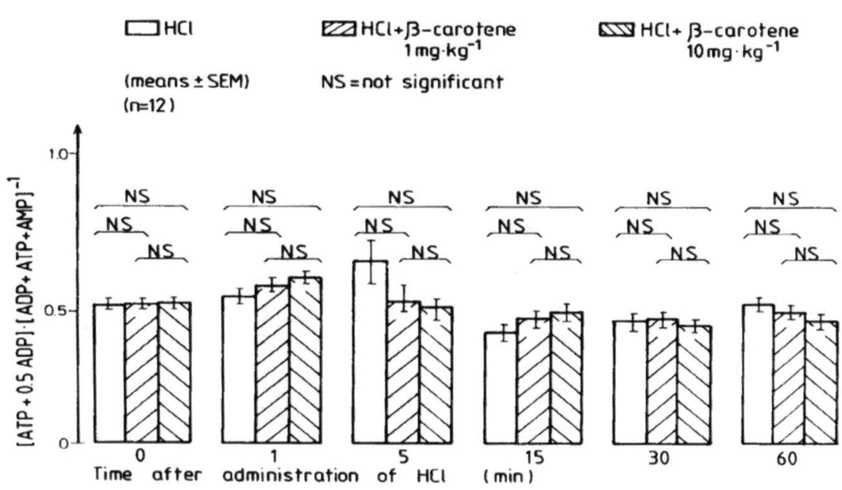

Figure 231. "Energy charge" in the rat gastric fundic mucosal level in HCl model before and after β-carotene treatment (means ± SEM). [Mózsik Gy. (2006). Molecular pharmacology and biochemistry of gastroduodenal mucosal damage and protection. In: Mózsik Gy. (Ed.) Discoveries in Gastroenterology (1960–2005). Akadémiai Kiadó, Budapest. pp. 139–224 (with kind permission).]

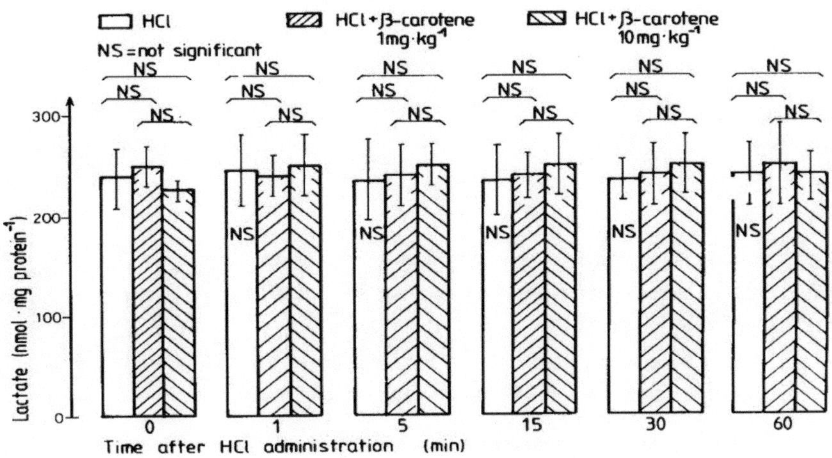

Figure 232. Tissue levels of lactate in the rat gastric fundic mucosa in HCl model before and after β-carotene treatment (means ± SEM). [Mózsik Gy. (2006). Molecular pharmacology and biochemistry of gastroduodenal mucosal damage and protection. In: Mózsik Gy. (Ed.) Discoveries in Gastroenterology (1960–2005). Akadémiai Kiadó, Budapest. pp. 139–224 (with kind permission).]

8.10.4. Mucosal-preventive effect of β-carotene versus changes in the gastric mucosal energy systems in ETOH model in rats

β-carotene showed gastric mucosal-preventive effect in ETOH model (Jávor et al., 1983; Mózsik and Jávor, 1981) (Figures 232–243).

The ED_{50} was also found for 1 mg/kg of β-carotene (i.g. given) (Figure 234). The gastric mucosal effect of β-carotene was also found in the later (from 15 to 60 min) time in order to number and severity of gastric mucosal damage (Figures 235–236). The ATP–ADP transformation was decreased, whereas the ATP–cAMP transformation was increased (Figures 237–241). No significant changes were obtained in the adenylate pool, "energy charge" and lactate (Figures 242, 243).

The results of our observations obtained from HCl- and ethanol-induced gastric mucosal damage and their gastric mucosal-preventive effects produced by PGI_2 and β-carotene (including the changes in the membrane-bound ATP-dependent energy systems) allowed us to evaluate the details of their mechanisms in the development of gastric mucosal damage (HCl and ethanol) and PGI_2 and β-carotene-induced gastric mucosal prevention (under animal experiments):

1. HCl and ethanol (as mucosal-damaging chemical agents with different chemical properties) produce the same macroscopic appearance of gastric mucosal damage after their applications;

http://dx.doi.org/10.5772/60505

2. The macroscopic appearance of gastric mucosal damage produced by HCl and ethanol indicated the same patterns of time sequences (in order of number and severity) of the development of gastric mucosal tissues;

3. PGI_2 and β-carotene exert gastric mucosal protection against HCl- and ethanol-induced gastric mucosal damage; however, their gastroprotective effects differ (from each other) in time after the administration of necrotizing agents: PGI_2 acts earlier (from 0 to 15 min), whereas β-carotene is gastroprotective and it can be detected later (from 15 to 60 min) after the administration of necrotizing agents;

4. The extent of ATP transformation into ADP is increased during the development of gastric mucosal damage produced by HCl and ethanol in the gastric fundic mucosa (in association with a small increase of gastric mucosal cAMP level) in both models;

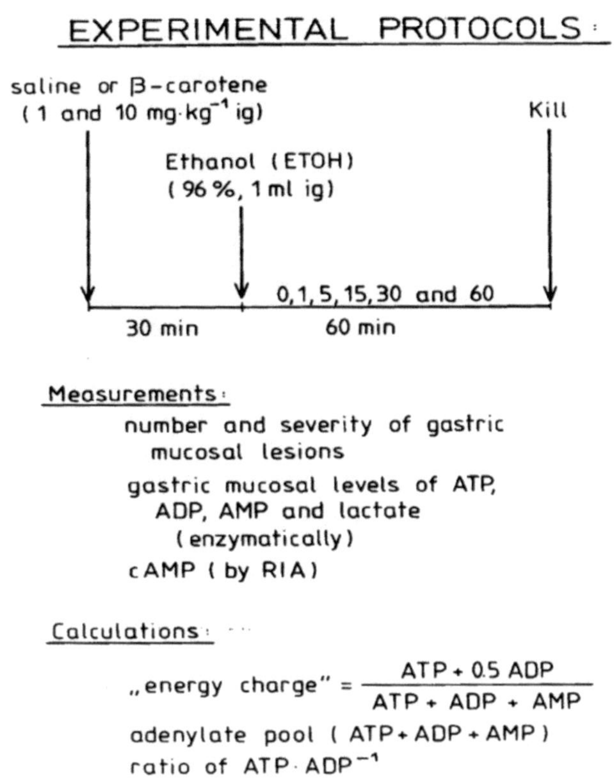

Figure 233. Experimental protocol for the study of gastric mucosal-protective effects and their biochemistry of β-carotene in ETOH model. [Mózsik Gy. (2006). Molecular pharmacology and biochemistry of gastroduodenal mucosal damage and protection. In: Mózsik Gy. (Ed.) Discoveries in Gastroenterology (1960–2005). Akadémiai Kiadó, Budapest. pp. 139–224 (with kind permission).]

5. The gastric mucosal-preventive effects of PGI_2 and β-carotene associate with the decrease of ATP transformation into ADP and increase of ATP transformation into cAMP in the rat gastric fundic mucosa;

6. PGI_2 and β-carotene produce dose-dependent biochemical responses in the rat gastric mucosa (ATP, ADP, AMP, cAMP and adenylate pool) during the development of gastric mucosal-preventive protection against the chemically induced gastric mucosal damage;

7. The biochemical mechanisms (changes in the membrane-bound ATP-dependent energy systems) of gastric mucosal-protective effects of PGI_2 and β-carotene are the same in the HCl- and ethanol-induced mucosa;

8. Biochemically, no presence of gastric hypoxemia was proved in the rat gastric fundic mucosa during the development of both gastric mucosal damage (by HCl and ethanol) and gastric mucosal protection of PGI_2 and β-carotene against HCl and ethanol.

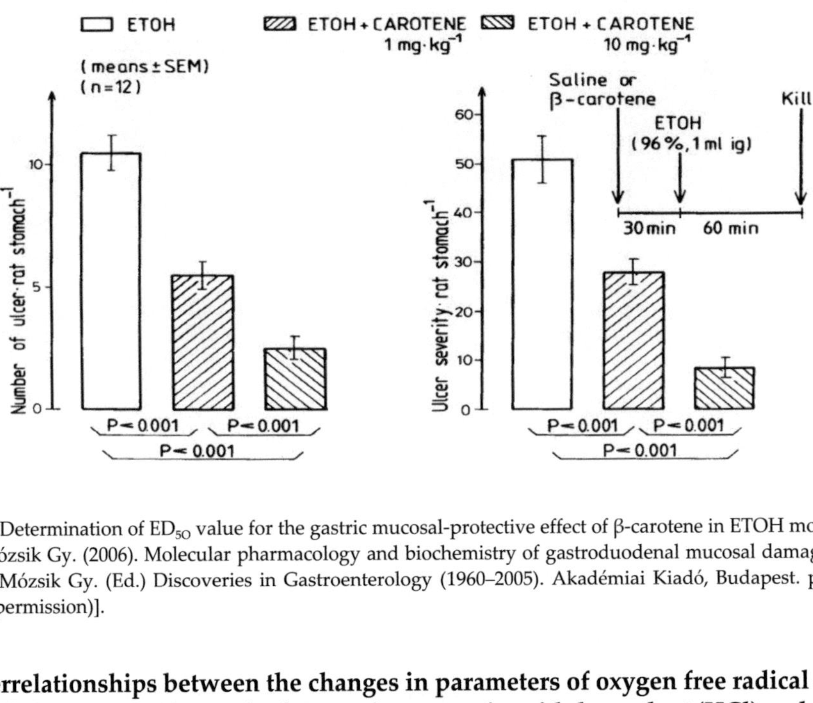

Figure 234. Determination of ED_{50} value for the gastric mucosal-protective effect of β-carotene in ETOH model (means ± SEM). [Mózsik Gy. (2006). Molecular pharmacology and biochemistry of gastroduodenal mucosal damage and protection. In: Mózsik Gy. (Ed.) Discoveries in Gastroenterology (1960–2005). Akadémiai Kiadó, Budapest. pp. 139–224 (with kind permission)].

8.11. Interrelationships between the changes in parameters of oxygen free radical systems versus cellular energy systems in the gastric mucosa in acid-dependent (HCl) and nonacid-dependent (ETOH) experimental models during the time of development of gastric mucosal damage and gastric mucosal prevention produced by PGI_2 and β-carotene

Many observations indicated clearly that the maintenance of good equilibrium (between the aggressive and defensive mechanisms) is an extremely complicated summary (result) in the living organs. We are able to learn and recognize different aspects of this extremely complicated equilibrium in the living organs, and our knowledge has changed over time.

http://dx.doi.org/10.5772/60505

The researchers are able to approach only some small piece from the whole, meanwhile many-many processes (regulatory pathways) are running beside each others. We are willing to hope that the selected piece(s) (to be used in the studies) is (are) an important field(s) for the whole screening method to understand the key point(s) in the keeping of this equilibrium between the aggressive and defensive factors.

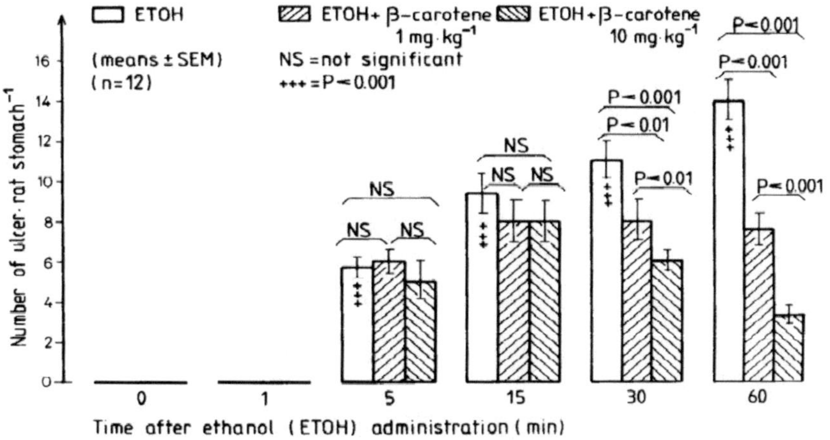

Figure 235. β-carotene-induced gastric mucosal-preventive effects on the rat gastric fundic mucosa (number) in ETOH model (means ± SEM). [Mózsik Gy. (2006). Molecular pharmacology and biochemistry of gastroduodenal mucosal damage and protection. In: Mózsik Gy. (Ed.) Discoveries in Gastroenterology (1960–2005). Akadémiai Kiadó, Budapest. pp. 139–224 (with kind permission).]

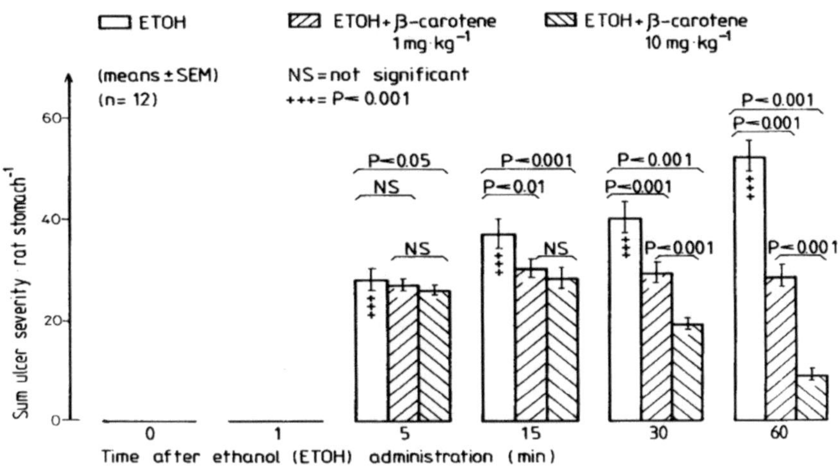

Figure 236. β-carotene-induced gastric fundic mucosal-preventive effect (on the severity) in ETOH model (means ± SEM). [Mózsik Gy. (2006). Molecular pharmacology and biochemistry of gastroduodenal mucosal damage and protection. In: Mózsik Gy. (Ed.) Discoveries in Gastroenterology (1960–2005). Akadémiai Kiadó, Budapest. pp. 139–224 (with kind permission).]

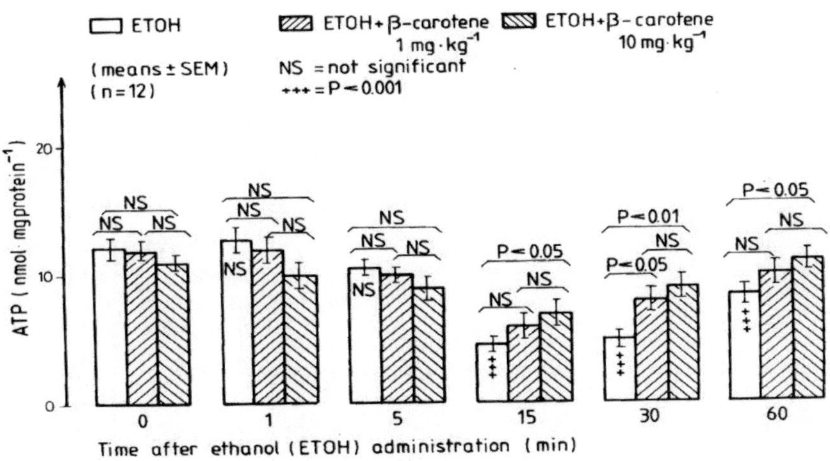

Figure 237. β-carotene-induced changes in the rat gastric fundic mucosal level of ATP in ETOH model (means ± SEM). [Mózsik Gy. (2006). Molecular pharmacology and biochemistry of gastroduodenal mucosal damage and protection. In: Mózsik Gy. (Ed.) Discoveries in Gastroenterology (1960–2005). Akadémiai Kiadó, Budapest. pp. 139–224 (with kind permission).]

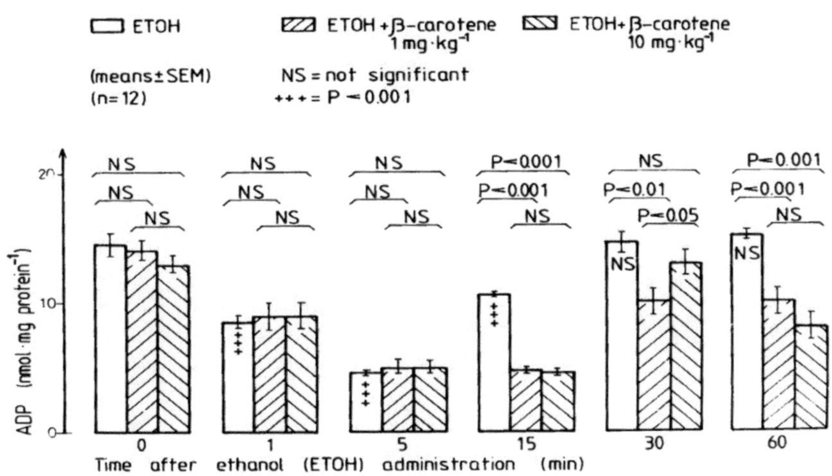

Figure 238. β-carotene-induced changes in the rat gastric fundic mucosal levels of ADP in ETOH model (means ± SEM). [Mózsik Gy. (2006). Molecular pharmacology and biochemistry of gastroduodenal mucosal damage and protection. In: Mózsik Gy. (Ed.) Discoveries in Gastroenterology (1960–2005). Akadémiai Kiadó, Budapest. pp. 139–224 (with kind permission).]

http://dx.doi.org/10.5772/60505

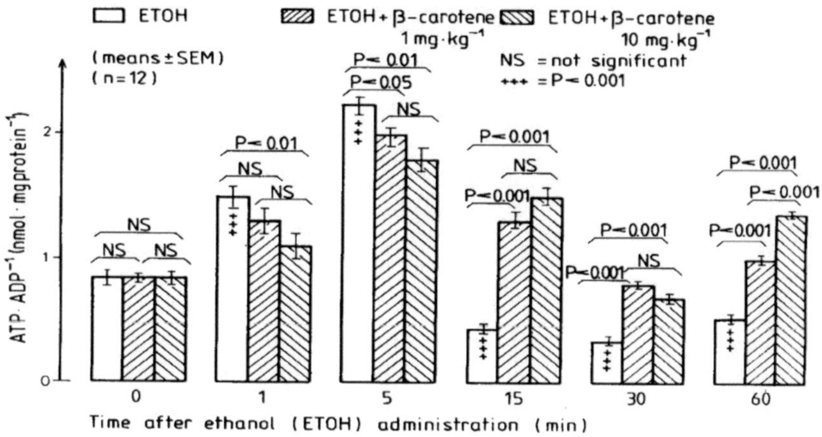

Figure 239. β-carotene-induced changes in ratio of ATP/ADP of the rat gastric fundic mucosa in ETOH model (means ± SEM). [Mózsik Gy. (2006). Molecular pharmacology and biochemistry of gastroduodenal mucosal damage and protection. In: Mózsik Gy. (Ed.) Discoveries in Gastroenterology (1960–2005). Akadémiai Kiadó, Budapest. pp. 139–224 (with kind permission).]

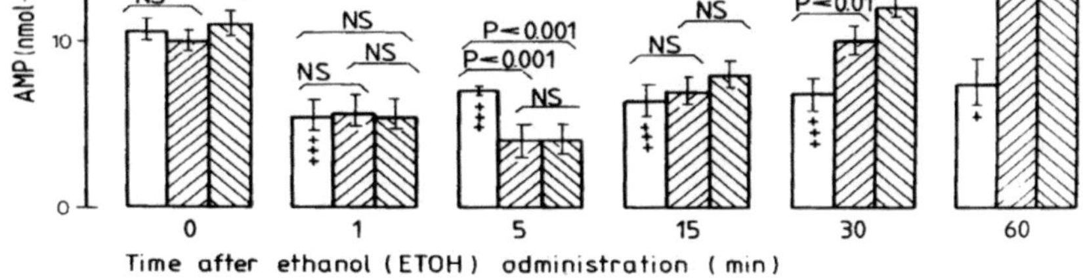

Figure 240. β-carotene-induced changes in the rat gastric mucosal levels of AMP in ETOH model (means ± SEM). [Mózsik Gy. (2006). Molecular pharmacology and biochemistry of gastroduodenal mucosal damage and protection. In: Mózsik Gy. (Ed.) Discoveries in Gastroenterology (1960–2005). Akadémiai Kiadó, Budapest. pp. 139–224 (with kind permission).]

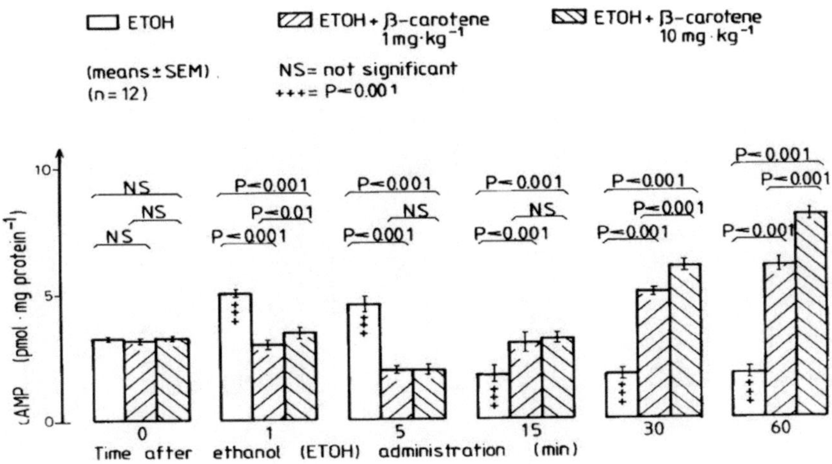

Figure 241. β-carotene-induced changes in the rat gastric fundic mucosal levels of cAMP in ETOH model (means ± SEM). [Mózsik Gy. (2006). Molecular pharmacology and biochemistry of gastroduodenal mucosal damage and protection. In: Mózsik Gy. (Ed.) Discoveries in Gastroenterology (1960–2005). Akadémiai Kiadó, Budapest. pp. 139–224 (with kind permission).]

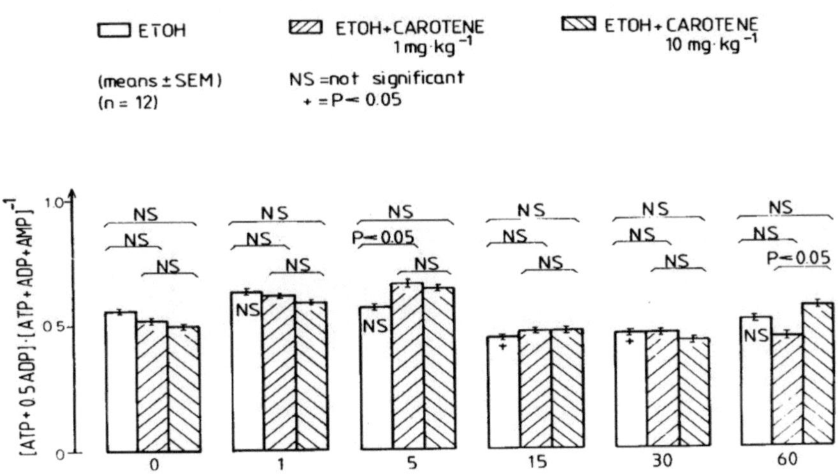

Figure 242. "Energy charge" in the rat gastric fundic mucosa with and without application of β-carotene in ETOH model (means ± SEM). [Mózsik Gy. (2006). Molecular pharmacology and biochemistry of gastroduodenal mucosal damage and protection. In: Mózsik Gy. (Ed.) Discoveries in Gastroenterology (1960–2005). Akadémiai Kiadó, Budapest. pp. 139–224 (with kind permission).]

http://dx.doi.org/10.5772/60505

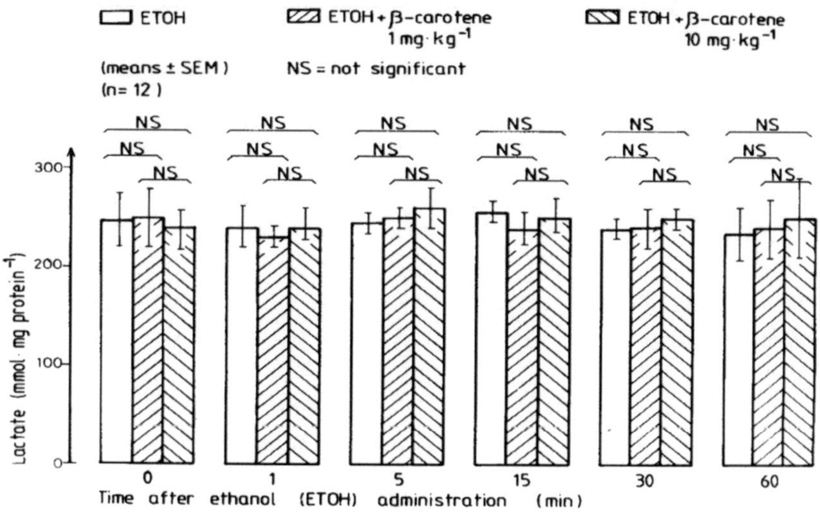

Figure 243. Lactate levels in the rat gastric fundic mucosa produced by β-carotene in ETOH model (means ± SEM). [Mózsik Gy. (2006). Molecular pharmacology and biochemistry of gastroduodenal mucosal damage and protection. In: Mózsik Gy. (Ed.) Discoveries in Gastroenterology (1960–2005). Akadémiai Kiadó, Budapest. pp. 139–224 (with kind permission).]

One of these fields is the oxygen free radical system, which incorporates different endogen enzyme systems (catalase, peroxidase, reduced glutathione peroxidase and superoxide dismutase) and many internal (vitamin C, vitamins A and E) and other external (chemical) components.

The production of oxygen free radicals and the compensation with different antioxidant compounds (scavengers) came into the focus of research. An excellent handbook was published (Laher, 2014), in which these problems were overviewed in the different organs (including the cellular, organ and body levels of living organisms).

We were also involved in this field of the studies (Bódis et al., 1995 a, b; 1996, 1997 a, b; 1998; 2000; Mózsik et al., 2001a; Szabó et al., 1996, 1997 a, b, c; 2000, 2012, 2014).

In these observations, systematic observations were carried out in the experimental models as those detailed in Section 8.10.

In the forthcoming sections, we demonstrate the tendencies of changes of oxygen free radical systems in comparison with the changes in the cellular energy systems in the gastrointestinal tract.

The superoxide dismutase (SOD) activity was determined according to the method of Misra and Fridovich (1972), which was modified by Matkovics et al. (1977). The glutathione peroxidase (GSH-px) activity was determined by the loss of reduced added to the supernatant and expressed as μmol GSH oxidized per minute (Flohe and Güzlei, 1984). The catalase (CAT) activity was measured using the method of Beers and Sizer (1952) and the glutathione (GSH) content was determined using Ellman's method (1959). The tissue level of malondial-

dehyde (MDA) was measured using a modification (Zsoldos et al., 1983) of the original method described by Fong et al. (1973). The protein content was assayed by the method described by Lowry et al. (1951). The biochemical results were expressed in accordance to 1.0-mg protein (means ± SEM).

These parameters were measured from the gastric mucosal tissues (and not from the sera). Furthermore, these studies were carried out in an acid-dependent (HCl) and nonacid-dependent (ETOH) ulcer model in rats. Additionally we applied to prevent the gastric mucosal damage an endogenous compound (PGI_2) (which has no scavenger property) and a scavenger compound (β-carotene). The main results of these observations are summarized briefly in the forthcoming sections.

8.11.1. Relationships between the changes in parameters of oxygen free radical systems versus cellular energy systems in the gastric mucosa of rats treated by intragastrically given HCl and ETOH

The observations were carried out in the morning. The gastric lesions were produced by intragastric administration of 1 mL of 96% ethanol or 1 mL of 0.6 M HCl. The animals were sacrificed at 0, 1, 5, 15, 30 and 60 minutes after giving the necrotizing agents.

The number and severity, parameters of the oxygen free radicals and the biochemical constituents of cellular energy systems were measured from the gastric fundic mucosa (the details of these measurements).

It is important to note that all measurements were carried out from the same tissue samples.

The detailed results are expressed in case of changes in the gastric fundic mucosa of rats, after the application of necrotizing agents on time sequence (Mózsik7et al., 1991 a).

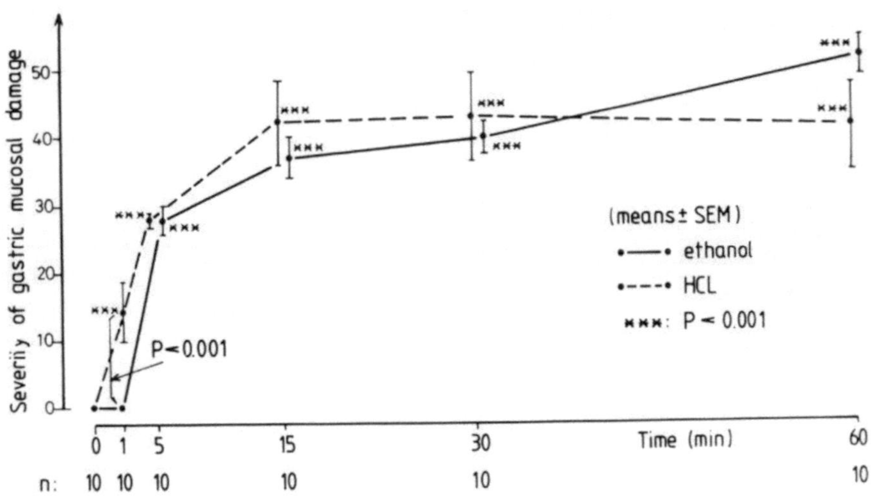

Figure 244. Changes in the severity of gastric mucosal damage of rats, produced by intragastrically applied ethanol (ETOH) and HCl, dependent on time after administration of necrotizing agents. [Mózsik, Sütő, Garamszegi, Jávor, Nagy, Vincze, Zsoldos: Eur. J. Gastroenterol. Hepatol. 3: 757–761, 1991 (with kind permission).]

http://dx.doi.org/10.5772/60505

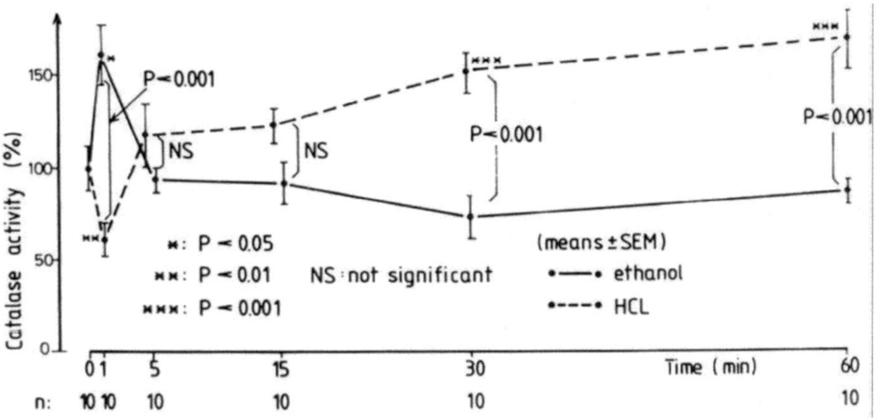

Figure 245. Changes in the catalase activity in the gastric fundic mucosa of rats, during the development of gastric mucosal damage produced by intragastrically applied ethanol or HCl, dependent on time after administration of necrotizing agents (100 = 0.60 Bergmeyer unit/mg protein). [Mózsik, Sütő, Garamszegi, Jávor, Nagy, Vincze, Zsoldos: Eur. J. Gastroenterol. Hepatol. 3: 757–761, 1991 (with kind permission).]

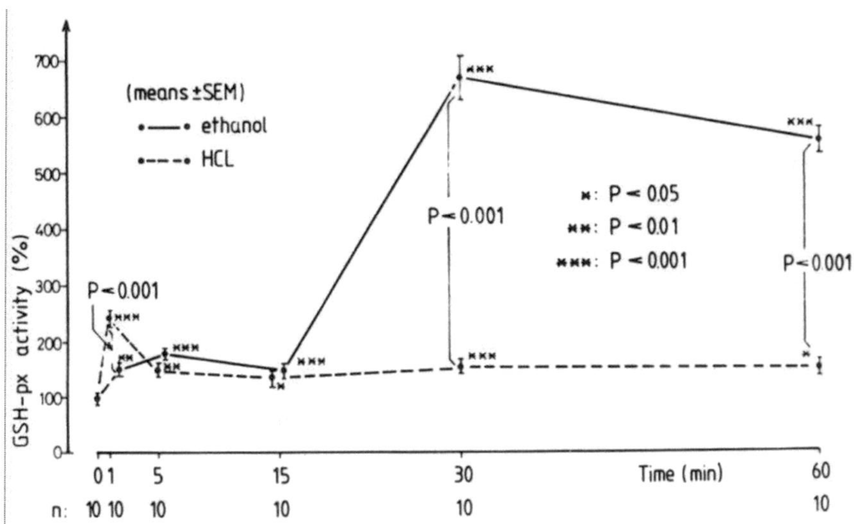

Figure 246. Changes in the glutathione peroxidase (GSH-px) activity in the gastric fundic mucosa of rats, during the development of gastric mucosal damage produced by intragastrically applied ethanol or HCl, dependent on time after administration of necrotizing agents (100 = 0.60 Bergmeyer unit/mg protein). [Mózsik, Sütő, Garamszegi, Jávor, Nagy, Vincze, Zsoldos: Eur. J. Gastroenterol. Hepatol. 3: 757–761, 1991 (with kind permission).]

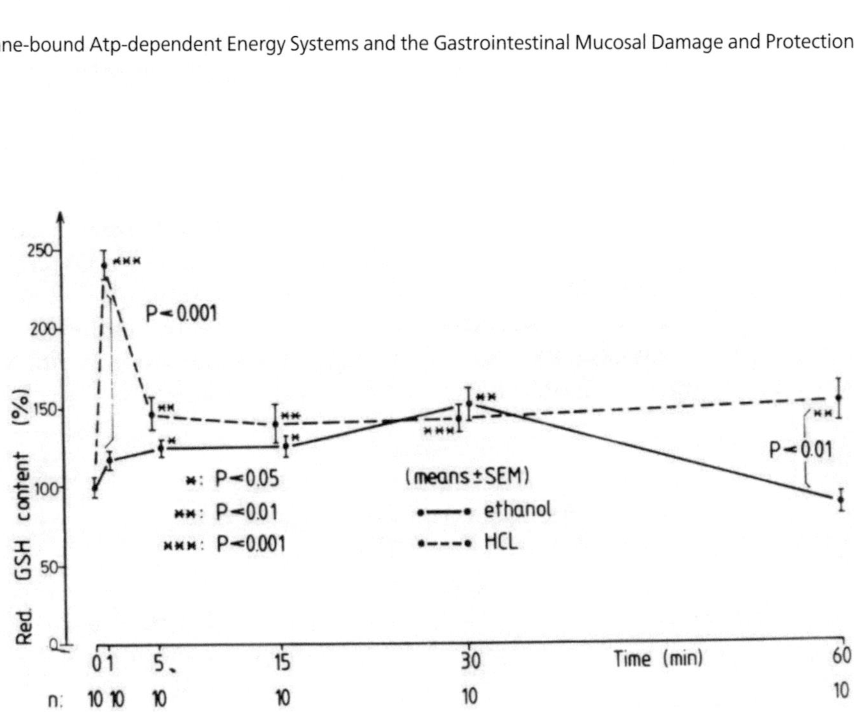

Figure 247. Changes in the tissue contents of reduced glutathione (GSH) from the gastric fundic mucosa of rats, during the development of gastric mucosal damage produced by intragastrically applied ethanol or HCl, dependent on time after administration of necrotizing agents (100 = 0.60 Bergmeyer unit/mg protein). [Mózsik, Sütő, Garamszegi, Jávor, Nagy, Vincze, Zsoldos: Eur. J. Gastroenterol. Hepatol. 3: 757–761, 1991 (with kind permission).]

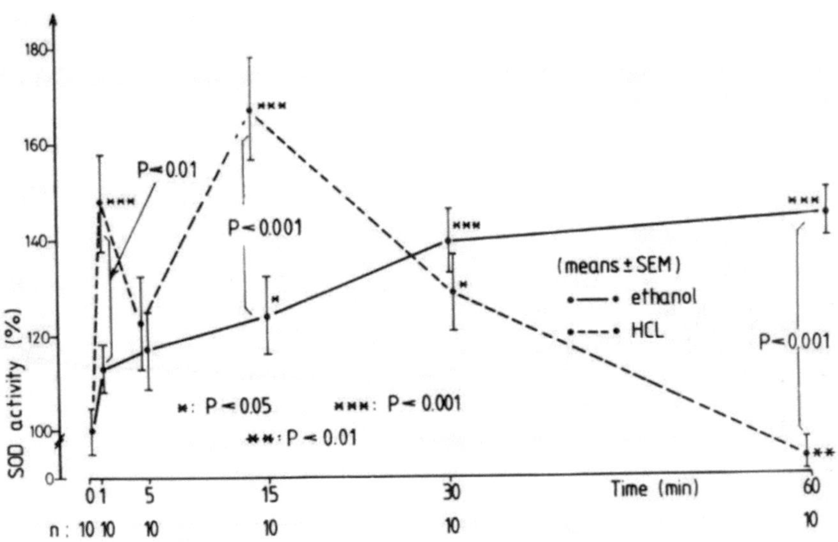

Figure 248. Changes in the superoxide dismutase (SOD) activity in the gastric fundic mucosa of rats, during the development of gastric mucosal damage produced by intragastrically applied ethanol or HCl, dependent on time after administration of necrotizing agents (100% = 20.0 U/mg protein). [Mózsik, Sütő, Garamszegi, Jávor, Nagy, Vincze, Zsoldos: Eur. J. Gastroenterol. Hepatol. 3: 757–761, 1991 (with kind permission)].

http://dx.doi.org/10.5772/60505

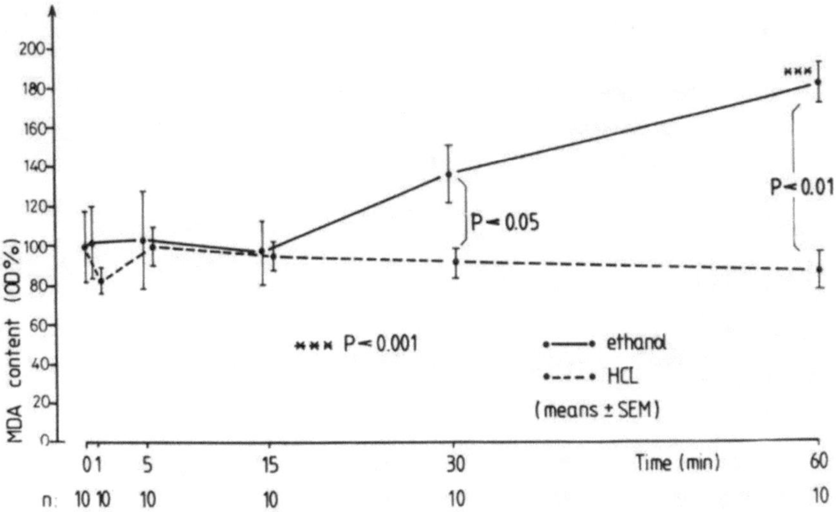

Figure 249. Changes in the tissue content of malondialdehyde (MDA) in the rat gastric fundic mucosa, during the development of gastric mucosal damage produced by intragastrically applied ethanol and HCl, dependent on time after administration of necrotizing agents (100% = 0.316 optical density/mg protein). [Mózsik, Sütő, Garamszegi, Jávor, Nagy, Vincze, Zsoldos: Eur. J. Gastroenterol. Hepatol. 3: 757–761, 1991 (with kind permission)].

	Ethanol-model					HCL - model				
Time (min)	1	5	15	30	60	1	5	15	30	60
Number of gastric lesions		↑↑↑	↑↑↑	↑↑↑	↑↑↑	↑↑↑	↑↑↑	↑↑↑	↑↑↑	↑↑↑
Severity of gastric lesions		↑↑↑	↑↑↑	↑↑↑	↑↑↑	↑↑↑	↑↑↑	↑↑↑	↑↑↑	↑↑↑
Gastric mucosal Catalase	↑					↓↓			↑↑↑	↑↑↑
Gastric mucosal GSH-px	↑↑	↑↑↑	↑↑↑	↑↑↑	↑↑↑	↑↑↑	↑↑	↑	↑↑↑	↑↑
Gastric mucosal GSH		↑	↑	↑↑		↑↑↑	↑↑	↑↑	↑↑↑	↑↑
Gastric mucosal SOD			↑	↑↑↑	↑↑↑	↑↑↑		↑↑↑	↑	
Gastric mucosal MDA					↑↑↑					

↑ = increase ↓ = decrease

↑(↓): $P < 0.05$; ↑↑(↓↓): $P < 0.01$; ↑↑↑(↓↓↓): $P < 0.001$

Figure 250. Summary of the changes in oxygen free radicals (catalase; glutathione peroxidase, GSH; reduced glutathione, GSH; superoxide dismutase, SOD and malondialdehyde, MDA) in the gastric fundic mucosa of rats treated with ethanol or HCl during the development of gastric mucosal damage dependent on time after administration of necrotizing agents. [Mózsik, Sütő, Garamszegi, Jávor, Nagy, Vincze, Zsoldos: Eur. J. Gastroenterol. Hepatol. 3: 757–761, 1991 (with kind permission).]

	TIME PERIODS AFTER ETOH (min)						TIME PERIODS AFTER HCl (min)					
	0	1	5	15	30	60	0	1	5	15	30	60
NUMBER		N	↑↑↑	↑↑↑	↑↑↑	↑↑↑		↑↑↑	↑↑↑	↑↑↑	↑↑↑	↑↑↑
SEVERITY		N	↑↑↑	↑↑↑	↑↑↑	↑↑↑		↑↑↑	↑↑↑	↑↑↑	↑↑↑	↑↑↑
ATP		N	N	↓↓↓	↓↓↓	↓↓↓		N	↓↓	↓↓↓	↓↓↓	↓↓↓
ADP		↓↓↓	↓↓↓	↓↓↓	N	N		↓↓↓	N	N	↑↑	↑↑↑
$ATP \cdot ADP^{-1}$		↑↑↑	↑↑↑	↓↓↓	↓↓↓	↓↓↓		↑↑↑	↓↓↓	↓↓↓	↓↓↓	↓↓↓
AMP		↓↓↓	↓↓↓	↓↓↓	↓↓↓	↓↓↓		↓↓	↓↓	↓↓	↓↓↓	↓↓↓
ADENYLATE POOL		↓↓↓	↓↓↓	↓↓↓	↓↓↓	↓		↓↓	↓↓↓	↓↓↓	↓	
"ENERGY CHARGE"			N	↓	↓	N		N	↑	↓	N	N
cAMP		↑↑↑	↑↑↑	↓↓↓	↓↓↓	↓↓↓		↑↑↑	↓↓↓	↓↓↓	↓↓↓	↓↓↓
LACTATE		N	N	N	N	N		N	N	N	N	N

↑ = increase ↓ = decrease

N: not changed ; ↑(↓) : $P < 0.05$; ↑↑(↓↓) : $P < 0.01$; ↑↑↑(↓↓↓) : $P < 0.001$

Figure 251. Summary of the changes in the biochemical parameters of cellular energy systems in the rat gastric fundic mucosa after intragastrically applied ethanol and HCl, dependent on time after administration of necrotizing agents (details are presented earlier). [Mózsik, Figler, Garamszegi, Jávor, Nagy, Sütő, Tárnok, Zsoldos, 1987c (with kind permission).]

The critical analyses of these results allowed us to conclude that:

1. The different changes in the experimentally measurable parameters (SOD, GSH-px, GSH, CAT and MDA) are present in gastric fundic mucosa of rats during the development of gastric mucosal damage produced by necrotizing agents, ETOH and HCl), however, these are not in a time-dependent manner;

2. The changes in the oxygen free radicals differ in the gastric fundic mucosa of rats treated with intragastrically applied necrotizing agents during the development of gastric mucosal damage, depending upon the extent of gastric mucosal damage and time after administration of necrotizing agents;

3. The measurable parameters of cellular energy systems are also detectable in the rat gastric fundic mucosa during the development of gastric mucosal damage produced by ETOH and HCl, dependent on time after necrotizing agents;

4. The changes in the parameters of cellular energy systems indicate in the same directions, however, there are differ from each other, on dependence of time after administration of necrotizing agents;

5. No close (which mathematically can be proven) the existing correlations are present in changes on experimentally measurable parameters of oxygen free radicals and of cellular energy systems in the gastric fundic mucosa of rats, treated by intragastrically applied ethanol and HCl on dependence severity (number) of gastric mucosa and on dependence of time after administrations of necrotizing agents (Mózsik et al., 1987c; Szabó et al., 2014).

8.10.2. Correlations between the oxygen free radicals and cellular energy systems in the gastric fundic mucosa of rats, during the development of gastric mucosal protection by prostacyclin (PGI_2) and β-carotene, on dependence of applied doses of protecting compounds, extent of mucosal protective effects and time after administration of EtOH and HCl

These observations were carried out in the gastric fundic mucosa of rats during the development of gastric mucosal protection produced by PGI_2 and β-carotene in which the gastric mucosal damage induced by intragastrically applied 1 mL of 0.6 M HCl and 1.0 of 96% EtOH in 1-hour observations. The results are presented in the forthcoming schematic summaries of Figures 252–255.

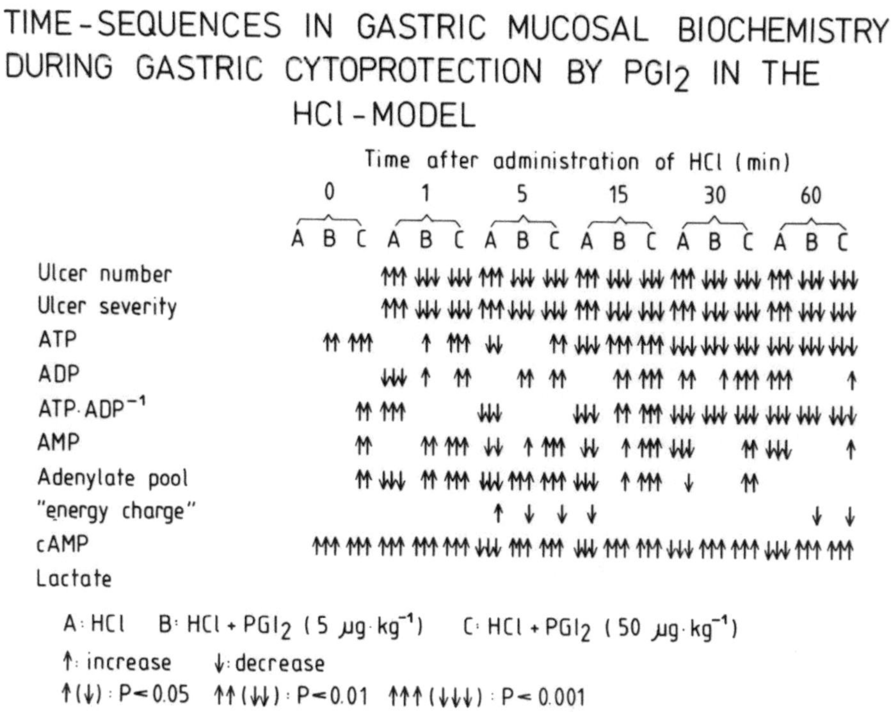

Figure 252. Summary of the changes in the parameters of cellular energy systems from the gastric fundic mucosa during the development of gastric mucosal protection of PGI_2 in rats, in which the gastric mucosal damage was produced by intragastric application of 1 mL of 0.6 M HCl (HCl model), depending upon the extents of mucosal protection, doses of PGI_2 dependent on time after administration of necrotizing and protecting agents. (Note that the PGI_2 was given 30 minutes before the HCl.) [(Mózsik, Garamszegi, Jávor, Sütő, Vincze, Tóth, Zsoldos: Mechanisms of gastric mucosal protection. In: Tsuchiya et al., 1988, Free Radical in Digestive Diseases. Elsevier Science Publishers, pp. 111–116 (with kind permission).]

Similar observations were carried out with the oxygen free radicals and cellular energy systems in the gastric fundic mucosa of rats, during the development of gastric mucosal protection of PGI_2 and β-carotene in rats, in which the gastric mucosal damage was produced by 1 mL of 96% ethanol given intragastrically in 1-hour time period. PGI_2 and β-carotene were applied 30 minutes before the application of ETOH.

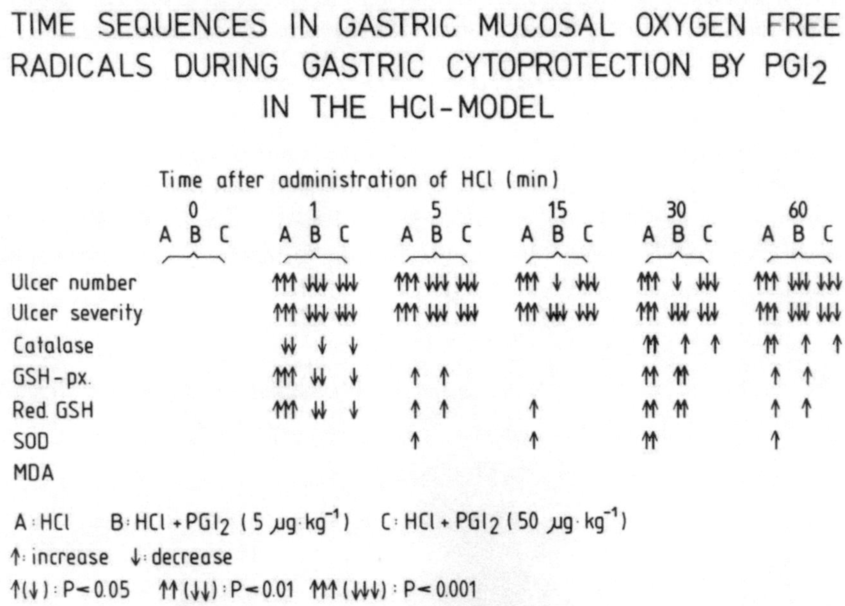

Figure 253. Summary of the changes in the parameters of oxygen free radicals in the gastric fundic mucosa during the development of gastric mucosal protection of PGI_2 in rats, in which the gastric mucosal damage was produced by intragastric application of 1 mL of 0.6 M HCl (HCl model), depending on the extents of mucosal protection, doses of PGI_2 and dependent on the time after administration of necrotizing and protecting agents. (Note that the PGI_2 was given 30 minutes before the HCl.) [Mózsik, Garamszegi, Jávor, Sütő, Vincze, Tóth, Zsoldos: Mechanisms of gastric mucosal protection. In: Tsuchiya et al., 1988, Free Radical in Digestive Diseases. Elsevier Science Publishers, pp. 111–116 (with kind permission).]

The results and correlations between the results in these experimental parameters were in ETOH model the same as those in HCl model with PGI_2 and β-carotene (these results are not presented in figures).

The following conclusions have been made from these observations:

1. The parameters of oxygen free radicals are involved in the gastric mucosa during the development of gastric mucosal-preventive effects of PGI_2 and β-carotene both in the HCl- and ETOH models in rats; however, there were no correlations depending on the doses of preventive drugs and on time after the application of necrotizing agents;
2. The changes in the parameters of cellular energy systems in the gastric fundic mucosa in HCl- and ETOH models, during the development of gastric mucosal-protective effects, are dose-dependent in the case of both PGI_2 and β-carotene depending on the extent of their mucosal-protective effects related to their characteristic to times of their different appearances, after the application of necrotizing agents;
3. The changes in both the parameters of oxygen free radicals and cellular energy systems from the rat gastric fundic mucosa, during the development of gastric mucosal damage – produced by HCl and ETOH – and the development of gastric mucosal prevention by

http://dx.doi.org/10.5772/60505

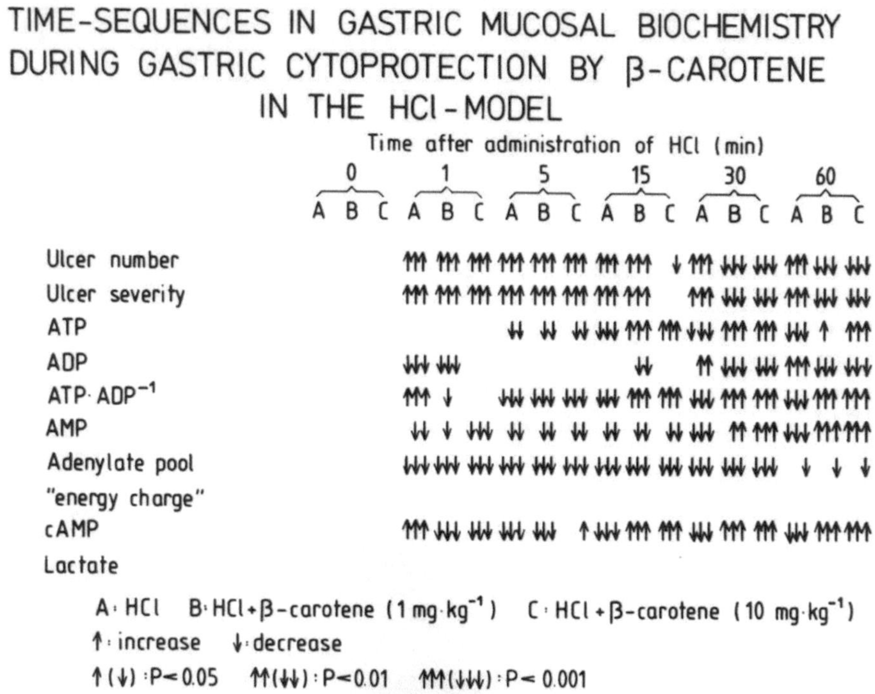

Figure 254. Summary of the changes in the parameters of cellular energy systems in the gastric fundic mucosa during the development of gastric mucosal protection of β-carotene in rats, in which the gastric mucosal damage was produced by intragastric application of 1 mL of 0.6 M HCl (HCl model), depending on the extents of mucosal protection, doses of PGI_2 and dependent on the time after administration of necrotizing and protecting agents. (Note that the PGI_2 was given 30 minutes before the HCl.) [Mózsik, Garamszegi, Jávor, Sütő, Vincze, Tóth, Zsoldos: Mechanisms of gastric mucosal protection. In: Tsuchiya et al., 1988, Free Radical in Digestive Diseases. Elsevier Science Publishers, pp. 111–116 (with kind permission).]

PGI_2 and β-carotene, are to be present; however, dose–response correlations are presented only in case of parameters of cellular energy systems versus development of mucosal damage and its prevention (in both HCl and ETOH models);

4. The changes in the parameters in oxygen free radicals and in cellular energy systems do not indicate close correlations in the gastric fundic mucosa of rats, during the development of mucosal damage produced by the intragastric administration of 1 mL of 0.6 M HCl or 1 mL of 96% ethanol and of mucosal-protective effects of PGI_2 and β-carotene in these models, depending on time after the administration of necrotizing agents and on different doses of mucosal-protective agents;

5. PGI_2 is a physiological regulatory component but not a scavenger in living bodies, while β-carotene is one of the typical scavengers; however, both of them are able to produce practically the same changes in the parameters of oxygen free radicals and in cellular energy systems in association with the gastric mucosal-protective effects on gastric

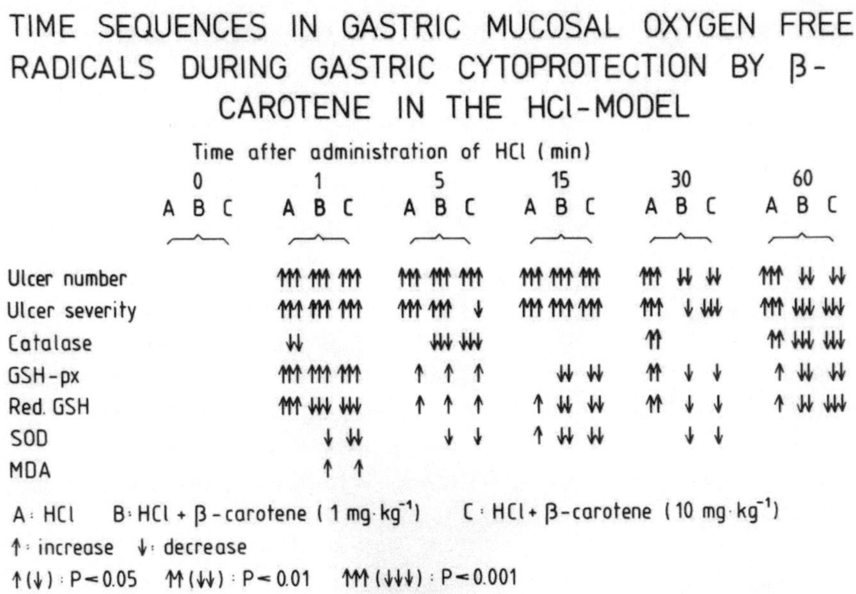

Figure 255. Summary of the changes in the parameters of oxygen free radicals in the gastric fundic mucosa during the development of gastric mucosal protection of β-carotene in rats, in which the gastric mucosal damage was produced by intragastric application of 1 mL of 0.6 M HCl (HCl model), depending on the extents of mucosal protection, doses of β-carotene dependent on the time after administration of necrotizing and protecting agents. (Note that the PGI_2 was given 30 minutes before the HCl.) [Mózsik, Garamszegi, Jávor, Sütő, Vincze, Tóth, Zsoldos: Mechanisms of gastric mucosal protection. In: Tsuchiya et al., 1988, Free Radical in Digestive Diseases. Elsevier Science Publishers, pp. 111–116 (with kind permission).]

mucosal damage produced by HCl and ETOH, suggesting that the changes run besides each other both in the development of gastric mucosal damage and its prevention.

8.12. Comparative cellular molecular pharmacology of development of gastric acid secretion in ethanol-induced gastric mucosal damage and in PGI_2-induced gastric mucosal prevention

Various drug actions and cellular mechanisms were demonstrated in the gastric fundic mucosa (especially in animal experiments). The changes of the cellular energy systems in the gastric fundic mucosa – in different animal models – suggested that "active metabolic adaptation" exists in the gastric tissues against the different ulcerogenic agents during the development of gastric mucosal damage.

There was no doubt that the prostacyclin also enhances mucosal biochemistry (including the cellular energy systems), when it was given to protect the gastric mucosal damage in rats. It is also clear that the gastric acid secretion is a consequence of an active metabolic process (involving the cellular energy systems).

In this chapter, the effects of different drugs having different subcellular mechanisms were studied in the following experimental models:

http://dx.doi.org/10.5772/60505

1. In gastric acid secretion of 4-hour pylorus-ligated rats;
2. In the development of gastric mucosal damage (number and severity) produced by 1 mL of 96% ethanol intragastrically applied in 1 hour; and
3. In the gastric mucosal prevention (number and severity) of prostacyclin (PGI_2; 5 μg/kg s.c. given at 30 minutes before the administration of 1 mL of 96% ethanol) as in point 2;

The inhibitory effects of different drugs having different subcellular mechanisms were observed in different experiments, and thereafter their affinity and intrinsic activity curves were calculated according to the methods of Csáky (1969). The value of atropine was taken to be equal to 1.0 in calculation of intrinsic activity ($\alpha_{atropine} = 1.0$).

The following drugs were used in these observations: atropine, actinomycin D, cimetidine, epinephrine, histamine, mannomustine, pentagastrin, PGI_2, ouabain and tetracycline (Table 43).

Drugs	Subcellular mechanisms
Atropine	Decrease of ATP transformation into ADP by membrane ATPase, Small increase of ATP transformation by adenylate Cyclase
Actinomycin D	Inhibition of RNA synthesis depending on DNA
Cimetidine	Inhibition of ATP-cAMP transformation by adenylate cyclase
Dinitrophenol	Inhibition of oxidative phosphorylation
Epinephrine	Decrease of ATPtransformation into ADP by membrane ATPase Increase of ATP-cAMP transformation by adenylate cyclase
Histamine	Increase of ATP-cAMP transformation by adenylate cyclase Decrease of ATP-ADP transformation by membrane ATPase
Mannomustine	Inhibition of *de novo* synthesis of DNA
Pentagastrin	Increase of ATP-cAMp transformation by adenylate cyclase Decrease of ATP transformation into ADP by membrane ATPase
PGI_2	Increase of ATP-cAMP transformation by adenylate cyclase Decrease of ATP-ADP transformation by membrane ATPase
Ouabain	Inhibition of ATP transformation by membrane ATPase
Tetacycline	Inhibition of protein translation

Table 43. Subcellular mechanisms of drugs used in the experiments. For detailed references for drug actions, see Mózsik and Jávor: Dig. Dis. Sci. 33:92–105, 1988 (with kind permission).

8.12.1. Affinity and intrinsic activity curves for drugs inhibition the gastric acid secretion in 4 hours pylorus ligated rats

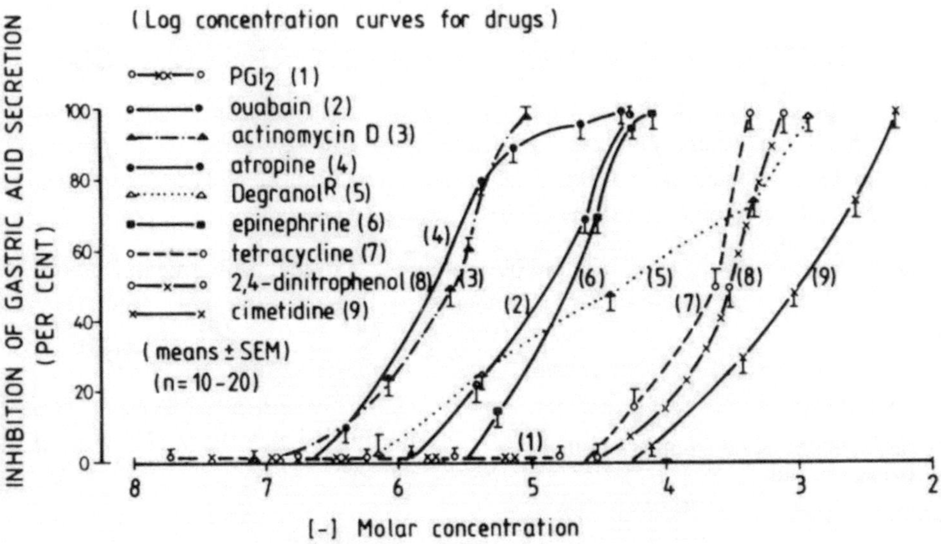

Figure 256. Affinity curves for the drugs inhibiting the gastric acid secretion in 4-hour pylorus-ligated rats. [Mózsik and Jávor: Dig. Dis. Sci. 33:92–105, 1988 (with kind permission).]

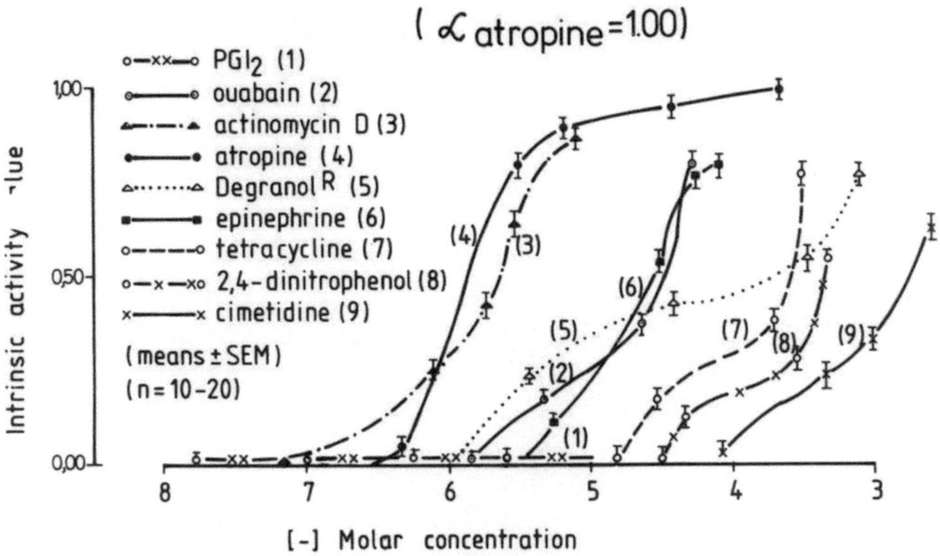

Figure 257. Intrinsic activity curves for the drugs inhibiting gastric acid secretion in 4-hour pylorus-ligated rats. [Mózsik and Jávor: Dig. Dis. Sci. 33:92–105, 1988 (with kind permission).] The values of pD_2 (dose necessary to produce 50% inhibition in the affinity curves) and of pA_2 (dose necessary to produce 50% inhibition in the intrinsic activity curves) were calculated from the affinity and intrinsic activity curves (Table 44).

http://dx.doi.org/10.5772/60505

Drugs	pD_2	α	pA_2
Atropine	5.75	1.00	5.80
Actinomycin D	5.63	0.87	5.86
Cimetidine	3.00	0.64	3.20
Mannomustine(Degranol)	4.25	0.78	4.90
Dinitrophenol	3.50	0.56	3.75
Epinephrine	4.95	0.80	4.75
PGI_2	0.00	0.00	0.00
Oaubain	4.75	0.80	4.50
Tetracycline	3.63	0.78	3.75

Table 44. Values of affinities (pD_2) and intrinsic acivities ($\alpha_{atropine}$ = 1.00 and pA_2) for drugs inhibiting the gastric acid secretion in 4-hour pylorus-ligated rats. Values are in [−] molar. [Mózsik and Jávor: Dig. Dis. Sci. 33: 92–105, 1988 (with kind permission).]

8.12.2. Affinity curves for the drugs inhibiting the development of ethanol-induced gastric mucosal damage in rats

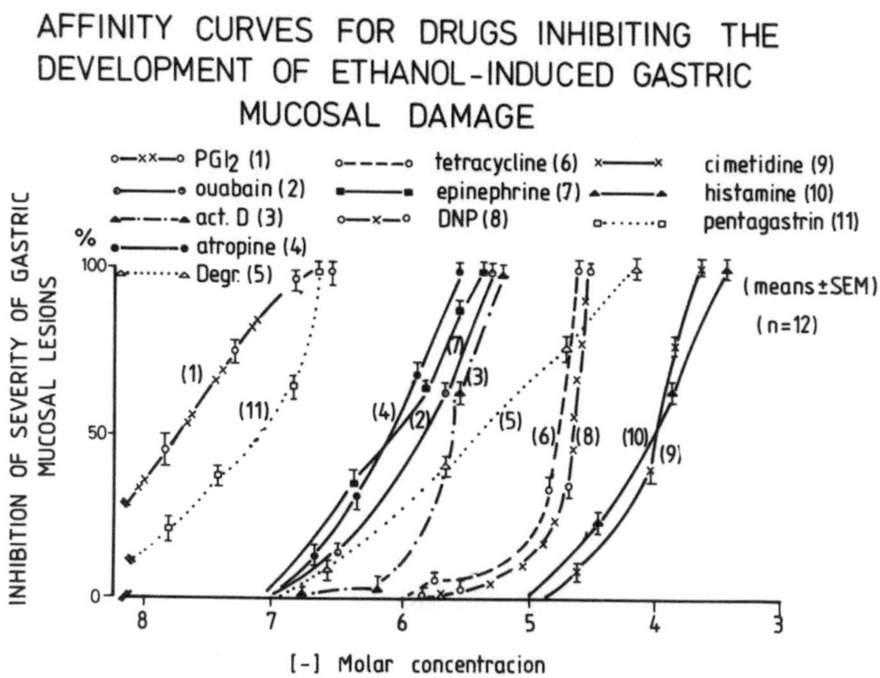

Figure 258. Affinity curves for the drugs inhibiting the development of gastric mucosal damage produced by ethanol administration in rat. [Mózsik and Jávor: Dig. Dis. Sci. 33: 92–105, 1988 (with kind permission).]

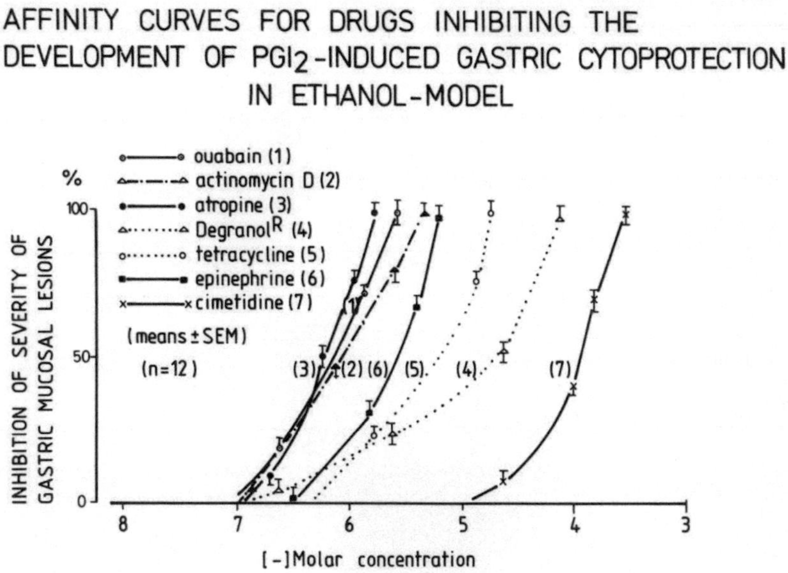

Figure 259. Intrinsic activity curves for the drugs inhibiting the development of gastric mucosal damage produced by ethanol administration in rats. [Mózsik and Jávor: Dig. Dis. Sci. 33: 92–105, 1988 (with kind permission).]

8.12.3. Affinity and intrinsic activity curves for the drugs inhibiting the PGI_2-induced gastric mucosal prevention on the gastric mucosal damage produced by ethanol in rats

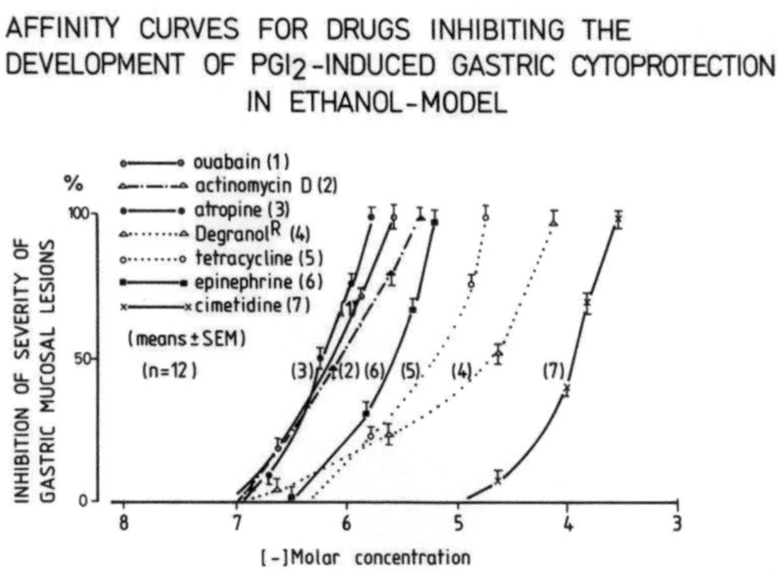

Figure 260. Affinity curves for the drugs inhibiting the PGI_2-induced gastric mucosal protection of the ethanol-produced gastric mucosal damage in rats.

http://dx.doi.org/10.5772/60505

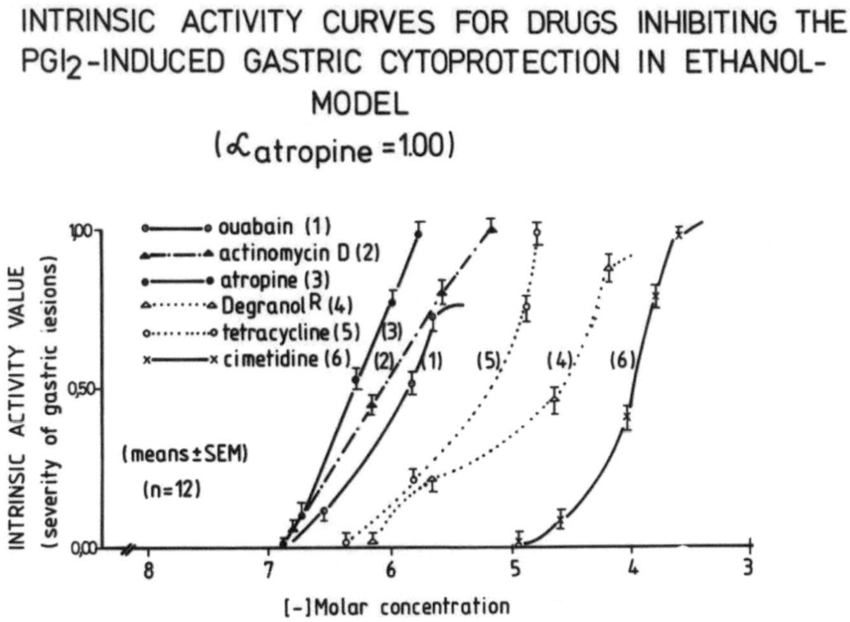

Figure 261. Intrinsic activity curves for the drugs inhibiting the PGI_2-induced gastric mucosal protection of the ethanol-produced gastric mucosal damage in rats.

8.11.4. Short discussion of results obtained from the observations presented in Sections 8.14.1–8.14.3

There were different unexpected results, when we practically noted that the examined drugs (with different subcellular mechanisms) were able to produce very similar actions on the inhibition of gastric acid secretion, ethanol-induced mucosal damage and PGI_2-induced gastric mucosal protection in the ethanol-produced gastric mucosal damage in rats (Figure 262).

The histamine, pentagastrin and dinitrophenol enhanced the PGI_2-induced gastric mucosal protection, and histamine and pentagastrin stimulated the gastric acid secretion in 4-hour pylorus-ligated rats. The contrary action of dinitrophenol (namely its inhibition of gastric acid secretion and its stimulation of the PGI_2-induced gastric mucosal protection) can be explained by the significant time difference of the experiments.

When the values of pD_2 and pA_2 were calculated, these values were practically in all of three different experimental models.

The same drugs were used to study the subcellular mechanisms of damage to the gastric mucosa by ethanol. Pentagastrin and histamine, while stimulating acid secretion, were able to reduce gastric mucosal damage due to ethanol. The effects of all drugs on both acid secretion and mucosal protection were dose-dependent. Furthermore, the molarities were similar in both types of experiments.

The following can be concluded:

1. The same subcellular mechanisms are involved in acid secretion and mucosal protection;
2. Active metabolic processes are involved in both;
3. Significant changes in membrane-bound ATP-dependent energy systems, oxidative phosphorylation, DNA and RNA synthesis, and *de novo* protein synthesis in both;
4. Ethanol-induced gastric mucosal injury can be prevented by drugs which inhibit active metabolism or those which increase active metabolic responses (histamine, pentagastrin);
5. No significant difference in effective doses on gastric acid secretion or protection against ethanol-induced mucosal injury was seen between drugs having different mechanisms of subcellular action;
6. The same subcellular mechanisms are involved in the PGI_2-induced gastric mucosal protection in ethanol-model.

SUMMARY OF DRUG EFFECT ON GASTRIC ACID SECRETION (A) DEVELOPMENT OF ETHANOL-INDUCED GASTRIC MUCOSAL DAMAGE (B) AND OF PGI_2-INDUCED GASTRIC CYTOPROTECTION IN ETHANOL-MODEL (C)

	A	B		C	
		NUMBER	SEVERITY	NUMBER	SEVERITY
Atropine	↓	↓	↓	↓	↓
Actinomycin D	↓	↓	↓	↓	↓
Cimetidine	↓	↓	↓	↓	↓
Degranol R	↓	↓	↓	↓	↓
Dinitrophenol	↓	↓	↓	↑	↑
Epinephrine	↓	↓	↓	↓	↓
Histamine	↓	↓	↓	↑	↑
Pentagastrin	↓	↓	↓	↑	↑
PGI_2	no effect	↓	↓	–	–
Ouabain	↓	↓	↓	↓	↓
Tetracycline	↓	↓	↓	↓	↓

↓ = decrease ↑ = increase

Figure 262. Schematic summary of the effects of different drugs having different subcellular mechanisms on the gastric acid secretion, development of ethanol-induced gastric mucosal damage and PGI_2-induced gastric mucosal protection in the ethanol-produced gastric mucosal damage in rats.

8.13. Epinephrine-model

As demonstrated earlier, epinephrine, given immediately after pylorus ligation, inhibited the gastric acid secretion and ulcer development (Nagy et al., 1976; Sethbakdi et al., 1970 a, b; Pfeiffer, 1971; Pfeiffer and Sethbakdi, 1971; Pfeiffer and Mózsik, 1990) (Figure 263).

http://dx.doi.org/10.5772/60505

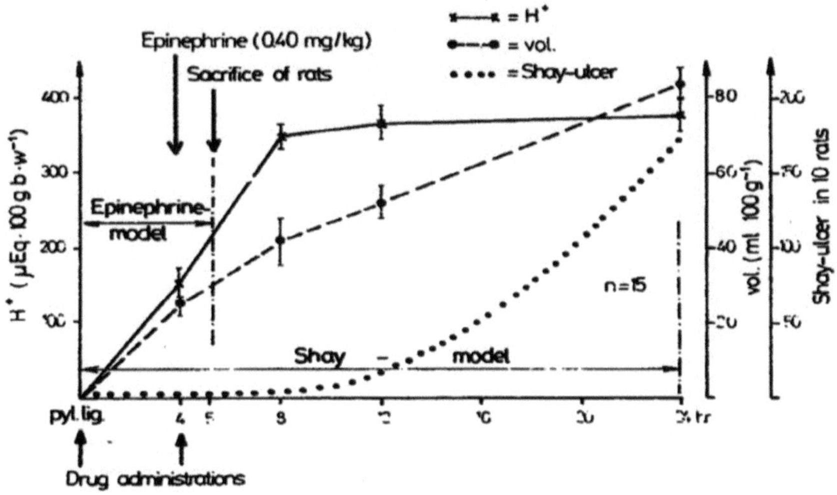

Figure 263. The schematic representation of the different ulcer provocations in pylorus-ligated rats and in epinephrine model. [Nagy, Mózsik, Tárnok, Jávor (1979) Drugs Exp. Clin. Res. 5, 87–96 (with kind permission).]

Sethbakdi et al. (1970 a, b) elaborated a new experimental model, "epinephrine model," in which the gastric ulceration appeared in the glandular stomach. Sethbakdi et al. (1970 a, b) applied epinephrine at 4 hours after pylorus ligation and the animals were sacrificed at 5 hours after the pylorus ligation. The biochemical analysis of this epinephrine model led to a new possibility to understand the mechanisms of this model (especially membrane-bound energy systems) (Mózsik and Pfeiffer, 1992).

Figure 263 indicates the time correlation between the 24-hour pylorus-ligated rats versus epinephrine model. Sethbakdi et al. found that the optimal dose of epinephrine is 0.4 mg/kg given at 4 hours after pylorus ligation, whereas the animals were sacrificed at 5 hours after pylorus ligation (that is 1 hour after the epinephrine application) (Nagy et al., 1976; 1981a; Mózsik, 1971) (Figure 264).

When we applied different doses (0.1, 0.4 and 1.0 mg/kg), the H^+ concentration, H^+ output and volume of gastric secretion dose-dependently decreased (Figure 263).

The peak of gastric mucosal injury was found after the application of 0.4 mg/kg, when different doses of epinephrine were given at 4 hours; however, the ulceration was smaller when epinephrine was given at a dose of 0.1 or 1.0 mg/kg (Figures 264, 265).

When the effect of epinephrine (given at the time of pylorus ligation) was studied (applied in a dose of 0.4 mg/kg), the tissue level of cAMP was significantly higher only in the pylorus-ligated rats; however, when epinephrine (in doses of 0.1, 0.4 and 1.0 mg/kg) was given at 4 hours after pylorus ligation, we could not notice any increase in the tissue level of cAMP (Mózsik and Pfeiffer, 1992) (Figures 267, 268). In other words, the different doses of epinephrine were not able to produce an elevation in the tissue cAMP. Therefore, cAMP-induced gastric mucosal-protective effects completely disappeared in 4-hour pylorus-ligated rats.

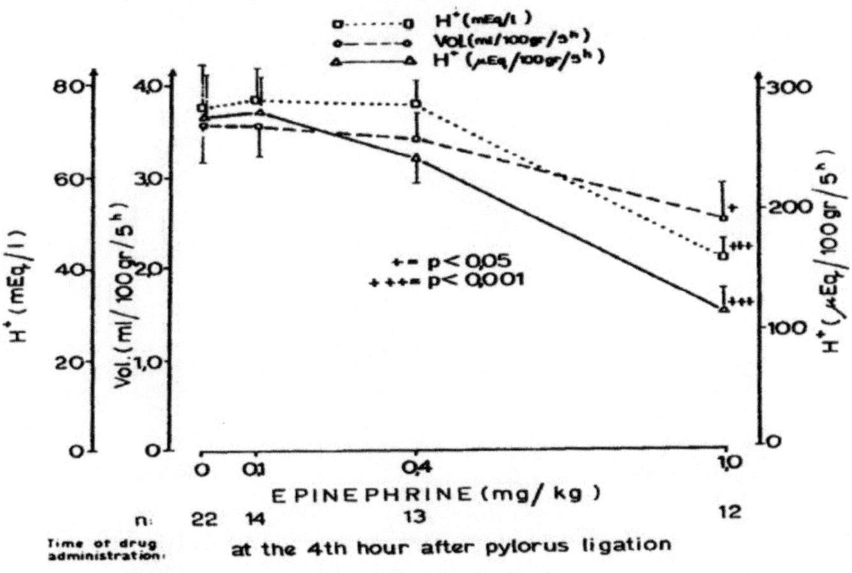

Figure 264. Dose–response curves for epinephrine on the gastric secretory responses (volumes H^+ output and H^+ concentration) in 5-hour pylorus-ligated rats, when the different doses of epinephrine were given at 4 hours after pylorus ligation. The animals were sacrificed one hour later (means ± SEM). [Nagy, Mózsik, Tárnok, Jávor (1979), Drugs Exp. Clin. Res. 5, 87–96 (with kind permission).]

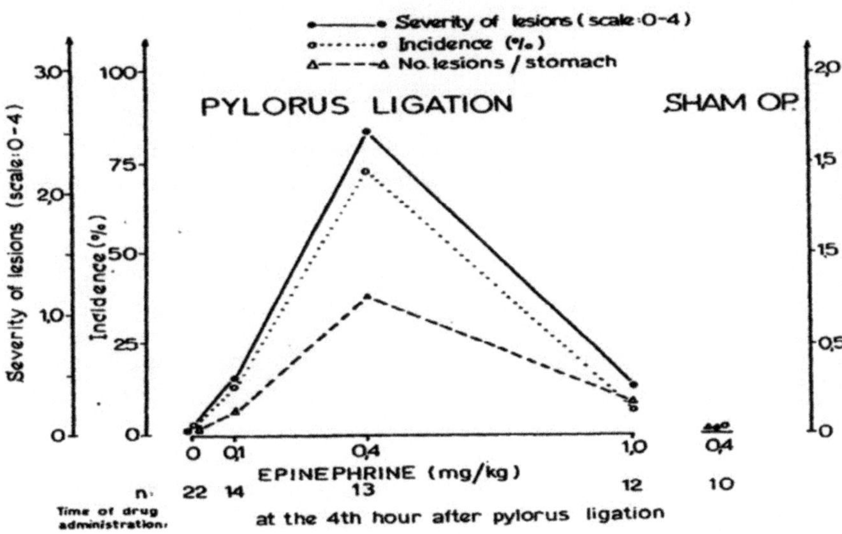

Figure 265. The extent of gastric ulcer provocation by epinephrine in 5-hour pylorus-ligated rats when the different doses of epinephrine were i.p. at 4 hours after pylorus ligation. The right side of the figure indicates epinephrine effect on the same parameters given at a dose of 0.4 mg/kg immediately after pylorus ligation (means ± SEM). [Nagy, Mózsik, Tárnok, Jávor (1979). Drugs Exp. Clin. Res. 5, 87–96 (with kind permission).]

http://dx.doi.org/10.5772/60505

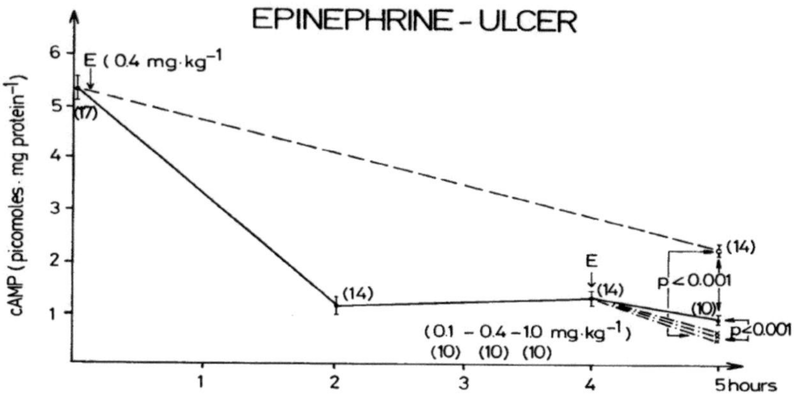

Figure 266. Changes in the tissue level of cAMP in pylorus-ligated rats when epinephrine (given at a dose of 0.4 mg/kg) was given immediately after pylorus ligation (E) and in different doses at 4 hours after pylorus ligation. The animals were sacrificed at 5 hours after pylorus ligation (means ± SEM). [Mózsik et al. (1981g). Acta Medica Acad. Sci. Hung. 36: 1–29 (with kind permission).]

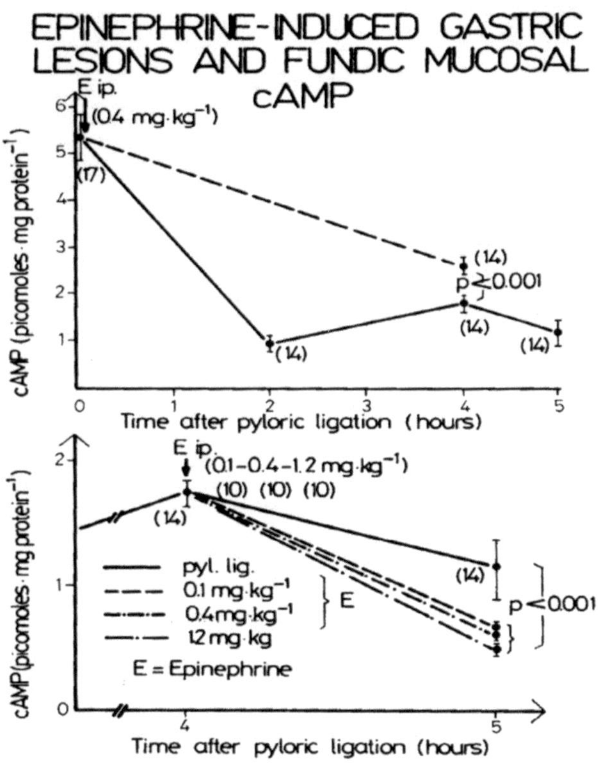

Figure 267. The epinephrine (E) induced changes in the rat gastric fundic mucosal levels of cAMP depending upon the time and doses (means ± SEM). [Mózsik et al. (1981g). Acta Medica Acad. Sci. Hung. 36: 1–29 (with kind permission).] For further explanation, see Figure 263.

8.14. Drug actions depend on the stomach cellular energy systems in dependence of different functional states of target organ

The Δ changes in the gastric fundic mucosal ATP, ADP, AMP and cAMP were detected by the application of different doses of epinephrine (0.1, 0.4 and 1.0 mg/kg) given in intact, 1 hour and 4 hours pylorus-ligated rats (Figures 268–271). These values differed significantly from each other. The largest action was obtained in intact animals, smaller in 1 hour and less values in 4-hour pylorus-ligated rats. These results together clearly indicate that the drug actions depend on the actual functional state of the target organ.

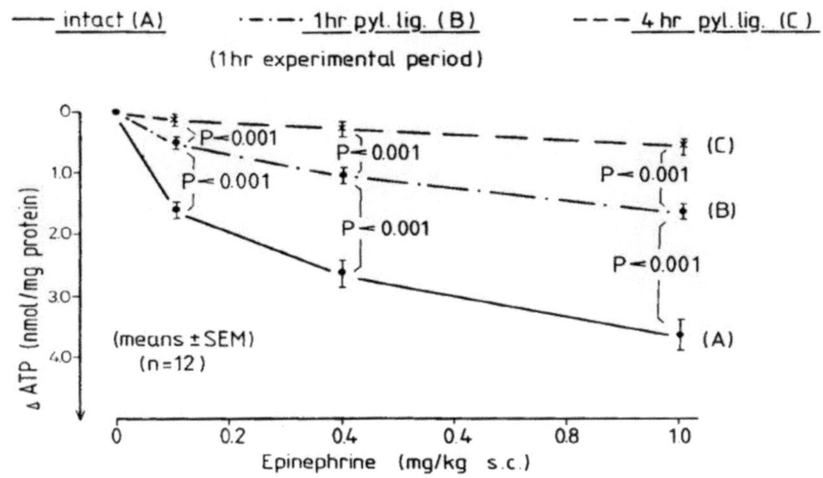

Figure 268. Δ changes in the epinephrine-induced gastric mucosal levels of ATP depending upon different functional activities of the rat gastric fundic mucosa (means ± SEM). [Mózsik and Pfeiffer, Exp. Clin. Gastroenterol 2, 190–194, 1992 (with kind permission).]

The results of observations presented in Sections 8.15 and 8.16 clearly indicate that the drug (epinephrine) effects significantly differ depending on different functional states of the target organ (presently, of stomach). Furthermore, the differences in the drug actions on the stomach – depending on the differences of its functional state – show dose-dependent actions.

In everyday medical practice, the clinicians never know exactly the etiology of peptic ulcer, when patients are diagnosed with the existence of the disease. These different conditions of the functional states of GI tract surely involved in the final efficiency of the medical treatments in patients with GI disorders as well as pathogenic roles of different noxious agents.

http://dx.doi.org/10.5772/60505

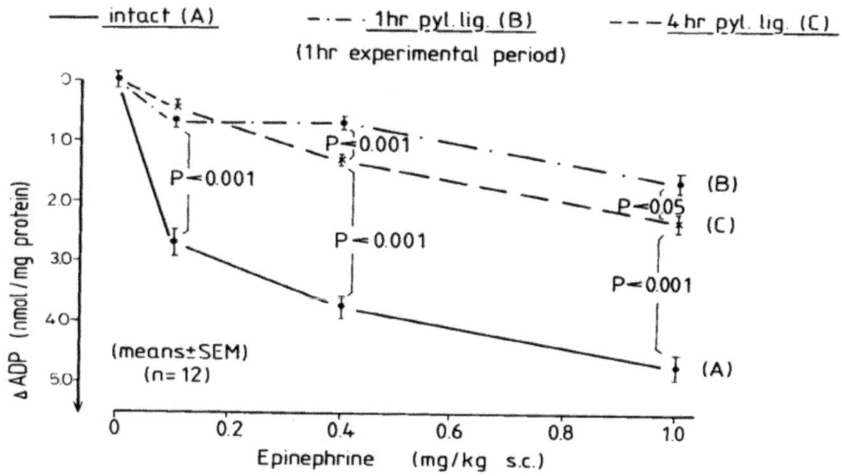

Figure 269. Δ changes in epinephrine-induced gastric mucosal level of ADP depending on different functional activities of the rat gastric fundic mucosa (means ± SEM). [Mózsik and Pfeiffer, Exp. Clin. Gastroenterol 2, 190–194, 1992 (with kind permission).] For further explanation, see Figure 263.

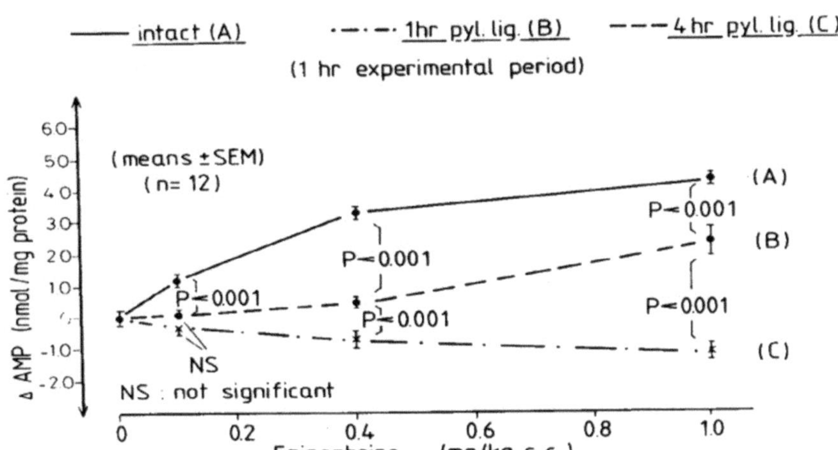

Figure 270. Δ changes in epinephrine-induced gastric mucosal levels of AMP depending upon different functional activities of the rat gastric fundic mucosa (means ± SEM). (Mózsik and Pfeiffer, Exp. Clin. Gastroenterol 2, 190–194, 1992). For further explanation, see Figure 263.

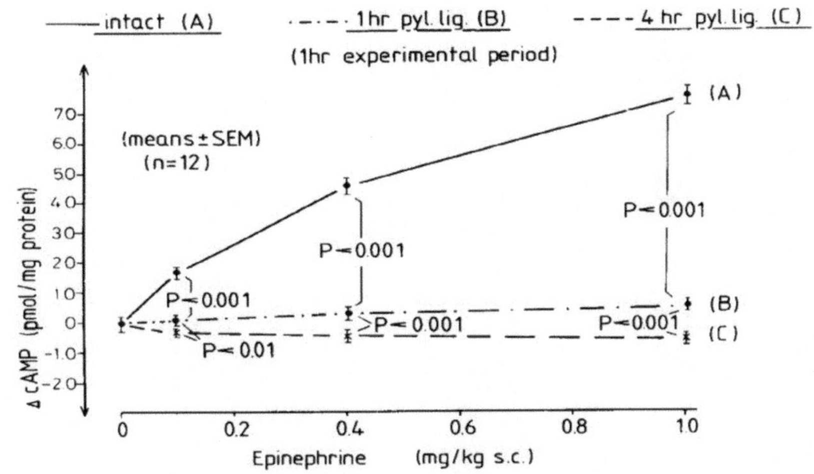

Figure 271. Δ changes in the epinephrine-induced gastric mucosal levels of cAMP depending upon different functional activities of the rat gastric fundic mucosa (means ± SEM). [Mózsik and Pfeiffer, Exp. Clin. Gastroenterol 2, 190–194, 1992 (with kind permission).] For further explanation, see Figure 263.

8.14. Surgical vagotomy and atropine-, cimetidine-, PGI_2- and ß-carotene-induced gastric mucosal damage in ETOH-model

There was no doubt after the works of Robert et al. (1979) that the small dose of PGI_2 (5 μg/kg) is able to prevent the chemically induced gastric mucosal damage.

Figure 272 clearly demonstrates that the ETOH-induced gastric mucosal damage was enhanced after bilateral surgical vagotomy. (Jávor et al., 1981; Mózsik et al., 1981a).

This observation was the first evidence to suggest that the intact vagal nerve is necessary not only in the aggression but also in the defense in the stomach (Jávor et al., 1981a; Mózsik et al., 1992 ; ütő et al.,;1989, 1992; Vincze et al.; 1992; 1993 a 1997; Király et al.,; 992 a b).

After bilateral surgical vagotomy, the gastric mucosal-protective effects of atropine (Figure 273), cimetidine (Figure 274) β-carotene (Figure 275) and PGI_2 (Figure 276) were not present.

Miller et al. (1983) published an excellent review paper on the PGs, which indicated that the gastric mucosal effect of PGs disappear after surgical vagotomy. In other papers written by his team (1983), our original observations were mentioned; however, those were completely forgotten later on in the literature (Henagan et al., 1983; Forte and Lee, 1977).

http://dx.doi.org/10.5772/60505

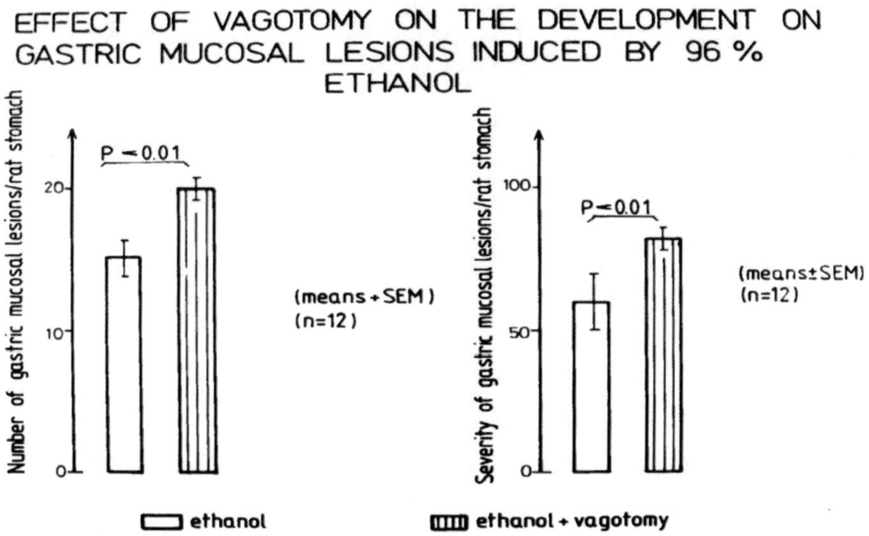

Figure 272. The ethanol-induced gastric fundic mucosal lesions (number and severity) with and without bilateral surgical vagotomy (means ± SEM). [Mózsik et al., Life Sciences 49, 1383–1388, 1991 (with kind permission).]

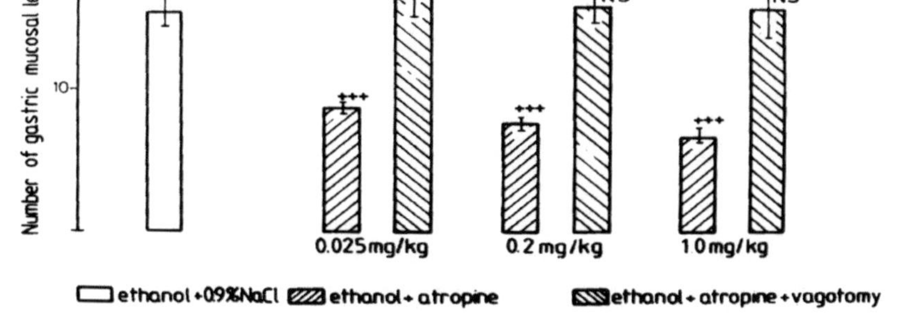

Figure 273. The atropine (given in cytoprotective and antisecretory doses)-induced gastric mucosal-preventive effects with intact vagal nerve, which disappeared completely after bilateral surgical vagotomy in ETOH model (means ± SEM). [Mózsik et al., Life Sciences 49, 1383–1388, 1991 (with kind permission).]

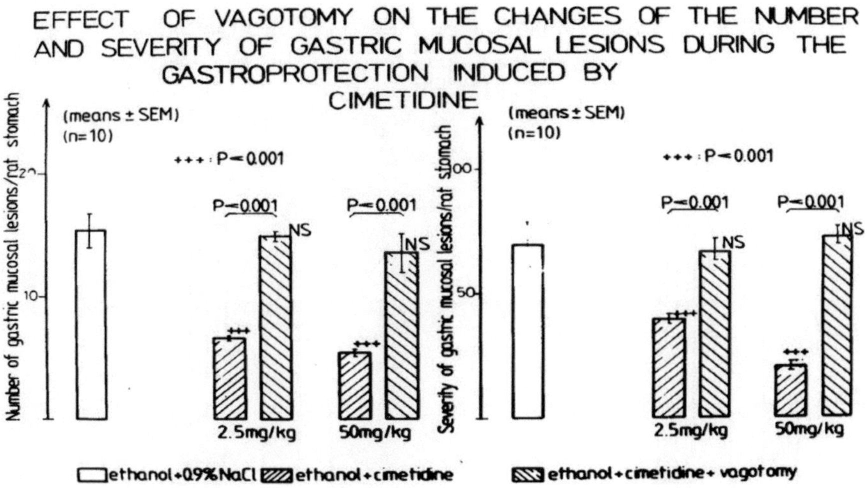

Figure 274. The cimetidine (given in cytoprotective and antisecretory doses)-induced gastric mucosal-preventive effects on the number and severity in the rat gastric fundic mucosa with intact vagal nerve and after bilateral surgical vagotomy (means ± SEM). [Mózsik et al., Life Sciences 49, 1383–1388, 1991 (with kind permission).]

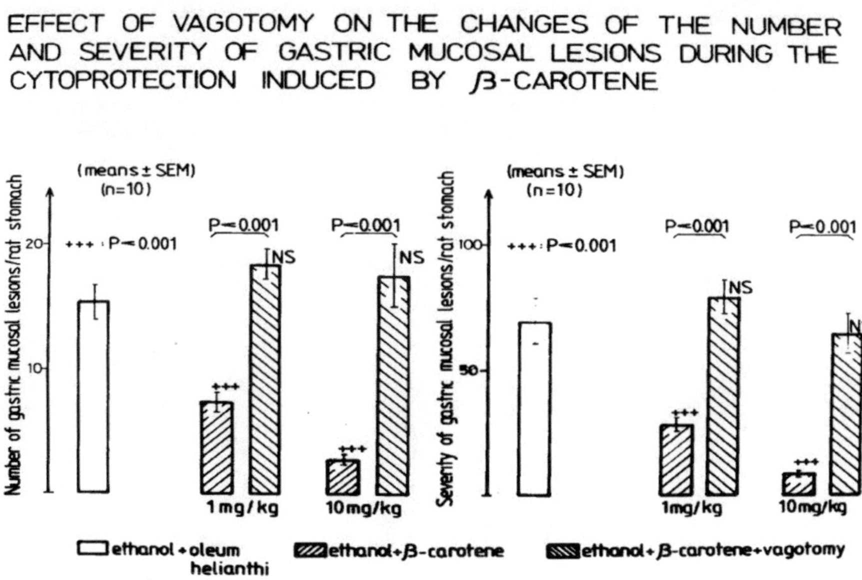

Figure 275. The β-carotene (given at doses of 1 mg and 10 mg/kg doses)-induced gastric mucosal-preventive effects on the number and severity in rats with intact vagal nerve and after bilateral surgical vagotomy in ETOH model (means ± SEM). [Mózsik et al., Life Sciences 49, 1383–1388, 1991 (with kind permission).]

http://dx.doi.org/10.5772/60505

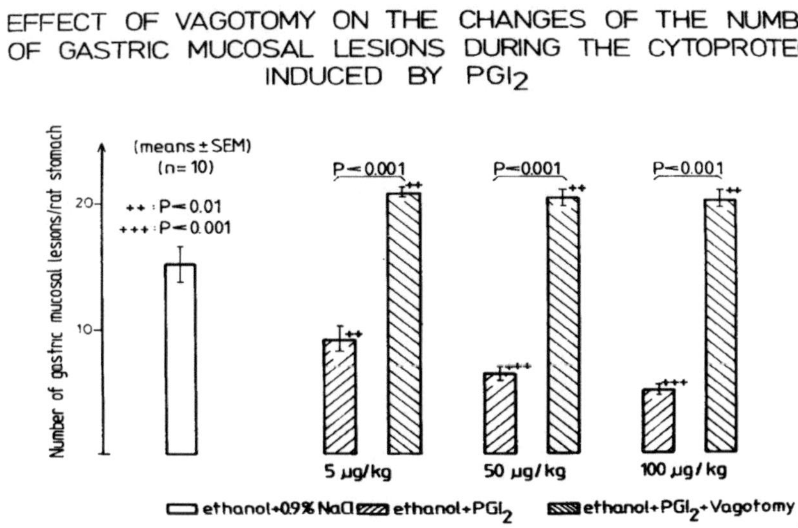

Figure 276. The PGI_2 (given at doses of 5, 50 and 100 µg/kg i.g.)-induced gastric mucosal-protective effect on the number in the rat gastric fundic mucosa treated with ETOH – in intact vagal nerve and after bilateral surgical vagotomy (means ± SEM). [Mózsik et al., Life Sciences 49, 1383–1388, 1991 (with kind permission).]

8.16. Gastric mucosal protective effects of ß-carotene and adrenals

Previously, β-carotene was used as a scavenger material. When the surgical vagotomy was able to neglegee β-carotene-induced gastric mucosal-preventive effect, we suggested that the intact adrenals are also important key factors for the development of its gastric mucosal-protective effects (Szabo et al., 1983; Sütő et al., 1989; Vincze et al., 1997).

No gastric mucosal-preventive effects of β-carotene were observed after the surgical removal of adrenals. When supplementation with glucocorticoid was performed, the gastric mucosal effects of β-carotene resumed. When supplementation with mineralocorticoid was performed, the gastric mucosal-protective effects of β-carotene did not appear.

This was another interesting observation, because the scavenger agent cannot act in rats without adrenals (Mózsik et al., 2001a).

8.16. Surgical vagotomy and tissue levels of PGE_2 and PGI_2

After surgical vagotomy, both PGE_2 and PGI_2 (6-keto-PGF-$_1\alpha$) significantly decreased (Sütő et al., 1992) (Figure 277).

The gastric mucosal-protective effect of β-carotene was dose-dependent; however, a significant difference was obtained between the effects (number) registered in animals with intact vagal nerve versus post bilateral surgical vagotomy (Figure 278).

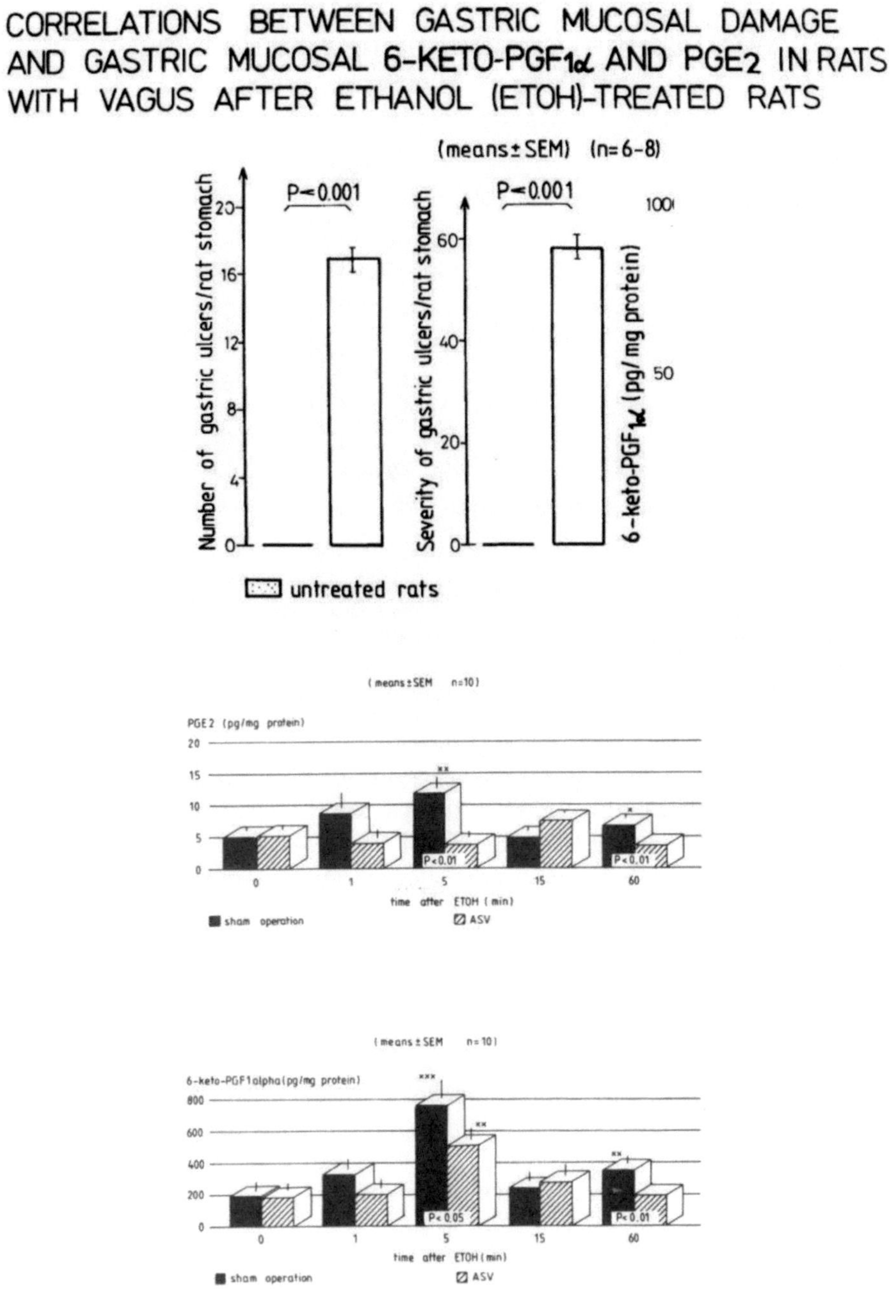

Figure 277. Surgical vagotomy-induced changes in ethanol-induced gastric mucosal damage without (untreated, sham-operated rats) and with surgical vagotomy (a) changes in levels of PGI_2, (b) 6-keto-$PGF_{1\alpha}$ (as the final product of) and (c) in the gastric mucosa (means ± SEM). [Sütő et al., Acta Physiol Hung 80, 205–211, 1992 (with kind permission).]

http://dx.doi.org/10.5772/60505

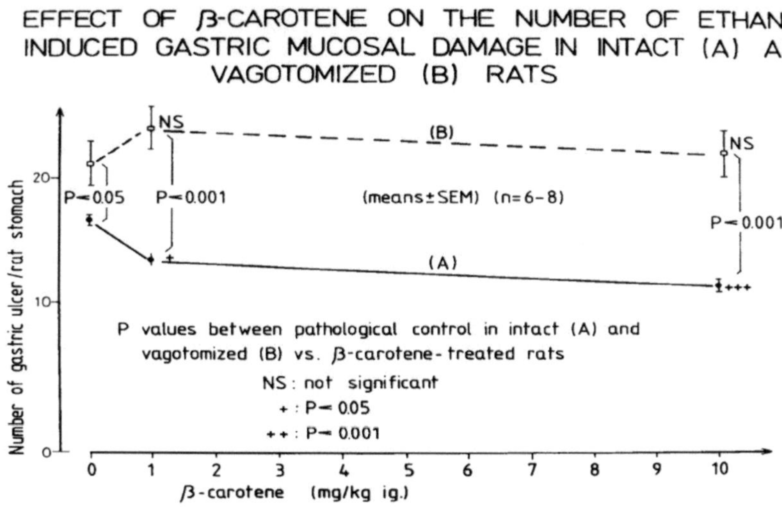

Figure 278. Dose–response curves for β-carotene in gastric mucosal damage (number) in rats treated with ETOH in animals with intact vagal nerve and after bilateral surgical vagotomy (means ± SEM). [Sütő et al., Acta Physiol Hung 85, 207–213, 1993 (with kind permission).]

8.17. Biochemical changes in the gastrointestinal tract and oxygen free radicals, scavengers in of intact vagal nerve, "surgical" and "chemical" vagotomy, intact adrenals, after adrenelectomy and supplemention of glucocorticoid and mineralocorticoid

There is no doubt that significant changes can be obtained in the oxygen free radicals during the development of the gastrointestinal mucosal damage (Mózsik et al., 1984 a, b, c). However, we expected the gastric mucosal-protective effects of retinoids in rats after surgical vagotomy (Jávor et al., 1983; Mózsik et al., 1988; Mózsik et al, 1991a; Mózsik and Jávor, 1991). Surprisingly, the gastric mucosal-protective effects of retinoids completely disappeared after bilateral surgical vagotomy (Mózsik et al., 1991a; Sütő et al., 1992). It was suggested that the presence of the intact vagal nerve and adrenals is necessary for the development of gastric mucosal-preventive effects of scavengers in animal observations.

Author details

Gyula Mozsik[1*] and Imre Szabó[2]

*Address all correspondence to: gyula.mozsik@aok.pte.hu

1 First Department of Medicine, Medical and Health Centre, University of Pécs, Hungary

2 Associate Professor at the First Department of Medicine, University of Pécs, Hungary

Chapter 9

Direct Action of Helicobacter pylori on the Freshly Isolated Rat Gastric Mucosa Cells (GMCs)

Gyula Mozsik and Imre Szabó

Additional information is available at the end of the chapter

http://dx.doi.org/10.5772/60103

9.1. General introduction

The etiological role of *H. pylori* has been suggested in the development of gastric and duodenal ulcer and it later advances to chronic atrophic gastritis and gastric cancer. Consequently, everyone tried to find suitable treatment for *H. pylori*-induced disorders. Finally, "evidence-based" therapeutic recommendations were established consisting of antibiotic combination, metronidazole and proton pump inhibitors (PPI). The efficacy of various therapeutic schemes differing by small modification has been widely studied by randomized, multiclinical, multinational studies and their meta-analysis (www.cancer.gov/cancertopics/factsheet/Risk/p-pylori-cancer; Wong et al., 1998; Molloy et al., 1998; Molloy and Sonneberg, 1997; Mabe et al., 2009).

The researchers all over the world can be divided into two groups based on their view of *H. pylori*'s importance. A larger group of researchers totally accepts the role of *H. pylori* in all abovementioned pathological conditions, including the etiological role and eradication treatment in these H. *pylori*-induced diseases. A smaller group of researchers shows a little skepticism toward the H. *pylori* as being a factor in gastric and duodenal ulcer, gastric atrophic gastritis and gastric cancer development (Mózsik et al., 2014). We did a critical analysis of gastric secretory responses (BAO, MAO) on patients with duodenal ulcer with respect to their age and duration of complaints ($n = 120$) (Mózsik et al., 1981f). Surprisingly, their MAO values remained the same in old age as those in the younger age, meanwhile the BAO values increased with respect to their age and duration of complaints. We had no information about the presence of Hel*icobacter pylori* infection at that time (for details, see Mózsik et al., 2014 a, b, c, d).

INTECH
open science | open minds

The aim of this chapter is to give a summary of the observations that are not in agreement with the main line of *H. pylori* infection and the necessity of its eradication treatment (Mózsik et al., 2014 a, b, c, d).

9.2. Testing of *Helicobacter pylori* (*H. pylori*) cultures on the isolated gastric mucosal cell

As the letters of Warren and Marshall in *Lancet* (1983) were published, a very active research chain was started throughout the world. Researchers tried to find the explanation on how *H. pylori* can lead to inflammation in the stomach and peptic ulcer.

The existence of *H. pylori* as the cause for direct damaging effect in the stomach was one of the possibilities. To answer the question, we analyzed the direct cellular effect of sonicated *H. pylori* cultured (at the level of membrane, mitochondrion and DNA) alone and with different combinations on the freshly isolated gastric mucosal cells of rat. The aggravation effect of this sonicated *H. pylori* was also examined in ethanol-induced cell injury model to evaluate the changes in cell resistance.

9.2.1. H. pyloric culture

Bacteria were obtained from human gastric and duodenal biopsy samples. Urease test and histological positivity were both required to be definite in the tissue samples. Bacterial suspensions (10^6 bacteria/mL in 20 Tris/HCl buffer, pH 7.0) were sonic on ice (30 W) in six consecutive treatments lasting 30 seconds.

9.2.2. Preparation of mixed Gastric Mucosal Cells (GMCs)

Gastric mucosal cells from 1 or 2 unfasted Sprague-Dawley strain rats were isolated by the method of Nagy et al. (1994). Briefly, the segments of glandular stomach without blood vessels surrounding the connective tissue were sequentially incubated in a physiological solution containing 0.5 mg/mL Pronase E (Type XXV Sigma Chemical Co.) and 10^{-3} EGTA. After washing for several times, the cells were resuspended and kept in shaking water bath at a temperature of 37°C in a solution (0.157 M, pH 7.4) freshly produced with the following ingredients: 98.0 mM NaCl, 5.8 mM KCl, 2.5 mM NaH_2PO_4, 5.1 mM Na pyruvate, 6.9 mM Na fumarate, 2 mM glutamine, 24.5 mM HEPES Na, 1.0 mM Trizma base, 11.1 mM D-glucose, 1.0 mM $CaCl_2$, 1.0 mM $MgCl_2$ and 2 mg/mL (w/v) bovine serum albumin. Mixed population of isolated rat GMCs contained at least three types of cells: parietal (20–25%), chief (40%) and epithelial cells (40–45%). An initial viability of 85–95% of the isolated cells was maintained for 6–7 hours. The examinations were carried out through the same media of solution.

9.2.3. Toxicological studies

9.2.3.1. H. pylori culture

Cells were incubated with sonicated *H. pylori* (10^6–10^8 bacteria /mL) for 30 minutes in the shaking water bath at 37°C. Equivalent volume of both diluted toxic agent and cell suspension were added. At the end of 30 minutes of incubation, the cells were separated from the

supernatant by centrifugation. Cell pellet was carefully resuspended and incubated for 10 minutes in the shaking water bath, before it was centrifuged again (500 g, 10 minutes) to obtain the toxic-agent-free supernatant. Cells were resuspended for further biochemical examinations.

9.2.3.2. Ethanol

Pretreated and washed cells of sonicated *H. pylori* were incubated with 15% ethanol (EtOH) for 5 minutes in shaking water bath at 37°C after the cells were treated as described above.

9.2.3.3. Indomethacin

Pretreated and washed cells were incubated with 10^{-8}–10^{-4} M indomethacin (IND) (Chinoin, Hungary) for 5 minutes in shaking water bath at 37°C. Then the cells were treated as described above.

9.2.3.4. Determination of cell viability by Trypan Blue exclusion test

Trypan Blue (TB) is excluded by viable cells, while being taken up by damaged cells, staining the cytoplasm blue (Bauer et al., 1972). A solution of 0.4% TB (Sigma Chemical Co., St Louis, USA) was mixed with the same volume of cell suspension, and 5 minutes later the rate of stained (dead) and unsustained (viable) cells were calculated as percentage of counting 100 cells in a hemocytometer.

9.2.3.5. Biochemical assays

9.2.3.5.1. Lactate dehydrogenase assay

The enzyme, lactate dehydrogenase (LDH) can be found in the cytoplasm of the cells. If it is present in the supernatant, it indicates membrane damage of cells. Its activity was determined in samples of both toxic-agent-free supernatant and the cell pellet destroyed by freezing. The calorimetric assay was based on the reduction of NAD^+ to NADH, catalyzed by LDH in the presence of lactate as a substrate (Bergmayer and Bern, 1972). The color produced by the reduction of phenazine methosulfate (Sigma Chemical Co., St. Louis, USA) and tetrazonium salt isinicotinic acid hydrazide (Sigma Chemical Co., St. Louis, USA) was measured at 520 nm by a Hitachi 124 spectrophotometer. The results were expressed as mU/min/10^6 cells.

9.2.3.5.2. Succinic dehydrogenase assay

The enzyme succinate dehydrogenase (SDH) can be found in the mitochondria. The mitochondrial integrity was tested in $2{\times}10^6$ previously treated and redispersed cells (Mosmann, 1983). The callus formazon product was quantified using a Hitachi 124 spectrophotometer at 500 nm and calculated as nmol/min/$2{\times}10^6$ cells.

9.2.3.5.3. Ethidium bromide-DNA flourescence assay

The nuclear damage of cells due to ethidium bromide–DNA-binding was assessed by nuclear rluorescence duey and Majumder, 1988) .To the ethinium bromide (EB) solution, 10^7 cells were mided withma Chemical Co., St. Louis, USA), and the fluorescence intensity was measured bny aHitachi F-3000 spectrophotometer at 325-–385 m (excitation-–emision). The results were expressed as arbitrary flouorencenceunits / 10^7clls.

9.2.3.6. Direct cellular effect of H. pylori, EtOH and IND

9.2.3.6.1. H. pylori culture alone

Sonicated 10^6–10^8 bacteria/mL had no direct cellular toxicity on freshly isolated rat GMCs by Trypan blue exclusion test (Figure 279), LDH activity (Figure 280) or ethinium bromide–DNA fluorescence (Figure 281) (Bódis et al., 1995 a, b; 1996, 2000; Mózsik et al., 1996c).

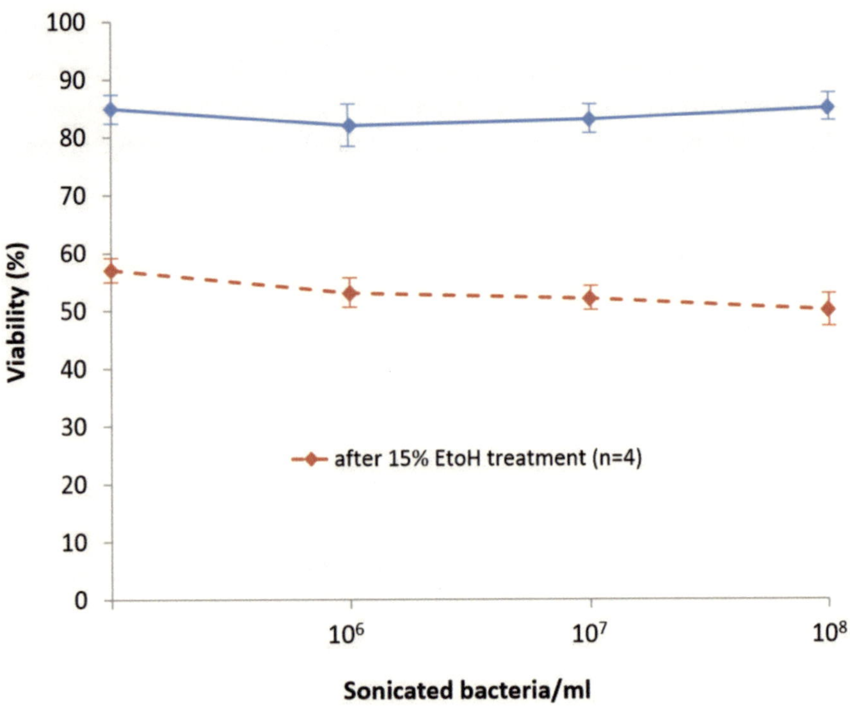

Figure 279. Effect of 30 minutes incubation with sonicated 10^6–10^8 bacteria/mL *H. pylori* on the viability of freshly isolated gastric mucosal cells of rat detected by Trypan blue exclusion test with or without 5 minutes of 15% ethanol treatment. [Bódis, Karadi, Voros, Mozsik (1995b): Has sonicated Helicobacter pylori any direct cellular effect? In: Bajtai A., Papp J., Rácz I., Simon L. (Eds.). Helicobacter pylori. Hungarian Society of Gastroenterology. Medicom, Budapest. pp. 137–142 (with kind permission).]

http://dx.doi.org/10.5772/60103

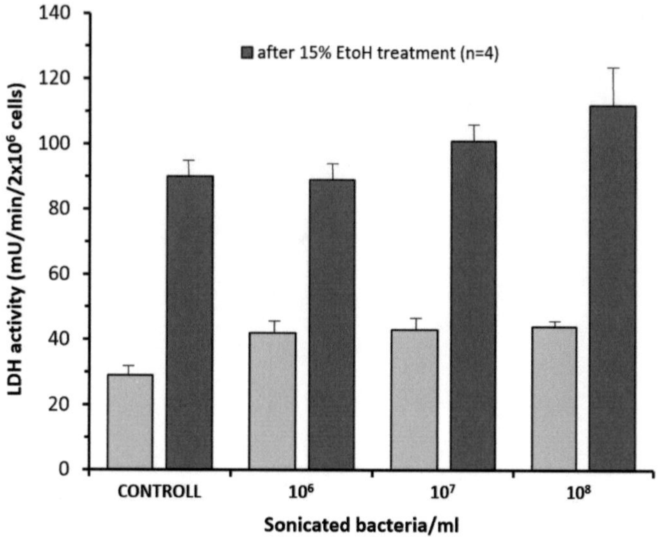

Figure 280. Changes in lactate dehydrogenase activity of freshly isolated gastric mucosal cells of rat after 30 minutes incubation with sonicated 10^6–10^8 bacteria/mLL *H. pylori* withoor without 5 minutes of 15% ethanol treatment. [(ódisBoKaradi, Voros, Mozsik (1995b): Has sonicated Helicobacter pylori any direct cellular effect? In: Bajtai A., Papp J., Rácz I., Simon L. (Eds.). Helicobacter pylori. Hungarian Society of Gastroenterology. Medicom, Budapest. pp. 137—142) with kind permission).]

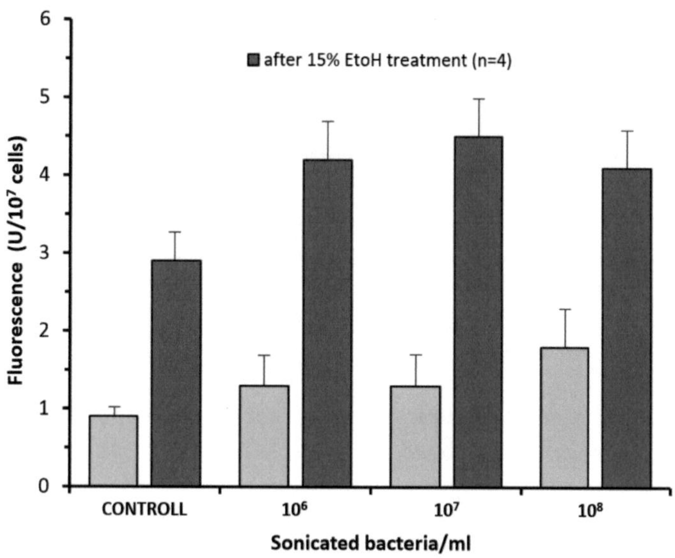

Figure 281. Changes in ethidium bromide–DNA fluorescence of freshly isolated gastric mucosal cells of rat after 30 minutes of incubation by sonicated 10^6–10^8 bacteria/mL *H. pylori* with or without 5 minutes of 15% ethanol treatment. [Bódis, Karadi, Voros, Mozsik (1995b): Has sonicated Helicobacter pylori any direct cellular effect? In: Bajtai A., Papp J., Rácz I., Simon L. (Eds.). Helicobacter pylori. Hungarian Society of Gastroenterology. Medicom, Budapest. pp .137–142 (with kind permission).]

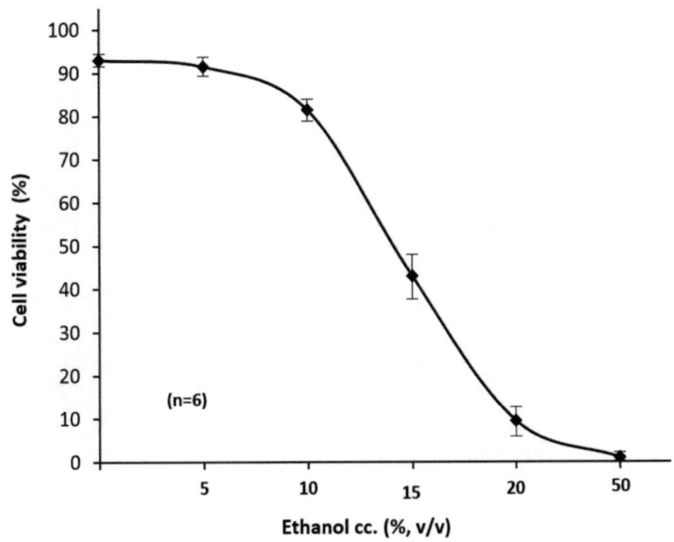

Figure 282. Changes in the viability of acutely (freshly) isolated rat gastric mucosal cells after 5 minutes incubation of 5–50% (v/v) ethanol detected by Trypan blue test. The EC_{50}=13.5%. [Bódis et.al., (1996): Dig.Dis.Sci.41:430; Bódis, Németh, Mózsik (1998). Akadémiai Kiadó, Budapest (with kind permission).]

9.2.3.6.2. Combined effect of H. pyloriand EtOH

Pre-incubation of cells with sonicated *H. pylori* (10^6–10^8 bacteria/mL) did not aggravate the 15% EtOH-induced cell injury detected by TB (Figure 282) and biochemical assays (Bódis et al., 1995b, 1996, 1997 a, b, 1998).

9.2.3.6.3. Combined effects of H. pylori and Indomethacin (IND)

After 5 minutes incubation of 10^{-8}–10^{-3} M indomethacin, only high doses (10^{-4}–10^{-3} M) of IND significantly decreased ($P< 0.01$) the number of viable cells (Figure 283).

When the IND and *H. pylori* (10^7 sonicated bacteria/mL) were applied in combination, the number of viable cells was not changed compared with IND treatments alone (Figure 283), and no changes were obtained by biochemical assays (Figures 284, 285).

9.2.3.6.4. Combined effect of EtOH and IND

Using these toxic agents, IND and all doses significantly aggravated the 15% EtOH-induced cell injury determined by Trypan blue exclusion (Bódis et al., 1995 a, b, 1996, 1998).

In these studies, the direct effects of sonicated *H. pylori* were examined under different experimental conditions (when it was given alone or in combination with EtOH and IND).

http://dx.doi.org/10.5772/60103

This model was suitable to eliminate the additional effect of immune systems, which is usually involved in a bacterial infection.

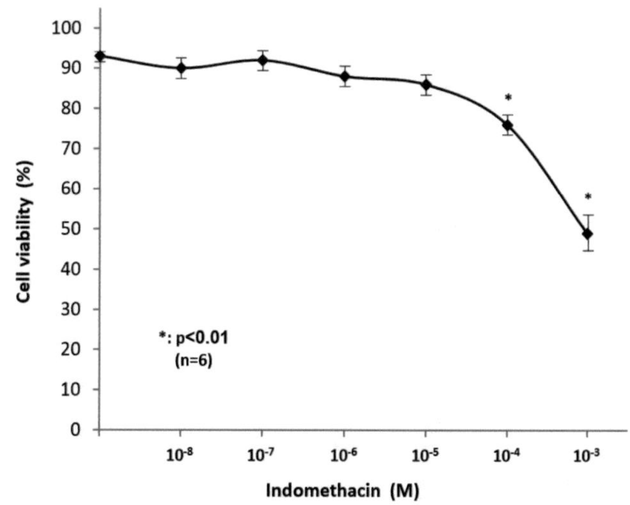

Figure 283. Changes in the viability of acutely (freshly) isolated rat gastric mucosal cells after 5 minutes incubation of 10^{-8}–10^{-3} M indomethacin (IND) detected by Trypan Blue exclusion test.*$P<0.01$ compared with untreated cells. [Bódis, Németh, Mózsik (1998). Akadémiai Kiadó, Budapest (with kind permission).]

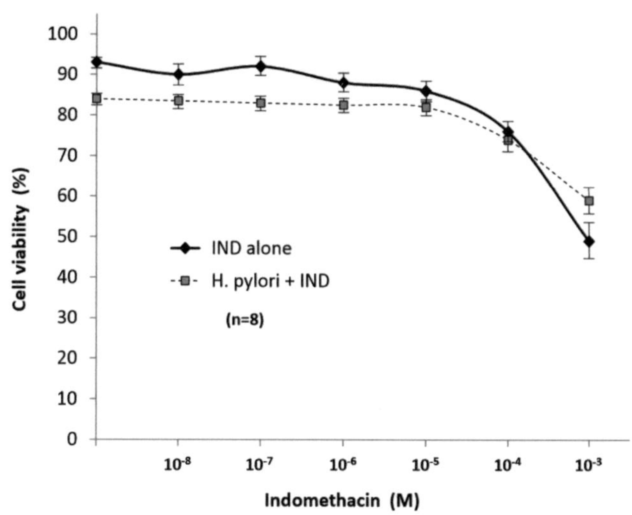

Figure 284. Effects of indomethacin (given in doses of 10^{-8}–to 10^{-3} M concentrations) with and without co-administration of sonicated *H. pylori* (given in a dose of 10^{7} bacteria/mL together with all doses of indomethacin) on the viability of acutely (freshly) isolated gastric rat mucosal cells by Trypan Blue test. The incubation time was 30 minutes in all cases. [Bódis, Németh, Mózsik 1998. Akadémiai Kiadó, Budapest (with kind permission).]

We found that sonicated *H. pylori* had no direct cellular toxicity.

These types of observations with freshly isolated gastric mucosal cells from rat stomach were widely used to study the direct actions of various aggressive and protective compounds under experimental conditions.

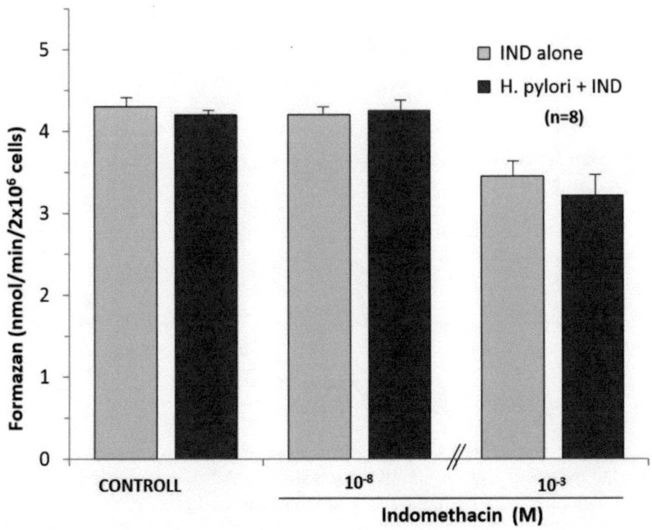

Figure 285. Effects of indomethacin (given in doses of 10^{-8}–10^{-3} M concentrations) alone and in co-administration with sonicated *H. pylori* (given in 10^7 bacteria /mL together with all doses of indomethacin) on the succinate dehydrogenase activity of acutely (freshly) isolated rat gastric mucosal cells. The incubation time was 30 minutes in all cases. [Bódis, Németh, Mózsik (1998). Akadémiai Kiadó, Budapest (with kind permission).]

For the correct understanding, the results obtained with H. pylori (given alone or in combinations with EtOH or IND) have to be emphasized:

1. Rat (as animal strain) might not be the best model to study the possible gastric mucosal damaging mechanisms involved in *H. pylori* infection. Mongolian gerbil might be a better animal model to evaluate the mechanisms of *H. pylori*-induced pathology (Takahashi et al., 1998);

2. This *in vitro* model is an excellent model to study the direct cellular reactions of different chemical and hormonal, natural compounds (EtOH, IND, pentagastrin, histamine, body protective compound, BPC, etc.);

3. This experimental model is widely used in the research for preclinical selection of various drug candidates (Nagy et al., 1994);

4. No absolute correlation exists between the direct cellular damaging and defending effects of different biological agents and chemical compounds obtained in freshly isolated gastric mucosal cells and *in vivo* observations (Bódis et al., 1998).

http://dx.doi.org/10.5772/60103

Author details

Gyula Mozsik[1*] and Imre Szabó[2]

*Address all correspondence to: gyula.mozsik@aok.pte.hu

1 First Department of Medicine, Medical and Health Centre, University of Pécs, Hungary

2 Associate Professor at the First Department of Medicine, University of Pécs, Hungary

Chapter 10

Studies on the Stable Cell Lines (Gastric Cancer, Hepatoma, Colorectal Cancer, Mouse Myeloma)

Gyula Mozsik and Imre Szabó

Additional information is available at the end of the chapter

http://dx.doi.org/10.5772/60104

10.1. Introduction

The original term "gastric cytoprotection" described by Robert in 1979 (Robert, 1979; Robert et al., 1979) has new meaning nowadays. The "cytoprotection" expression has been limited to the level of cells, and new concepts have been defined, such as histoprotection and organo-protection (gastroprotection), which are widely accepted and recently studied in experiments searching for other fields of gastroenterology (e.g., hepatology). In these *in vivo* investigations, many environmental factors, such as central nervous system (Grijalva and Novin, 1990), vagal nerve (Mózsik et al., 1993 a, b, 1992 a, b, c, d), blood flow (Szabó et al., 1985; Guth et al., 1984), vascular permeability (Szabo et al., 1985) and rapid epithelial restitution of neck cell (Lacy et al., 1984), were studied as a part of defense mechanisms of the gastric mucosa.

The *in vivo* and *in vitro* experiments essentially differ from each other. *In vitro* investigations on isolated cells have many advantages. Ali of the environmental effects originated from other organs, tissues can be eliminated, so the behavior of a single cell can purely be examined. Unfortunately, these kinds of studies might have harmful consequences. The acutely isolated cells are less suitable for pharmacological studies than the gastric mucosa *in vivo* experiments because of their isolation procedure (Nagy et al., 1994).

The stress may reduce the cell responsiveness; surface receptors are damaged during the digestive stages of the isolation procedure. These effects are eliminated by using stable cultured cells in the experiment, though they are few in number and some properties of the tumor origin can be seen in their behavior.

Ethanol (EtOH) is widely used as a toxic agent in the gastric cytoprotection investigations *in vivo* (Nagy et al., 1994; Djahanguiri, 1969; Brodie et al., 1970; Karádi et al., 1994; Lacy et al., 1982). Indomethacin (IND) is also generally used for experiments (Djahanguiri, 1969; Brodie et al., 1970; Nagy et al., 1994). It inhibits prostaglandin synthesis, which is responsible for the maintenance of gastric mucosal integrity due to the stimulation of mucosal blood flow,

preservation of cellular-ion transport and protection of the mucosal proliferative zone (Lacy and Ito, 1982). These chemical agents have been widely studied *in vivo* experiments, but only a few experiments have been carried out *in vitro* on isolated cells or cell lines with these toxic agents.

Various chemicals have been known and used as cytoprotective agents in the investigation of gastric, liver, pancreatic and large bowel protection; quite a few of them are scavengers (β-carotene, DMSO, DMPO, GSH and mannitol).

10.2. The aims of this present study were the followings

- To analyze the toxic effect of 5-minute EtOH treatment *in vitro* on acutely isolated mixed gastric mucosal cells (GMC) and on stable cultured cell lines;
- To compare the differences between the GMC and stable cultured cells – myeloma (Sp2/0-Ag14) and hepatoma (Hep G2) cell lines;
- To evaluate the differences between the myeloma (Sp2/0-Ag14) and hepatoma (Hep G2) cell lines;
- To study the effect of IND on GMC and Sp2/0-Ag14 cells;
- To examine the combined effect of EtOH and IND on these two types of cells;
- To analyze the toxic effect of EtOH after an alcohol-dehydrogenase enzyme inhibitor treatment (we used pyrazole for inhibition);
- To examine the scavenger effect of dimethyl sulfoxide (DMSO), glutathione (GSH) and β-carotene on these two types of stable cultured cells.

10.3. Materials and methods

10.3.1. Preparation of mixed gastric mucosal cells

Gastric mucosal cells from Sprague-Dawley rats were isolated by the method of Nagy et al. (1994). The segments of the glandular stomach were separated from the blood vessels and the surrounding connective tissue and were incubated in a physiological solution containing 0.5 mg/mL pronase E (type XXV, Sigma Chemical Co.) and 10^{-3} mol/L EGTA. After several washings, the cells were resuspended in a solution (0.157 mol/L, pH 7.4) produced freshly with the following ingredients: 98.0 mmol/L NaCl, 5.8 mmol/L KCl, 2.5 mmol/L Na_2P0_4, 5.1 mmol/L sodium pyruvate, 6.9 mmolJL sodium fumarate, 2.0 mmol/L glutamine, 24.5 mmol/L HEPES-Na, 1.0 mmol/L Trizma base, 11.1 mmol/L D-glucose, 1.0 mmol/L $CaCl_2$, 1.0 mmol/L $MgCl_2$ and 2.0 mg/mL (w/v) bovine serum albumin. AH examinations were carried out in this solution.

10.3.2. Stable cultured cells

Sp2/0-Ag14 (CRL 1581) is a non-secreting mouse myeloma; Hep G2 is a human hepatocellular carcinoma cell line obtained from the American type culture collection (ATCC). Cells were

http://dx.doi.org/10.5772/60104

cultured and the examinations were carried out in Dulbecco's modified Eagle's medium containing 10% fetal calf serum in a humidified incubator that held 95% air and 5% CO_2 at 37°C.

10.3.3. Toxicological studies

The cells were incubated with different concentrations of EtOH (1, 5, 10, 15, 20 and 50%) (v/v), IND (10^{-8}–10^{-3} mol/L dissolved in 5% $NaHC0_3$, pH 7.4 with 5 N HCI) and their combination (15% EtOH and 10^{-3} mol/L IND) for 5 minutes in a shaking water bath at 37°C. Each study used 10^5 cells. Alcohol-dehydrogenase inhibitor pyrazol was used during and after the EtOH treatment in the concentration of 10^{-5} mol/L. After 5 minutes of incubation, the cells were separated from the supernatant by centrifugation (500 g, 10 minutes), washed out (10 minutes water bath and centrifugation again) and resuspended in a toxic-free medium.

10.3.4. Cytoprotective studies

In the cytoprotective studies, the DMSO was used in the concentration of 10^{-3} mol/L. The GSH was applied to our medium in two concentrations: 10^{-4} mol/L and 10^{-3} mol/L. The 10% water-soluble β-carotene from Sigma was used in three concentrations: 10^{-8}, 10^{-7} and 10^{-6} mol/L.

1.3.5. Trypan blue exclusion test

Trypan blue is taken up by damaged cells, staining the cytoplasm blue; viable cells can resist this staining. Trypan blue (0.2%) was mixed with the same volume of cell suspension and, after 5-minute latency, the numbers of stained (dead) and unstained (viable) cells were calculated as percentages in a hemocytometer. In comparison with stable cultured cells, we examined the viability for longer periods (5 minutes, 60 minutes, 4 hours and 24 hours) after the 5-minute EtOH incubation.

Statistics

Values in figures and text are expressed as means ± SEM. Comparisons were performed using the unpaired Student's *t*-test, and *P*-values were considered significant at $P < 0.05$.

10.4. Results

10.4.1. Result of the toxicological studies

10.4.1.1. Effect of EtOH on GMC

EtOH (1, 5, 10, 15, 20 and 50%) concentration-dependently decreased the viability of GMC. The EC_{50} was 13.5% (Figure 286).

10.4.1.2. Effect of EtOH on the Sp2/0-Ag14 cell line

The EtoH decreased the viability of the stable cultured cells in concentration- dependently. In the case of Sp2/0-Ag14 cells, there is no significant difference between the viability values

obtained at 5 and 60 minutes, but 4 hours after the incubation with 10 and 15% of EtOH, a significant cell loss (secondary cell destruction) could be detected (Figure 287).

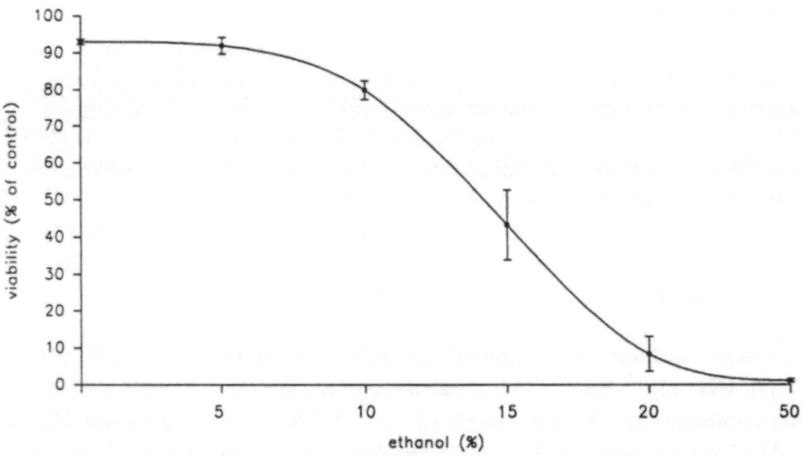

Figure 286. Changes in the viability of acutely isolated rat gastric mucosal cells after 5 minutes of incubation with 1–50% ethanol, detected by Trypan blue exclusion test (percentage of control). The results are expressed as means ± SEM ($n = 5$).

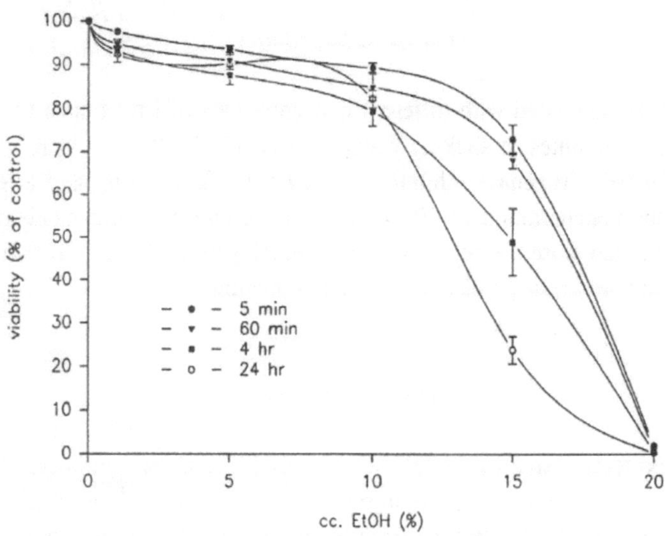

Figure 287. Changes in the viability of Sp2/0-Ag14 cells after 5 minutes of incubation with 1–20% ethanol (EtOH) counted at 5 minutes, 60 minutes, 4 hours and 24 hours by Trypan blue exclusion test. The results are expressed as means ± SEM (n=5). * : $P < 0.01$ compared to 4-hour value. [Szabo et al. (1997a) Inflammopharmacology 5:20–28 (with kind permission).]

http://dx.doi.org/10.5772/60104

10.4.1.3. Effect of EtOH on the Hep G2 cell line

In the case of Hep G2 cell line, a higher resistance was found up to 15% of EtOH concentration than in the case of Sp2/0-Ag14 cells. Above that concentration, a similar level of cell destruction occurred. During the 5-minute incubation of Hep G2 cells with various concentration of EtOH (1–20%), secondary cell destruction could not be detected (Figure 288).

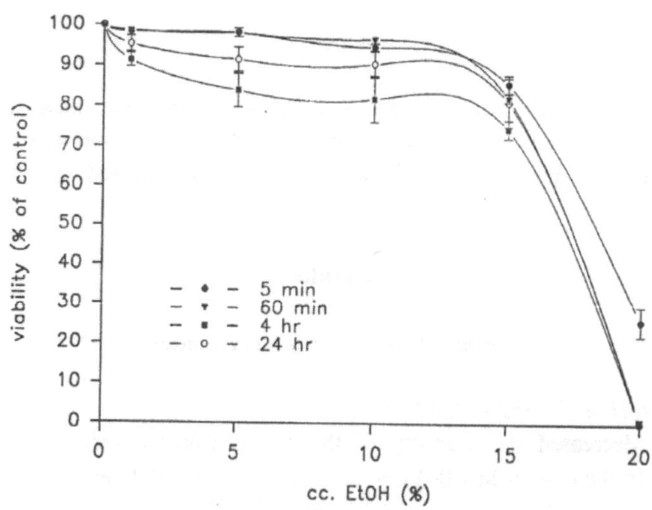

Figure 288. Changes in the viability of Sp2/0-Ag14 cells after 5 minutes of incubation with 1–20% ethanol (EtOH) counted at 5 minutes, 60 minutes, 4 hours and 24 hours by Trypan blue exclusion test. The results are expressed as means ± SEM (*n*=5). * : $P < 0.01$ compared to 4-hour value. [Szabo et al. (1997a) Inflammopharmacology 5:20–28 (with kind permission).]

10.4.1.4. Comparing gastric mucosal cells(GMCs) and stable cultured cells

At all concentrations, the EtOH decreased the viability of GMC much more potently than the viability of the stable cultured cells. The EC_{50} for GMC was 13.5%; the EC_{50} for Sp2/0-Ag14 was 16% (Figures 287 and 288).

10.4.1.5. Effect of IND

Five minutes of incubation with 10^{-8}–10^{-3} mol/L IND had no effect on the viability of Sp2/0-Ag14 cells. In the case of GMC, only the highest dose (10^{-3} mol/L) of IND decreased the number of viable cells significantly ($P < 0.02$) (Figure 289).

10.4.1.6. Combined effect of EtOH and IND

After the combined treatment, greater cell destruction could be detected. While using different concentrations, the 10^{-3} mol/L dose was the most aggressive; the amount of necrotic cell loss

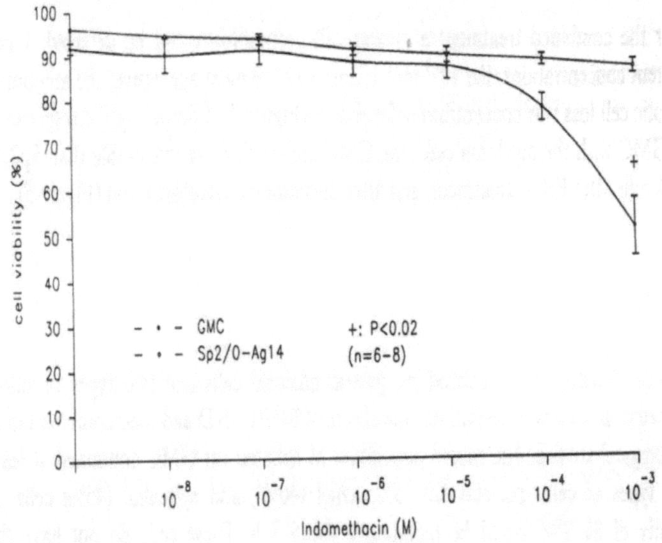

Figure 289. Changes in the viability of GMC and Sp2/0-Ag14 cells after 5 minutes of incubation with 10^{-8}–10^{-3} mol/L indomethacin, detected by Trypan blue exclusion test (percentage of control). The results are expressed as means ± SEM (n = 6–8). * :$P < 0.02$ compared with GMC. [Szabo et al. (1997a) Inflammopharmacology 5:20–28 (with kind permission).]

was concentration-dependent (Figure 290). Comparing the response of the GMC with the myeloma cells, the GMC are much more vulnerable than Sp2/0-Ag14 cells after the EtOH treatment and after the combined treatment too (Figure 291).

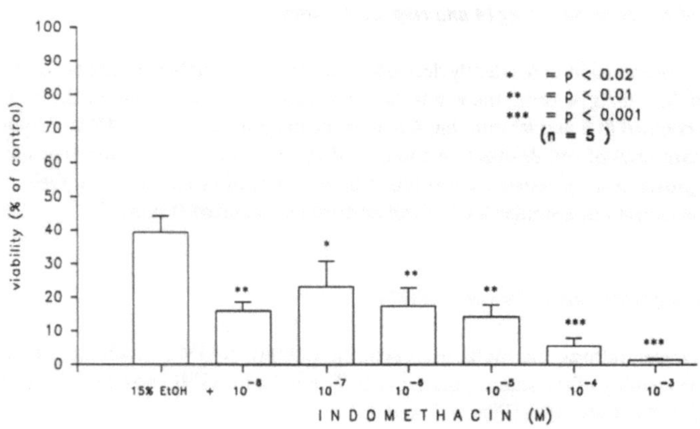

Figure 290. Changes in the viability of gastric mucosal cells (GMCs) after combined incubation with 15% ethanol and 10^{-8}–10^{-3} mol/L indomethacin, detected by Trypan blue exclusion test (percentage of control). The results are expressed as means ± SEM (n = 5). * : $P < 0.02$, ** : $P < 0.01$, *** : $P < 0.001$ compared with 15% EtOH alone. [Szabo et al. (1997a) Inflammopharmacology 5:20–28 (with kind permission).]

http://dx.doi.org/10.5772/60104

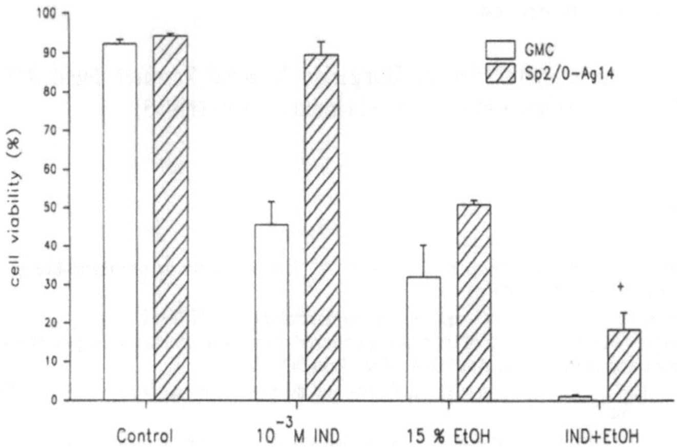

Figure 291. Changes in the viability of GMC and Sp2/0-Ag14 cells after 5 minutes of incubation with 15% ethanol (EtOH), 10^{-8}–10^{-3} mol/L indomethacin (IND) and 15% EtOH and 10^{-3} mol/L IND combined, detected by Trypan blue exclusion test (percentage of control). The results are expressed as means ± SEM (n = 6–8). + $P < 0.01$ compared with GMC. [Szabo et al. (1997a) Inflammopharmacology 5:20-28] with kind permission).]

10.4.1.7. Comparison of myeloma (Sp2/0-Ag14) cells and hepatoma (Hep G2) cells after pyrazole treatment

The viability values of the Sp2/0-Ag14 cells, compared to the values of EtOH treatment, did not change during the 5-minute co-incubation of the alcohol-dehydrogenase inhibitor pyrazole and EtOH (Figure 292).

In the case of Hep G2 cells, adding pyrazole to the incubation medium decreased the viability values, subduing the high resistance observed during the EtOH incubation (Figure 293).

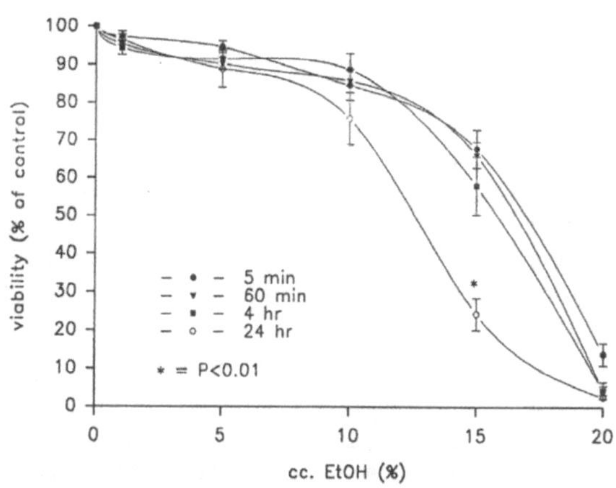

Figure 292. Changes in the viability of Sp2/0-Ag14 cells after 5 minutes of incubation with 1–20 % ethanol (EtOH) and continuous 10^{-5} mol/L pyrazole treatment counted at 5 minutes, 60 minutes, 4 hours and 24 hours by Trypan blue exclusion test. The results are expressed as means ± SEM (n = 5).

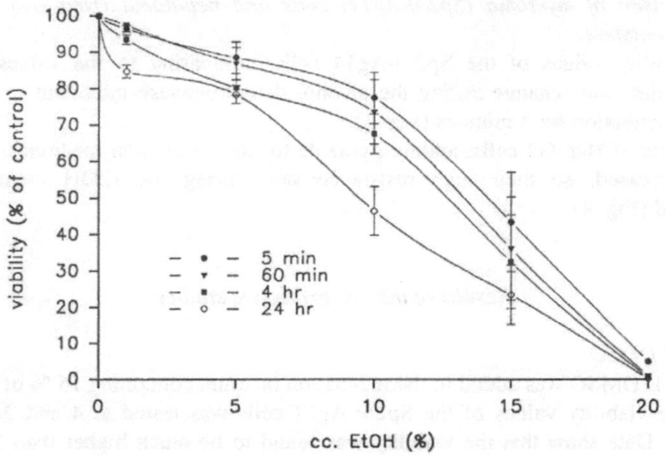

Figure 293. Changes in the viability of Hep G2 cells after 5 minutes of incubation with 1–20% ethanol (EtOH) and continuous 10^{-4} mol/L pyrazole treatment counted at 5 minutes, 60 minutes, 4 hours and 24 hours by Trypan blue exclusion test. The results are expressed as means ± SEM (n = 5). [Szabo et al. (1997a) Inflammopharmacology 5:20-28] with kind permission).]

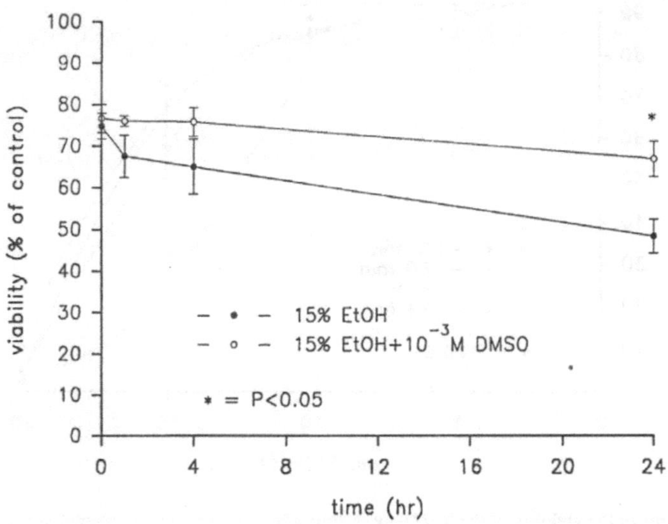

Figure 294. Changes in the viability of Sp2/0-Ag14 cells after 5 minutes of incubation with 15% ethanol (EtOH) and continuous 10^{-3} mol/L dimethyl sulfoxide (DMSO) counted at 5 minutes, 60 minutes, 4 hours and 24 hours by Trypan blue exclusion test. The results are expressed as means ± SEM (n = 5). *$P < 0.05$ compared to 24-hour value of 15% EtOH incubation. [Szabo et al. (1997b) Usage of scavengers on stable cultured (Sp2/0-Ag14 and Hep G2) cell lines as an approach to reveal the mechanisms of cytoprotection. In: Mózsik Gy., Nagy L., Király Á. (Eds). *Twenty Five Years of Peptic Ulcer Research in Hungary (1971–1995)*. Akadémiai Kiadó, Budapest. pp. 275–283 (with kind permission).]

http://dx.doi.org/10.5772/60104

10.4.2. Results of the cytoprotective studies

10.4.2.1. Effect of DMSO

A 10^{-3} mol/L DMSO was added to the incubation medium containing 15% of EtOH (for 5 minutes); the viability values of the Sp2/0-Ag14 cells were tested at 4 and 24 hours of incubation. The 10^{-3} mol/L DMSO significantly decreased the secondary cell destruction of the Sp2/0-Ag14 cell line (Figure 294).

10.4.2.2. Effect of GSH

Both concentrations (10^{-4} and 10^{-3} mol) of GSH used during and after the EtOH incubation significantly increased the viability of the Sp2/0-Ag14 cells at the time period of 4-hour toxic-free incubation (Figure 295). Four hours after the incubation of EtOH, the GSH effect to protect was lost, probably due to its short-life span.

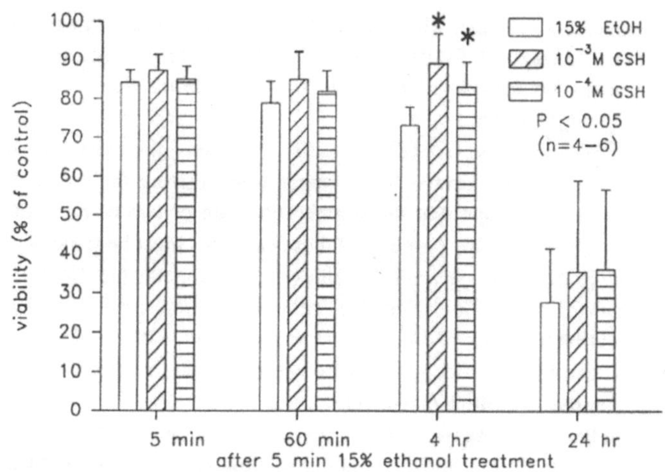

Figure 295. Changes in the viability of Sp2/0-Ag14 cells after 5 minutes of incubation with 15% ethanol (EtOH) and continuous 10^{-4}–10^{-3} mol/L glutathione counted at 5 minutes, 60 minutes, 4 hours and 24 hours by Trypan blue exclusion test. The results are expressed as means ± SEM (n = 4–6). *$P < 0.05$ compared to 4-hour value of 15% EtOH incubation. [Szabo et al. (1997b) Usage of scavengers on stable cultured (SP2/0-Ag14 and Hep G2) cell lines as an approach to reveal the mechanisms of cytoprotection. In: Mózsik Gy., Nagy L., Király Á. (Eds). *Twenty Five Years of Peptic Ulcer Research in Hungary (1971–1995).* Akadémiai Kiadó, Budapest. pp. 275–283 (with kind permission).]

10.4.2.3. Effect of β-carotene

During the co-incubation with 15% of EtOH and 10^{-8}–10^{-6} mol/L – β-carotene, we could not find any protective effect. The viability values of the Sp2/0-Ag14 cells were much lower than they were obtained in the 15% EtOH incubation. The 10^{-7} mol/L dose of β-carotene significantly aggravated the 15% EtOH-induced cell destruction of the myeloma cells ($P < 0.01$) (Figure 296).

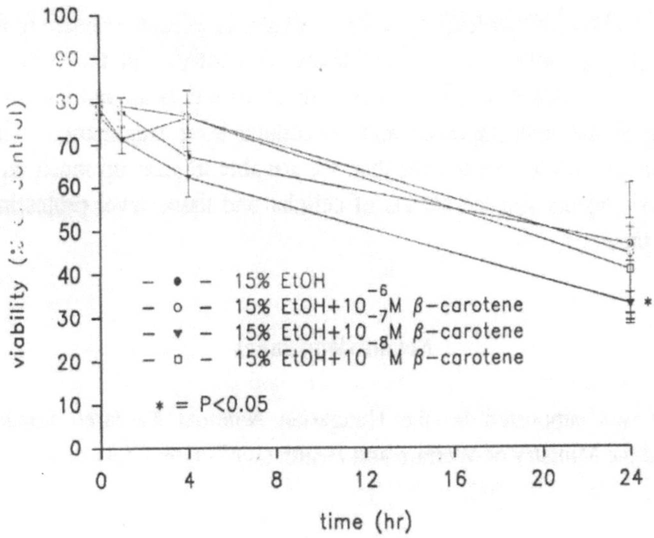

Figure 296. Changes in the viability of Sp2/0-Ag14 cells after 5 minutes of incubation with 15% ethanol (EtOH) and continuous 10^{-8}–10^{-6} mol/L β-carotene counted at 5 minutes, 60 minutes, 4 hours and 24 hours by Trypan blue exclusion test. The results are expressed as means ± SEM ($n = 6$). $^*P < 0.05$ compared to 24-hour value of 15% EtOH incubation. [Szabo et al. (1997b) Usage of scavengers on stable cultured (SP2/0-Ag14 and Hep G2) cell lines as an approach to reveal the mechanisms of cytoprotection. In: Mózsik Gy., Nagy L., Király Á. (Eds). *Twenty Five Years of Peptic Ulcer Research in Hungary (1971–1995)*. Akadémiai Kiadó, Budapest. pp. 275–283 (with kind permission).]

10.5. Discussion

In these studies freshly isolated rat gastric mucosal cells and two types of stable cultured cells were used to evaluate the effects of EtOH, IND and their combination in toxicological studies. The mixed population of isolated rat GMC contained at least three types of cells: parietal (20–25%), chief (40%) and epithelial (45%). A viability of 80–95% could be maintained for 6–7 hours. These cells do not have the potential for proliferation. Cultured cells were always kept in the same conditions, tests are reproducible and cells can survive for a longer time. During the calculation of viability, it must be remembered that the two cell lines have different proliferation rates. In particular, this should be borne in mind during the interpretation of the different viability values of longer incubation times. Our results indicate that the acutely isolated cells are more vulnerable than cultured cells. After EtOH treatment, in the case of Sp2/0-Ag14 cells, the EC_{50} (16%) was higher than that of GMC (13.5%). IND had no damaging effect on stable cultured cells. The combined treatment reduced the viability in both types of cells, but this effect was much smaller in Sp2/0-Ag14; almost all the GMC were destroyed. These results show that cultured cells are more resistant to toxic agents than acutely isolated cells. Though different types of cells were used in this study, the differences in behavior may derive from the differences in isolation procedure rather than their differences in type. *In vivo* experiments have shown that gastrointestinal ulceration can be produced by IND administration (Nagy et al., 1994; Djahanguire et al., 1969). It is known that IND inhibits the activity of cyclooxygenase, producing less prostaglandins and excessive vasoconstrictor leukotrienes (Rainsford, 1992),

http://dx.doi.org/10.5772/60104

and decreases the mucosal level of adenosine triphosphate (Rainsford, 1987). These factors reduce the gastric mucosal resistance to acid. In the *in vitro* study described here, IND was applied without any other aggressive factor, such as EtOH, and was not toxic for these cells. However, after the combination treatment, cell viability was considerably decreased compared with the effect of EtOH alone. It is likely that the decreased levels of endogenous prostaglandins might play a role in the enhanced toxic effect of EtOH. These results are in good agreement with those of Tarnawski et al. (1988) who observed a protective effect of exogenous prostaglandins on human-isolated gastric glands against IND and EtOH injury.

In our experiment, two types of stable cultured cells were used for cytoprotective studies with DMSO, GSH and β-carotene. In our experiment, when the Hep G2 cells were incubated with an alcohol-dehydrogenase inhibitor, their higher resistance against ethanol disappeared. This observation indicates that the alcohol- dehydrogenase enzyme might have an important role in the high resistance of the Hep G2 cells.

In the case of the Sp2/0-Ag14 cells, a great cell loss (secondary cell destruction) was derived after a long period (4 and 24 hours of incubation time). In the background of this phenomenon, the role of oxygen-free radicals had been suspected and proved (Bódis et al., 2000). Therefore, we tested the effect of the applications of some commonly known scavengers. Dimethyl sulfoxide and glutathione were effective, but the 10% water-soluble β-carotene had no cytoprotective effect. It was possible that the β-carotene with high molecular weight did not have enough time to be taken up by the cells in our experiments. In order to support this assumption, we have studied the effect of a 24-hour preincubation of 10^{-7} mol/L β-carotene, but in this case, we also found similar toxic behavior.

The tissue level (organoprotection) and cellular level (cytoprotection) mechanisms of the stomach "cytoprotection" have many similarities, but they also have many differences (e.g., dosages). The details of these differences are not clearly known yet. If we accomplish the tissue and cellular level examinations by choosing different toxic and protective agents, then we will easily be able to understand the effects of toxic agents and the cellular and tissue level protecting reactions generated by them.

Author details

Gyula Mozsik[1*] and Imre Szabó[2]

*Address all correspondence to: gyula.mozsik@aok.pte.hu

1 First Department of Medicine, Medical and Health Centre, University of Pécs, Hungary

2 Associate Professor at the First Department of Medicine, University of Pécs, Hungary

Chapter 11

Discussion

Gyula Mozsik and Imre Szabó

Additional information is available at the end of the chapter

http://dx.doi.org/10.5772/60105

In the discussion, we will focus our attention on different main points of our present work:

11.1. Etiological and terminological problems of gastrointestinal mucosa (ulcers in humans);

11.2. Clinical pharmacology;

11.3. Biochemical results of the human gastrointestinal tract;

11.4. Results of biochemical–pharmacological studies in animal experiments;

11.5. Direct cellular damaging effects of ethanol, indomethacin and *Helicobacter pylori* on freshly isolated rat gastric mucosal cells;

11.6. Observations with stable cell lines;

11.7. General conclusions;

11.8. Present and future observations.

11.1. Etiological and terminological problems of gastrointestinal mucosa damage (ulcers in humans)

The developmental mechanisms of the acute (dominantly in experimental models) and chronic antral, duodenal and jejunal ulcers are unknown. Before the use of the term "gastroduodenal ulcer" – without any recognition of the causative factor(s) – we used the term "genuine ulcer" "(in about 80% of total number of patients with GI ulcer).

After the publications of Waren and Marshall (1983) and Marshall and Waren (1983), most gastroenterologists accepted the presence of *Helicobacter pylori* as the real cause of PUD – an infectious disease; however, some experts are of the opinion that the presence of *Helicobacter pylori* is only one of the different causative factors (hyperacidity, physical and chemical stress, drugs, psychical status, trauma, different diseases of central nervous system, etc.). These

problems of the etiological role of *Helicobacter pylori* in peptic ulcer disease have been reviewed very recently [Buzas Gy. (Ed.) *Helicobacter pylori*: a Worldwide Perspective 2013. Bentham Science Publishers. Sharjah, UAE – Oak Park, IL, USA]. The overall role of *Helicobacter pylori* infection in peptic ulcer disease has been emphasized after Barry James Marshall and John Robin Warren (Royal Perth Hospital, Australia) received the Nobel Prize. The experimental approach to ulcer development and prevention was based on different physiological, pathological and pharmacological fields (with the exception of experimental observations with Mogolian gerbils which is sensitive to *Helicobacter pylori* infection) (Takahashi et al., 1998). Hence, there is a contradiction between the etiologies of human gastric and duodenal ulcers and experimental ulcers in animals.

Changes in the suggested etiological factors of ulcer diseases appeared in the actual levels of applied drugs in the medical treatment of peptic ulcer patients (parasympatholytics, antacid compounds, histamine$_2$ receptor blockings, antigastrin compounds, proton pump inhibitors and the eradication treatment since 1980s).

It is important to clarify that the "classical histological definition of peptic ulcer diseases" is given by the presence of gastrointestinal mucosal damage which can be histologically characterized as a mucosal defect reaching the muscularis mucosae.

The term "secondary ulcer" was introduced as peptic ulcer disease associated with stress, burn, chronic liver, kidney and pulmonary diseases (in about 20% of patients with GI ulcer).

The connotation and use of the term PUD changed significantly in the past decade, when NSAID-induced gastrointestinal mucosal injury was found to be the cause of GI bleedings (ulcers) in patients in everyday medical practice. A couple of years ago, the term "non-ulcer disease" (NUD) was published by Scandinavian researchers, which indicated clinically the same symptoms as active peptic ulcer, however, without any endoscopic and histologic features.

Earlier it was thought that the primary cause for peptic ulcer disease (PUD) was unknown in patients. Furthermore, the inhibition of gastric acid secretion was taken as the primary tool for the treatment of PUD.

The classically used experimental ulcer models practically do not accept the histological definition of gastrointestinal ulcers (these models are widely used in the research on ulcer).

The peptic ulcer disease is similar to the infectious disease caused by *Helicobacter pylori* – in terms of classical (and old) terminology of this disease – which can be accepted partially, and now classical eradication treatment seems to be successfully used in the medical treatment (for details, see Mózsik et al., 2014 a, b, c, d). No clear histological evidence has been given by international experts that the infections caused by *Helicobacter pylori* produce histologically "classical" ulcer.

However, there is no doubt that many results of classical human observations were given earlier, and these results remained with us after Garrick and Warren received the Nobel Prize in 2005 [for the etiological role of *Helicobacter pylori* infection as a causative (or main) factor to human peptic ulcer disease]. During that time, the attention of physicians was only focused

http://dx.doi.org/10.5772/60105

on reality to prove the role of *Helicobacter pylori* infection. This approach suggested two different important points, namely, a). the eradication treatment was widely accepted in every medical practice and b). the results of classical gastroenterological research were forgotten after 2005 (when Warren and Garrick received the Nobel Prize for their research with *Helicobacter pylori*) in our everyday medical practice.

Clinicians have very frequently met patients with gastrointestinal mucosal damage, who obtained different drugs (dominantly non-steroidal anti-inflammatory compounds). The histological features of these drug-induced gastric mucosal damages do not indicate the classical ulcer structures.

The term "peptic ulcer" is not used in everyday medical practice. The characterization of ulcer by the name of "peptic" potentially suggested the overproduction and function of pepsin in the development of ulcer diseases.

11.2. Clinical pharmacology

Our interest in peptic ulcer disease started in the 1960s. We studied different clinical symptoms, functional parameters of the stomach and small intestine, "actual traditional medical treatment", and efficiency of different drugs used in the medical treatment of peptic ulcer (gastric ulcer, duodenal ulcer, typical complaints of detectable symptoms resembling hyperacidity; however, no ulcer was detectable).

In the 1960s, there was no methodology to approach these complicated fields of gastroenterology; however, there was hope that a new tool would be invented.

The basic problems of human clinical pharmacology are the following: measurements of absorption, metabolism, excretion of different drugs, serum levels of drugs and to find correlations between the obtained clinical pharmacological parameters and drug actions (inhibition of gastric acid secretion, gastric emptying, healing rate, side effects). Our studies started with the establishment of methodology for parasympatholytics in the 1960s. These observations enabled in excluding different drugs from the human "classical medical treatment," because these compounds were not absorbed from the gastrointestinal tract.

The classical pharmacological research tried to produce new quaternary ammonium compounds (instead of tertiary ammonium compounds). The theoretical background of these research works was as follows:

1. To produce drugs having long-lasting drug actions (the therapeutic time interval of atropine is 4–5 hours) in the medical therapy;
2. The tertiary ammonium compounds can pass across the hemato-encephalic barrier, while the quaternary ammonium compounds cannot pass over across this barrier;
3. The quaternary ammonium compounds produced have stronger blocking effects on peripheral neural ganglions than those produced by tertiary ammonium compounds.

Clinical pharmacological studies have proved clearly that the absorption of quaternary ammonium compounds from the human gastrointestinal tract is bad (or not absorbed). We

received a clear explanation for why some drugs are without any objective effects in the human medical therapy (so we received another explanation from our observations why different indications resulted in gastric surgery for peptic ulcer). We had a quaternary ammonium compound (Gastropin®) in our medical practice (at that time) which is absolutely not absorbed from human GI tract (e.g., 1000 pills given orally); however, when this drug was given as injection, we were able to detect its serum level and excretion of the drug in the same person.

On the contrary, the results of our previous clinical pharmacological examinations demonstrated clearly that the results of experimental pharmacological research cannot be applied directly to the human medical therapy.

One of the most important results was (obtained by clinical pharmacology) that the duodenal ulcer completely healed during classical atropine treatment in patients with duodenal ulcer; however, the gastric acid secretory responses of these patients were unchanged (1965). It was also important to emphasize that the clinical pharmacological parameters of atropine treatment were also unchanged.

Another important question was in medical therapy (especially after establishing the clinical pharmacological methodology). "What kind of therapy" can be taken as "basic therapeutic state"? In other words, what happens to patients who are not given an effectively acting drug (or compounds)? Halter and coworkers published a paper in gastroenterology (Scheurer et al., 1977), which described that gastric and duodenal ulcers were able to heal without the administration of any drug (however, the description of this placebo compound – without any pharmacological actions – was not clearly defined chemically in the aforementioned paper).

In our clinical pharmacological practice, we used an antacid tablet (without the neutralization capacity of gastric acid secretion) as placebo drug (aluminum hydroxide).

In randomized and prospective studies, the efficiencies of atropine (3 × 1–2 tablets/day orally given), cimetidine (1.0 g/day orally given), carbenoxolone (3 × 100 mg/day orally given for 2 weeks and 3 × 50 mg/day orally given for 3rd and 4th weeks) and placebo (3 × 1 placebo tablet/day orally given) for one month was analyzed. Different laboratory examinations, such as gastrofiberoscopic examinations (the presence of ulcer was detected, and the measurement of ulcer size was carried out planimetrically), were carried out at the beginning, 2nd and 4th weeks of the study, while dairy card observations (complaints, appetite, body weight,, etc.) were recorded day to day from patients with duodenal ulcer during the whole time period of the study (Tárnok et al., 1989).

The results of this study clearly indicated the following:

1. The beneficial effects of atropine, cimetidine and carbenoxolone were superior to that of placebo in a multicenter, randomized, prospective and comparative study in duodenal ulcer (DU) patients;

2. No significant difference was obtained in the beneficial effects of atropine versus cimetidine versus carbenoxolone in DU patients;

http://dx.doi.org/10.5772/60105

3. Because the carbenoxolone has no inhibitory action of gastric acid secretion in DU patients, the ulcer healing effects (due to stimulation of mucus) could be considered independent of any effect on gastric acid production (Tárnok et al., 1979; Mózsik et al., 2011).

Thus, these and earlier demonstrated studies of chronic atropine treatment in DU patients (during the 1960s–1970s) were performed before the classical concept of "gastric cytoprotection" was formulated by André Robert, yet it is clear now in retrospect that we had been observing acid-independent gastroduodenal protection with atropine and other drugs before Robert et al. had defined gastric cytoprotection (1979).

On the contrary, these observations clearly indicated us that the beneficial effects of different drugs (or drug candidates) were compared to that of placebo effect. This was the first step in the gastrointestinal clinical pharmacology, when the effects of different drugs (compounds) were compared to that of placebo. In our days, the basic requirement for new drug production is that the suggested beneficial effect should be better than that of the most effective drug in different medical fields.

Clinical pharmacology offers a new possibility to suggest a proof for the development of tolerance (Mózsik et al., 1965 a, b, 1966 a, b, c, 1969 a, b, c, d, e, f) and cross-tolerance (Mózsik and Jávor, 1968 a, b, 1969 a, b, c, d, e, f) without any inhibition in gastric basal and supraliminal (but submaximal) stimulated gastric secretory responses in patients with chronic GI ulcers (Mózsik et al., 1966, a, b, c, 1970 a, b, c). In other words, the PUD healed without any inhibition of gastric acid outputs (so clearly the PUD healed just on the dependence of gastric mucosal protective mechanisms).

The facts for the existence of "gastric cytoprotection" were generally and clearly indicated by the works of Robert et al. (1979) in experimental observations in rats. This phenomenon was proved specifically to prostaglandins in rat observations (Grossmann, 1979).

The gastric mucosal healing without any inhibition of gastric acid secretion was proved by our team with anticholinergic cimetidine and retinoids in animal observations (Jávor et al., 1981; Mózsik, 2005; Mózsik et al., 1967c, 1969a; Morón et al., 1984c) and in patients (Rumi et al., 1997, 2001 a, b).

We also demonstrated – in randomized multiclinical, multicentric and prospective study in gastric ulcer patients – that vitamin A (3 × 50.000 IU/day orally given) has an ulcer healing effect in GU patient (without any gastric acid inhibitory action) (Patty et al., 1982, 1983; Mózsik et al., 1986). Vitamin A is an important nutritional component having scavenger properties (Mózsik et al., 2005, 2007).

To the best of our knowledge, this study was first carried out in multiclinical, randomized and prospective study with nutritional components (as scavenger) in patients worldwide.

Clinical pharmacology studies helped us in comparing the beneficial effects of different drugs in gastric and duodenal ulcers in patients. The key roles in these clinical pharmacological studies were the follow-up of changes in the incidence of ulcer sizes at different times of randomized, multiclinical, prospective and multiclinical studies. To understand and evaluate

the dynamism of ulcer healing rates of different drugs, clinical pharmacological studies of the changes of ulcer sizes in incompletely healed patients are necessary.

The general hypothesis (the increased side of aggression, that is, the overproduction of HCl secretion) responsible for the development of GI ulcers in patients was applied for many years. As we can see from the literature and our observations, this standpoint has been invalid both in animal experiments and in patients (Mózsik et al., 1985).

11.3. Biochemical results of the human gastrointestinal tract

After obtaining the new clinical pharmacological results in patients with gastric and duodenal ulcer, it was another important standpoint that the classical gastric and duodenal ulcers develop as a result of tissue hypoxia (like myocardial infarction). However, it was also interesting to note that many drugs (used in the medical treatment of peptic ulcer) inhibit the biochemical metabolism of gastrointestinal mucosa (parasympatholytic drugs, $histamine_2$ receptor blockers, later the proton pump inhibitions). As it is well known, these compounds inhibit the breakdown of energy storage molecule (adenosine triphosphate, ATP). In other words, these drugs inhibit the liberation of energy (by splitting up of ATP into ADP). However, it was (and is) suggested that the resynthesis of ATP can be inhibited under hypoxemic conditions in GI mucosal tissues. Therefore, we medically applied different drugs in the medical treatment of peptic ulcer, which was a priori able to inhibit the metabolic adaptation. Our primary aims were to stimulate positive metabolic adaptation. The aims of medical treatment and suggestions in the development and healing of gastric and duodenal ulcers are absolutely in contradiction. These (and other) arguments and counter-arguments (or suggestions) led us to start with the biochemical examinations of gastrointestinal mucosal tissues.

It is important to learn the basic methodologies applied in the biochemical examinations in GI mucosal tissues. We tried to follow up the updated, so-called general, trends in the biochemical observations. We have to emphasize that the progression of biochemical research (in detail) is practically an impossible challenge for clinicians. In consequence of many circumstances, we started with simple biochemical examinations of gastrointestinal mucosa from 1966. We spent more time in learning these biochemical methodologies in animal experiments (see Chapters 3, 4 and 5).

Our basic standpoints were, during the "learning" period, to learn and demonstrate the involved cellular mechanism of gastrointestinal mucosal damage and prevention. The results of many of our biochemical observations proved that the cell membrane, mitochondrion, proteins, RNA and DNA are involved in the development of gastric mucosal damage and prevention in animal experiments.

Probably the best representative key moments in these tissue reactions were to understand the details of the changes in cellular energy systems under different pathological and experimental conditions. The acid-soluble inorganic and organic phosphates were measured in GI mucosa. The components of acid-soluble organic phosphates were not known in the earlier times (in the 1960s–1970s). Later, we could separate adenosine triphosphate (ATP), adenosine diphosphate (ADP), adenosine monophosphate (AMP) and adenine–adenosine from the acid-soluble

http://dx.doi.org/10.5772/60105

organic phosphates. Consequently, we were able to not only follow up with the changes to the extent of ATP transformation into ADP but also approach the possible extent of rephosphorylation. Similar observations were made by Atkinson (1968) to approach the general metabolism of living cells, including some calculation index from the results of measurements [such as ATP/ADP, adenylate pool (ATP+ADP+AMP), "energy charge" (ATP + 0.5 ADP)/(ATP+ADP +AMP)]. The calculated values of "energy charge" give information on the extent of phosphorylation (and dephosphorylation). When the value of "energy charge" is equal to 1, then all adenosine compounds are phosphorylated (e.g., in the form of ATP); however, if its value is 0, then all adenosine compounds are in dephosphorylated form (e.g., practically not in the form of ATP). The results of these observations gave us a possibility to prove (or to exclude) the presence of tissue hypoxemia (which was a key point in the development of mucosal damage during ulceration).

Biochemical observations from the resecates of human gastrointestinal tract after the surgical intervention in patients with peptic ulcer were carried out in the 1970s (see Chapter 7 for details). These biochemical examinations were performed under the nationally accepted medical practice, our scientific knowledge and ethical laws; however, our methodological abilities were limited by the current knowledge in medicine (e.g., no possibility for cAMP).

From the evaluation of these biochemical examinations, we emphasize the following:

1. Simultaneously 6–10 biochemical measurements were performed (from the same resecate obtained from a patient);
2. All biochemical examinations (measurements of ATP, ADP, AMP, lipid phosphates, RNA and DNA preparation of membrane ATPase) – from the tissue of one patient – were simultaneously carried out;
3. Tissue samples obtained by biopsy were not suitable enough for simultaneously carried measurements (the technical problems of the measurements were excluded by these simultaneously carried out biochemical examinations).

All biochemical examinations from the gastric tissues (obtained from one patient) were also simultaneously carried out.

There are different important points applicable from the biochemical methodology from 1969–1970, when we learned the existence of the details of the specific sodium pump (substrate enzyme with its classic biochemical behaviors) and "second messenger" systems in other tissues (as GI tract). Because we succeeded in preparing the classical Na^{+}–K^{+}-dependent ATPase and adenylate cyclase from rat heart muscle, rat and human gastric mucosa, we received an absolutely new possibility to understand some parts of regulations of cellular energy systems (Mózsik and Øye, 1969; Mózsik, 1969 a, b, 1970; Mózsik et al., 1970 a, b).

We were the first authors to prove the presence of Na^{+}–K^{+}-dependent ATPase (Mózsik and Øye, 1969; Mózsik, 1969 a, b) and adenylate cyclase (Mózsik et al., 1970) in rat and human gastric fundic mucosa (Gheorghui, 1976; Mózsik et al., 1975 a, b, 1976 a, b, 1978 a, 1982 a, b).

These observations were carried out in earlier time period under different *in vitro* conditions to describe the existence of feedback system between two membrane-bound ATP-dependent

energy systems (Mozsik, 1969 a, b, 1970 a, b). We also measured the changes in these energy supply systems by the direct *in vivo* measurements of different adenosine compounds by different enzymatic kits and RIA method (such as ATP, ADP, cAMP, AMP) in the gastrointestinal tract. (We did not have these conditions at the time of our human biochemical examinations.)

Because no systematic biochemical examinations from the human gastrointestinal tract were carried out and published, out attention is focused on the results obtained from GI resecates of human GI tract obtained at the time of surgical intervention (treatment) in peptic ulcer patients.

There are important notes to the evaluation of human biochemical results obtained from the GI resecates of patients with peptic ulcer:

1. We had no information (at the time of gastric resection) on the suggested etiological factors for this disease;
2. The gastric secretory responses (basal acid output, BAO; maximal acid output, MAO) were – as the gastric secretory responses and the suggested main aggressive factor for peptic ulcer disease – permanently measured in these patients. The extents of these secretory responses were used to create different groups of biochemically evaluated patients;
3. We had no information on the presence of *Helicobacter pylori* infection in these patients. Now we know well that practically all DU patients were infected with *Helicobacter pylori,* and its infection rate is less in GU patients. In our days, we had no knowledge on *Helicobacter pylori* infection in jejunal ulcer patients (after Billroth II-type surgical intervention);
4. We had no information on the details of medical treatment (applied drugs, time periods of medical treatments) on GI mucosal cells in the ulcerated and control animal and patients' tissues;
5. The necessary indication for surgical intervention was done based on a special consultation between the internist and the surgeons; however, we did not participate personally in this process;
6. In the critical evaluation of ATP, membrane ATPase, and ADP, the possible role(s) was used as an energy supply system (namely energy liberation) for different regulations of enzymes and a critical biochemical parameter of GI tissues to prove (or to exclude) the presence of tissue hypoxemia (by the measurements of dephosphorylation and oxidative phosphorylation). This enzyme system exists in all animals tissues;
7. We wanted to know more on the biochemical structure of cells in the human GI tract in peptic ulcer patients.
8. An important fact is that the Na^+–K^+-dependent ATPase and H^+–K^+–ATPase differ from each other; however, the ATP is a common substrate for the function of both enzymes (see Chapter 5);

http://dx.doi.org/10.5772/60105

9. The activity of membrane ATPase (ATP transformation into ADP by Na^+–K^+–ATPase) and its extent can be used as an important energy biochemical marker function related to the functional state and to the general buildup of target organs;

10. The H^+–K^+–ATPase is located only in the parietal cells of the stomach (see Chapter 5) and not in other cells of the GI mucosal tissue.

The results of human biochemical examinations (from the resecates of GI tract) indicated clearly that:

1. A very close and positive correlation exists between the Na^+–K^+-dependent ATPase activity (liberated quantities of inorganic phosphate from ATP by Na^+–K^+-dependent ATPase, measured in *in vitro* conditions) versus gastric basal acid output (BAO)($r = 0.88$; regression line: $Y = 0.49 + 0.39.X$; $n = 45$) (Mózsik et al., 1974d).;

2. The Na^+–K^+–ATPase system (from the human gastric fundic mucosa) works without any trouble under cholinergic influences (Mózsik et al., 1974c) and its activity can be inhibited by parasympatholytics, histamine, pentagastrin, PGE_1 and PGE_2 (Mózsik et al., 1974b; Mózsik et al., 1974a), epinephrine (Mózsik, 1969 a, b).;

3. There are positive and significant correlations between the BAO, MAO values and members of ATPase systems (Na^+–K^+-dependent ATPase activity, tissue levels of ATP and ADP in the human gastric fundic mucosa – including the positive correlations between these biochemical parameters) (Mózsik et al. 1981).;

4. The ATP transformation into ADP by Na^+–K^+–ATPase system can be regulated by drugs, hormones and mediators in smaller molar concentrations than the ATP transformation into cAMP by adenylate cyclase, and the drug actions are contraregulatory in these energy systems (Mozsik et al. 1997c).

5. The gastric acid secretion depends on the activation of Na^+–K^+-dependent ATPase and stimulation of adenylate cyclase, besides the activation of function of H^+–K^+–ATPase in human beings.

6. The active transport functions across the gastric mucosal cells depend on different cellular (however, ATP-dependent membrane-bound) energy systems (such as Na^+–K^+-dependent ATPase-, adenylate cyclase- and H^+–K^+-dependent ATPase systems) in human beings.

7. Biochemical and energetic gradients exist in the gastric fundic, antral, duodenal (jejunal) mucosal tissues dependent on the gastric basal acid secretory responses in patients with hyperacidity and normacidity; however, these gradients disappear in patients with hypoacidity (Mózsik— et al., 1976).;

8. The extents of ATP transformation into ADP by membrane ATPase are significantly higher in the mucosal tissues around the gastric (antral), duodenal and jejunal ulcer patients than those in their identical normal (non-ulcerated) mucosal tissues (in the same patients) (the values of "energy charge" remained unchanged in these tissue specimens). These results together proved clearly that the oxidative phosphorylation is intact in the ulcerated mucosa, which cannot be obtained in the presence of hypoxemic damage in the tissues.

For understanding these results, we have to mention different points:

1. We had no information on the existence of classical ulceration in the antrum, duodenum and jejunum in patients;

2. We had no information on the kinds (and their time periods) of medical treatments;

3. We did not receive any information on the reasons for the indication of surgical intervention in these patients;

4. We also had no suggestion on the possible healing processes of ulceration in these patients without any surgical intervention;

5. During surgical interventions, we did not hear anything on the presence of *Helicobacter pylori* infection; however, now it is clear that the incidence of *Helicobacter pylori* infection differs in the case of duodenal ulcer and gastric ulcer (no data are available on *Helicobacter pylori* infection in jejunal ulcer after surgical intervention in patients). Based on our opinion on these, we suggested that the presence of *Helicobacter pylori* infection is independent of these biochemical observations;

9. Our human biochemical results (obtained in the ulcerated and non-ulcerated mucosa) suggest the positive metabolic adaptation against ulcer development in the antral, duodenal and jejunal mucosa. The extent (capacity) of the metabolic adaptation depends on the general biochemical buildup of the tissues. There is no doubt that the highest metabolic activity can be obtained in the gastric fundic mucosa in patients with gastric hyperacidity and normacidity (because of the existence of biochemical and energetic gradients in these mucosal tissues). Consequently, the exhaustion of antral, duodenal and jejunal mucosa will appear in a shorter time than that in corpus mucosa. Probably that suggestion gives a real explanation for why we applied drugs (having metabolic blocking effect) for the medical treatment of peptic ulcer disease in patients.

We established a uniform biochemical explanation for the development and location of "genuine" gastric, duodenal and jejunal ulcers in patients (Mózsik, et al., 1997b).

9. These results, demonstrated earlier (Figures 67–71), clearly indicated that the extent of ATP–ADP breakdown is significantly higher in the ulcerated antral, duodenal and jejunal mucosa specimens than in the control (non-ulcerated) mucosa specimens. This fact can be proven by the increased membrane ATPase activity and increased level of ADP in association with significant increase in the tissue level of ATP. The following facts are found in the background:

    a. No impaired oxidative phosphorylation can be found in ulcerated mucosa specimens, which can be proven by increased tissue levels of ATP in time when the ATP–ADP breakdown was significantly increased (significantly higher membrane ATPase activity and increased level of ADP);

    b. The tissue levels of ATP and ADP are significantly higher in the ulcerated mucosa than those in the non-ulcerated mucosa (in the same patients);

http://dx.doi.org/10.5772/60105

c. The membrane ATPase activity is also significantly higher in the ulcerated mucosa than that in the non-ulcerated GI mucosa (Mózsik et al., 1979);

d. The higher ATP tissue levels (in time when the ATP breakdown was increased in both directions) can only be obtained by the intact oxidative phosphorylation pathway;

e. The biochemical components of gastric mucosal tissue were expressed in accordance to 1.0 mg DNA, which represents the same number of cells (Figure 157). The values of adenine–adenosine, ATP, ADP and AMP were increased in the gastric fundic mucosa in patients with increased gastric secretory responses (BAO, MAO) and in the mucosa around chronic antral, duodenal and jejunal ulcer (Mózsik et al., 1979 a, b, d, f, h, 1981 a, b, 1987 a, b; Nagy et al., 1978, 1981b);

f. No physiological data exist in the literature to prove the presence of decreased GMBF in the gastric fundic mucosa in patients with gastric hyperacidity; nobody found an increased tissue level of lactate. Experts accept the increased energy turnover (increased capacities of ATP–ADP and ATP–cAMP transformation) in these gastric fundic mucosa specimens.

The chemical comparison of the biochemical results obtained in the human gastric fundic mucosa with different gastric acid secretory responses and non-ulcerated and ulcerated antral, duodenal and jejunal mucosa in patients is shown in Figure 297. The results are expressed as amounts of biochemical parameters/1 mg DNA.

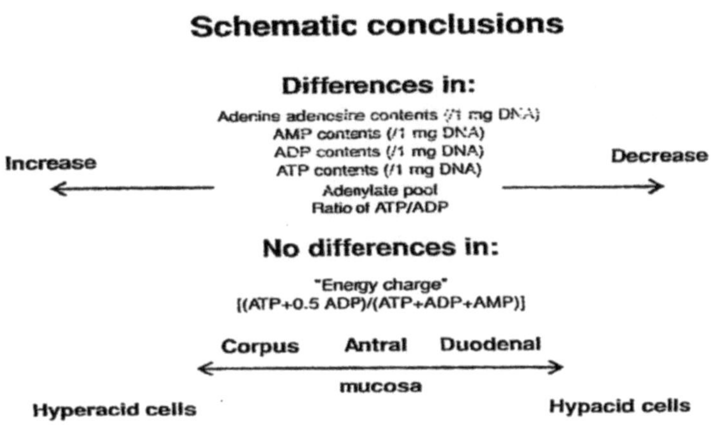

Figure 297. The schematic presentation of biochemical buildup of human gastrointestinal mucosa in patients with different gastric acid secretory responses. All of the adenine and adenosine compounds increased significantly (meanwhile the stream of ATP breakdown enhanced in both directions) in the gastric corpus mucosa in comparison with those results obtained in corpus mucosa patients with hyperacidity. The same biochemical parameters were obtained in the ulcerated antral, duodenal and jejunal mucosa in patients with chronic antral, duodenal and jejunal mucosa. So the biochemical structure of human chronic antral, duodenal and jejunal mucosa is the same as that obtained in the corpus fundic mucosa in patients with gastric hyperacidity. [Mózsik, Abdel-Salam, Király, Morón, Nagy, Sütő, Tárnok, Jávor (1997) in Mózsik Gy., Nagy L., Király Á. (eds) Twenty Five Years of Peptic Ulcer Research in Hungary: From Basic Sciences to Clinical Practice (1971–1995) pp. 159–170., Akadémiai Kiadó, Budapest; Mózsik, 2006. In: Discoveries in Gastroenterology (1960–2005). Akadémiai Kiadó. Pp. 139–224 (with kind permission).]

The biochemical buildup (chemical composition) of cells in the human gastric fundic mucosa with hyperacidity and in the ulcerated antral, duodenal and jejunal mucosa in patients are significantly different from that in gastric fundic mucosa with hypoacidity and in non-ulcerated antral, duodenal and jejunal mucosa. In consequence of these facts, the physiological, neural, hormonal and pharmacological regulations of these cells in the human gastric fundic mucosa in patients with hyperacidity and in ulcerated antral, duodenal and jejunal mucosa also differ (quantitatively) as those in the cells in gastric fundic mucosa with hypoacidity and in non-ulcerated antral, duodenal and jejunal mucosa in peptic ulcer. The physiological, pharmacological and pathological regulations of membrane-bound ATP-dependent energy systems had essential roles in these processes.

How can we explain the contradictions of the presence and absence of ulcerated gastrointestinal mucosa in animals and patients with peptic ulcer?

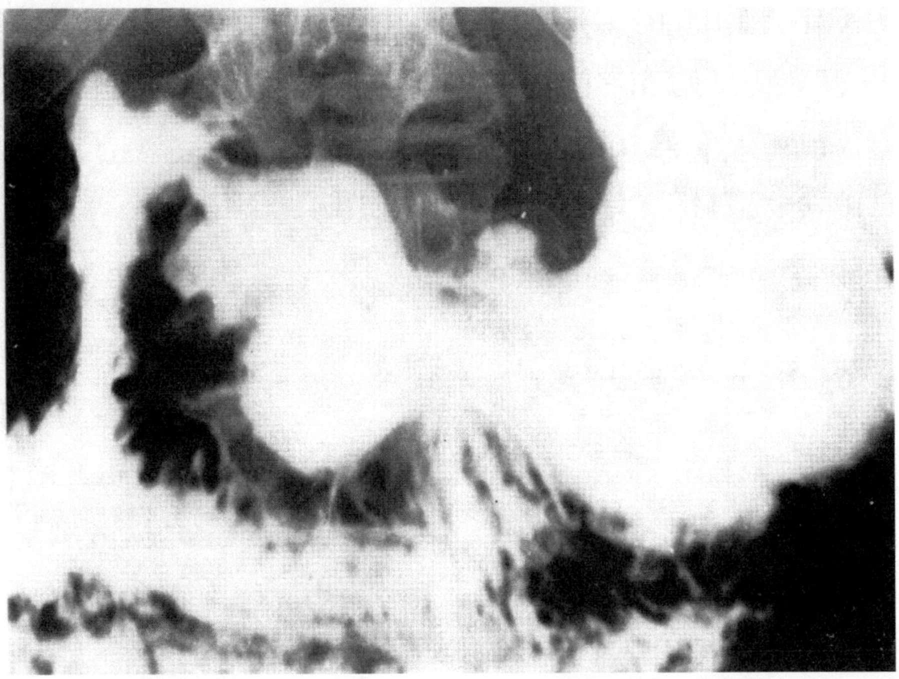

Figure 298. Roentgenogram of gastric ulcer localized on the lesser curvature of the stomach of a 56-year-old patient. The X-ray examination was performed by Z.Molnár M.D. at the Radiological Department, University of Medical School, Pécs, Hungary, in 1970. [Mozsik, Nagy, Tárnok , Jávor (1971): In: Pfeiffer C.J. (Ed). Peptic Ulcer. Munksgaard, Copenhagen – Lippincott, Philadelphia. pp. 323–328 (with kind permission).]

1. The results of experimental measurements in the animal gastrointestinal mucosa (used different – dominantly physiological – different experimental conditions, but not under the development of mucosal damage) and there bewer were proved the causative correlation between the physiologically measured decrease of GMBF versus insufficiency of oxidative phosphorylation in the same tissue samples in the same time (Kitajima, 1989);

http://dx.doi.org/10.5772/60105

2. The experimental evidence of decrease in tissue ATP has been based on the observations of Menguy et al. (1974 a, b, c, d); however, the examined animals had a severe blood loss in the experiments. No similar changes of blood circulation existed in other experimental models (used by different experts all over the world);

3. The measurement of the tissue level of gastrointestinal mucosal tissues alone cannot give a scientific evidence for the existence of impaired oxidative phosphorylation (see Mózsik and Vizi, 1976 a, b; Mózsik et al., 1983). We have to measure the tissue levels of ATP, ADP, AMP and cAMP together (with the simultaneous measurement of lactate) in the same tissue samples in the same time;

4. The biochemical structures of the human gastric fundic mucosa with increased gastric acid basal (BAO) and maximal (MAO) secretory responses are the same as those obtained in the ulcerated antral, duodenal and jejunal mucosa in patients with peptic ulcer;

5. The tissue levels of ATP in the antral, duodenal and jejunal ulcerated mucosa are much higher than those in the non-ulcerated (control) mucosa. On the contrary, the tissue levels of ADP – in these tissue samples – are the same as ATP. However, the membrane (transport) ATPase (Mg^{2+}-dependent, Mg^{2+}–Na^{+}–K^{+}-dependent and Na^{+}–K^{+}-dependent) activities are also significantly higher in the ulcerated mucosal tissues than those in the control (non-ulcerated) ones.

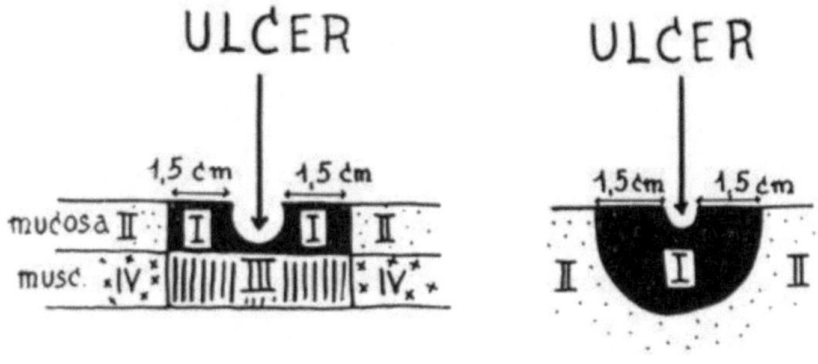

Figure 299. Schematic presentation of separation of gastric tissue surrounding a gastric ulcer localized on the lesser curvature of the stomach (same patients as in Figure 298). The left-hand side figure shows the transaction of the gastric wall; the right-hand side figure indicates the surface of the gastric mucosa. The gastric mucosa was separated from the muscular layer, and both layers were separated into two parts: gastric mucosa up to 1.5 cm around the gastric ulcer (I); gastric mucosa without ulcer (II); "callus" (III) i.e., the muscular layer under the gastric ulcer; and muscular layer (IV), i.e., the muscular layer under the gastric tissue without ulcer. These specimens of gastric tissues were used for the preparation of Na^{+}–K^{+}-dependent ATPase. [Mózsik, Nagy, Tárnok, Jávor (1971): In: Pfeiffer C.J. (Ed). Peptic Ulcer. Munksgaard, Copenhagen – Lippincott, Philadelphia. pp. 323–328 (with kind permission).]

The following main biochemical events are incorporated by these observations:

a. The increased membrane (transport) ATPase in the ulcerated antral, duodenal and jejunal mucosa produces an increased tissue level of ADP in these tissue samples;

b. The increased tissue levels of ATP in the ulcerated antral, duodenal and jejunal mucosa were compared with those in the non-ulcerated (control) mucosa tissue specimens;

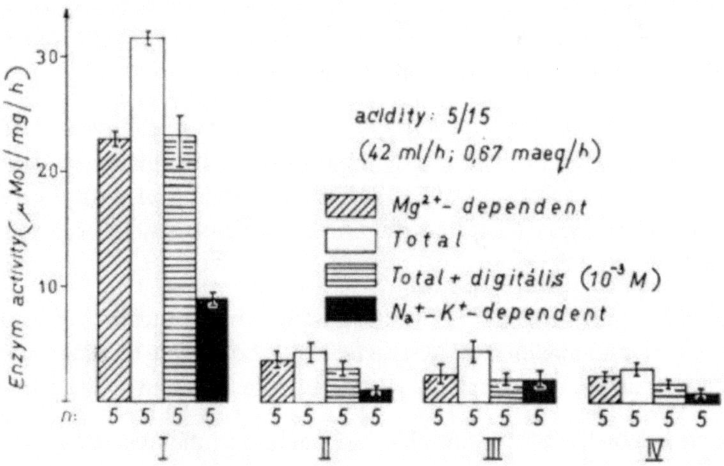

Figure 300. Alterations of the Na^+–K^+-dependent ATPase (transport) ATPase in the gastric tissues around the gastric ulcer in a patient. The ATPase activity was measured by the liberation of inorganic phosphorus and expressed in μMol/mg "dried membrane material"/hour. Secretory characteristics of the patient: volume of gastric secretion: 42 mL/hour; acidity, 0.67 mEq/hour or 5/15 clinical units, unstimulated; n, number of examinations (results presented as means ± SEM of five experiments). [Mozsik, Nagy, Tárnok, Jávor (1971): In: Pfeiffer C.J. (Ed). Peptic Ulcer. Munksgaard, Copenhagen – Lippincott, Philadelphia. pp. 323–328 (with kind permission).]

c. The existence of increased tissue levels of ATP with ADP and increased membrane (transport) ATPase activity gave a clear evidence for the increased (not impaired) oxidative phosphorylation in the ulcerated antral, duodenal and jejunal mucosa tissue specimens (excluding the presence of tissue hypoxia in the mucosal tissues around the antral, duodenal and jejunal ulcers in patients).

6. The GMBF increases with the increase in gastric acid secretory responses in human beings (Jávor, 1968).

The first molecular-pharmacological–biochemical examinations in gastric ulcer of patients with gastric ulcer was internationally demonstrated by us in 1970 at the 4th World Congress of Gastroenterology which was located in Copenhagen, Denmark (Mózsik et al.., 1971b). The forthcoming figures show these memory presentations (Figures 298–301). (Note: we did not mention – at that time – that the transformation of ATP into cAMP is probably also present in cases of higher molecular doses of atropine for the real explanation in the form of atropine-induced-inhibitory action curve on the Na^+–K^+–ATPase activity.)

11.4. Results of biochemical-pharmacological studies in animal experiments

The animal observations were carried out simultaneously with human observations. The rats were used for these observations (under the national law regulatory conditions). A majority of animal experiments were used as acute models, while the characteristics of peptic ulcer were used for chronic experimental models (in dogs dominantly) (see Table 45).

http://dx.doi.org/10.5772/60105

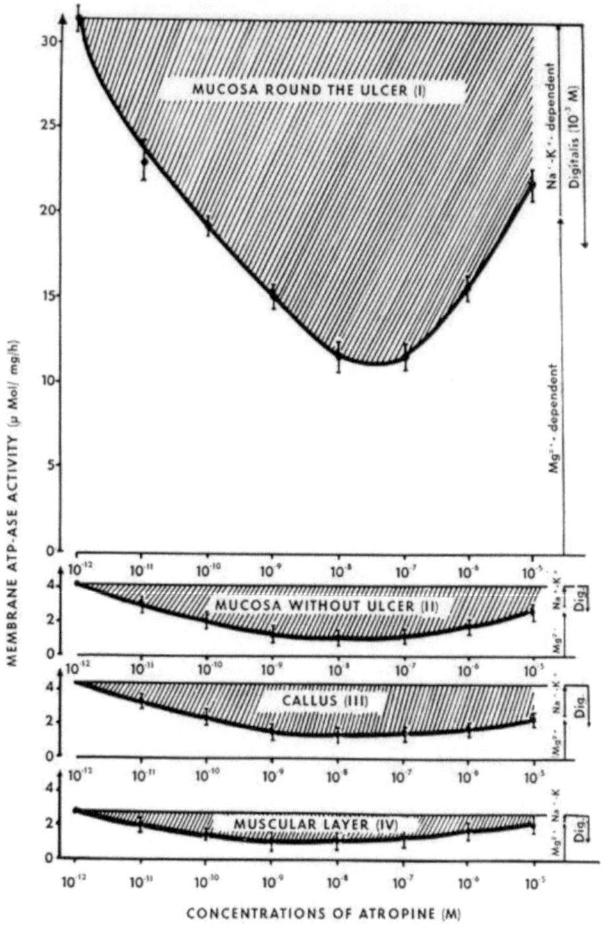

Figure 301. Inhibitory effect of atropine on Na^+–K^+-dependent ATPase activity prepared from different regions of gastric tissue around the gastric ulcer in the patient. The ordinate shows the ATPase activity by liberated, inorganic P, in μMol /mg dried "membrane material"/hour, atropine. Each point on the curves represents the means ± SEM of 5 experiments. The arrows on the right-hand side of the figure indicate the increased membrane ATPase by Na^+ (80 mM) and K^+ (33 mM) and the decreased activity of membrane ATPase by ouabain (10^{-3} M). [Mózsik, Nagy, Tárnok, Jávor (1971): In: Pfeiffer C.J. (Ed). Peptic Ulcer. Munksgaard, Copenhagen – Lippincott, Philadelphia. pp. 323–328] (with kind permission).]

To elucidate the pathomechanism of human peptic ulcer, and to find effective drugs to treat patients, a series of animal models have been devised to mimic the natural history of ulcer disease. Unfortunately, the results contained – if not all – in these techniques do not process the main characteristics of human ulcer disease.

In spite of important differences, we do not have better direct methods for tackling the problems of ulcerogenesis than to use animal models. Generally, we use the expression of "experimental ulcer" for all sorts of experimentally induced gastric mucosal lesion irrespective of the true nature of the damage (erosion, acute and chronic ulcer). However, it is highly

Main characteristics of Peptic ulcer disease	Experimental chronic gastric ulcers
- Appears unexpectedly	- No spontaneous gastric ulcer in animals
- May heal spontaneously	- Rapid healing after withdrawal of The ulcerogenic agent
- Reappear unexpectedly	- Do not reappear
- Gastric ulcre are solitary	- Mostly multiple
-Antral localization (mainly)	- Mainly in the fundus
- Role of Helicobacter pylori duodenal ulcers	- No proofs of Helicobacter pylori influence

Table 45. Natural history of human ulcer disease and the experimental techniques, which do not process the main characteristics of the human disease.

important to differentiate between these three types of gastric lesions in both animal and man as their pathomechanisms are different. Erosions and acute ulcers differ from the chronic ones due to the underlying cause, which is mostly known. If properly treated, they disappear rapidly and do never become chronic. This does not mean that they represent harmless conditions; sometimes it might be difficult to treat them, and they may cause massive bleeding, perforation or even death.

The rat stomach is, however, quite different from that of the man, and the same is true for guinea pigs and other small rodents. The animals best suited for ulcer research are monkey, pigs and dogs. Even in these animals, there are some peculiarities that hamper the evaluation of the results, but with some precautions, the data obtained with some methods might be extrapolated to man. We had possibilities to do experimental observations only in rats, and consequently we were able to carry out acute observations. Biochemical pharmacological observations were carried out in rats under different experimental conditions.

Our attention was focused on evaluating the following:

1. The changes in the biochemical parameters of gastric tissues before the development of gastric mucosal lesions (produced by surgical intervention or administration of different drugs and chemicals) without and with administration of any protective drugs;

2. The study of interrelationships of the Na^{+}–K^{+}-dependent (transport) ATPase system (ATP transformation into ADP by membrane ATPase) and "second messenger system" (ATP transformation into cyclic 3′,5′-adenosine monophosphate by adenylate cyclase) in gastric tissues during the development of mucosal damage and its protection;

http://dx.doi.org/10.5772/60105

3. The study of the role of vagus nerve of "surgical" and "chemical vagotomy" in mucosal protection against different drugs and chemicals;

4. The time-sequence study for the evaluation of oxygen free radicals and scavengers in the gastric tissues in acid-dependent and non-acid-dependent gastric ulcer models;

5. The presence (or absence) of tissue hypoxia in gastric tissues under different experimental conditions;

6. The comparative study for the actions of different drugs with different well-known subcellular mechanisms in gastric acid secretion, in the ethanol-induced model and prostacyclin-induced gastric mucosal protection in the ethanol-induced model.

The methodological problems (designs) and biochemical assays were detailed in some chapters.

We indentified very simple questions to clear these different scientific problems in the chapters, and we tried to give correct(s) answers to our previous questions in acute experiments. We are sure that we cannot give correct answers to the questions asked after chronic biological and pathological processes. We had to learn these methodological and scientific problems from human clinical pharmacology and human biochemical examinations of the resecated tissues of gastrointestinal tract (in patients who underwent the gastric surgery because of peptic ulcer disease). We tried to collect some important information from the ulcer research (including the results in animal experiments and human observations) in animal experiments.

Main discussion points of animal experiments are as follows:

1. The significant changes of membrane-bound ATP-dependent energy systems appear earlier in time in the rat gastric mucosa than those in the development of peak value of gastric acid hypersecretion of an ulcer development in 24-hour pylorus-ligated rats. The extent of ATP transformation into ADP by membrane ATPase increased, in association with decreased ATP transformation into cyclic AMP by adenylate cyclase in the gastric (fundic mucosa and forestomach) tissues in above-mentioned times of experiments (for further information, see Section 8.1.1).

When ouabain (as a specific drug to inhibit the Na^+–K^+–ATPase) was used in this experimental model, we found significant inhibition on both gastric acid secretion and ulcer development. Furthermore, these actions of ouabain also appeared in the same time as those in the untreated animals.

The results of these observations clearly proved the following:

a. The Na^+–K^+-dependent ATPase system (e.g., ATP transformation into ADP by membrane ATPase) plays a key role in the development of gastric acid hypersecretion and ulcer and in the inhibition (prevention) of gastric mucosal hypersecretion and ulcer production in 24-hour pylorus-ligated rats;

b. The gastric acid hypersecretion response by gastric fundic mucosa appears before the ulcer development of forestomach (rumen), and the inhibition of gastric acid secretion is

also associated with ulcer development in the forestomach (rumen) in 24-hour pylorus-ligated rats;

c. The biochemical changes in the gastric fundic mucosa and rumen – during the development of gastric hypersecretion together with ulcer development and prevention of gastric hyperacidity and ulcer development – indicated similar directions (different in their quantitative values) in both parts of the rat stomach.

2. The surgical vagotomy-induced decrease of gastric acid hypersecretion and the prevention of ulcer development are associated with decreased ATP transformation into ADP by Na^+–K^+-dependent ATPase in 24-hour pylorus-ligated rats.

These results suggest the following:

a. The breakdown of gastric mucosal ATP (both in directions of ATP transformation into ADP by membrane ATPase and of ATP transformation into cAMP by adenylate cyclase) is a basic biochemical background to the development of gastric acid hypersecretion and gastric ulceration and to their inhibitions by surgical vagotomy (for further information, see Section 8.1.2);

b. The measurement of tissue level of ATP (without measurements of tissue ADP, cAMP, AMP) does not give correct information on the approach of the actual levels of cellular energy systems (extents of dephosphorylation and oxidative phosphorylation, presence of tissue hypoxia);

c. The development of ulcer in the forestomach is only a hyperacid secretion process, independently from that of the ulcer location (in this experimental model), and is not related to human pathology of peptic ulcer disease in humans.

The gastric ulcer is located in the antrum of patients with peptic ulcer (which also has no acid secretory ability).

d. The results of the biochemical results (especially to energy supply systems of rat gastric fundic mucosa and forestomach) of 24-hour pylorus-ligated rats indicate a similarity to the biochemical background of the development of human antral ulcer, namely, the biochemical constituents (in terms of energy supply system, which significantly differs in the human gastric fundic mucosa vs. antrum in patients with gastric hyperacidity and normacidity). No antral ulcer can be found in the literature and in our practice (from 1960 to 2014) for the existence of antral location in patients with gastric hypoacidity. The results of biochemical examinations in rats and human gastric (fundic and antral mucosa tissues) give a very closed and acceptable biochemical explanation for antral ulcer development in patients as well as the forestomach of pylorus-ligated rats. These results explain that the gastric ulceration appears as a consequence of gastric hypersecretion (and not after *Helicobacter pylori* infection), which clinically appears after a significantly increased metabolic (energetic) adaptation in gastric tissues (antrum in humans and forestomach in rat). The level of metabolic adaptation in the energy supply systems is limited by the different biochemical structures (and their energetic background) of different parts of the stomach (in both humans and rats). Probably a similar (or the same) explanation is true

http://dx.doi.org/10.5772/60105

for the biochemical explanation of the location of duodenal ulcer in patients (dominantly with hyperacidity) (see results presented in Sections 7.9.2 and 7.10) and jejunal ulcer after Billroth II gastric resection in patients.

3. Molecular pharmacological background of different drug actions in the gastric mucosa of intact gastric tissues under different pathological conditions.

The applications and uses of different drugs were widely used in the physiological, biochemical as well as in the pharmacological research. These methods have been applied to evaluate the characteristics of the effects of new compounds, or physiological events, by the modification in their effects. The atropine application is used to indicate the cholinergic influence and its participation in different physiological phenomena and development of new drugs.

The key points of these studies with "standard drugs" were to measure their actions at the level of final physiological (pathological) effects; however, we have no knowledge on the background of these drug actions. We studied the biochemical background of these "basic drugs" as well as the commonly used experimental standard pathological events (such as pylorus-ligated rats without the administration of any drugs or ethanol-induced gastric mucosa in rats). Our attention was focused on the changes in the membrane-bound ATP-dependent energy systems of the cells.

It was interesting to note that the *in vivo* observations of the interrelationships (extents) between the ATP transformation into ADP and the ATP transformation into cyclic AMP were changed from time to time (in hours in pylorus-ligated rats, in minutes in ethanol-induced model), and there were also absolutely contradictory changes (increased and decreased) between them. The results of these *in vivo* measurements were the same as those obtained by *in vitro* measurements due to the interrelationship of the cellular energy systems.

We had no knowledge on the cellular effects (on membrane-bound ATP-dependent energy systems) of atropine and epinephrine in the gastric mucosa. It was interesting to note that the biochemical background of atropine and epinephrine is very similar to each other; however, their molecular weights differ from each other.

The results of these biochemical pharmacological examinations offered a further explanation for the understanding of significantly different actions of the same drug after its administration during the actual functional (biochemical) state of the target organ (see Sections 8.12. and 8.13.).

4. The biochemical background of aspirin-induced gastric mucosal damage was studied in 4-hour pylorus-ligated rats. Aspirin (200 mg) was dissolved in 2 mL of 150 mmol HCl and intragastrically administered immediately after pylorus ligation. The ATP transformation into ADP significantly increased after pylorus ligation (without the administration of aspirin), while the extent of ATP-cAMP transformation decreased under this experimental condition. After aspirin administration, no metabolic adaptation both in ATP-ADP and in ATP-cAMP system, which can be explained by the direct damaging effect of non-ionized acetylsalicylic acid (as consequence of the presence of weak acid in presence of strong – gastric acid - , and it can to precipitate the membrane of cells), and by partly no

presence of any drug, which would be able to modify the membrane enzyme functions (Figure 90).

The administration of atropine (in doses of 0.1, 0.5 and 1.0 mg/kg) can stimulate ATP transformation into cAMP, which further inhibits the Na^+–K^+-dependent ATPase (besides the direct inhibitory effect of atropine on the Na^+–K^+-dependent ATPase). This active metabolic adaptation of the gastric mucosal tissue (increase in tissue level of cAMP) can produce a protective effect against aspirin (Figures 91–98). It is interesting to note that this metabolic adaptation is only dependent on the ATP–cAMP transformation (without the active participation of ATP–ADP transformation).

Vitamin A and β-carotene are important nutritional components in animals and humans; however, they have no antisecretory properties on the gastric acid secretion (Jávor et al., 1983; Mózsik et al., 1986). These compounds are also present in the aspirin-induced gastric mucosa damage (without any gastric acid inhibitory effects) (Figures 99–110 and Table 40). The biochemical background of these compounds is also similar to that of atropine, namely the ATP–cAMP transformation increased significantly by the application of vitamin A and β-carotene, which produce direct inhibitory action of Na^+–K^+-dependent ATPase (by the increased level of cAMP and AMP). Probably the actual level of ATP can reach to a critical level in the tissues, which can determine the ATP splitting processes by membrane-bound ATP-dependent enzymes.

The contradictory evaluation pathways of these results (obtained with aspirin administration in 4-hour pylorus-ligated rats alone and in combination with atropine, vitamin A and β-carotene) are given in the following:

a. The aspirin-induced gastric mucosal damage is a consequence of any positive metabolic adaptation in the cellular energy systems. The primary explanation given by Davenport (1965), namely the primary role of increased gastric H^+ back diffusion in the aspirin-induced mucosal damage, can be modified by the consequence of the absence of any active metabolic adaptation in the cellular energy systems (which is produced by non-ionized weak acetylsalicylic acid on the cell membranes);

b. If we can produce some active metabolic adaptation by membrane-bound ATPase-dependent energy systems, we can prevent the damaging effect of aspirin (independently on the presence or absence of gastric acid secretion).

5. The observation with indomethacin in different combinations offered further interesting results in the field of experimental ulcer research.

The indomethacin (20 mg/kg s.c. given) causes gastric mucosal damage in fundic mucosa in 4 hours time period. During this time period, the extent of ATP transformation into ADP increased significantly (together with the decreased extent of ATP transformation into cAMP) in the gastric fundic mucosa of rats (without the application of any protective agents).

http://dx.doi.org/10.5772/60105

The atropine and cimetidine doses together decreased the ulcer development caused by indomethacin in 4 hours time period; however, the biochemical background of the preventive effects of atropine and cimetidine significantly differs in the rat gastric fundic mucosa.

Vitamin A also increases the IND-induced gastric mucosal damage, which is associated with the increased ATP–cAMP transformation. Similar types of observations were made with β-carotene in IND-induced model. With the biochemical background of these observations, we analyzed in detail the correlations between the changes in tissue levels of PGE_2 (its tissue level is inhibited by the application of indomethacin), cAMP, development of IND-induced mucosal damage and prevention of β-carotene. We have observed the following:

a. There was no direct correlation between the tissue levels of PGE_2 versus IND-induced mucosal damage and its prevention by β-carotene;

b. There was a very close correlation between the decreased tissue level of cAMP versus gastric mucosal damage produced by indomethacin (at 1 and 4 hours after indomethacin administration);

c. There was no significant difference between the decreased tissue levels of cAMP at 1 and 4 hours;

d. The indomethacin-induced decrease of tissue level of PGE_2 indicated a tendency to return to the normal level (in untreated animals) during the 4-hour experimental period;

e. The β-carotene-induced gastric mucosal protective effects are dose dependent and closely associated with the increase in tissue levels of cAMP (but not with changes in tissue levels of PGE_2);

f. The gastric mucosal protective effect of β-carotene differs from the prostaglandin system; however, it depends on the positive metabolic biochemical membrane-bound ATP-dependent energy systems.

6. The increased ATP transformation into cAMP (in association with the decreased ATP transformation into ADP) was observed during the development of stress-induced and reserpine-induced gastric mucosal damage in rats. It is also important to note that these changes in the membrane-bound ATP-dependent energy systems are detectable before the macroscopic appearance of gastric mucosal damage;

7. The observations with chemical (96% EtOH, 0.2 M NaOH, 0.6 M HCl and 25% NaCl solution)-induced models allowed us to conclude the following:

   a. The gastric mucosal damage by different chemicals in rats produced the same macroscopic features in the fundic part of the rat stomach, which appears at the same time after the application of necrotizing agents;

   b. There was no difference between the gastric mucosal features (and their characteristics in time and macroscopic pictures) produced by acid-dependent (HCl model) and non-acid-dependent (EtOH model) gastric ulcer models in rats;

c. The ED_{50} doses of PGI_2 (5 μg/kg) and β-carotene (1 mg/kg) (which produce 50% prevention of gastric mucosal damage produced by intragastric administration of 0.6 M HCl and 96% ethanol) were identified in animal experiments. These doses and higher doses were used for studies to evaluate the correlations between the gastric mucosal damage, gastric mucosal biochemistry (ATP, ADP, AMP, cAMP, adenylate pool, "energy charge," ATP/ADP, lactate) and oxygen free radicals (catalase activity, glutathione peroxidase, superoxide dismutase, reduced glutathione and malondialdehyde) in the rat gastric fundic mucosa (see Figures 251–255). These observations were carried out at the same time and the same tissue samples were used for biochemical examinations. The results of these observations showed us the following facts:

- The gastric mucosal preventive effects of PGI_2 appear earlier (from 0 to 15 minutes), and β-carotene-induced gastric mucosal effects appear later (from 15 to 60 minutes) after the administration of necrotizing agents in both acid-dependent and non acid-dependent experimental models;
- The increased ATP–ADP transformations by membrane ATPase were obtained in the gastric fundic mucosal tissue (in association with the decreased extents of ATP–cAMP transformation) by both PGI_2 and β-carotene. These changes in the biochemical parameters of gastric fundic tissues were dose dependent and these appeared at the time of detectable characteristics of gastric mucosal preventions;
- The changes in the parameters of oxygen free radicals also were well detectable; however, the changes were not found to be dose-dependent actions.

We concluded the following from these observations:

a. There is a close and mathematically significant correlation between the protection of gastric mucosal damage by both PGI_2 and β-carotene and the changes in the biochemical parameters of membrane-bound ATP-dependent energy systems (with respect to extents in their changes and appearance in time). These correlations between the above-mentioned parameters were not dose-dependent and mathematically significant;

b. No differences were obtained in the appearance of gastric mucosal damage caused by acid-dependent (0.6 M HCl) and non acid-dependent (96% ethanol) mucosal damage, and their mucosal protective actions caused by a non scavenger (PGI_2) and a scavenger (β-carotene) have the same characteristics in these animal models;

c. The preventive actions of scavengers against tissue injuries involve significant changes in experimentally measurable parameters of oxygen free radicals; however, we suggest that the changes in the membrane-bound ATP-dependent energy systems have key roles in the development of tissue protective effects;

8. Selye (1936) emphasized the non-specificities of different stress reaching the living organs. The reactions of target organs give specific replies.

http://dx.doi.org/10.5772/60105

We noted the results of the observations with 0.2 M NaOH, 25% NaCl, 96% ethanol and 0.6 M HCl (given orally), in the study of the development of mucosal damage, its biochemical background (Figures 181–183) and the development of prostacyclin-induced gastric mucosal damage (Figures 193–199). These results also clearly indicate its principal role and its action of stress theory established by Hans Selye (Szabo et al., 2012);

9. The epinephrine model offered a very special experimental opportunity to understand the possible action of one mediator (epinephrine) under different functional states of the target organ (target organ with different functional states). The epinephrine inhibited the development of gastric acid secretion and ulcer development in 24-hour pylorus-ligated rats; however, the epinephrine (given is in a suitable dose) at 4 hours later after pylorus ligation produces ulcer development. The biochemical background of the significant actions of epinephrine depend on the actual levels of membrane-bound energy systems, that is, the tissue level of ATP is normal immediately after pyloric ligation (therefore epinephrine produces a significant increase in the tissue level of cAMP); however, it was impossible at 4 hours after pylorus ligation when the tissue level of ATP was extremely low, and consequently the epinephrine application was not able to produce an increase in the tissue level of gastric fundic mucosal level of cAMP.

These results concluded the following:

a. The functional and regulatory steps of the feedback systems between the Na^+–K^+-dependent ATPase and adenylate cyclase systems work in a regulatory manner in the gastric tissues;

b. The regulatory mechanism, between the Na^+–K^+-dependent ATP and adenylate cyclase systems can be separated in some way under pathological conditions.

10. The results of animal experiments clearly indicated that the biochemical components differ significantly in the glandular stomach in comparison with the values measured in the forestomach (Mózsik et al., 1967 a, b, 1969 a, b, c, d; Mózsik et al., 1970). When we analyzed the time sequence and biochemical changes of the development of gastric hyperacidity and ulcer, in 24-hour pylorus-ligated rats, it was found that the gastric hyperacidity developed before ulcer, and the changes in the gastric mucosal biochemistry in both parts of the stomach appeared before the development of gastric hyperacidity(Mózsik and Vizi, 1976 a, b).

A significant biochemical gradient was biochemically proved in the gastric fundic, antral, duodenal and jejunal mucosa dependent on the gastric secretory responses (BAO, MAO) (Mózsik et al., 1976 a, b, 1979 a, b, c, e, f, g, h, 1981e).

The presence of tissue hypoxia was proved by Menguy et al. (1974 a, b, c) and Menguy and Master (1974) by hemorrhagic shock (Kitajima, 1989; Pihan et al., 1989). Pihan et al. (1989) explained the stasis of blood flow after the administration of chemicals. Under our experimental conditions, we could not prove the presence of tissue hypoxia (no elevation was obtained in the tissue levels of lactate, and the extent of phosphorylation was intact) (Mózsik

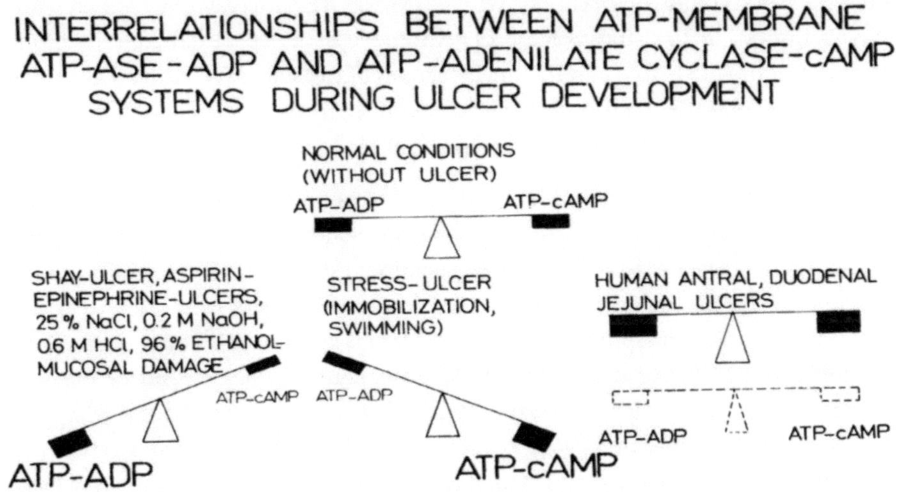

Figure 302. Changes in equilibrium between the ATP–ADP and ATP–cAMP transformations during the development of different experimental models (under significantly different experimental conditions). (For further details, see Chapters 7 and 8).

et al., 1971 a, b; Mózsik et al., 1979 b, f, h, 1981 e; Mózsik and Jávor, 1988e; Mózsik et al., 1990a, 1992c; Mózsik and Pfeiffer, 1992).

The application of biochemical–pharmacological methods in the peptic ulcer research offered a possibility to approach the developmental mechanisms (oxygen supply, biochemical changes, oxygen free radicals, vagal nerve, drug actions, scavenger actions, gastric mucosal secretory responses, ulcer development, drug-and chemical-induced GI mucosal changes) of aggressive and defensive factors in the GI mucosa. Our attention was dominantly focused on the actions of drugs acting at the mucosal level or efferent nerves. These studies analyzed the tissue reactions and not the programmed death of cells (apoptosis). The definition of tissue reactions differs from that of apoptosis.

Modern observations deal with the cellular mechanisms of apoptosis (Bódis et al., 1998; Pai et al., 2000, 2002; Szabó et al., 1996, 1997 a, b, 2000; Szabo, 2004; Tarnawski and Szabó, 2001).

In the future, we need to keep the integrity of living cells, tissues, animals and humans. We lost this integrity by receiving a great deal of detailed information. Our studies dealing with the membrane-bound ATP-dependent energy systems offered an excellent possibility to understand the integrity of these energy supply systems from the point of physiology, biochemistry, pharmacology and pathology.

11. Probably one of the most interesting results was obtained in surgical vagotomy when we observed that the PGI_2-induced gastric cytoprotective effect disappeared after bilateral surgical vagotomy (Jávor et al., 1981; Mózsik et al., 1982). The results of these observations first proved that the intact vagal nerve is necessary for gastric mucosal defense (not only for the gastric acid secretion). Similar results were published by Miller (1983). Unfortu-

http://dx.doi.org/10.5772/60105

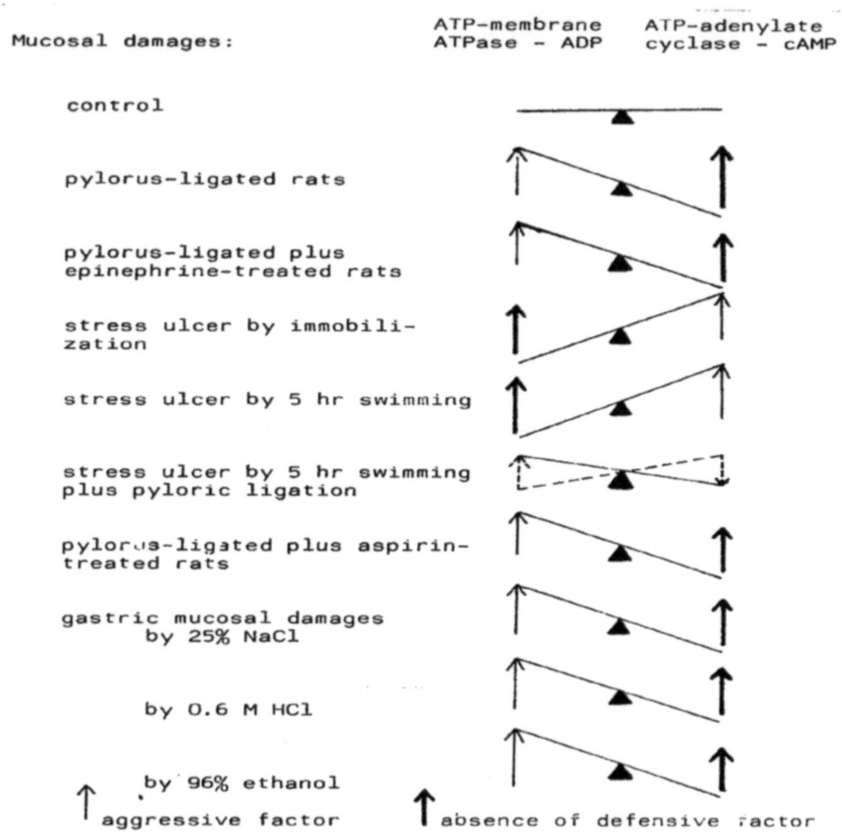

Figure 303. Correlations between the aggressive and defensive mechanisms during the development of gastric mucosal damage in different experimental models (a schematic summary of animal experiments). [Mózsik, Figler, Nagy, Patty, Jávor (1981). In: Mózsik Gy., Hänninen O., Jávor T. (Eds.) Advances in Physiological Sciences. Vol. 29. Gastrointestinal Defence Mechanisms. Pergamon Press, Oxford- Akadémiai Kiadó, Budapest. pp. 213–276 (with kind permission).]

nately, the necessary role of intact vagal nerve for the mucosal protection is known worldwide from the publication of Miller (we published this new observation earlier).

Later, Karádi and Mózsik (2000) studied surgical and chemical vagotomy (atropine treatment) in rats treated with indomethacin in detail, under different acute and chronic experimental conditions in the stomach, small intestine and large bowel. The indomethacin-induced mucosal damage (in the stomach and small intestine) enhanced after surgical vagotomy but not after "chemical vagotomy" (atropine treatment), and the small dose of atropine (cytoprotective effect) disappeared after surgical vagotomy.

Similar results were demonstrated with atropine, cimetidine, PGI_2 and β-carotene due to their failures in gastric mucosal protection after surgical vagotomy (see Section 8.17). The tissue levels of PGE_2 and PGI_2 (or its metabolite 6-keto-$PGF_{1\alpha}$) significantly decreased in the rat gastric mucosa after surgical vagotomy (see Section 8.17); however, we were of the opinion that these

facts (namely, decrease of PGE_2 and PGI_2) can only partially explain the disappearance of gastric mucosal protective effects of atropine, cimetidine, PGE_2, PGI_2 and β-carotene by surgical vagotomy (we emphasize better the roles of neural regulation of intact vagal nerve on cellular energy systems).

12. The actions of atropine, actinomycin D (inhibitor of RNA synthesis dependent on DNA), dinitrophenol (inhibitor of oxidative phosphorylation), epinephrine, histamine, mannomustine (Degranole^R) (inhibitor of *de novo* synthesis of DNA), pentagastrin, PGI_2, ouabain (specific inhibitor of Na^+–K^+-dependent ATPase enzyme) and tetracycline (inhibitor of protein translation) were studied and their dose–response curves were identified under three different experimental models, namely, in 4-hour pylorus-ligated rats (HCl secretion), ethanol-induced gastric mucosal damage and prostacyclin-induced gastric mucosal protection (see Section 8.14).

The affinity and intrinsic activity (α) curves were calculated from the obtained results (the doses of these drugs are given in [−] molarities), and the values of ED_{50}, intrinsic activity and pA_2 were calculated. These molecular pharmacological results are able to approach the importance of different subcellular mechanisms involved in the development of gastric acid secretion, ethanol- and prostacyclin-induced gastric mucosal damage in rats.

The results (including the values of ED_{50} and intrinsic activities and their pA_2 values) indicated practically the same results. It is tough to evaluate these results in understanding the cellular mechanisms of gastric mucosa under these experimental conditions.

13. The biochemical background of epinephrine ulcer (Section 8.15) clearly proved that the membrane-bound ATP-dependent energy systems (namely Na^+–K^+-dependent ATPase and adenylate cyclase) can be separated from each other depending on different functional states of target organs (Figures 263–267), which can give a schematic explanation for the gastric mucosal damage and prevention (Figures 302, 303). Similar conclusions can be drawn from the results of Figures 268–271.

14. The results of biochemical examinations in gastric mucosal tissues (in animals and humans) offered a general biochemical approach to the main biochemical cellular events (during the development and protection of mucosal damage). Changes in many mechanisms (at the levels of functions, cell membrane, mitochondrion, nucleic acids) are involved in these pathological and therapeutic processes of the mucosa of gastrointestinal tract.

There were and are many researchers who worked (or still working) on the study of gastrointestinal tract (pathologists, biochemists, physiologists, pharmacologists, internists, gastroenterologists, etc.) and they emphasized the importance of different fields from their research. An increased biochemical research has provided information on many cellular events in these target reactions, and we have to learn to evaluate the importance of these observations (dominantly done in animal experiments and isolated cells, cell lines).

The observation of the background of gastrointestinal mucosal damage and protection mechanisms shows that intact cellular energy systems are present in these processes.

http://dx.doi.org/10.5772/60105

The results of our observations (done in humans and animals) show the key roles of membrane-bound ATP-dependent energy systems in different cell functions (under intact and different pathological conditions, without and with any drug treatments). These membrane-bound ATP-dependent energy systems also differ in the target organ under these investigational conditions.

We have described many observations in this book to understand different cellular reactions based on the key roles of membrane-bound ATP-dependent energy systems in both gastrointestinal mucosal damage and protection of patients and animals.

The chemicals can enhance or cause injury to the gastric mucosa (Figure 304). So a well-defined, regulated and dynamic system exists between the positive and negative metabolic adaptations to different (physical, chemical) stress. Furthermore, the GI mucosal injury can be healed (or some to extent prevented) by the positive and negative influences of the mediators, hormones and drugs (see Sections 5.7.1. and 5.7.2).

The mediator-, hormone- and drug-induced regulatory functions depend on the affinity and intrinsic activity curves of the membrane-bound ATP-dependent energy systems. The most important scientific information can be obtained by the comparison of values of pD_2 and pA_2 (when the doses are expressed in molarities).

Figures 303 and 304 demonstrate the presence of an active metabolic adaptation of gastric mucosa in rats and patients to increased gastric secretory responses and to chemical loadings. This metabolic adaptation is directed to ATP–ADP and to ATP–cAMP transformation in the cell membrane (with mitochondrial ATP). These facts suggest the existence of equilibrium between the two enzyme systems. This equilibrium is regulated by mediators, hormones, drugs (as first messengers) and different intracellular events. The different steps of these regulatory pathways were analyzed by the studies conducted on different acute animal models.

The PUD development is an acid- and biochemical (energetic)-dependent active metabolic adaptation; however, both membrane-bound ATP-dependent energy systems are involved in this active metabolic adaptation. These results suggest that the acid-dependent "genuine" ulcers appear as consequence of exhaustion of the metabolic adaptation (Mózsik et al., 1979 a, b, d, f, h, 1981a, 1982 a, b, 1987 a, b; Nagy et al., 1976, 1978, 1981 a, b) (Figure 73). The existence of the extremely high metabolic adaptation excludes the presence of tissue hypoxia.

11.5. Direct cellular damaging effects of ethanol, indomethacin and *Helicobacter pylori*

In this chapter, freshly isolated gastric mucosal cells were analyzed and the results were obtained. The effects of different mucosal damaging agents (such as *Helicobacter pylori* cultures, ethanol, indomethacin) were studied at the levels of cell membrane, mitochondrion and DNA, when these agents were administered individually and in combination).

This chapter concludes that the *Helicobacter pylori* alone does not produce any damage at the levels of cell membrane, mitochondrion and DNA, and it will not change by the administration of indomethacin.

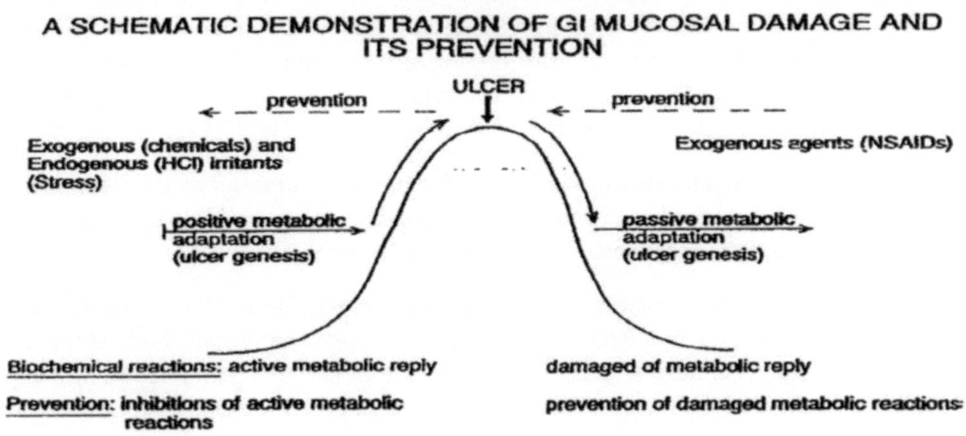

Figure 304. A schematic demonstration of gastrointestinal mucosal damage and prevention including human and experimental observations, summed from about 40000–50000 experiments. For further explanation, see Figure 303.

These results were surprising, because the presence of *Helicobacter pylori* in the gastric mucosa is the real cause for the development of peptic ulcer (gastric and duodenal ulcers) and chronic atrophic gastritis in patients.

The freshly isolated gastric mucosal cells are widely used to test the harmful and beneficial effects of different drugs (or drug candidates) in the experimental research of ulcer. It is well known that the rat (as experimental animal) is not the best experimental model to study and test the actions of *Helicobacter pylori* (see Chapter 9).

11.6. Observations with stable cell cultures

In earlier days, cell line cultures were widely available for research, because most of these cultures originated from human tissues. This fact suggests that the results obtained from these cell cultures are nearest to humans than those with rats (see Chapter 10).

The results of these observations were used to compare the results obtained from freshly isolated gastric mucosal cells and stable cell cultures. The mouse myeloma cell line is used as a "general cell line" in different fields of research, because this cell line has no secretory property.

The results obtained from these stable lines indicated different important notes to us:

1. The mechanisms of "cytoprotection" and "organoprotection" differ to some extent;
2. The freshly isolated gastric mucosal cells are more vulnerable than the stable cell culture lines against different chemicals (drugs, drug candidates);
3. The results obtained in the experiments with stable cell cultures can be accepted with a good criticism.

http://dx.doi.org/10.5772/60105

11.7. General conclusions

It is very difficult to summarize the above-mentioned results (presented in the book). Furthermore, this study involves more serious work for clinicians than for people working just on experimental research. However, we have to mention a few points to explain this:

1. Patients with the same clinical diagnosis do not represent the same characteristics (such as their ages, body weights, life conditions, nutritional habits and states, genetics, etc.), whereas researchers have used the same animal strains (clearly identified their body weight, nutritional state, standard living conditions, genetic background, etc.);

2. The levels of clinical observations and animal experiments significantly differ from each other;

3. Clinical observations (exception of laboratory measurements from the blood samples) just can be done (owing many medical and ethical conditions and laws) in the before noon;

4. The conditions for carrying out clinical observations in human beings (patients) and animals cannot be compared to each other;

5. The clinicians know the borders of their knowledge in the everyday medical practice, but they practically are not able to carry out different research steps to solve these problems;

6. The clinicians do not have enough knowledge (from the modern biological research methods) and suitable conditions to carry out modern medical observations (exceptions are the clinical methods which depend on the modern diagnostic equipment, and these can be used for modern human research);

7. The fields of clinicians and researchers vary, and they have different conditions to do a well-planned research;

8. The clinicians have no correct information on the onset of diseases;

9. The fields of experimental research (in some meaning) are different from the problems of clinicians, and furthermore there are no collaborations between them;

10. Clinicians have consider important results of multiclinical, randomized, prospective, studies in their everyday medical practice (which somewhat depends on business), and there is no possibility to evaluate the background of clinical problems in patients' service;

11. General information (TV, radio, newspapers, Internet) on the so-called new observations are given by researchers (who are as far from the reality of clinicians and patients), and they are not participants in clinical realizations of experimentally discovered results (including the required time, economical support, etc.).

Earlier, it was an excellent practice for young physicians to learn more on the possibilities of methodologies (including new methods, general research laws, laws of presentations, etc.) when they stayed for years in research institutes before and after entering clinical practice. They learned much from the research institutes (e.g., the ways to approach different scientific problems). The postgraduate education offered an excellent possibility for them to recognize

the main problems of clinical practice (especially the details of medical treatments) and to plan the possibility pathways to scientifically approach them.

The authors worked as internists; however, they worked for 2–3 years in research institutes (in Europe and USA).

The following topics in the human and experimental research were:

1. We participated (as pioneers) in establishing the human clinical pharmacology in patients with peptic ulcer. This methodology offered us to do comparative clinical pharmacological studies of different drugs, to demonstrate the existence of drug tolerance (to the drug used chronically in the treatment of patients and to other chemically similar drugs that were not used in the treatment) together with the development of "pharmacological denervation phenomenon" in peptic ulcer patients – during a chronic drug therapy – however, these noted (proved) pharmacological observations disappeared in 6–10 days after cessation of drug therapy. These studies were carried out in the 1960–1970s, when we had the opportunity to use parasympatholytic drugs in the treatment of peptic ulcer.

Many observations were made later by us, which indicated that the surgical vagotomy was a harmful medical intervention in the treatment of patients with peptic ulcer. Many of our results clearly proved that the long-lasting effects of surgical and chemical vagotomy differ significantly in the gastric mucosa. It is important to note that "chemical vagotomy" can produce reversible pharmacological actions (development of tolerance to the medically used drug with "pharmacological denervation phenomenon") during the medical treatment of patients with peptic ulcer. The results of these observations proved clearly that the efficiency of the therapeutically used drugs decreased, and the complaints of patients increased during that time; however, these pharmacological effects can be reversed by the interruption of drug treatment (for 6–10 days). In other words, the sensitivity (efficiency) of the drug to the target organ can be tested clinically and pharmacologically by the administration of drugs intermittently in a long-lasting medical treatment of peptic ulcer patients. In contrast to the effects of chemical vagotomy, surgical vagotomy produces the final effects (including the compositions of gastric mucosal damage, the significant actions of their extra- and intracellular regulatory mechanisms, disappearance of gastric mucosal defensive actions by drugs and scavengers, changes in the tissue preventive effects of scavengers, etc.) on the target organs.

We applied the results of our observations in the chronic intermittent atropine treatment of patients with peptic ulcers, and the number of surgical innervations decreased significantly (from 160–170 patients to 2–5 patients in 1-year period in our surgical department). We followed up these patients for 10 years. Surgical intervention was not necessary in these patients as there was no complication.

It is true that we were away from the scientific problems of chronic atropine treatment in peptic ulcer patients; however, we learned the general problems of medical treatment with different modern drugs.

2. We noted the theoretical contradiction between the effects of therapeutically applied drugs (all of them inhibited the active metabolic adaptation of gastric tissues, while the

http://dx.doi.org/10.5772/60105

ulcer disease appeared as a result of hypoxemic mucosal damage) and their desired actions, but we were not able to solve this significant contradiction in peptic ulcer treatment.

These problems were not studied in detail by the actually and traditionally known pathways in the 1970s. We had no concrete knowledge on the biochemical background of the development of gastric mucosal damage and prevention in both animal experiments and patients. This was the reason why we tried to start with the biochemical examination of gastric mucosal tissues.

The preliminary results of our biochemical observations in the gastric mucosa clearly indicated that significant changes can be found in the biochemical components of cell membrane, mitochondrion, proteins and nucleic acids.

It was observed that the changes in the biochemical composition of peripheral parts of cells (cell membrane, mitochondrion) are much more higher than those in proteins and nucleic acids.

In the early period of our biochemical observation, there was no internationally accepted methodology to approach the changes in the mitochondrial functions in detail (energy-dependent processes).

3. The preparations of Na^+–K^+-dependent (transport) ATPase and adenylate cyclase were carried out in the rat and human gastric mucosa. We noted that the functions of these enzymes can be regulated by mediators, hormones and drugs. Furthermore, the ATP is a common substrate for both the enzymes in the presence of Mg^{2+}. A very complex intra- and extracellular feedback mechanism system was proved to exist between the Na^+–K^+-dependent ATPase adenylate cyclase system under normal (physiological) and different pathological conditions. The significant changes in the equilibrium of regulation of the feedback system (Na^+–K^+-dependent ATPase and adenylate cyclase) are deeply involved in both development and prevention of gastrointestinal mucosal damage in animals and patients.

4. The results of measurements of tissue levels of lactate and the calculation of "energy charge" [(ATP+05 ADP)/(ATP+ADP+AMP)], together with simultaneous measurements of ATP, ADP, cAMP and AMP, are able to exclude the presence of impaired oxidative phosphorylation in the gastrointestinal mucosal tissues in both animal experiments and patients with peptic ulcer.

5. The cellular mechanisms of surgical and "chemical" vagotomy significantly differ in the rat gastrointestinal tract. The intact vagal nerve is basically necessary for gastric mucosal protection produced by PGE_2, prostacyclin, scavengers (vitamin A, β-carotene) and drugs (atropine, cimetidine).

6. *Helicobacter pylori* alone and in combination with indomethacin cannot cause any damage at the levels of cell membrane, mitochondrion and DNA on freshly isolated gastric mucosal cells.

7. A cellular biochemical explanation was given to the development and prevention of gastrointestinal mucosal damage in different animal models and humans.

11.8. Present and future observations

In the last decade, we summarized and reviewed our results obtained from our animal experiments and human observations for some actual scientific problems in different fields of biochemical pharmacological results (Mózsik, 2006), oxygen free radicals, antioxidants (Szabo et al., 2014) and role of *Helicobacter pylori* in the development of peptic ulcer disease in patients (Mózsik et al., 2014).

The actions (effects) of capsaicin on the gastrointestinal tract of animals since 1980 (Mózsik et al., 1997) and healthy human subjects and patients with different gastrointestinal disorders since 1997 were studied, with permission from the Hungarian Pharmaceutical Institute and Regional Ethical Committee of Pécs University (Hungary) since 1997 (Mózsik et al., 2009). These results clearly proved that the capsaicin (given in small doses) protects the development of gastrointestinal mucosal damage via the capsaicin-sensitive afferent nerves. These studies were conducted in collaboration with different institutes (Department of Pharmacology and Pharmacotherapy, Institute of Pharmaceutical Chemistry, Pécs University, Hungary) and therapeutic departments (Department of Gastroenterology, Petz Aladár Teaching Hospital, Győr, Department of Gastroenterology, Markusovszky Teaching Hospital, Szombathely, Hungary).

We observed the animal, preclinical and human examinations with capsaicin for innovative pharmacological and pharmaceutical research (since 2005).

We analyzed in detail the actions of different doses of capsaicin in animal experiments and stimulatory (small) doses on capsaicin-sensitive afferent nerves in healthy human beings and patients with different gastrointestinal disorders, principal problems of capsaicin chronic toxicology, preclinical dossier, basic problems of clinical pharmacology of capsaicin (tolerability, presence or absence of desensitization of afferent nerve to capsaicin during a chronic treatment), international (and national) permission of therapeutically (orally) applicable natural capsaicin preparation, classical clinical pharmacological phases I and II in order to produce new orally applicable drugs or combination of drugs in patients. These results were summarized and published recently (Szabo et al., 2012; Mózsik, 2014, Mózsik et al., 2014 a, b, c). Capsaicin-containing drugs are used alone or in different combinations in healthy human beings and patients with different gastrointestinal disorders.

12. Epilogue

The authors of this monograph are internists, who have been involved in various researches (physiological, pharmacological, molecular biological), from Hungary and other foreign countries (Norway, USA) either before or after becoming internists, gastroenterologists or clinical pharmacologists.

http://dx.doi.org/10.5772/60105

The authors have focused on various aspects (including symptomatology, suggested etiologies, pharmacological and dietetical treatments, endoscopy and follow-up of patients for a long time period) of peptic ulcer disease, since the 1960s. Our knowledge, of course, has changed significantly from time to time in the above-mentioned fields. We joined the clinicians with some research questions (problems) in the field of peptic ulcer disease.

The clinical research study was conducted dominantly by surgeons in the first part of the last century. The possibility of surgical treatment of patients with peptic ulcer was emphasized dominantly by Germanian surgeons in the last part of the 19th century.

The use of different experimental (animal) models has internationally appeared to understand and approach the various problems (such as etiology, development mechanisms at different levels, prevention or treatment) of human peptic ulcer disease in the second half of the 20th century.

Professor Carl. C. Pfeiffer (Philadelphia, USA) was the pioneer researcher who organized an international workshop on peptic ulcer (in connection with the 4th World Congress of Gastroenterology) in 1970 at Copenhagen, Denmark. This workshop offered the "last opportunity" for the personal meeting of world famous (though older) researchers with the representative members of young generation. This workshop was named later as the "First International Conference on Experimental Ulcer" (Pfeiffer, 1971).

Following this conference, an international series of conferences on experimental ulcers has been established [Cologne (Germany), 1972; Parádfürdő (Hungary), 1976; Tokyo (Japan), 1980; Boston (USA), 1985; Jerusalem (Israel), 1988; Berlin (Germany), 1991; Kyoto (Japan), 1994; Hong Kong (China), 1997; Budapest- Pécs (Hungary), 2000; Dubrovnik (Croatia), 2003; Osaka (Japan), 2006; Split (Croatia), 2009; Tokyo (Japan), 2012 and the forthcoming conference will be located at Ottawa, Canada (2015)].

The Standing Committee of International Conference on Experimental Ulcer was officially established in 1976 [(C.J. Pfeiffer (Blackburg (USA) general secretary; members are T. Gheoghiu (Cologne, Germany), Gy. Mozsik (Pécs, Hungary), A. Robert (Kalamazoo, USA) and S. Umehara (Tokyo, Japan)]. One of the authors (Gy. Mozsik) was a member of the Standing Committee up to 2000, and he was general secretary of the Standing Committee from 2000 to 2009) (for details, see Mózsik 2006)].

Other series of international conferences (symposia) were established in connection with International Union of Pharmacology (currently with the name "International Union of Pharmacology, Basic and Clinical Pharmacology"). The Gastrointestinal Section of International Union of Pharmacology (GI Section of IUPHAR) was officially established in 1994 at Montreal, Canada. Before that, different satellite symposia were organized in connection with World Congress of Pharmacology (International Union of Pharmacology) in 1984 in London (UK), in 1990, in Amsterdam (the Netherlands) and in Pécs (Hungary) (1984, 1990). After the official establishment of GI Section of IUPHAR, special symposia dealing with GI pharmacology were incorporated in the program of main congresses [Munich (Germany) 1998, San Francisco (USA) 2002, Beijing (China) 2006, Copenhagen (Denmark) 2010, Cape Town (South African Republic) 2014; different satellite symposia were also organized in these main world

congresses of pharmacology [Pécs (Hungary) 1998; Honolulu, Hawaii (USA); Osaka (Japan) 2006]. Some other symposia of GI Section of IUPHAR were also organized in different parts of the world [Pécs (Hungary), 1995; Sperlonga (Italy), 1996; Kyoto (Japan) 2004; Honolulu, Hawaii (USA) 2012; Zagreb (Croatia), 2013; Budapest (Hungary), 2014].

One of the authors (Gy. Mozsik) was one of the establisher experts, member of different committees, the President (2002–2026) of the GI Section of IUPHAR and, of course, he organized several symposia in Hungary and other countries (see for details, Mozsik, Szabo, Takeuchi, 2006).

During the last four decades, we participated in establishing the processes of different international congresses:

1. Cell/Tissue Injury and Cytoprotection/Organoprotection in the Gastrointestinal Tract;
2. World Congress on Inflammation, Antirheumatics, Analgetics, Immunomodulators [Venice (Italy) 1984; Monte Carlo (Prinicipality of Monaco) 1986 and 1989; Geneva (Switzerland) 1995];
3. International Symposia of International Brain-Gut Society (Lake Arrowhead (Los Angeles) (USA) 1988; Pécs (Hungary) 1990; Florence (Italy) 1993; Pécs (Hungary) 1996)] (two symposia of this series were organized by Hungarian experts);
4. The First International Symposium on Gastrointestinal Cytoprotection was organized (established a new international series in this field) by Gy. Mozsik at Pécs (Hungary) in 1983, thereafter in 1987, 1991, 1995 and 2000;
5. World Congress of International Union of Physiological Sciences (Budapest, Hungary, 1980).

Summarizing our participation in the international flow of sciences, it can be interpreted that we tried to build up a functional bridge between the members working in Western countries and in Eastern (Central) European countries in the time period 1970–1995. This work was very difficult, but we believed that our work would result in a successful interaction between Western countries and Eastern (central) European countries in the field of scientific organizations and hopefully in their scientific activities. During that time, one of the authors (Gy. Mozsik) was the head of the First Department of Medicine, University of Pécs, Hungary (from 1993 to 2003), and his pupils spent approximately 51 years studying in foreign laboratories. We are proud that all colleagues who worked in Western countries returned to Hungary after finishing their research/study period.

Finally, we would like to summarize our scientific activities in the field of gastrointestinal research (focused mostly on peptic ulcer disease). We present this retrograde review of five decades starting from the 1960s; however, different observations and research were done in different clinical, instrumental conditions and research conditions. Consequently, we had to consider the actual time, when we made those observations and to give these critical (but, in some meaning, subjective) evaluations on our scientific activities.

http://dx.doi.org/10.5772/60105

12.1. Clinical pharmacology of parasympatholytic drugs in patients with peptic ulcer

In the 1960s, the efficiency of medical treatment of patients with peptic ulcer was analyzed. The physicians had no objective methodology for the critical evaluation of efficiency of medical treatment of patients with peptic ulcer hade success of medical treatments ofpatients with peptic ulcer wereapproached only by the "subjective" signs of patients (to follow the changes in patients' complaints, body weight, appetite, etc.). These observations were given by the retrospective notes of the above- mentiond parameters.

The treatment of patients with peptic ulcer was done partly by internists (the so-called conservative treatment) and by surgeons. The indications for gastric surgery were dominantly based on the failure of medical treatments, which was one of the most important standpoints to us, the reason why we wanted to know more (in detail) about medical (pharmaceutical) treatments.

One of the most important questions was how to obtain objective data on the gastrointestinal absorptions of various drugs. Only the parasympatholytic drugs (atropine, scopolamine and some other tertiary and quaternary ammonium compounds) were used in clinical practice to decrease the suggested gastric acid hypersecretion.

No chemical methodology was found in clinical practice for the determination of parasympatholytics from different biological samples (serum, urine, bile) of treated patients. The biological methodology was used in our studies for the determination and measurements of different parasympatholytic drugs (in different biological samples) in patients treated with orally and parenterally applied doses of various drugs (see Chapter 2.).

The parasympatholytics (as water-soluble compounds) are not linked to albumin in the serum of patients; consequently, these compounds are excreted in the urine (after some metabolic processes) at the time of administration during the medical treatment. The liver (as the main metabolic organ) was suggested for the metabolization of drugs; so the results of this metabolic process could be followed by the detection of these drugs in the bile.

When the same dose of different parasympatholytics was applied orally and parenterally, we were able to identify the ratio of oral/parenteral dose of the drugs in the same patients. These results offered to control the suitable laws on the applicability of the "experimental pharmacology" in human medical treatment (no similar observations were carried out before in patients).

After careful systematic results from parasympatholytics in patients with peptic ulcer offered us to establish a "complete methodology for clinical pharmacology of parasympatholytics" in peptic ulcer patients (in 1960–1970), we received the possibilities for the identification of the following clinical pharmacological parameters:

a. Absorption from the gastrointestinal tract;

b. Ratio of oral/parenteral rate of different drugs;

c. Linkage of drugs to albumin;

d. Time course of drug actions by their urinary excretion;

e. Changes in the serum levels of different drugs during administration of different drugs.

These observations clearly indicated the following:

1. Different parasympatholytic drugs (dominantly quaternary ammonium compounds) are not absorbed from the gastrointestinal tract in patients with peptic ulcer;

2. The challenge of pharmacologists (namely to discover more new quaternary ammonium compounds to obtain longer blocking effects on the peripheral nervous system under experimental conditions) would help in clinical medicine (from the viewpoint of clinical pharmacology);

3. The failure of medical treatment (by quaternary ammonium compounds) does not give a real indication of gastric surgery (since these compounds are not absorbed from the human gastrointestinal tract).

12.2. Problems of chronic parasympatholytic drug in patients with peptic ulcer: Development of tolerance to drugs and together with appearance of "pharmacological denervation phenomenon" in patients with peptic ulcer

The decrease of gastric acid secretion was the main goal of medical treatment in parasympatholytics (in the 1960s) during a chronic (in about 4 weeks) treatment.

Systematic clinical observations were made in patients with chronic duodenal ulcer during chronic atropine treatment (4 weeks), when the gastric acid secretory responses (basal and secretory answer to superluminal but submaximal dose of histamine) and the ulcer healing (controlled by X-ray examination) were studied before and after the medical treatment.

It was surprising that the ulcers healed in patients with chronic duodenal ulcer, while no changes (no decreases) were found in the gastric acid secretion before and after a chronic atropine treatment (of course, without acute administration of atropine) (Mózsik et al., 1965). We could not interpret these results at the time of completion of these observations, since the "key role of gastric hypersecretion" was not present in these patients in order to heal duodenal ulcer in patients. These results are absolutely contradictory to the internationally suggested etiological standpoint of ulcer development (and healing) in patients with duodenal ulcer.

The theory of "cytoprotection" (e.g., existence of the gastric mucosal protection without any inhibitory action on the gastric acid secretion) was discovered and named by André Robert (1979), based on animal observations. Consequently, the existence of cytoprotection ("ulcer healing action without any decrease in gastric secretion") was proved in patients with chronic duodenal ulcer in 1965.

The inhibitory actions of the same doses of atropine were measured (from the viewpoint of clinical pharmacology) in these patients with duodenal ulcer before and after a chronic atropine treatment. Atropine was intramuscularly given (so the changes in the absorption were excluded). The magnitudes of the inhibitory effect of parenterally applied atropine significantly decreased the gastric basal and stimulated (given superluminal, but submaximal dose – 0.5 mg – histamine s.c.) dose after chronic atropine treatment.

http://dx.doi.org/10.5772/60105

Thereafter, as atropine was orally given (before and after a chronic atropine), its levels were measured in the sera, bile and urine in patients who had no changes in these parameters. We concluded from these observations that no changes are present in the absorption, metabolism and excretion of atropine (in case of oral application) in the treated patients, during a chronic atropine treatment.

The vagal nerve is partially involved in the innervation of human parotid gland. The extents of salivary secretion of parotid gland were studies, using a coaxial capsule, during an acute administration of atropine (given orally or parenterally), and the inhibitory time indicated the same time as the excretion of drug from patients (when the titration of atropine in biological samples was parallel with the measurement of salivary excretion). When we injected patients with different agents (such as acetylcholine, epinephrine and histamine) before and after a chronic atropine treatment, the excretion of the basic salivary secretion significantly increased to acetylcholine (but not to epinephrine and histamine). These results focused our attention on the development of "pharmacological denervation supersensitivity" during a chronic atropine treatment.

In other words, "tolerance to atropine" and "pharmacological denervation supersensitivity" to acetylcholine appeared in patients with duodenal ulcer during the chronic atropine treatment. These phenomena (namely the development of tolerance to atropine and "pharmacological denervation supersensitivity" to acetylcholine) existed only together (for details, see Chapter 2). It was important from a clinical point of view that both the tolerance to atropine and "pharmacological denervation supersensitivity" and the tolerance to acetylcholine disappeared in 6–10 days after cessation of atropine treatment. We were the first researchers to demonstrate the existence of the development of tolerance to atropine and the "pharmacological denervation supersensitivity" to acetylcholine during a chronic parasympatholytic treatment in patients with peptic ulcer. In consequence of our observation, we applied only the intermittent atropine treatment in the medical treatment in patients with peptic ulcer.

12.3. Comparative clinical pharmacology in patients with peptic ulcer

The methodology of clinical pharmacology offered us to carry out randomized, prospective, multicentric and comparative clinical pharmacological studies with different therapeutically applied drugs (as an actual clinical examination) in patients with chronic gastric and duodenal ulcer (for details see Chapter 2). These studies were carried out with the permission of Regional Ethical Committee of Pécs University, Hungary. Different objectives, laboratories and subjective parameters were noted during the treatment of patients with peptic ulcer. The changes in the ulcer sizes were also calculated in the examined patients (before 2 and 4 weeks of treatments).

The most important note was from these observations that vitamin A produced gastric ulcer healing effect that was not less than those produced by other antisecretory drugs.

Earlier we suggested these observations that the antisecretory effect of drugs played the key role in medical treatment; however, vitamin A is a classical scavenger biological molecule

(without any antisecretory properties). Consequently, the phenomenon of gastric cytoprotection exists in patients with chronic gastric ulcer.

12.4. General biochemical examinations in the rat stomach under different experimental conditions

General biochemical examinations of the gastric mucosa (and other parts) were done in animals with different experimental conditions (effects of surgical and chemical vagotomy in acute experiments and in chronic observations) (for details, see Sections 4.2 and 4.3). These results clearly indicated that the "surgical" and chemical" vagotomy produced significantly different biochemical changes in the tissues of rat stomach. The key roles of cellular energy systems have also been suggested from these examinations.

12.5. Membrane-bound ATP-dependent energy systems in the gastrointestinal mucosa in animals and humans

These studies opened an absolutely new avenue for us to study the biochemical mechanisms and their regulations by mediators, hormones and drugs (*in vitro* and *in vivo* observations) (for details, see Chapter 6).

The classical Na^+–K^+-dependent ATPase and adenylate cyclase enzymes were first prepared from rat and human gastric mucosa by us. The examination of these enzymes gave an excellent possibility to study critically the changes of the membrane-bound ATP-dependent energy systems in the gastric mucosal tissues.

These types of observations are especially interesting (and important), because the ATP is a common substrate molecule for both Na^+–K^+-dependent ATPase and adenylate cyclase in the presence of Mg^{2+}. The actual level of ATP is also a limiting factor for the functions of Na^+–K^+-dependent ATPase. The ATP level decreases by the functions of membrane-bound enzyme systems; however, ATP resynthesis can be obtained only under intact oxidative phosphorylation. The measurements of tissue ATP (*in vivo* observations) performed alone do not give a correct argument to prove or to exclude the presence of tissue hypoxia. This question is a basic problem in the ulcer development (under experimental conditions of patients).

The results of these observations proved the existence of a very complex regulatory (feedback) mechanism system between the Na^+–K^+-dependent ATPase and adenylate cyclase in *in vitro* and *in vivo* conditions by mediators, hormones, drugs and by the actual level of tissue ATP in the gastric mucosa. Furthermore, the function of Na^+–K^+-dependent ATPase can be modified by smaller concentrations of these compounds, in comparison with those of adenylate cyclase. It is also interesting and important to note that the regulatory actions of these regulatory compounds produce contradictory directions (stimulation vs. inhibition or inhibition vs. stimulation) on the Na^+–K^+-dependent ATPase and adenylate cyclase from gastric mucosal tissues. We have to emphasize the extents of energy liberation by the transformations of ATP into ADP, and ATP and cAMP also differ from each other in terms of energy liberation.

The ATP–ADP transformation by Na^+–K^+-dependent ATPase represents the first-line metabolic adaptation of the gastric mucosal cells to different influences (drugs, hormones, media-

http://dx.doi.org/10.5772/60105

tors), while the ATP–cAMP transformation by adenylate cyclase indicates the secondary metabolic adaptation of the cells in the gastric mucosa. The term "second messenger system" has been defined by Sutherland, who received the Nobel Prize in Physiology (Medicine) in 1971 for the discovery of ATP–cAMP transformation by adenylate cyclase in liver slides.

12.6. Biochemical measurements in the gastrointestinal mucosa of patients with peptic ulcer who underwent gastric surgery for ulcer disease

The gastric partial resection (dominantly according to Billroth II intervention) was frequently applied in the treatment of patients with peptic ulcer, because of the failure in "medical" (pharmacological, dietetic) treatment carried out by internists.

We never emphasized the importance of surgical treatment of peptic ulcer because we observed many early (dumping syndrome, diarrhea, etc.) and late (malabsorption syndrome, osteoporosis, stump cancer) complications of gastric surgery. These medical problems led us to evaluate the reason(s) why the "medical treatment" failed in these (1960s) years. These facts stimulated us to start with the critical analysis of the problems of pharmacological treatment in patients with peptic ulcer, and the methodology of clinical pharmacology appeared in consequence of these facts. The number of patients with peptic ulcer was 160–170/year who underwent surgical intervention at the First Department of Surgery, Pécs University, Hungary; however, after our clinical pharmacological results were introduced into everyday medical treatment, the number of surgically treated patients with peptic ulcer decreased to 2–3 patients per year in a very short time.

The necessity of gastric surgery was not indicated by internists, but by surgeons. Our biochemical observations were carried out on the resecates of human gastrointestinal tract obtained during surgical intervention.

The gastrointestinal resecates (obtained after surgical intervention) were biochemically studied (for details, see Chapter 7). Our biochemical examinations (using the internationally accepted methodology during the first half of 1970–1975) were expressed in relation to 1.0 mg DNA (representing the same number of cells).

The Na^+–K^+-dependent ATPase differs from the H^+–K^+–ATPase (for details, see Chapter 5); however, about 50–60% of Na^+–K^+–ATPase is incorporated into H^+–K^+–ATPase. The H^+–K^+–ATPase is located only in the parietal cells of stomach, while the Na^+–K^+-dependent ATPase can be found in all types of cells. Interestingly, the ATP is a common substrate molecule for both enzymes. (Note: We have to emphasize that we had no possibility to measure the cAMP directly from the surgically obtained resecates of the GI tract of patients with peptic ulcer at the time of gastric surgery.)

The gastric basal (BAO) and maximal (MAO) secretory responses were used as objective parameters for the stomach (these observations were carried out before the surgical intervention).

The biochemical results obtained from the gastric fundic mucosa and ulcerated antral, duodenal and jejunal mucosa must be observed.

These results were very surprising, since they were the same (note that the results were calculated as 1.0 mg DNA). The levels of ATP and ADP were higher in the gastric fundic mucosa with increased gastric acid secretory responses (together with the increased activity of Na^{+}–K^{+}-dependent ATPase). The same results were obtained in the ulcerated antral, duodenal and jejunal mucosa (1.5–2.0 cm around to ulcer), while these parameters were significantly lower (in the same patients) in the non-ulcerated (control) antral, duodenal and jejunal mucosa. The increased level of tissue ATP can be obtained by the increased oxidative phosphorylation, while the increased splitting (turnover) of ATP into ADP can be found by the increased Na^{+}–K^{+}-dependent ATPase in these tissue specimens. These results gave clear evidence for the exclusion of the presence of tissue hypoxia (impaired oxidative phosphorylation) in the ulcerated antral, duodenal and jejunal mucosa in patients with antral, duodenal and jejunal ulcers.

If we carefully observe the biochemical structures of corpus (fundus), antrum, duodenum in patients with peptic ulcer, we can notice that different energetic and biochemical gradients are present between fundic, antral and duodenal mucosa in these patients.

After a very careful analysis of these results, we can suggest that the clinically detectable appearance of antral, duodenal and antral ulcer is a consequence of a very active (increased) metabolic process (and not of decreased tissue metabolism). The possibility of adaptation to increased metabolic processes is determined by the original biochemical and energetic structures of fundus, antrum, duodenum and jejunum in patients with peptic ulcer. These structures, of course, depend on the general activity (such as gastric secretory parameters) of the stomach in humans (patients with peptic ulcer).

There are some problems with the critical evaluation of the presence of tissue hypoxia:

a. The decrease in gastric mucosal blood flow measured by different physiological methods does not prove the presence of tissue hypoxia in the ulcerated tissues in patients with peptic ulcer;

b. No clear and easily used methods were available in the case of humans (especially to measure the gastric mucosal blood flow (GMBF) in patients with peptic ulcer in time just before the development of ulcer);

c. The increased level of tissue level of lactate is one of the two main arguments to prove the existence of tissue hypoxia; the second one is the decreased tissue level of ATP due to impaired oxidative phosphorylation.

12.7. Messages of biochemical examinations in different ulcer models

Many animal observations were carried out to understand the changes in the gastric mucosa with and without mucosal damage and ulcer. A wide scale of biochemical methods were used in these animal studies (for details, see Sections 4.2 and 4.3) and different necrotizing agents (aspirin, indomethacin, ethanol, NaOH, HCL, concentrated NaCL solution and other drugs such as epinephrine, reserpine and stress situation) (or surgical intervention) were administered to cause gastric mucosal damage. The biochemical examination was done in a time-

http://dx.doi.org/10.5772/60105

dependent manner after the administration of different necrotizing agents; consequently, we were able to study the biochemical mechanisms before the macroscopic appearance of gastric mucosal damage, and, of course, during the time of macroscopic appearance of gastric mucosal damage. The critical analyses of these results (obtained in different experimental models) helped in understanding the suggested key biochemical events responsible for the development of gastric mucosal damage (for details, see Chapter 8).

Our attention was focused on the changes in the members of membrane-bound ATP-dependent energy systems (e.g., ATP, ADP, AMP, cAMP) in connection with the measurements of tissue lactate levels in gastric mucosa. All biochemical measurements were carried out in the same tissue samples at the same time. The key goal was to understand the problems of tissue hypoxia in the development of gastric mucosal damage (in very different experimental conditions).

In other observations, we administered various drugs (atropine, cimetidine, drugs interfering with different subcellular mechanisms and vitamin A and β-carotene – as typical nutritional scavengers – prostacyclin) to prevent the development of mucosal damage produced by different chemicals or stress. The biochemical examinations were conducted under the same experimental conditions as those in the previous models.

We have concluded the following from the analyses of the results obtained from these biochemical examinations in different experimental models:

a. The ATP breakdown (by membrane-bound ATPase and adenylate cyclase) increased practically in all models, with the exception of aspirin-induced mucosal damage and pylorus ligation by after surgical vagotomy).

b. The changes in energy systems in cells appear before the macroscopic appearance of gastric mucosal damage, while these changes in the cellular energy systems can be prevented by the administration of different mucosal protective agents in the same time period as in the case of the development of mucosal damage.

c. The existence of feedback mechanism can be proven in different experimental models, in terms of development of mucosal damage and prevention.

d. The presence of tissue hypoxia can be excluded by biochemical observations in the gastric mucosa with the development of gastric mucosal damage.

e. The mucosal protection by drugs and scavengers, or biological agents (such as prostaglandins), exists in animals only in conditions of intact vagal nerve, while the gastric mucosal protection ("cytoprotection") disappears after surgical vagotomy, but not in the case of "chemical vagotomy." Consequently, the "surgical" vagotomy and "chemical" vagotomy differ significantly from each other. We were pioneers, who demonstrated first that the intact vagal nerve is involved in the increase of aggressive factors in the stomach, because no gastric mucosal protection exists after surgical vagotomy.

f. The gastric mucosal protection produced by scavengers appears in pathways of the changes in parameters of oxygen free radical system (peroxidase, glutathione peroxidase,

superoxide dismutase, reduced glutathione, MDA) and in the parameters of membrane-bound ATP-dependent energy system (ATP, ADP, AMP, cAMP). Interestingly, the mucosal protecting effects of scavengers (vitamin A, β-carotene) produced dose-dependent changes in the membrane-bound ATP-dependent energy system but not in the parameters of oxygen free radicals. It is important to note that these actions are associated with the changes of membrane-bound ATP-dependent energy system and oxygen free radical system; however, without the biochemical presence of tissue hypoxia in the gastric mucosa (in both the time of development of gastric mucosal damage and prevention by scavengers).

g. The mucosal aggressive and protective effects of different drugs (or other compounds) depend on the functional states of effector organ (including their biochemical background). The observation of these facts is an important factor in the medical treatment by different drugs (compounds). The clinicians have enough information on the onset of the disease and functional states of effector organ. Observing these facts, probably, we can better understand the efficiencies of various therapeutic drugs, but these suggestions are also true in the case of mucosal producing drugs.

It is well known that these experimental models cannot be interpreted in human pathology without criticism; however, we received more information in this field from experimental ulcers.

12.8. Observations on freshly isolated gastric cells from the rat gastric mucosa

The special cellular biochemical examinations were carried out on gastric mucosal cells freshly isolated from gastric mucosa of rat (for details, see Chapter 9). These methodologies were able to demonstrate the cellular damaging effects of different agents at the levels of cell membrane, mitochondrion and DNA.

The effects of ethanol, indomethacin and sonicated *Helicobacter pylori* cultures (obtained from the cultured strains of *Helicobacter pylori* isolated from the gastric mucosa in patients with duodenal ulcer) were studied.

It was very surprising to note that sonicated *Helicobacter pylori* were given alone in doses of 10^8 to 10^6 germs/mL, indomethacin and its combination had no actions at any level of cell membrane, mitochondrion or DNA of freshly isolated cells (for details, see Chapter 9). This experimental methodology is internationally used to screen the cellular mucosal damaging and protecting effects of compounds.

One of the authors (Gy. Mozsik) observed that gastric cancer did not develop in patients, who originally suffered from the classical duodenal ulcer (from 1960 to 2014), without gastric surgical intervention (Mózsik Szabó and Czimmer, 2014). It is well known that most patients with duodenal ulcer are infected with *Helicobacter pylori*. We are of the opinion that the presence of *Helicobacter pylori* infection is only one of many causes, which are able to produce gastrointestinal mucosal damage. It seems that researchers have forgotten the results of classic GI research when the role of *Helicobacter pylori* became emphasized. However, we have to

http://dx.doi.org/10.5772/60105

remember the possibility that the single isolated cells from rat gastric mucosa are not able to produce prostaglandins.

12.9. Experimetal studies with different compounds on the stable cell lines

The tendency of drug (and some meaning physiological) research with stable cell cultures significantly increased during the last decades. We also used different stable cell lines to study the effect of various chemicals on cells and to do some toxicological examinations (for details, see Chapter 10).

The results obtained with different compounds in stable cell lines are important; however, these effects are not the same as those in living organs.

12.10. The "Take Home Messages" from the authors.

Several different mechanisms (existing at different levels of living organisms) run parallelly beside each other during the development of damage and protection at the levels of organisms, organs, tissues, cells or different subcellular particles (besides the genetic control in the whole living organisms). The researchers have many possibilities to modify a separated mechanism from this extremely large number of mechanisms. We can prove some correlation(s) between the examined parameters versus different phenomena. We believe that we are right and we discovered some new mechanism(s) in our field. Other researchers are in the same position to discover the actually studied phenomenon versus main problems of results in the field, and they also believed that they discovered some other new mechanism(s). Unfortunately, these new results together are not able to help to understand the human medical problems.

We are not able to understand the deep mechanisms, when we observe the whole organism; however, as we observe the very small pieces of cellular and subcellular mechanisms, we might lose the whole organism. This contradiction is also permanently present between clinicians and basic researchers.

Our attention was focused on the existing cellular regulatory mechanisms in the biochemical changes of gastric (gastrointestinal in patients) mucosa in patients with peptic ulcer and gastric mucosa in different experimental models (including the different subcellular particles) under basic (normal and different pathological conditions, without and with the application of different biologically active compounds, drugs).

We have faced the actual challenges of peptic ulcer disease in patients, namely, critical evaluation of the efficiency of medical treatment, principal role of gastric hypersecretion in ulcer development in patients, establishing the human clinical pharmacology, biochemical constitutes of gastric fundic mucosa with different gastric acid secretory responses, the presence of hypoxia in the ulcerated antral, duodenal, jejunal tissues around the ulcer, other detailed biochemical mechanisms of gastric ulcer in the human gastrointestinal mucosa under different conditions (fundic, antral, duodenal and jejunal) and in tissues (with and without ulcer).

A wide scale of experimental ulcers has been applied (together with different experimental conditions). The main attention was focused on the changes of cellular energy (membrane-bound ATP-dependent energy) systems versus the presence of tissue hypoxia (the lactate levels were measured together with other biochemical examinations to prove/to exclude the presence of impaired oxidative phosphorylation in the gastric mucosal tissues). The observations were done at the time of development of damage and its protection by different chemical compounds (drugs).

Answers to our (main) scientific problems are the following in the last half of the century:

a. Without clinical pharmacology, we were not able to critically evaluate the efficiencies (and their background) of the drugs used in the treatment of patients with peptic ulcer. We obtained an excellent reconfirmation by the international clinical pharmacological research to pioneer our work in establishing methodology of clinical pharmacology in patients with peptic ulcers.

The established clinical pharmacology gave scientifically based observations to understand the different medical questions and compare the efficiencies of drugs (with different actions of mechanisms).

b. The key role of decrease of gastric acid secretion (by therapeutically applied drugs) is not necessary for the healing of gastric and duodenal ulcer in patients. In other words, the phenomenon of "cytoprotection" exists in patients with both chronic duodenal and jejunal ulcers.

c. The development of "development of tolerance" to parasympatholytic drugs together with the "development of pharmacological denervation phenomenon" is one of the clinical pharmacological explanations for the existence of "cytoprotection" in patients with chronic atropine treatment. This explanation was never given for the existence of "gastric (duodenal) cytoprotection" in patients with chronic gastric and duodenal ulcer. However, it is also clear that the "gastric cytoprotection" is an existing phenomenon in patients with chronic gastric ulcer (for details, see Chapter 2) (without this clinical pharmacological explanation, vitamin A has really gastric mucosal damage, but without its inhibitory action on gastric acid secretion).

d. The presence of gastric hypoxia in the ulcerated antral, duodenal and jejunal mucosa (e.g., of impaired oxidative phosphorylation) biochemically can be excluded in the presence of gastric antral, duodenal and jejunal mucosa around chronic ulcer in patients with chronic peptic ulcer (because the biochemical compositions of these ulcerated mucosal tissues are the same as those in the gastric fundic mucosa with gastric hyperacidity).

e. The successful preparation of Na^+–K^+-dependent ATPase and adenylate cyclase by us opened an absolutely new gate to study and understand the classic biochemical mechanism of the equilibrium between different parameters of cellular energy system (ATP, ADP, AMP, cAMP) under normal (intact) and different pathological conditions).

The axis of cellular ATP–ADP–cAMP–AMP–ATP breakdown by the membrane-bound ATPase splitting enzymes (membrane ATPase, adenylate cyclase),– ATP resynthesis (under

http://dx.doi.org/10.5772/60105

intact oxidative phosphorylation), tissue levels of lactate, gastric acid hypersecretion, the development of gastric (gastrointestinal) mucosal damage (ulcer), intact vagal nerve, damaging and protective effects of different drugs, decrease of gastric acid secretion and the protection of GI mucosal damage cover the main topics of gastrointestinal physiology, pathophysiology and pathology in animals and humans. The obtained results in this axis can be critically evaluated in respect with the results of the above-mentioned cellular parameters.

The drugs (and other compounds) represent the "first messengers," while the intracellular mechanisms together indicate the details of "second (intracellular) mechanisms" in the cellular energy systems in both normal (intact) and different pathological conditions, without and with the application of any drug (compounds). We have to emphasize that the changes in the cellular energy systems are in very close correlation with other intracellular mechanisms (for details, see Chapter 5). The details of these different mechanisms presented by international experts (over the world) are related closely to this axis. Our molecular pharmacological examination with the drugs interfering with different cellular mechanisms clearly indicated that the functions of the levels of cell membrane, mitochondrion, protein synthesis, RNA and DNA are involved in the development of gastric acid hypersecretion, mucosal damage and mucosal protection produced by PGI2 and scavengers (vitamin A, β-carotene) (for details, see Section 8.12).

The actions of first messengers and their intracellular changes in the energy systems depend on the actual functional levels of target organ (including other intracellular mechanisms) at the time after the onset of different pathological (drugs) processes.

f. The existence of "gastrointestinal cytoprotection" and drugs produced by different compounds (scavengers, drugs, other compounds) disappears after surgical vagotomy; however, it remains intact in the case of "chemical vagotomy." This is a great criticism on the clinical application (practice) of surgical vagotomy in the treatment of patients with chronic peptic ulcer.

g. The results of the observations obtained from freshly isolated gastric mucosal cells and stable cells lines (gastric cancer, hepatoma, colorectal cancer, mouse myeloma) gave important scientific information for researchers (clinicians); however, it is also important to note that these results differ – in some meaning – from those obtained in living organs;

h. The observations with capsaicin (in respect to all of the very strict international laws of clinical pharmacology) offer a new pathway for the medical treatment of patients with peptic ulcer and for the prevention of drug-induced gastrointestinal mucosal damage by the stimulation of capsaicin-sensitive afferent nerves via the stimulation of capsaicin receptor (TRPV1) and liberation of different neuropeptides (calcitonin gene-related peptide, CGRP; substance P, SP; somatostatin; glycagon).

Newer research fields in gastroenterology, such as the research with capsaicin or newer neural mediators, opened a new window to further approach the mechanism of gastrointestinal mucosal damage and prevention.

The clinicians have followed the theoretical and practical advantages of clinical medicine with the simultaneous development of basic research. It has been very difficult for clinicians to maintain this position (we have tried to live two lives in the last half century). We were basically clinicians; however, apart from that we foray into the experimental research, thus accepting the actual scientific questions of basic research in gastroenterology.

There are general problems that no critical and scientific communications exist between the clinicians and basic researchers in gastroenterology.

The following list of references includes (incorporates) the most selective list of references, the detailed list of references is incorporated in the original publications.

Acknowledgements

The authors express their thanks to all Hungarian and Foreign coworkers.

These studies were supported by the grants of Hungarian Ministry of Health (ETT-735/93, ETT-03660/93, ETT-385/96, ETT-34/2000, ETT-595/2003), Hungarian Research Funds (T-307, T-2466, T-016945, T-020098) and National Office for Research and Technology ["Pázmány Péter programme" (RET-II 08/2005) and "Baros Gábor Programme" (REG_DKI_ O, CAPSATAB, 2009-2012)].

Author details

Gyula Mozsik[1*] and Imre Szabó[2]

*Address all correspondence to: gyula.mozsik@aok.pte.hu

1 First Department of Medicine, Medical and Health Centre, University of Pécs, Hungary

2 Associate Professor at the First Department of Medicine, University of Pécs, Hungary

References

[1] Albers R. W. (1967) Biochemical aspects of active transport. Ann. Rev. Biochem. 36: 727–756.

[2] Andrási F. (1997) Search for new antiulcer molecules at the IDR between 1971-1996 (The omeprazole-story). In: Mózsik Gy., Nagy L., Király Á. (eds) Twenty Five Years of Peptic Ulcer Research in Hungary: From Basic Sciences to Clinical Practice (1971-1995). Akadémiai Kiadó, Budapest. pp. 411–416.

http://dx.doi.org/10.5772/60105

[3] Asano S., Yoshida A., Yashiro H., Kobayashi Y., Morisato A., Ogowa H., Tageuchi N., Morii M. (2003) The cavity structure for blocking the K+-competitive inhibitors in the gastric proton pump. J. Biol. Chem. 279: 13968–13975.

[4] Askari A. (1974) Properties and functions of Na^{+}-K^{+}-activated adenosine-triphosphate Ann. N. Y. Acad. Sci. 242: 1–741.

[5] Atkinson D. E. (1968) The energy charge of the adenylate pool as a regulatory parameter. Interaction with feedback modifiers. Biochemistry 7: 3030–4034.

[6] Bauer H., Kasperek S., Pfaff E. (1972) Criteria of viability of liver isolated cells. Z. Physiol. Chem. 356: 827–838.

[7] Beers R. F., Sizer J. W. (1952) A spectrophotometric method for measuring the hydrogen peroxidase by catalase. J. Biol. Chem. 95: 133–140.

[8] Bergmayer H. U., Bern T. E. (1972) Calorimetric assay with L(+)lactase, NAD, phenazone methosulphate and INT. In: Bergmayer H. U. (ed) Methods in Enzymatic Analysis. Academic Press, New York. pp. 579–582.

[9] Bódis B., Abdel-Salam O. M. E., Karádi O., Mozsik Gy. (1995a) Protective effect of prostacyclin against indomethacin on isolated gastric mucosal cell. Z. Gastroenterol. 33: 282.

[10] Bódis B., Karádi O., Voros S., Mozsik Gy. (1995b) Has sonicated Helicobacter pylori any diect cellular effect? In: Bajtai A., Papp J., Rácz I., Simon L. (eds) Helicobacter pylori. Hungarian Society of Gastroenterology. Medicom, Budapest. pp. 137–142

[11] Bódis B., Karádi O., Abdel-Salam O. M. E., Vörös S., Nagy L., Mózsik Gy. (1996) Direct cellular effect of Helicobacter pylori alone and with cotreatments of ethanol and indomethacin in mixed isolated rat gastric mucosa cell. Dig Dis. Sci. 41: 430.

[12] Bódis B., Karádi O., Abdel-Salam O. M. E, Faludi R., Nagy L., Mózsik Gy. (1997a) Organoprotection and cytoprotection of histamine differ in rats. Inflammopharmacol. 5: 29–41.

[13] Bódis B., Karádi O., Nagy L., Mózsik Gy. (1997b) Aggressive and protective agents in organo- and cytoprotection in the stomach. In: Mózsik Gy., Nagy L., Király Á. (eds) Twenty Five Years of Peptic Ulcer Research in Hungary: From Basic Sciences to Clinical Practice (1971-1995) . Akadémiai Kiadó, Budapest. pp. 255–263.

[14] Bódis B., Németh P., Mózsik Gy. (1998) Organoprotection and Cytoprotection in the Stomach. Akadémiai Kiadó, Budapest.

[15] Bódis B., Karádi O., Szabo I., Németh P., Belágyi J., Mózsik Gy. (2000) Evidence for the involvement of oxygen free radicals in the ethanol-induced late cellular injury in mouse myeloma cells. J. Physiol. Paris 94: 67–70.

[16] Bowen J. B., Fairchild R. B. (1984) Oxygen in gastric mucosal protection. In: Allen A, Flemström A. G., Garner A., Silen W., Turnberg L. A. (eds) Mechanisms of Mucosal Protection in the Upper Gastrointestinal Tract. Raven Press, New York. pp. 57–64.

[17] * The list of references includes (incorporates) the most selective list of references, the detailed list of references is incorporated in the original publication.

[18] Brodie D. A., Cook P. G., Bauer B. J. (1970) Indomethacin-induced intestinal lesions in the rat. Toxicol. Appl. Pharmacol. 17: 615–624.

[19] Bunnier M. (2008) Sodium in Health and Disease. CRC Press. Broca Raton, Fl. USA.

[20] Butcher R. W. (1966) Cyclic 3′,5′-AMP and the lipolytic effects of hormones on adipose tissue. Pharmacol. Rev. 18: 237–247.

[21] Butcher R. W. and Sutherrland E. W. (1962) Adenosine 3′,5′-phosphate in biological materials. I. Purification and properties of cyclic 3′,5′-nucliotide phosphodiesterase and use of this enzyme to characterize adenosine 3′,5′-phosphate in human urine. J. Biol. Chem. 237: 1244–1250.

[22] Butcher R. W., Sutherland E. W. (1965) Adenosine 3′5′- monophosphate in biological materials. II. The measurement of cyclic 3′,5′-AMP in tissues and the lipolytic response of tat to epinephrine. J. Biol. Chem. 240: 4515–4523.

[23] Calderon D. P., Fremont R., Kraenzlin F., Khodakhah K. (2011) The neuron substances of rapid-onset dystonia Parkinsonism. Nature Neuroscience 14: 357–365.

[24] Cannon C. (2004) Paying the Price at the Pump: dystonia from mutations in a Na^{+}-K^{+}-ATPase. Neuron 43: 153–154. (http:/www.cell.com/neuron/retrive/pii/S089662730400426X)

[25] Chang H., Saccomani G., Rabon E., Schachmann R., Sachs G. (1977) Proton transport by gastric membrane vesicles. Biochim. Biophys. Acta 464: 313–327.

[26] Chaudhury T. K., Jacobson E. D. (1978) Prostaglandin cytoprotection of gastric mucosa. Gastroenterology 74: 59–63.

[27] Csáky T. Z. (1969) Introduction to General Pharmacology, Appleton-Century Crofts Educational Division, New York. pp.17–34

[28] Davenport H. M. (1965) Damage to gastric mucosa: effects of salicylates and stimulation. Gastroenterology 49: 487–499.

[29] De Jongh D. K., Proosdij-Hartzema E. G., Jannsen P. (1955) Substituted phenylpropamides. II. Pharmacological properties of basis butironitriles and butiramides. Arch. Int. Pharmacodyn. 103: 100–109.

[30] Dey C., Majumder G. C. (1988) A simple quantitative method of estimation of cell-intactness based on ethidium bromide fluorescence. Biochem. Int. 17: 367–374.

http://dx.doi.org/10.5772/60105

[31] Djahanguiri B. (1969) The production of acute gastric ulceration by indomethacin in the rat. Scand. J. Gastroenterol. 4: 265–267.

[32] Dunbar L. A., Caplan M. J. (2001) Ion pumps in polarized cells: sorting and regulation of Na^{+}-K^{+}- and H^{+}-K^{+}-ATPases. J. Biol. Chem. 276: 29617–29620.

[33] Ellman G. (1959) Tissue sulfhydryl groups. Arch. Biochem. Biophys. 195: 133–140.

[34] Emmelin N. (1952) "Paralytic secretion" of saliva. A sample of supersensitivity after denervation. Physiol. Rev. 32: 21–46.

[35] Emmelin N. (1961) Supersensitivity following "pharmacological denervations". Pharmacol. Rev. 13: 17–37.

[36] Emmelin N., Muren A. (1951a) Paralytic secretion in cats after prolonged treatment with atropine. Acta Physiol. Scand. 22: 277–280.

[37] Emmelin N., Muren A. (1951b) Effects of prolonged administration of atropine and pilocarpine on the submandibular gland of the cat. Acta Physiol. Scand. 24: 128–143.

[38] Emmelin N., Muren A. (1952) The sensitivity of submaxillary glands to chemical agents?

[39] Emmelin N., Rosenblueth A. (1951) The Supersensitivity of Denervated Structures. McMillan Co.

[40] Faller L. D., Malinowska D. H., Rabon E., Smolka A., Sachs G. (1982) Mechanistic studies of gastric H^{+}-K^{+}-ATPase. Prog. Clin. Biol. Res. 73: 153–179.

[41] Fehér O. (1960) The role of acetylcholine-cholinesterase system in the synaptic transmission process. Ph.D. Dissertation. University of Debrecen, Hungary.

[42] Figler M., Tárnok F., Nagy L., Patty I., Mózsik Gy. (1985) Biochemical background of the effect of atropine on the gastric mucosal damage produced by intragastric application of aspirin in pylorus-ligated rats. Digestion 31:145–146.

[43] Figler M., Jávor T., Nagy L., Patty I., Tárnok F., Mózsik Gy. (1986) Biochemical background of the development of gastric mucosal damage in pylorus-ligated plus aspirin-treated rats. Int. J. Tiss. Reac. 8: 15–22.

[44] Figler M., Szabó I., Mózsik Gy. (1999) Effects of pectin-induced passive linkage of gastric H^{+} on the gastric acid secretion and on the development of ethanol- and salicylate-induced gastric mucosal lesions in rats. J. Physiology (Paris) 93: 495–499.

[45] Flohe L., Güzlei W. S. (1984) Assay of glutathione peroxidase. In: Pocher I. (ed) Methods in Enzymology. Academic Press, New York. pp. 114–121.

[46] Fong K. L., McKay P. B., Polyer J. L. (1973) Evidence that peroxidation of lyposomal membranes is initiated by hydroxyl free radicals produced by flavin enzyme activity. J. Biol. Chem. 248: 7792–7797.

[47] Forrest M. D., Wall M. J., Press D. A., Feng J. (2012) The sodium-potassium pump controls the intrinsic firing on the intrinsic firing of the cerebellar Purkinje neuron. (https://dx.plos.org/10.1371/jopurnal.phone.0051169).

[48] Forte J. C., Lee H. C. (1977) Gastric adenosine triphosphatase: a review of their possible role in HCl secretion. Gastroenterology 73: 921–926.

[49] Gaginella T. S., Mózsik Gy., Rainsford K. D. (1997) (eds) Biochemical pharmacology as an approach to gastrointestinal disorders. In: Basic Science to Clinical Perspectives. Kluwer Academic Publishers, Dordrecht, Boston, London.

[50] Ganser A. L., Forte J. G. (1973) K^+-standard ATPase perfused microsomes of bullfrog oxyntic cells. Biochim. Biophys. Acta 307: 169–180.

[51] Garamszegi M., Jávor T., Sütő G., Vincze Á., Tóth Gy., Mózsik Gy. (1989) Effect of atropine, PGF_2 and cimetidine on the ß-carotene-induced gastric cytoprotection in ethanol-treated rats. Acta Physiol. Hung. 73: 221–224.

[52] Garamszegi M., Tárnok F., Patty I., Nagy L., Németh A., Pakodi F., Mózsik Gy. (1997) Comparison of different antisecretory and protective agents in the treatment of gastric ulcer patients. In: Mózsik Gy., Nagy L., Király Á. (eds). Twenty Five Years of Peptic Ulcer Research in Hungary (1971-1995). Akadémiai Kiadó, Budapest. pp. 361–366

[53] Gasztonyi B., Király Á., Sütő G., Vincze Á., Karádi O., Mózsik Gy. (1996) A comparative study on the adenine nucleotide metabolism of the acid-dependent and non acid-dependent acute gastric mucosal injury in the rats. Inflammopharmacology 4: 351–360.

[54] Gheorghui T. H. (1976) (ed) Experimental Ulcer Models, Methods and Clinical Validity. Gerhard, Wizstrock Publishers. Baden-Baden, Bruxelles-Cologne.

[55] Glynn I. M. (1964) The action of cardiac glycosides on ion movements. Pharmacol. Rev. 16: 381–407.

[56] Graff G. L. S., Hudson A. J., Strickland P. K. (1965a) Biochemical changes in denervated skeletal muscle. I. The effect of denervation atrophy on the main phosphate fractions of rat gastrocnemius muscle. Biochim. Biophys. Acta 104: 524–531.

[57] Graff G. L. S., Hudson A. J., Strickland P. K. (1965b) Biochemical changes in denervated skeletal muscle. II. Labelling patterns of the main phosphate fractions in normal and denervated rat gastrocnemius muscle using $^{32}P_i$ as indicator. Biochim. Biophys. Acta 104: 532–542.

[58] Graff G. L. S., Hudson A. J., Strickland P. K. (1965c) Biochemical changes in denervated skeletal muscle. III. The effect of denervation atrophy on the concentration and ^{32}P labelling of the individual phospholipids of the rat gastrocnemius. Biochim. Biophys. Acta 104, 542–553.

http://dx.doi.org/10.5772/60105

[59] Gregory R. A (1962) Secretory mechanisms of the gastrointestinal tract. Monogr. Physiol. Soc 11. Edward Arnold, London.

[60] Grenell R. G., Mullins L. J. (1956) Molecular Structures and Functional Activity of Nerve Cells. Series of International Book Series, Washington.

[61] Grijalva C.V., Novin D. (1990) The role of the hypothalamus and dorsal vagal complex in the gastrointestinal function and pathophysiology. Ann. N.Y. Acad. Sci. 597: 207–222.

[62] Grossmann I. M. (1979) Protection of gastric mucosa by prostaglandins. Gastroenterology 77: 593–594

[63] Gustafson J., Welling D. (2010) "No acid, no ulcer" – 100 years later: a review of the history of peptic ulcer disease. J. Amer. Coll. Surg. 210: 110–116.

[64] Guth P. H., Aures D., Paulsen G. (1979) Topical aspirin plus HCl gastric lesions in the rat. Cytoprotective effect of prostaglandin, cimetidine and probanthine. Gastroenterology 76: 88–93.

[65] Guth P. H., Paulsen G., Nagata H. (1984) Histologic and microcirculatory changes in alcohol-induced gastric lesions in the rat: effects of prostaglandin cytoprotection. Gastroenterology 87: 1083–1090.

[66] Gyermek L. (1951) Studies on the cholinergic blocking substances. I. Sites of action of compounds of the atropine group. Acta Physiol. Hung. 2: 511–517.

[67] Gyermek L. (1953) Studies on the cholinergic blocking substances. IV. Correlations between structure and effect of quaternary derivates of bensoyltropine and bensoyl tropine compounds. Acta Physiol. Hung. 4: 333–340.

[68] Gyermek L., Nádor K. (1952) Studies on the cholinergic blocking substances. II. Correlations between structures and the effect in antimuscarine, ganglion blocking and curare-like actions of mono- and bis-quaternary ammonium compounds. Acta Physiol. Hung. 3: 183–193.

[69] Gyermek L., Nádor K. (1953a) Studies on the cholinergic blocking substances. III. Neuromuscular blocking tropines. Acta Physiol. Hung. 4, 159–174.

[70] Gyermek L., Nádor K. (1953b) Studies on the cholinergic blocking substances. V. The pharmacology of monoquaternary tropines acting on vegetative ganglia. Acta Physiol. Hung. 4: 341–354.

[71] Győrffy Á., Mózsik Gy., Dobi S., Jávor T. (1964) Clinical-pharmacological investigations with parasympatholytic drugs. 7e Congress International de Gastro-Enterologie (A.S.N.E.M. G.E.) Resumes des communications (Bruxelles), p. 22.

[72] György L., Dóda M., Nádor K. (1961) The significance of quaternary groups of various steric configurations for the parasympatholytic and ganglion blocking effect of tropines. Arzneimittel-Forsch 11: 444–449.

[73] Hall J. E., Guyton A. C. (2006) Textbook of Medical Physiology. Elsevier Saunders, St. Louis, Mo, USA.

[74] Hansson L. E., Nyrén O., Hsing A. W., Bergström R., Joseffsonn S., Cwow W. H., Frumeni F. F., Adam H. O. (1996) The risk of stomach cancer in patients with gastric and duodenal ulcer diseases. N. Eng. J. Med. 107: 242–249.

[75] Henagan J. M., Seidel E. R., Miller T. A. (1983) Evidence that cytoprotection may be vagally mediated. Gastroenterology 84: 1186.

[76] Henion W. F., Sutherland E. W. (1955) Immunological differences of phosphorylase. J. Biol. Chem. 176: 169–170.

[77] Howard C., Gleeson P., Attwell D. (2012) Updated energy budgets for neural computation in the neocortex and cerebellum. J. Cereb. Blood Flow Metab. 32: 1222–1232.

[78] Hunyady B. (1997) Clinical and clinicopharmacological applications of the 24-hour intragastric pH-metry. In: Mózsik Gy., Nagy L., Király Á. (eds) Twenty Five Years of Peptic Ulcer Research in Hungary (1971-1995). Akadémiai Kiadó, Budapest. pp. 383–397

[79] Ihász M. (1980) Vagotomia (Vagotomy). Akadémiai Kiadó, Budapest.

[80] in cats under various conditions over long periods. Acta Physiol. Scand. 2, 221–238.

[81] Jávor T. (1968) The roles of gastric secretion, gastric emptying and blood flow supply in the development of peptic ulcer. Sc. D. Thesis of Debrecen University, Hungary.

[82] Jávor T., Győrffy Á., Mózsik Gy., Dobi S., Nagy Gy. (1965) Clinical pharmacology of some parasympatholytic drugs. Acta Medica Hung. 21: 271–277.

[83] Jávor T., Mózsik Gy., Krausz M. (1967) Clinical pharmacological methods for the study of intestinal drugs absorption. IV. Conferentia Hungarica pro Therapia et Investigatione in Pharmacologia. Akadémiai Kiadó, Budapest. pp. 563–565.

[84] Jávor T., Mózsik Gy., Szokola J., Vigh V., Rajnai E., Rauth J., Tárnok F. (1970) Gastric secretion and ulceration inhibitory effects by drugs interfering with some subcellular functions. In: Riis P., Anthonisen P., Baden H. (eds) Advance Abstracts, 4th World Congress of Gastroenterology. The Danish Gastroenterological Association. Copenhagen. p. 309.

[85] Jávor T., Bata M., Kutor G., Lovász L., Mózes Gy., Mózsik Gy. (1981) Gastric mucosal resistance to physical and chemical stress. In: Mózsik Gy., Hänninen O., Jávor T. (eds) Advances in Physiological Sciences. Vol. 29. Gastrointestinal Defense Mechanisms. Pergamon Press, Oxford – Akadémiai Kiadó, Budapest. pp. 141–159.

[86] Jávor T., Bata M., Lovász L., Morón F., Nagy L., Patty I., Szabolcs J., Tárnok F., Tóth Gy., Mózsik Gy. (1983) Gastric cytoprotective effect of vitamin A and other carotenoids. Int. J. Tiss. Reac. 5: 289–296.

http://dx.doi.org/10.5772/60105

[87] Karádi O., Mózsik Gy. (2000) Surgical and Chemical Vagotomy on the Gastrointestinal Mucosal Defense. Akadémiai Kiadó, Budapest.

[88] Kasbekar D. K., Durbin RP (1965) Adenosine triphosphatase from frog gastric mucosa Biochim. Biophys. Acta (Amsterdam) 105: 472–482.

[89] Király Á., Matus Z., Sütő G., Vincze Á., Mózsik Gy. (1992a) Correlation between the β-carotene-induced gastric cytoprotective effect and its gastric mucosal level in indomethacin-treated rats. Acta Physiol. Hung. 80: 215–220.

[90] Király Á., Sütő G., Vincze Á., Jávor T., Mózsik Gy. (1992b) Effect of acute (ASV) and chronic (CSV) surgical vagotomy on the vascular permeability of the gastric mucosa after 96% ethanol (ETOH) treatment in rats. Acta Physiol. Hung. 80: 221–226.

[91] Kitajima M. (1989) Gastric mucosal vascular architecture and mucosal blood flow in rats during stress. In: Szabó S., Pfeiffer C. J. (eds) Ulcer Disease: New Aspects of Pharmacogenesis and Pharmacology. CRC Press, Boca Raton.

[92] Klainer L. M., Chi Y. M., Freiidberg S. L., Rall T. W., Sutherland E. W. (1962) Adenyl cyclase. IV. Effects of neurohormones on the formation of adenosine 3′,5′-phosphate by preparation from brain and other tissues. J. Biol. Chem. 237: 1239

[93] Koenderink J. B., Swarts H. P., Hermsen H. H., De Pont J.P.H.H.M. (1999) The β-subunits of Na^+-K^+-ATPase and gastric H^+-K^+-ATPase have a high preference for their own α-subunit and affect the K^+ affinity of these enzymes. J. Biol. Chem. 274: 11604–11610.

[94] Kühlbrandt W. (2004) Biology, structure and mechanism of P-type ATPases. Nat. Rev. Mol. Cell Biol. 5: 282–295.

[95] Lacy E. E., Ito S. (1982) Microscopic analysis of ethanol damage to rat gastric mucosa after treatment with a prostaglandin. Gastroenterology 83: 619–625.

[96] Lacy E. R., Ito S. (1984) Rapid epithelial restitution of the rat gastric mucosa after ethanol injury. Lab. Invest. 51: 573–583.

[97] Laher I. (2014) (ed) Systems Biology of Free Radicals and Antioxidants. Springer, Berlin, Heidelberg.

[98] Lee S., Simpson G., Sachs G. (1974) ATPase of dog gastric microsomes. Changes of outer pH in suspensions of membrane vesicles. Biochem. Biophys. Res. Commun. 60: 825–864.

[99] Lee K., Jung J., Kim M., Gdotti G. (2001) Interaction of the alpha subunit of Na^+-K^+-ATPase with cofilin. J. Biol. Chem. 353: 377–385.

[100] Levine R. A. (1971) The role of cyclic AMP in gastric secretion. Ann. N.Y. Acad. Sci. 185, 363–375.

[101] Li Z., Cai T., Tian J. (2009) Na-Ktide, a Na^{+}-K^{+}-derived peptide Scr inhibitors, antagonises ouabain-activated signal transduction in cultured cells. J. Biol. Chem. 284: 21066–21076.

[102] Lowry O. H., Rosenbrough N. J., Farr A. L., Randal R. J. (1951) Protein measurement with folin phenol reagent. J. Biol. Chem. 193: 265–275.

[103] Mabe K., Takahashi M., Oizumi H., Tsukuma H., Shibata A., Fukase K., Matsuda T., Takeda H., Kawanta S. (2009) Does Helicobacter pylori eradication therapy for peptic ulcer prevent gastric cancer. World J. Gastroenterol. 14: 4290–4297.

[104] Maclennan D. H., Brandt C. J., Korczak B., Green N. M. (1985) Amino acid sequence of a Ca^{++} + Mg^{2+}-dependent ATPase from rabbit muscle sarcoplastic reticulum, deducted from its complementary DNA sequence. Nature 316: 696–700.

[105] Marshall B. J., Warren R. J. (1983) Unidentified curved bacilli in the stomach of patients with peptic ulcer. Lancet I: 1311–1315.

[106] Matkovics B., Novak R., Rank H. D., Szabo I., Varga Sz. I., Zalesna G. (1977) A comparative study of some more important experimental animal peroxidase metabolisms enzymes. Chem. Biochem. Physiol. 568: 31–34.

[107] Menguy R., Desbaillets L., Master Y. F. (1974a) Mechanisms of stress ulcer. I. Influence of hypovolemic shock on energy metabolism in the gastric mucosa. Gastroenterology 66: 46–55.

[108] Menguy R., Master Y. F. (1974b) Mechanism of stress ulcer. II. Differences between the antrum, corpus and fundus on gastric energy metabolism. Gastroenterology 66: 509–516.

[109] Menguy R., Master Y. F. (1974c) Mechanism of stress ulcer. III. Effects of hemorrhagic shock on metabolism in the antrum, corpus and fundus of the rabbit stomach. Gastroenterology 66: 1168–1176.

[110] Menguy R., Master Y. F. (1974d) Mechanism of stress ulcer. IV. Influence of fasting on the tolerance of gastric mucosal energy metabolism to ischemia and on the incidence of stress ulcer. 66: 1177–1186.

[111] Miller J. A. (1983) Protective effect of prostaglandins against gastric mucosal damage current knowledge and proposed mechanisms. Am. J. Physiol. 245: G601–G623.

[112] Misra H. P., Fridovics I. (1972) The role of superoxide anion in the autoxidation of epinephrine and a single assay for superoxide mismutase. J. Biol. Chem. 247: 3170–3175.

[113] Molloy R. M., Sonneberg A. (1997) Relationship between gastric cancer and previous peptic ulcer disease. Gut 40: 247–252.

[114] Morón F., Jávor T., Bata M., Figler M., Mózsik Gy. (1982) The relationships between the indomethacin-induced gastric ulcer, ulcer protection by cimetidine and prostacy-

http://dx.doi.org/10.5772/60105

cline and the cAMP system of the gastric fundic mucosa in rats. Acta Physiol. Acad. Sci. Hung. 60: 149–153.

[115] Morón F., Cuesta E., Bata M., Mózsik Gy. (1983) Cytoprotective effect of cimetidine: experimental evidence in the rat gastric mucosal lesions induced by intragastric administration of necrotizing agents. Arch. Int. Pharmacodyn. 265: 309–319.

[116] Morón F., Mózsik Gy., Jávor T. (1984a) Effects of cimetidine administered in cytoprotective and antisecretory doses on the membrane-bound ATP-dependent energy systems in the rat gastric mucosal lesions induced by HCl in rats. Acta Physiol. Hung. 64: 293–299.

[117] Morón F., Mózsik Gy., Nagy L., Patty I., Tárnok F., Jávor T. (1984b) Evidence for cytoprotective effect of atropine and cimetidine in human gastric mucosa. Acta Physiol. Hung. 64: 367–372.

[118] Morón F., Pena C., Cuesta E., Mózsik Gy., Jávor T. (1984c) Comparative study of the cytoprotective effects of anticholinergic agents on the gastric mucosal lesions produced by intragastric administration of 0.6 M HCl in rats. Acta Physiol. Hung. 64: 247–252.

[119] Morón F., Mózsik Gy., Nagy L., Patty I., Tárnok F., Jávor T. (1986) Evidence of the gastric cytoprotective effect of atropine and cimetidine in humans. Acta Physiol. Hung. 65: 367–372.

[120] Mosmann T. (1983) Rapid colorimetric assay for cellular growth and survival. Application to proliferation and cytotoxicity assay. J. Immunol. Methods 17: 367–374.

[121] Mózsik Gy. (1969a) Data to the action of mechanism of anticholinergic agents in patients and animals. Dissertation for Ph.D. pp. 1–255. Pécs University, Hungary.

[122] Mózsik Gy. (1969b) Some feedback mechanisms by drugs in the interrelationships between the active transport and adenyl cyclase system localized in the cell membrane Eur. J. Pharmacol. 7: 319–327.

[123] Mózsik Gy. (1970) Direct inhibitory effect of adenosine monophosphates on Na^{+}-K^{+}-dependent ATPase from human gastric mucosa Eur. J. Pharmacol. 9: 207–210.

[124] Mózsik Gy. (1971) In discussion of vascular impairment – an etiological factor in peptic ulcer? Pfeiffer C. J. (ed) Peptic Ulcer. Lippincott Company, Philadelphia – Munksgaard, Copenhagen. p. 220

[125] Mózsik Gy. (1975) Cellular mechanisms involved in the gastric acid secretion and ulcer development. Dissertation for Scientific Degree of the Hungarian Academy of Sciences. Pécs University. pp. 1–372.

[126] Mózsik Gy. (2005) Neural, hormonal and pharmacological regulations of retinoids-induced gastrointestinal mucosal protection. Recent Res. Develop. Life Sci. 3, 131–202.

[127] Mózsik Gy. (2006a) Molecular pharmacology and biochemistry of gastroduodenal mucosal damage and protection. In: Mózsik Gy. (ed) Discoveries in Gastroenterology: From Basic Science to the Clinical Perspectives (1960–2005). Akadémiai Kiadó, Budapest. pp. 139–224.

[128] Mozsik Gy. (2006b) History of the International Conferences on Ulcer Research (1970-2006). University Press of Pécs, Hungary.

[129] Mózsik Gy. (2010) Gastric cytoprotection 30 years after its discovery by André Robert: a personal perspective. Inflammopharmacology 18, 209–221.

[130] Mózsik Gy. (2014) Capsaicin as new orally applicable gastroprotective and therapeutic drug alone or in combination with nonsteroidal anti-inflammatory drugs in healthy human subjects and in patients.In: Adbel-Salam O. M. E. (ed) Capsaicin as a Therapeutic Molecule. Progress in Drug Research. Vol. 68. Springer, Basel. pp. 209–258.

[131] Mózsik Gy., Jávor T. (1965a) Clinical pharmacological analysis of Priamide. Magyar Belorvosi Archivum (Hung. Med. Arch.) 18: 42–49.

[132] Mózsik Gy., Jávor T. (1965b) Effects of parasympatholytics on the secretory responses of parotid glands and of stomach in humans (New clinical pharmacological test method). Kísérletes Orvostudomány (Experimental Medicine) 17: 213–218.

[133] Mózsik Gy., Jávor T. (1966a) Clinical pharmacology of parasympatholytic drugs. In: Borsy J. (ed) Experimental and Clinical Aspects of Ulcer Disease. Hungarian Society of Pharmacology, Budapest. pp. 81–94.

[134] Mózsik Gy., Jávor T. (1966b) Clinical pharmacological study of development of drug tolerance in chronic atropine treatment in patients. In: Borsy J. (ed) Current States of Absorption, Metabolism and Excretion of Drugs. Hungarian Society of Pharmacology, Budapest. pp. 56–65.

[135] Mózsik Gy., Jávor T. (1966c) Clinical-pharmacological testing for parasympatholytic drugs. Med. Pharmacol. Exp. 14: 183–190.

[136] Mózsik Gy., Jávor T. (1968a) Clinical pharmacological and pharmacodynamic problems of atropine treatment in patients suffering from peptic ulcer. In: Gregor O., Riedl O. (eds) Modern Gastroenterology. F. K. Shattauer Verlag, Stuttgart, New York. pp. 292–294

[137] Mózsik Gy., Jávor T. (1968b) Development of drug cross-tolerance in patients treated with atropine chromically. In: Gregor O., RiedO. (eds) Modern Gastroenterology. F. K. Shattauer Verlag, Stuttgart, New York. pp. 295–297

[138] Mózsik Gy., Jávor T. (1969) Development of drug cross-tolerance in patients treated chronically with atropine. Eur. J. Pharmacol. 6: 169–174.

http://dx.doi.org/10.5772/60105

[139] Mózsik Gy., Jávor T. (1988) A biochemical and pharmacological approach to the genesis of ulcer disease. I. A model study of ethanol-induced injury to gastric mucosa in rats. Dig. Dis. Sci. 33: 92–105.

[140] Mózsik Gy., Jávor T. (1991) Therapy of ulcers with sulfhydryl and nonsulfhydryl antioxidants. In: Swabb E. A., Szabó S. (eds) Ulcer Disease. Investigation and Basis for Therapy. Marcel Dekker, New York, Basel, Hong Kong. pp. 321–341.

[141] Mózsik Gy., Pfeiffer C. J. (1992) A biochemical and pharmacological approach to the genesis of ulcer disease. III. A model study of epinephrine–induced injury to gastric mucosa in rats. Exp. Clin. Gastroenterol. 2: 190–194.

[142] Mózsik Gy., Øye I. (1969) The preparation of Na^+-K^+-dependent ATPase from human gastric mucosa. Biophys. Biochim. Acta (Amsterdam) 183: 640–641.

[143] Mózsik Gy., Vizi F. (1976a) Examination of stomach wall Mg^{2+}-Na^+-K^+-dependent ATPase, ATP and ADP in pylorus-ligated rats. Amer. J. Digest. Dis. 21: 649–654.

[144] Mózsik Gy., Vizi F. (1976b) Surgical vagotomy and stomach wall ATP and ADP in pylorus-ligated rats. Amer. J. Digest. Dis. 22: 1072–1075.

[145] Mózsik Gy., Györffy Á., Dobi S., Jávor T. (1965a) Comparative clinical pharmacology study of atropine and Priamide. In: III. Conferentia Hungarica pro Therapia et Investigatione in Pharmacologia. Akadémiai Kiadó, Budapest. pp. 497–506.

[146] Mózsik Gy., Jávor T., Dobi S. (1965b) Clinical pharmacological analysis of long term parasympatholytic treatment. In: Magyar I. (ed) Acta Terii Conventus Medicinae Internae. Gastroenterologia. Akadémiai Kiadó, Budapest. pp. 709–715.

[147] Mózsik Gy., Jávor T., Dobi S., Petrássy K., Szabó A. (1967a) Development of "pharmacological denervation phenomenon" in patients treated with atropine. Eur. J. Pharmacol. 1: 391–395.

[148] Mózsik Gy., Szabó A., Krausz M., Jávor T. (1967b) Biochemical analysis of the stomach wall in normal rats. Scand. J. Gastroenterol. 2: 321–325.

[149] Mózsik Gy., Szabó A., Krausz M., Jávor T. (1967c) Biochemical analysis of vagotomized stomach wall in rats. Scand. J. Gastroenterol. 2: 326–332.

[150] Mózsik Gy., Vizi I., Jávor T. (1967d) Objective comparative clinicalpharmacological analysis of parasympatholytic drugs. Recent Advances of Gastroenterology. Third World Congress of Gastroenterology, Tokyo. Vol. 1. pp. 681–684.

[151] Mózsik Gy., Kiss B., Jávor T., Krausz M. (1968) Data for biochemical meaning of cholinergic nerve function in the stomach. In: Gregor O., Riedl O. (eds) Modern Gastroenterology. F. K. Shattauer Verlag, Stuttgard, New York. pp. 561–563.

[152] Mózsik Gy., Berstad A., Myren J., Setekleiv J. (1969a) Absorption and urinary excretion of oxyphencyclamine HCl in patients before and after a prolonged oxyphencyclimide treatment. Med. Exp. 19: 10–16.

[153] Mózsik Gy., Hauck M., Kóródy I., Szepesi Zs. (1969b) Base alterations of nucleic acids in the stomach wall after prolonged atropine treatment. Eur. J. Pharmacol. 7: 73–79.

[154] Mózsik Gy., Kiss B., Jávor T., Krausz M. (1969c) Some cellular effects of prolonged treatment with atropine in the stomach wall of the rats. (A biochemical-pharmacological approach of the effects of vagal exclusion – vagotomy and atropine treatment – on cellular molecular level). Eur. J. Pharmacol. 7: 66–72.

[155] Mózsik Gy., Kiss B., Jávor T., Krausz M., Tóth E. (1969d) Effect of a cholinesterase inhibitor treatment on the phosphorus and nucleic acid metabolism in the stomach wall. Pharmacology 2: 45–49.

[156] Mózsik Gy., Kiss B., Krausz M., Jávor T. (1969e) A biochemical- cellular- morphological-explanation for anticholinergic effects of parasympatholytics and of surgical vagotomy. Scand. J. Gastroenterol. 4: 641–651.

[157] Mózsik Gy., Kiss B., Krausz M., Jávor T. (1969f) A cellular- biochemical-morphological-explanation of the development of gastric ulcer in Shay rats. Scand. J. Gastroenterol. 4: 633–640.

[158] Mózsik Gy., Jávor T., Daróczy É. (1970a) Alterations in stomach wall ATP – ADP induced by atropine treatment. Pharmacology 4: 113–119.

[159] Mózsik Gy., Morón F., Jávor T. (1970b) Examination of adenyl cyclase system prepared form human gastric mucosa. In: Riis P., Anthonisen P., Baden H. (eds) Advance Abstracts, 4th World Congress of Gastroenterolology. Copenhagen. The Danish Gastroenterological Association. p. 381.

[160] Mózsik Gy., Jávor T., Hauck M., Karsai T. (1971a) On some cellular mechanisms of ulcer development in pylorus-ligated rats. In: Pfeiffer C. J. (ed) Peptic Ulcer. Lippincott Company, Philadelphia – Munksgaard, Copenhagen. pp. 171–184.

[161] Mózsik Gy., Nagy L., Tárnok F., Jávor T. (1971b) Examination of the cholinergic nervous transmission processes to cell of tissue around the gastric ulcer in patients. A molecular-pharmacological study. In: Pfeiffer C. J. (ed) Peptic Ulcer. Lippincott Company, Philadelphia-Munksgaard, Copenhagen. pp. 323–328.

[162] Mózsik Gy., Tárnok F., Nagy L., Vizi F. (1972) Na^{+}-K^{+}-dependent ATPase and adenyl cyclase systems in the human gastric mucosa. In: Greengard P., Robinson G. A., Paoletti R. (eds) Advances in Cyclic Nucleotide Research. Vol. 1. Physiology and Pharmacology of Cyclic AMP. Raven Press Publishers, New York. p. 582.

[163] Mózsik Gy., Nagy L., Tárnok F., Jávor T., Kutas J., Myren J., Berstad A. (1973a) On some molecular-pharmacological background of gastric secretory responses by pentagastrin, histamine and 2-pyridil-thio-acetamide (GYKI-43023) in patients. In: Borsy J., Mózsik Gy. (eds) Gastrin and its Antagonists. Akadémiai Kiadó, Budapest. pp. 97–111.

[164] Mózsik Gy., Tárnok F., Nagy L., Szokola J., Kutas J., Hauck M., Karsai T., Horváth L. (1973b) Biochemical approach to peptic ulcer. In: Jávor T., Mózsik Gy. (eds) Ten

Years Research of Peptic Ulcer in Hungary (1960-1970). Akadémiai Kiadó, Budapest. pp. 219–256.

[165] Mózsik Gy., Kutas J., Nagy L., Németh Gy. (1974a) Inhibition of Mg^{2+}-Na^{+}-K^{+}-dependent ATPase system from human gastric mucosa by prostaglandin E_1 and E_2. Eur. J. Pharmacol. 29: 133–137.

[166] Mózsik Gy., Nagy L., Jávor T., Kutas J. (1974b) Effects of histamine on transport (Na^{+}-K^{+}-dependent) ATPase system from the human gastric mucosa. Pharmacology 12: 193–200.

[167] Mózsik Gy., Nagy L., Kutas J., Tárnok F. (1974c) Interaction of cholinergic function with Mg^{2+}-Na^{+}-K^{+}-dependent ATPase system of cells in the human gastric fundic mucosa. Scand. J. Gastroenterol. 9: 741–745.

[168] Mózsik Gy., Nagy L., Tárnok F., Vizi F., Kutas J. (1974d) H^{+} secretion and Na^{+}-K^{+}- dependent ATPase system from human gastric mucosa. Experientia (Basel) 30: 1024–1025.

[169] Mózsik Gy., Szokola J., Vigh V., Rajnai E., Tárnok F., Jávor T. (1975a) Evidence for etiological role of active transport system of cell during gastric ulceration by pyloric ligation. In: Gheorghui T. (ed) Experimental Ulcer. Models, Methods and Clinical Validity. Gerhard Witzstrock Publishers, Baden-Baden, Brussels, Cologne. pp. 348–353.

[170] Mózsik Gy., Vizi F., Jávor T. (1975b) Prevention of gastric hypersecretion and ulceration in pylorus-ligated rats by cytostatics. In: Gheorghui T. (ed) Experimental Ulcer Models, Methods and Clinical Validity. Gerhard Witzstrock Publishers, Baden-Baden, Brussels, Cologne. pp. 238–245.

[171] Mózsik Gy., Vizi F., Beró T., Kutas J. (1976a) Biochemical evaluation of mucosa tissues around the gastric, duodenal, and jejunal ulcer in patients. In: Mózsik Gy., Jávor T. (eds) Progress of Peptic Ulcer. Akadémiai Kiadó, Budapest. pp. 265–285.

[172] Mózsik Gy., Vizi F., Kutas J. (1976b) A cellular-biochemical evaluation of gastric body mucosa and muscular layer in patients with different basal acid outputs. Scand. J. Gastroenterol. 11: 205–211.

[173] Mózsik Gy., Vizi F., Nagy L., Beró T., Kutas J. (1976c) Na^{+}-K^{+}-dependent ATPase system and the gastric H^{+} secretion by the human gastric mucosa. In: Mózsik Gy., Jávor T. (eds.) Progress in Peptic Ulcer. Akadémiai Kiadó, Budapest. pp. 37–72.

[174] Mózsik Gy., Beck Zs., Füzesi Zs., Kiss J., Nagy L., Palotai Z., Szilágyi A., Tárnok F., Tóth E., Vizi F. (1978a) Cellular mechanisms of gastric hypersecretion in pylorus-ligated rats. Acta Physiol. Scand. Special Suppl. 187–198.

[175] Mózsik Gy., Kutas J., Nagy L., Tárnok., Vizi F. (1978b) Interrelationships between the cholinergic influences, gastric mucosa Na^{+}-K^{+}-dependent ATPase, ATP, ADP, ions of

gastric juice and basal secretion in patients. Acta Physiol. Scand. Special Suppl. 199–208.

[176] Mózsik Gy., Nagy L., Tárnok F. (1978c) Interrelationships between the gastric mucosal cAMP and gastric H^+ secretion in pylorus-ligated rats. Gastroenterology 75: 164 (research letter).

[177] Mózsik Gy., Figler M., Lőrincz P., Nagy L., Tárnok F. (1979a) The role of ATP adenylate cyclase – cAMP system and its pharmacological regulation in the development of gastric hypersecretion and ulceration. Acta Medica Acad. Sci. Hung. 36: 427–448.

[178] Mózsik Gy., Kutas J., Nagy L., Tárnok F. (1979b) Biochemical and energetical gradients in the mucosa of stomach and duodenum in patients with antral ulcer. Acta Medica Acad. Sci. Hung. 36: 449–457.

[179] Mózsik Gy., Kutas J., Nagy L., Tárnok F. (1979c) Comparative molecular pharmacological study of drugs inhibiting Na^+-K^+- dependent ATPase separated from human gastric fundic mucosa. Acta Medica Acad. Sci. Hung. 36: 459–466.

[180] Mózsik Gy., Kutas J., Nagy L., Tárnok F. (1979d) Biochemistry of antral ulcer in patients. Acta Medica Acad. Sci. Hung. 37: 39–49.

[181] Mózsik Gy., Lovász L., Kutor G., Nagy L. (1979e) Experimental evidence for cytoprotective effect of atropine on rat gastric mucosa. Acta Medica Acad. Sci. Hung. 37: 401–405.

[182] Mózsik Gy., Nagy L., Tárnok F. (1979f) Cellular mechanisms of ulcer development in patients with antral, duodenal and jejunal ulcers. Drugs Exp. Clin. Res. 5: 27–42.

[183] Mózsik Gy., Nagy L., Tárnok F. (1979g) Ten years results of the intermittent treatment with atropine in patients with duodenal ulcer. Drugs Exp. Clin. Res. 5: 185–195.

[184] Mózsik Gy., Nagy L., Tárnok F., Vizi F. (1979h) Energetical systems of the gastric tissues and their neural, hormonal and pharmacological regulations in order to gastric H^+ secretion and ulcer development. An experimental and clinical biochemical review. Acta Medica Acad. Sci. Hung. 36: 1–29.

[185] Mózsik Gy., Lovász L., Kutor G., Nagy L., Tárnok F. (1980) Experimental evidence for cytoprotective effect of atropine on the rat gastric mucosa. Acta Medica Acad. Sci. Hung. 37: 401–405.

[186] Mózsik Gy., Figler M., Nagy L., Patty I., Tárnok F. (1981a) Gastric and small intestinal energy metabolism in mucosa damage. In: Mózsik Gy., Hänninen O., Jávor T. (eds) Advances in Physiological Sciences. Vol. 29. Gastrointestinal Defense Mechanisms. Pergamon Press, Oxford-Akadémiai Kiadó, Budapest. pp. 213–276.

[187] Mózsik Gy., Nagy L., Tárnok F. (1981b) Feed-back mechanism systems between the ATP - adenylate cyclase – cAMP and ATP – Na^+-K^+-dependent ATPase – ADP in the rat and human gastric fundic mucosa in relation to gastric acid secretion. In: Gáti T., Szollár L., Ungváry Gy. (eds). Advances in Physiological Sciences. Vol. 12. Nutrition,

http://dx.doi.org/10.5772/60105

Digestion, Metabolism. Pergamon Press, Oxford – Akadémiai Kiadó, Budapest. pp. 157–173.

[188] Mózsik Gy., Morón F., Jávor T. (1982) Cellular mechanism of the development of gastric mucosal damage and of gastroprotection induced by prostacyclin in rats. A pharmacological study. Prostagland. Leucot. Med. 9: 71–84.

[189] Mózsik Gy., Nagy L., Tárnok F., Kutas J. (1981e) Biochemistry of chronic jejunal ulcer in patients. Acta Medica Acad. Sci. Hung. 38: 129–134.

[190] Mózsik Gy., Venter E., Schmelzer M., Kutas J., Nagy L., Tárnok F. (1981f) A critical analysis of the gastric secretory responses of patients with duodenal ulcer in dependence of their age and duration of complaints. Acta Medica Acad. Sci. Hung. 38: 117–128.

[191] Mózsik Gy., Tárnok F., Kutas J. (1981) In: Gáti, Szollár and Ungváry (Eds.) Advances in Physiological Sciences. Vol. 12. Pergamon Press, Oxford- Akadémiai Kiadó, Budapest. pp. 117–128.

[192] Mózsik Gy., Figler M., Nagy L., Patty I., Tárnok F. (1982a) Is there anoxia in the gastric and small intestinal mucosa during the development of ulceration? In: Umehara S., Ito H. (eds) Advances of Experimental Ulcer. Proceedings of the 4th International Conference on Experimental Ulcer. Tokyo. pp. 414–427.

[193] Mózsik Gy., Figler M., Nagy L., Tárnok F. (1982b) Feed-back mechanisms between the ATP-membrane ATPase – ADP and ATP – adenylate cyclase – cAMP systems in the gastric tissues during gastric hypersecretion and ulcer development in rats. In: Umehara S., Ito H. (eds) Advances of Experimental Ulcer. Proceedings of the 4th International Conference on Experimental Ulcer. Tokyo. pp. 460–471.

[194] Mózsik Gy., Morón F., Jávor T. (1982c) Cellular mechanism of the development of gastric mucosal damage and of gastroprotection induced by prostacyclin in rats. A pharmacological study. Prostagland. Leucot. Med. 9: 71–84.

[195] Mózsik Gy., Morón F., Figler M., Jávor T., Nagy L., Patty I., Tárnok F. (1983a) Interrelationships between membrane – bound ATP – dependent energy systems, gastric mucosal damage produced by NaOH, hypertonic NaCl, HCl, and alcohol and prostacyclin – induced gastric cytoprotection in rats. Prostaglan. Leucot. Med. 12: 423–436.

[196] Mózsik Gy., Morón F., Figler M., Jávor T., Nagy L., Patty I., Tárnok F. (1983b) Membrane – bound ATP–dependent energy systems and gastric cytoprotection by prostacyclin, atropine and cimetidine. Int. J. Tiss. React. 5: 263–278.

[197] Mózsik Gy., Nagy L., Patty I., Tárnok F. (1983c) Cellular energy systems and reserpine ulcer in rats. Acta Physiol. Hung. 62: 107–112.

[198] Mózsik Gy., Bata M., Figler M., Jávor T., Nagy L., Patty I., Tóth Gy., Tárnok F. (1984a) Interrelationships between the membrane-bound ATP – dependent energy systems of the gastric mucosa and the gastric cytoprotective effect of ß-carotene on the devel-

opment of gastric mucosal damage produced by 0.6 M HCl in rats. Acta Physiol. Hung. 64: 301–307.

[199] Mózsik Gy., Jávor T., Tóth Gy., Tigyi A. (1984b) Interrelationships between the gastric cytoprotective effects of vitamin A and ß-carotene and the gastric mucosal superoxide dismutase activity in rats. Acta Physiol. Hung. 64: 315–318.

[200] Mózsik Gy., Jávor T., Zsoldos T., Tigyi A. (1984c) The interrelationships between the development of ethanol-, HCl-, NaOH-, NaCl-induced gastric mucosal damage and the gastric mucosal superoxide dismutase activity in the rats. Acta Physiol. Hung. 64: 309–314.

[201] Mózsik Gy., Bertelli A., Deák G., Nagy L., Patty I., Simon L., Tárnok F., Jávor T. (1985) Some aspects of the critical evaluation of peptic ulcer therapy in patients. Int. J. Clin. Pharmacol. Res. 5: 447–455.

[202] Mózsik Gy., Moron F., Nagy L., Ruzsa Cs., Tárnok F., Jávor T. (1986) Evidence of the gastric cytoprotective effects of vitamin A, atropine and cimetidine on the development of gastric mucosal damage produced by administration of indomethacin in healthy subjects. Int. J. Tiss. React. 8: 85–90.

[203] Mózsik Gy., Figler M., Jávor T., Morón F., Nagy L., Patty I., Tárnok F. (1987a) Correlations between the membrane-bound ATP-dependent energy systems and ulcer treatment in the rat and man. In: Szabó S., Mózsik Gy. (eds) New Pharmacology of Ulcer Disease. Experimental and New Therapeutic Approaches. Elsevier Science Publishers, New York. pp. 11–27

[204] Mózsik Gy., Figler M., Morón F., Nagy L., Patty I., Tárnok F. (1987b) Molecular biochemistry and pharmacology of peptic ulcer treatment (review) Acta Medica Acad. Sci. Hung. 44: 3–29.

[205] Mózsik Gy., Pihan G., Szabo S., Jávor T., Czeglédi B., Tigyi A., Tárnok F., Zsoldos T. (1987c) Free radicals, non-sulfhydryl antioxidants, drugs and vitamin sin acute gastric mucosal injury and protection. In: Szabo S., Mózsik Gy. (eds) New Pharmaology of Ulcer Disease: Experimental and New Therapeutic Approaches. Elsevier Science Publishers, New York. 197–207.

[206] Mózsik Gy., Figler M., Garamszegi M., Jávor T., Nagy L., Sütő G., Vincze Á., Zsoldos T. (1988) Correlations between the oxygen free radicals, membrane-bound ATP-dependent energy systems in relation to development of ethanol- and HCL-induced gastric mucosal damage and of β-carotene-induced gastric cytoprotection. In: Tsuchiya M., Kawai K., Kondo M., Yoshikawa T. (eds) Free Radicals in Digestive Diseases. Elsevier Science Publishers, Amsterdam. pp. 111–116

[207] Mózsik Gy., Figler M., Garamszegi M., Jávor T., Nagy L., Sütő G., Vincze Á., Zsoldos T. (1989a) Mechanisms of gastric mucosal protection. I. Time-sequence analysis of gastric mucosal membrane-bound ATP-dependent energy systems, oxygen free radicals and macroscopically appearance of gastric cytoprotection by PGI_2 and β-caro-

tene in HCl-model of rats. In: Hayashi E., Niki M., Kondo M., Yoshikawa T. (eds) Medical, Biochemical, and Chemical Aspects of Free Radicals. Elsevier Science Publishers, Amsterdam. pp. 1421–1425.

[208] Mózsik Gy., Figler M., Garamszegi M., Jávor T., Nagy L., Sütő G., Vincze Á., Zsoldos T. (1989b) Mechanisms of gastric mucosal protection. II. Time-sequence analysis of gastric mucosal membrane-bound ATP-dependent energy systems, oxygen free radicals and macroscopically appearance of gastric cytoprotection by PGI_2 and β-carotene in ethanol-model of rats. In: Hayashi E., Niki M., Kondo M., Yoshikawa T. (eds) Medical, Biochemical, and Chemical Aspects of Free Radicals. Elsevier Science Publishers, Amsterdam. pp. 1427–1431

[209] Mózsik Gy., Garamszegi M., Jávor T., Nagy L., Sütő G., Tóth Gy., Vincze Á., (1989c) Cellular energy status of the gastric mucosa and gastric mucosal prevention by vitamin A in indomethacin treated rats. Int. J. Tiss. Reac. 11: 65–71.

[210] Mózsik Gy., Garamszegi M., Sütő G., Vincze Á., Jávor T. (1989d) A pharmacological approach to cellular mechanisms of PGI_2-induced gastric cytoprotection on ethanol-induced gastric mucosal damage in rats. Physiol. Hung. 73: 207 211.

[211] Mózsik Gy., Sütő G., Vincze Á., Zsoldos T. (1989e) Correlations between the free radicals and membrane-bound energy systems in ethanol-induced gastric mucosal damage in rats. In: Szabo S., Pfeiffer C. J. (eds) Ulcer Disease: New Aspects of Pathogenesis and Pharmacology. pp. 15–27. CRC Press, Inc. Boca Raton, USA.

[212] Mózsik Gy., Garamszegi M., Jávor T., Nagy L., Patty I., Sütő G., Vincze Á. (1990a) A biochemical and pharmacological approach to the genesis of ulcer disease. II. A model study of stress induced injury to gastric mucosa in rats. Ann. N. Y. Acad. Sci. 517, 264–281.

[213] Mózsik Gy., Garamszegi M., Jávor T., Nagy L., Németh A., Sütő G., Vincze Á. (1990b) Chemicals (alcohol, NaOH, NaCl, HCl)-induced changes in the gastric mucosal membrane bound ATP-dependent energy systems. Acta Physiol. Hung. 75: (Suppl), 217–218.

[214] Mózsik Gy., Király Á., Garamszegi M., Jávor T., Nagy L., Németh A., Sütő G., Vincze Á. (1990c) Gastric cytoprotection mediating in SH groups is failed by surgical vagotomy. Acta Physiol. Hung. 75: (Suppl), 219–220.

[215] Mózsik Gy., Király Á., Garamszegi M., Jávor T., Nagy L., Sütő G., Tóth Gy., Vincze Á. (1991a) Failure of prostacyclin, carotene, atropine and cimetidine to produce gastric cyto- and general mucosal protection in surgically vagotomized rats. Life Sciences 49, 1383–1389.

[216] Mózsik Gy., Sütő G., Garamszegi M., Nagy L., Vincze Á., Zsoldos T. (1991b) Oxygen free radicals and gastric mucosal damage in rats treated with ethanol and HCl. Eur. J. Gastroenterol. Hepatol. 3: 757–761.

[217] Mózsik Gy., Garamszegi M., Karádi O., Király Á., Nagy L., Sütő G., Vincze Á. (1992a) Correlation between the gastric mucosal biochemistry, vascular permeability and mucosal protection produced vs. cytoprotective and antisecretory doses of atropine and cimetidine in rats treated with indomethacin. Exp. Clin. Gastroenterol. 3: 205–215.

[218] Mózsik Gy., Király Á., Garamszegi M., Jávor T., Nagy L., Németh A., Sütő G., Vincze Á. (1992b) Mechanisms of vagal nerve in the gastric mucosal defence: unchanged gastric emptying and increased vascular permeability. J. Clin. Gastroenterol. 14: 140–144.

[219] Mózsik Gy., Király Á., Sütő G., Vincze Á. (1992c) ATP breakdown and in the development of gastrointestinal mucosal damage and its prevention in animals and human (An overview of 25 years ulcer research studies) Acta Physiol. Hung. 80: 39–80.

[220] Mózsik Gy., Sütő G., Vincze Á. (1992d) Correlation between the acute chemical and surgical vagotomy-induced gastric mucosal biochemistry in rats. J. Clin. Gastroenterol. 14: 135–139.

[221] Mózsik Gy., Karádi O., Király Á., Matus Z., Sütő G., Vincze Á., Tóth Gy. (1993a) Retinoids as scavengers and gastric cytoprotection in animals, human beings and patients with peptic ulcer. In: Mózsik Gy., Emerit I., Fehér J., Matkovics B., Vincze Á. (eds) Oxygen Free radicals and Scavengers in the Natural Sciences. Akadémiai Kiadó, Budapest. pp. 330–338.

[222] Mózsik Gy., Karádi O., Király Á., Matus Z., Tóth Gy., Vincze Á. (1993b) Vagal nerve and the gastric mucosal defense. J. Physiology (Paris) 87: 329–334.

[223] Mózsik Gy., Hunyady B., Garamszegi M., Németh A., Pakodi F., Vincze A.(1994) Dynamism of cytoprotective and antisecretory drugs in patients with unhealed gastric and duodenal ulcers. J. Gastroenterol. Hepatol. 9: S88–S92.

[224] Mózsik Gy., Abdel-Salam O. M. E., Bódis B., Karádi O., Király Á., Sütő G., Rumi Gy., Szabó I., Vincze Á. (1996a) Gastric mucosal preventive effects of prostacyclin and ß-carotene and their biochemical effects in rats treated with ethanol and HCl in dependence their doses and of time after administration of necrotizing agents. Inflammopharmacology 4: 361–378.

[225] Mózsik Gy., Abdel-Salam O. M. E., Bódis B., Karádi O., Nagy L., Szolcsányi J. (1996b) Role of vagal nerve in defense mechanisms against NSAIDs-induced gastrointestinal mucosal damage. Inflammopharmacology 4: 151–172.

[226] Mózsik Gy., Bódis B., Karádi O., Nagy L., Vörös S. (1996c) The action of Helicobacter pylori on the viability in freshly isolated rat gastric mucosal cells. Hung. Weekly Med. J. 137: 1749–1752.

[227] Mózsik Gy., Abdel-Salam O. M. E., Király Á., Morón F., Nagy L., Sütő G., Tárnok F., Jávor T. (1997a) The development and prevention of peptic ulcer disease in light of gastrointestinal mucosal biochemistry. In: Mózsik Gy., Nagy L., Király Á. (eds)

Twenty Five Years Of Peptic Ulcer Research in Hungary: From Basic Sciences to Clinical Practice (1971-1995). Akadémiai Kiadó, Budapest. pp. 159–170.

[228] Mózsik Gy., Bódis B., Juricskay I., Karádi O., Kövesdy Cs., Nagy L. (1997b) A new uniform biochemical explanation for the development and location of "genuine" gastric, duodenal and jejunal ulcers in patients. In: Gaginella T., Mózsik Gy., Raindford K. D. (eds) Biochemical Pharmacology as Approach to Gastrointestinal Diseases: From Basic Science to Clinical Perspectives. Kluwer Academic Publishers, Dordrecht, Boston, London. pp. 313–334.

[229] Mózsik Gy., Debreceni A., Juricskay I., Karádi O., Nagy L. (1997c) Biochemical energetical backgrounds and their regulations in the gastric corpus mucosa in patients with different gastric secretory responses. In: Gaginella T., Mózsik Gy., Raindford K. D. (eds) Biochemical Pharmacology as Approach to Gastrointestinal Diseases: From Basic Science to Clinical Perspectives. Kluwer Academic Publishers, Dordrecht, Boston, London. pp. 199–223.

[230] Mózsik Gy., Nagy L., Pár A., Rainsford K. D. (1997d) (eds) Cell Injury and Protection in the Gastrointestinal Tract: From Basic Sciences to Clinical Perspectives. Kluwer Academic Publishers, Dordrecht, Boston, London.

[231] Mózsik Gy., Bódis B., Karádi O., Király Á., Nagy L., Rumi Gy., Sütő G., Szabó I. (1998) Cellular mechanisms of ß-carotene-induced gastric cytoprotection in indomethacin-treated rats. Inflammopharmacol 6: 27–40.

[232] Mózsik Gy., Rumi Gy., Bódis B., Figler M., Király Á., Sütő G., Vincze Á. (1999) Effects of indomethacin, with vitamin A or ß-carotene, on the rat gastric mucosa: extra- and intracellular membrane-bound ATP mechanisms. Inflammopharmacology 7: 287–295.

[233] Mózsik Gy., Figler M., Rumi Gy. (2000) Membrane-bound ATP-dependent energy systems and tissue hypoxia in human gastric mucosa (Editorial). J. Gastroenterol. Hepatol. 15: 105–108.

[234] Mózsik Gy., Bódis B., Figler M., Király Á., Karádi O., Pár A., Rumi Gy., Sütő G., Tóth Gy., Vincze Á. (2001a) Mechanism of action of retinoids in gastrointestinal mucosal protection in animals, human healthy subjects and patients. Life Sciences 69: 3103–3112.

[235] Mózsik Gy., Karádi O., Király Á., Debreceni A., Figler M., Nagy L., Pár A., Pár G., Sütő G., Vincze Á. (2001b) The key-role of vagal nerve and adrenals in the cytoprotection and general gastric mucosal integrity. J. Physiology (Paris) 95: 229–237.

[236] Mózsik Gy., Gasztonyi B., Juricskay I., Pár A., Szolcsányi J. (2003) Direct evidence for the exclusion of desensitization to capsaicin during two weeks treatment in human healthy subjects. Inflammopharmacology 11: 546–547.

[237] Mózsik Gy., Rumi Gy., Dömötör A., Matuz Z., Figler M., Gasztonyi B., Papp E., Pár A., Pár G., Melegh B. (2005) Involvement of serum retinoids and activated protein C

in patients with oesophageal, gastric, liver, pancreatic and colorectal cancers in Hungary. World J. Gastroenterol. 11: 7646–7650.

[238] Mózsik Gy., Szabo S., Takeuchi K. (2006) History of the Gastrointestinal Section of the International Union of Pharmacology (IUPHAR GI Section) (1984-2006). University Press of Pécs, Hungary.

[239] Mózsik Gy., Dömötör A., Rumi Gy., Szekeres Gy. (2007) Gastrointestinal cytoprotection: from basic science to clinical perspectives. Inflammopharmacology 15: 49–60.

[240] Mózsik Gy., Dömötör A., Past T., Vas V., Perjési P., Kuzma M., Blázics Gy., Szolcsányi J. (2009) Capsaicinoids: From Plant Cultivation to the Production of the Human Medical Therapy. Akadémiai Kiadó, Budapest.

[241] Mózsik Gy., Szabo I.L., Czimmer J. (2011) Approaches to gastrointestinal cytoprotection: from isolated cells, via animal experiments to healthy human subjects and patients with different gastrointestinal disorders. Curr. Pharm Des. 17: 1556–2572.

[242] Mózsik Gy., Dömötör A., Czimmer J., Szabo I.L., Szolcsanyi J. (2014a) Capsaicin-sensitive afferent nerves and the human gastrointestinalTract. In: Mózsik Gy., Abdel-Salam O. M. E., Takeuchi K. (eds) Capsaicin-Sensitive Neural Afferentation and the GastrointestinalTract: From Bench to Bedside. INTECH Publishers, Rijeka. pp. 213–261.

[243] Mózsik Gy., Past T., Habon T., Keszthelyi Zs., Perjési P., Kuzma M., Abdel-Salam O.M.E., Szolcsányi J. (2014b) Capsaicin is a new gastrointestinal mucosal protecting drug candidate in humans – pharmaceutical development and production based on clinical pharmacology. In: Mozsik Gy., Abdel-Salam O.M.E., Takeuchi K. (eds) Capsaicin-Sensitive Neural Afferentation and the Gastrointestinal Tract: From Bench to Bedside. INTECH Publishers, Rijeka. pp. 265–364.

[244] Mózsik Gy., Past T., Habon T., Keszthelyi Zs., Szabo I., Sándor B., Szolcsányi J., Szalai M. (2014c) Orally given capsaicinoids do not modify the absorption, metabolism and excretion of aspirin and its platelet aggregation in human male subjects (human clinical pharmacological phase I. examinations). J. Adv. Clin. Pharmacol. 1, 34–61.

[245] Mózsik Gy., Szabo I. L., Czimmer J. (2014d) Vulnerable points of the Helicobacter pylori story – based on animal and human observations (1975-2112). In: Buzas Gy. M. (ed) Helicobacter pylori: A Worldwide Perspectives 2013. Bentham Science Publishers. Sharjah-Oak Park. pp. 449–480.

[246] Murad F., Chi Y. M., Rall T. W., Sutherland E. W. (1962) The effects of chatecolamines and cholin esters on the formation of adenosine-3′,5′-phosphate by preparations from cardiac muscle and liver. J. Biol. Chem. 237: 1233.

[247] Myren J. (1968) Gastric secretion following stimulation with histamine, histology and gastrin in man. In: Semb L., Myren J. (eds) The Physiology of Gastric Secretion. Universitetforlaget, Oslo. pp. 413–428.

http://dx.doi.org/10.5772/60105

[248] Myren J. and Semb L. (1968) The number of parietal cells and the rates of gastric secretion before and after subcutaneous injection of large doses of histamine. Gastroenterologia (Basel) 98: 207–216.

[249] Nagy L., Szilágyi A., Füzesi Zs., Tóth E., Németh Á., Mózsik Gy. (1976) Pharmacological aspects of the epinephrine-induced gastric lesions in the rat. In: Mózsik Gy., Jávor T. (eds) Progress in Peptic Ulcer. Akadémiai Kiadó, Budapest. pp. 485–507.

[250] Nagy L., Mózsik Gy., Tárnok F., Jávor T. (1979) Effects of histamine H_1 and H_2 receptor antagonists on gastric secretion and epinephrine-induced gastric erosions in pylorus-ligated rats. Drugs Exp. Clin. Res. 5: 87–96.

[251] Nagy L., Figler M., Jávor T., Mózsik Gy. (1981a) Role of acute starvation on the development of different experimental ulcers in rats. In: Mózsik Gy., Hänninen O., Jávor T. (eds) Advances in Physiological Sciences. Vol. 29. Gastrointestinal Defence Mechanisms. Pergamon Press, Oxford-Akadémiai Kiadó, Budapest. pp. 117–126

[252] Nagy L., Mózsik Gy., Fiegler M., Jávor T. (1981b) Role of functional state of the gastric mucosa in relation to development of epinephrine effects on rat stomach. In: Mózsik Gy., Hänninen O., Jávor T. (eds) Advances in Physiological Sciences. Vol. 29. Gastrointestinal Defense Mechanisms. Pergamon Press, Oxford-Akadémiai Kiadó, Budapest. pp. 89–100.

[253] Nagy L., Mózsik Gy., Figler M., Gerber E., Past T., Ruzsa Cs., Vezekényi Zs., Jávor T. (1982) Effects of drugs on the production of stress ulcer in the rat. Acta Physiol. Acad. Sci. Hung. 60: 219–227.

[254] Nagy L., Figler M., Mózsik Gy., Németh M., Ruzsa Cs., Gerber E., Jávor T. (1983) Some metabolic and biochemical alterations during the development of stress ulcer in rats forced to swim. Int. J. Tiss. Reac. 5: 363–371.

[255] Nagy L., Szabo S., Morales R. E., Plebani M., Jenkins J. M. (1994) Identification of subcellular targets and sensitive tests of ethanol-induced damage in isolated rat gastric mucosal cells. Gastroenterology 107: 907–914.

[256] Nagy L., Nagy Gy., Rácz I., Simon L., Solt I., Patty I., Tárnok F., Mózsik Gy., Jávor T. (1997) Multicentre Clinical investigation of Tisacid® (Al-Mg-hydoxy-carbonate) in duodenal ulcer. In: Mózsik Gy., Nagy L., Király Á. (1997) (eds) Twenty Five Years of Peptic Ulcer Research in Hungary (1971-1995). Akadémiai Kiadó, Budapest. pp. 367–395.

[257] Øye I., Butcher R. W. (1967a) The mode of action of adrenaline in the isolated rat heart. Universitetsforlaget, Oslo.

[258] Øye I., Butcher R. W. (1967b) Glycogen phosporylase: a specific secondary target system for adrenaline action in the heart. Acta Physiol. Scand. 69: 270–275.

[259] Øye I., Sutherland E. W. (1966) The effect of epinephrine and other agents on adenylcyclase in the cell membrane of avian erythrocytes. Biochim. Biophys. Acta (Amsterdam) 127: 347–354.

[260] Øye I., Butcher R. W., Morgan H. E., Sutherland E. W. (1964) Epinephrine and 3′,5′-AMP levels in working rat heart. Fed. Proc. 23: 262–268.

[261] Pai R., Soregham B., Szabó I., Pavelka M., Baatar D., Tarnawski A. S. (2002) Prostaglandin E_2 transactivates EGF receptor: A novel mechanism for promoting colon cancer growth and gastrointestinal hypertrophy. Nature Medicine 8: 289–293.

[262] Pai R., Szabó I., Sorenghan B., Tarnawski A. S. (2000) Indomethacin inhibits endothelial cell proliferation by suppressing cell cyclic proteins and PRB phosphorylation. A key to its antiangiogenic action? Mol. Cell Biol. Res. Commun. 4: 111–116.

[263] Patty I., Benedek Sz., Deák G., Jávor T., Kenéz P., Nagy L., Simon L., Tárnok F., Mózsik Gy. (1982) Controlled trial of vitamin A therapy in gastric ulcer. The Lancet II: 876.

[264] Patty I., Benedek Sz., Deák G., Jávor T., Kenéz P., Moron F., Nagy L., Simon L., Mózsik Gy. (1983) Cytoprotective effect of vitamin A and its clinical importance in the treatment of patients with chronic gastric ulcer. Int. J. Tiss. React. 5: 301–307.

[265] Patty I., Jávor T., Tárnok F., Deák G., Nagy L., Mózsik Gy. (1987) Comparative short-term clinical study of gastric ulcer treatments in patients. In: Szabo S., Mózsik Gy. (eds) New Pharmacology of Ulcer Disease: Experimental and New Therapeutic Approaches. Elsevier Science Publishers, New York. pp. 92–102.

[266] Pfeiffer C. J. (1971) (ed) Peptic Ulcer. Lippincott Company, Philadelphia Munksgaard, Copenhagen.

[267] Pfeiffer C. J., Sethbakdi S. (1971) Vascular impairment – An etiological factor in pepticulcer? In: Pfeiffer C. J. (ed) Peptic Ulcer. Lippincott Company, Philadelphia-Munksgaard, Copenhagen. pp. 207–220.

[268] Pfeiffer C. J., Mózsik Gy. (1990) Epinephrine-induced gastric damage in rats ultrastructural analysis of vascular changes .Pharmacodynamics Therapeutics (Life Sci Adv) 9, 29-36.

[269] Pihan G., Szabó S., Trier S. J. (1989) The role of the micovasculature in acute gastric mucosal damage and protection. In: Szabó S., Pfeiffer C. J. (eds) Ulcer Disease: New Aspects of Pathogenesis and Pharmacology. CRC Press, Boca Raton. pp. 135–144.

[270] Post R. H., Albright C. D. (1961) Membrane adenosine triphosphatase system as a part of system for active sodium and potassium transport. In: Kleinzeller A., Kotyk A. (eds) Membrane Transport and Metabolism. Academic Press, New York and Publishing House of the Czechoslovak Academy of Sciences, Praha. pp. 219–227.

[271] Proosdíj-Harzema E.G., Jannsen P.G., de Joungh D.K. (1955) Substituted phenylamines. III. Anticholinergic activity of quaternary ammonium bases Derived from R

http://dx.doi.org/10.5772/60105

55 / 2,2-diphenyl-4-diiso- propylamino-methyliodide. Arch. Int. Pharmacodyn. 103: 120–146.

[272] Rall T. W., Sutherland E. W. (1958) Formation of a cyclic ribonucleotide by tissue particcles. J. Biol. Chem. 232: 1065–1076.

[273] Rall T. W., Sutherland E. W., Berthet J. (1957) The relationship of epinephrine and glycacon to liver phosphorylase. J. Biol. Chem. 224: 463–475.

[274] Rainsford K.D. (1992) Mechanism of NSAD-induced ulcerogenesis: structural properties of drugs, focus on the microvascular factors and novel approaches for gastrointestinal protection. Acta Physiol. Hung. 80: 23–38.

[275] Reece J., Campbell N. (2002) Biology. Benjamin Cummings, San Francisco.

[276] Robert A. (1979) Cytoprotection by prostaglandins. Gastroenterology 77: 761–767.

[277] Robert A., Nemasis E. J., Lanchaster C., Hauchar J. (1979) Cytoprotection of gastric necrosis produced by alcohol, HCl, NaOH, hypertonic NaCl and thermal injury. Gastroenterology 77: 433–443.

[278] Robinson G. A., Bucher R. W., Sutherland E. W. (1971) Cyclic AMP. Academic Press, New York, London.

[279] Rumi Gy., Kovács K., Matus Z., Tóth Gy., Vincze Á., Mózsik Gy. (1997) Is only vitamin A activity of carotenoids necessary to the chemopreventive effect in gastrointestinal malignant diseases? In: Mózsik Gy., Nagy L., Király Á. (eds) Twenty Five Years in Peptic Ulcer Research in Hungary (1971-1995). Akadémiai Kiadó, pp. 377–382.

[280] Rumi Gy., Matus Z., Tóth Gy, Szabó I, Mózsik Gy (2001a) Changes of serum carotenoids in patients with esophageal, gastric, hepatocellular, pancreatic and colorectal cancer. J. Physiology Paris 95: 239–242.

[281] Rumi Gy., Pár A., Matus Z., Rumi Gy., Mózsik Gy. (2001b) The defensive effects of retinoids in the gastrointestinal tract (Animal experiments and human observations). Akadémiai Kiadó, Budapest.

[282] Ruoff H. J., Sewing K. F. (1974) Rat mucosal cAMP following cholinergic and histamine stimulation. Eur. J. Pharmacol. 28: 338–343.

[283] Saccomani G., Chang H. H., Spisni A., Helander H. F., Spitzer H. Z., Sachs G. (1979a) Effect of phospholipase A_2 on purified gastric vesicles. J. Supramol. Struct. 11: 429–444.

[284] Saccomani G., Helander H. F., Crago S., Chang H. H., Dailey D. W.,Sachs G. (1979b) Characterization of gastric mucosal membranes. X. Immunological studies of gastric (H^+-K^+)-ATPase. J. Cell Biol. 83: 271–283.

[285] Sachs G. (1977) H^+ transport by non electrogenic gastric ATPase as a model for acid secretion. Rev. Physiol. Biochem. Pharmacol. 79: 133–162.

[286] Sachs G. (1987) The gastric proton pump: the H^+-K^+-ATPase. In: Johnson L. R., Christensen J., Jackson M., Jacobson E. D., Walsh J. H. (eds). Physiology of Gastrointestinal Tract. Vol. 1. Chapter 28. (2nd Edition). Raven Press, New York. pp. 865–881.

[287] Sachs G., Shah G., Strych A. (1972) Properties of ATPase of gastric mucosa. III. Distribution of HCo3-stimulated ATP-ase in gastric mucosa. Biophys. Biochim. Acta (Amsterdam) 266: 625–638.

[288] Sachs G., Berglindl T., Rabon E., Stewart H. B., Barcellona M. L., Wallmark B., Saccomani G. (1980) Aspects of parietal cell biology: cells and vesicles. Ann. N.Y. Acad. Sci. 341: 312–334.

[289] Sachs G., Shin J. M., Briving C., Wallmark B., Hersey S. (1995) The pharmacology of the gastric acid pump: the H^+-K^+-ATPase. Ann. Rev. Pharmacol. Toxicol. 35: 277–305.

[290] Salganik R. I., Bersimbaev R. I. (1976) Integration of biochemical functions of different cells of rat gastric mucosa for hydrocholic acid secretion. Molec. Cell Biochem. 12: 181–191.

[291] Scheurer F., Witzel L., Halter F. Keller H. M., Huber R., Galeazzi R. (1977) Gastric and duodenal ulcer healing under placebo treatment. Gastroenterology 72, 838–846.

[292] Schmidt G., Tannhauser S. J. (1945) Method for determination of deoxyribonucleic acid,ribonucleic acid and phosphoproteins in animal tissues. J. Biol. Chem. 161: 83–89.

[293] Schwartz A., Lindenmayer G. E., Allen C. J. (1975) Sodium-potassium-adenosine-triphosphatase: pharmacological, physiological and biochemical aspects. Pharmacol. Rev. 27: 3–134.

[294] Selye J. (1936) Syndrome produced by diverse noxious agents. Nature 138: 32–45.

[295] Sethbakdi S., Pfeiffer C. J., Roth J. L. (1970a) Gastric mucosal ulceration following vasoactive agents. A new experimental model. Amer. J. Digest. Dis. 15: 261–270

[296] Sethbakdi S., Roth J. L., Pfeiffer C. J. (1970b) Gastric mucosal ulceration after epinephrine. A study of etiological mechanisms. Amer. J. Digest. Dis. 15: 1055–1065.

[297] Semb L., Myren J. (1968) (eds) The Physiology of Gastric Secretion. Universitatsforlaget, Oslo.

[298] Shay H., Komarov S. A., Fels S. S., Merance D., Gruenstein M., Siplet H. (1945) A simple method for the uniform production of gastric ulcer in the rat. Gastroenterology 5: 43–61.

[299] Shull G. E., Schwartz A., Lingrel J. B. (1985) Amino acid sequence of the catalytic subunit of the Na^+-K^+ ATPase deducted from a complementary DNA. Nature 316: 691–695.

http://dx.doi.org/10.5772/60105

[300] Skou J. C. (1957) The influence of some cations on an adenosine triphosphatase from peripheral nerves. Biochim. Biophys. Acta 23: 394–401.

[301] Skou J. C. (1965) Enzymatical basis for active transport of Na^+ and K^+ across cell membrane. Physiol. Rev. 45: 596–617.

[302] Stoll A. H., Berglinch T. (1987) Physiology of isolated gastric glands and parietal cells: receptors and effectors regulating function. In: Johnson L. R., Christensen J., Jackson M. J., Jacobson E. D., Walsh J. H. (eds) Physiology of Gastrointestinal Tract. Vol. 1. Chapter 29. (2nd Edition) Raven Press, New York. pp. 883–909

[303] Sutherland E. W. (1962) The biological role of adenosine 3′,5′-phosphate. Harvey lecture. Academic Press, New York, London. pp. 17–33.

[304] Sutherland E. W. (1972) Studies on the mechanism of hormone. Science 177: 401–408.

[305] Sutherland E. W., Rall T. W. (1957) The properties of an adenosine ribonucleotide produced by with cellular particles, ATP, Mg^{2+} and epinephrine or glucagon. J. Amer. Chem. Soc. 79: 3608–3615.

[306] Sutherland E. W., Rall T. W. (1958) Fraction and characterization of a cyclic adenine ribonucleotide formed by tissue particles. J. Biol. Chem. 232: 1077–1097.

[307] Sutherland E. W., Rall T. W. (1960) The relation to adenosine 3′,5′-phosphate and phosphorylase to actions of catecholamines and other hormones. Pharmacol. Rev. 17: 265–299.

[308] Sutherland E. W., Robison G. A. (1966) The role of cylic 3′,5′-AMP in response to catecholamines and other hormones. Pharmacol. Rev. 18: 145–161.

[309] Sutherland E. W., Rall T. W., Berthel J. (1957) The relationship of epinephrine and glucacons to liver phosphorylase. IV. Effect of epinephrine and glycagon on the activation of phosphorylase in liver homogenates. J. Biol. Chem. 224: 463–475.

[310] Sutherland E. W., Rall T. W., Menon T. (1962) Adenyl cyclase. I. Distribution, preparation and properties. J. Biol. Chem. 237: 1220–1227.

[311] Sutherland E. W., Øye I., Butcher R. W. (1965) Action of epinephrine and the role of the adenylate cyclase system in hormone action. Recent Progress in Hormone Research 21: 623–646.

[312] Sutherland E. W., Robison G. A., Butcher R. W. (1968) Some aspects in the biological role of the adenosine 3′,5′-monophosphate (cyclic AMP). Circulation 37: 279–306.

[313] Sütő G., Király Á., Garamszegi M., Jávor T., Nagy L., Vincze Á., Tóth Gy., Mózsik Gy. (1989) Neural and hormonal influences on ß-carotene-induced gastric mucosal cytoprotection in rats. In: Proceedings of 3rd Interscience World Conference on Inflammation, Antirheumatics, Analgetics, Immunomodulators. Monte Carlo. p. 236.

[314] Sütő G., Király Á., Vincze Á., Jávor T., Mózsik Gy. (1992) Effects of acute surgical vagotomy (ASV) on the mucosal content of 6-keto-PGF1α, PGE2 and glutation (GSH) after intragastric 96% ethanol treatment in rats. Acta Physiol. Hung. 85: 207–213.

[315] Szabó I. (2004) Approaching the mechanisms of indomethacin delaying gastric restitution and gastric cancer growth. Ph.D Thesis, University of Pécs. Hungary.

[316] Szabó I., Bódis B., Nagy L., Mózsik Gy. (1996) Evidence for the direct protective and toxic effect of ethanol, prostacyclin and indomethacin in isolated gastric mucosal mixed cells. Hung. Weekly Med. J. 137: 2687–2689.

[317] Szabó I., Bódis B., Nagy L., Mózsik Gy. (1997a) Comparative studies on isolated mucosal mixed cells and hepatoma, myeloma cell lines with ethanol, indomethacin and their combination. Inflammopharmacology 5: 21–28.

[318] Szabó I., Bódis B., Németh P., Mózsik Gy. (1997b) Usage of scavengers on stable cultured (Sp2/0-AG14 and HEP G2) cell lines as an approach to reveal the mechanisms of cytoprotection. In: Mózsik Gy., Nagy L., Király Á. (eds) Twenty Five Years of Peptic Ulcer Research in Hungary: From Basic Sciences to Clinical Practice. Akadémiai Kiadó, Budapest. pp. 275–283.

[319] Szabó I., Rumi Gy., Bódis B., Németh P., Mózsik Gy. (2000) Gastrin and pentagastrin enhance the tumor proliferation of human stable cultured gastric adenocarcinoma cells. J. Physiology (Paris) 94: 405–409.

[320] Szabó I. L., Czimmer J., Mózsik Gy (2012) From mucosal energy metabolism Capsaicin –Strategies for understanding mucosal protection. In: Filaretova L. P., Takeuchi K. (eds) Cell/Tissue Injury andCytoprotection/Organoprotection in the Gastrointestinal Tract: Mechanisms, Prevention and Treatment. Front Gastrointinal Research. Vol. 30. Karger, Basel. pp. 230–241.

[321] Szabó IL., Czimmer J., Mózsik Gy. (2014) Translational research on the roles of free radicals and anti-oxidants in gastrointestinal disorders. In: Laher I. (ed) Systems Biology of Free Radicals and Antioxidants. Springer Berlin, Heidelberg. pp. 1729–1755.

[322] Szabó S., Mózsik Gy. (1987) (eds) New Pharmacology of Ulcer Disease. Experimental and New Therapeutic Approaches. Elsevier Science Publishers, New York.

[323] Szabo S., Gallagher G., Horner H.C., Frankel R. H., Underwood R. H., Konturek S. J., Brozowski T., Trier J. S. (1983) Role of adrenal cortex in gastric mucosal protection by prostaglandins, sulfhydryls, and cimetidine in the rat. Gastroenterology 85: 1384–1390.

[324] Szabo S., Trier J.S., Broown A., Schoor J.(1985) Early vascular injury and increased vascular permeability in the gastric mucosa caused by ethanol in the rat. Gastroenterology 88: 228–236.

http://dx.doi.org/10.5772/60105

[325] Szabo S., Taché Y., Somogyi A. (2012) The lagacy of Hans Selye and the origins of stress research: a retrospective 75 years after his landmark brief "Letter" to the Nature. Stress 15: 472–478.

[326] Takahashi S., Keto Y., Fujima H., Muramatsu H., Nishinko T., Okabe S. (1998) Pathological changes in the formation of Helicobacter pylori-induced gastric lesions in Mongolian gerbils. Dig. Dis. Sci. 43: 754–765.

[327] Tárnok F., Mózsik Gy., Nagy L., Ivánfy F., Sáfrány B., Jávor T., Kutas J. (1970) Membrane ATPase activity of gastric ulcer tissues in patients. In: Riis P., Anthonisen P., Baden H. (eds) Advance Abstracts, 4th World Congress of Gastroenterology. The Danish Gastroenterological Association. Copenhagen. p. 381

[328] Tárnok F., Mózsik Gy., Nagy L., Jávor T. (1973) Effect of immunosuppressive drugs on active transport Na^+-K^+-dependent ATPase system from human gastric mucosa. In: Borsy J., Mózsik Gy. (eds) Gastrin and Its Antagonists. Akadémiai Kiadó, Budapest. pp. 113–121.

[329] Tárnok F., Jávor T., Mózsik Gy., Nagy L., Patty I., Rumi Gy., Solt I. (1979) A prospective multiclinical study comparing the effects of placebo, carbenoxolone, atropine, cimetidine in patients with duodenal ulcer. Drugs Exp. Clin. Res. 5: 157–166.

[330] Tárnok F., Mózsik Gy., Jávor T., Patty I., Deák G., Nagy L., Lőrincz P., Figler M., Laczkó T., Szilvás Á., Rumi Gy., Solt I. (1997) Comparative short-term clinical-pharmacological studies and maintenance treatment in patients with duodenal ulcer. In: Mózsik Gy., Nagy L., Király Á. (eds.) Twenty Five Years of Peptic Ulcer Research in Hungary (1971-1995). Akadémiai Kiadó, Budapest. pp. 345–360.

[331] Tarnawski A. S., Szabo I. (2001) Apoptosis-programmed cell death and its relervance to gastrointestinal epithelium: survival signals from the matrix (Editorial). Gastroenterology 120: 294–298.

[332] Thompson W. J., Chang L. K., Jacobson E. D. (1977a) Activation of rat gastric mucosal adenylyl cyclase by secretory inhibitors. Gastroenterology 72: 251–254.

[333] Thompson W. J., Chang L. K., Jacobson E. D. (1977b) Rat gastric mucosal adenylate cyclase. Gastroenterology 72: 244–250.

[334] Tian J., Chai T., Yuan Z. (2006) Binding of Scr to Na^+-K^+-ATPase forms a functional signaling complex. Mol. Biol. Cell 17: 317–326.

[335] Vincze Á., Király Á., Sütő G., Mózsik Gy. (1992) Acute surgical vagotomy (ASV) is an aggressor of gastric mucosa with and without indomethacin treatment? Acta Physiol. Hung. 80: 197–205.

[336] Vincze Á., Király Á., Sütő G., Mózsik Gy. (1993a) Changes of gastric mucosal biochemistry in ethanol-treated rats with and without acute surgical vagotomy. J. Physiology (Paris) 87, 339–341.

[337] Vincze Á., Matus Z., Tóth Gy., Mózsik Gy. (1993b) Changes of the serum carotenoid levels in patients with malignant diseases. In: Mózsik Gy., Emerit I., Fehér J., Matkovics B., Vincze Á. (eds) Oxygen Free radicals and Scavengers in the Natural Sciences. Akadémiai Kiadó, Budapest. pp. 323–329.

[338] Vincze Á., Király Á., Sütő G., Karádi O., Mózsik Gy. (1997) Role of neurohumoral and local mucosal factors in β-carotene-induced gastroprotection in the rat. In: Mózsik Gy, Nagy L, Király Á (eds) Twenty Five Years of Peptic Ulcer research in Hungary: From Basic Sciences to Clinical Practice. Akadémiai Kiadó, Budapest. pp. 265–273.

[339] Warren J. R., Marshall B. J. (1983) Unidentified curved bacilli on gastric epithelium in active chronic gastritis. Lancet I: 1273–1375.

[340] Wong B. C. Y., Ching C. K., Lam S. K., Li Z. L., Chen B. W., Liu J. B., Wang B. E., Yuan S. Z., Xu C. P., Hou X. H., Zang A. T., Zheng Z. T. (1998) Differential North to South gastric cancer – duodenal ulcer gradient in China. J. Gastroenterol. Hepatol. 13: 1050–1057.

[341] Wright L. F. and Hirschowitz B. I. (1976) Gastric secretion. Amer. J. Digest. Dis. 21: 409–418.

[342] Yao X. and Forte J. G. (2003) Cell biology of acid secretion by the parietal cell. Ann. Rev. Physiol. 65: 103–131.

[343] Young E. A., Fowler C. D., Kidd G. J., Chang A., Rudick R., Fisher E., Trapp B. H. (2008) Imaging correlates of decreased axonal Na^+/K^+-APase in chronic sclerosis lesions. Ann. Neurol. 63: 428–435.

[344] Yuan Z., Cai T., Cian J., Ivanov A. V., Giovannucci D. R., Xie Z. (2005) Na/K-ATPase tethers phospholipase C and IP3 receptor into a calcium-regulated complex. Mol. Biol. Cell 16: 4034–4045.

[345] Zsoldos T., Tigyi A., Monsko T., Puppi A. (1983) Lipid peroxidation in the membrane damaging effect of silica-containing dust on rat lunge. Exp. Path. 23: 72–78.

Chapter 12

Abbreviations

Gyula Mozsik and Imre Szabó

Additional information is available at the end of the chapter

http://dx.doi.org/10.5772/60496

ADP, adenosine diphosphate;

Adenylate pool, ATP+ADP+AMP;

ATP, adenosine triphosphate

AMP, adenosine monophosphate

cAMP, cyclic 3',5'-adenosine monophsophate;

CAT, catalase enzyme;

BAO, basal acid output;

COX, cyclo-oxygenase enzyme;

DNA, deoxyribonucleic acid;

DU, duodenal ulcer;

"energy charge", [(ATP+0.5 ADP)/(ATP+ADP+AMP)];

ETOH (EtOH), ethanol;

GMCs, gastric mucosal cells;

GMBF, gastric mucosal blood flow;

GSH-px, glutathione peroxidase;

GSH-red., reduced glutathione;

GU, gastric ulcer;

HCl, hydrochlorid acid;

Hep G2 cell line, human hepatoma cell line;

H. pylori, Helicobacter pylori;

IND, indomethacin;

IP3, inositol triphosphate;

JU, jejunal ulcer;

6-keto-$PGF_{1\alpha}$, metabolite of prosptacyclin;

LDH, lactate dehydrogenase;

MAO, maximal acid ouput;

MARK, mitogen-avtivated proptein kinase;

NaOH, sodim hydroxyde;

MDA, malondialdehyde;

NOSAIDs, non-steroidal anti-inflammatory compounds;

NUD, non ulcer dyspepsia;

PGE_2, prostagladin E_2,

PGI_2, prostacyclin;

PGs, prostaglandins;

PUD, peptic ulcer disease;

RNA, nuleic acids;

ROS, reactive oxydative species;

SOD, superoxide dismutase;

Sp2/0-Ag14 cell line, mouse myeloma cell line.

Author details

Gyula Mozsik[1] and Imre Szabó[2]

1 First Department of Medicine, Medical and Health Centre, University of Pécs, Hungary

2 Associate Professor at the First Department of Medicine, University of Pécs, Hungary

Chapter 13

Subject Index

Gyula Mozsik and Imre Szabó

Additional information is available at the end of the chapter

http://dx.doi.org/10.5772/60497

INTECH
open science | open minds

        - During ulcer development
        - During gastric mucosal protection produced by atropine
        - During gastric mucosal protection by vitamin A and β-carotene
- Indomethacin ulcer model
    - Biochemical backgrounds
    - Cellular mechanisms,
        - During gastric ulcer development,
        - During gastric mucosal protection
            - by atropine,
            - by cimetidine,
            - β-carotene,
            - by vitamin A,
        - Gastric mucosal cAMP vs gastric mucosal damage,
        - Gastric mucosal cAMP vs, gastric mucosal protection,
        - Prostaglandin system vs gastric mucosal protection by β-carotene,
- Reserpine ulcer model
- NaOH, NaCl, HCl and ethanol-induced gastric mucosal damage
    - Time-sequence between the mucosal damage vs. introduction of chemical agents,
    - Biochemical mechanisms vs. mucosal damage,
    - Acid-dependent ulcer model vs. gastric mucosal biochemistry,
    - Non- acid-dependent ulcer model vs. mucosal biochemistry,
    - Gastric mucosal protection by PGI_2
    - Gastric mucosal protection by β-carotene
    - Gastric mucosal damage vs. oxygen free radicals
    - Gastric mucosal protection vs. oxygen free radicals,
- Evidence-based medicine
- Problem-orientated medice,
- Human clinical pharmacology,
    - Acute comparative clinical pharmacology in patients,
    - Chronic atropine treatment in patients with duodenal ulcer
        - Development of tolerance to atropine
        - Development of drug tolerance to parasympatholytics,
        - Pharmacological denervation phenomenon,
- Cytoprotection
    - In patients with duodenal ulcer,
    - In patients with gastric ulcer,
    - In experimental circumstances,
        - Prostaglandins,

http://dx.doi.org/10.5772/60497

Stable cell lines

- Mouse cell myeloma cell line (Sp2/0-Ag14 cell line),
- Human hepatocellular carcinoma cell line (Hep G2),

„surgical" and „ chemical „ vagotomy

- Gastric acid secretion,
- Gastric mucosal protection,
  - Biochemistry in the gastric mucosal biochemistry,

Biochemistry of „use" and „disuse" in the rat gastric mucosa,

Chronic atropine treatment

- In patients with chronic duodenal ulcer
- In rats

Chronic treatment of rats with Neostigmine (choline)

Author details

Gyula Mozsik[1] and Imre Szabó[2]

1 First Department of Medicine, Medical and Health Centre, University of Pécs, Hungary

2 Associate Professor at the First Department of Medicine, University of Pécs, Hungary